EPIDEMIOLOGY AND OF PREVENTION VACCINE- PREVENTABLE DISEASES

13TH EDITION

This book was produced by the Communication and Education Branch, National Center for Immunization and Respiratory Diseases, Centers for Disease Control and Prevention, who is solely responsible for its content. It was printed and distributed by the Public Health Foundation. For additional copies, contact the Public Health Foundation at 877-252-1200 or website http://bookstore.phf.org/.

Slide sets to accompany this book are available on the CDC Vaccines and Immunization website at http://www.cdc.gov/vaccines/pubs/pinkbook/index.html.

E-mail address for comments, questions or suggestions about the contents of this book: nipinfo@cdc.gov.

Edited by:
Jennifer Hamborsky, MPH, MCHES
Andrew Kroger, MD, MPH
Charles (Skip) Wolfe

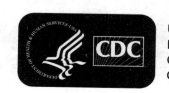

**U.S.Department of
Health and Human Services**
Centers for Disease
Control and Prevention

On the cover

This illustration depicts the influenza virus.
Graphic created by Dan J. Higgins, Division of Communication Services, CDC

Suggested Citation:
Centers for Disease Control and Prevention.
Epidemiology and Prevention of Vaccine-Preventable Diseases.
Hamborsky J, Kroger A, Wolfe S, eds. 13th ed. Washington D.C.
Public Health Foundation, 2015.

The editors would like to thank Dr. William L. Atkinson, who summarized, standardized and compiled CDC's vaccine-preventable disease and vaccine teaching materials to create the Pink Book.

"He just thought it up and did it." – Apocalypse Now

Milestones in the History of Vaccination

400 BCE	1100s	1721	1796
Hippocrates describes diphtheria, epidemic jaundice, and other conditions	Variolation for smallpox first reported in China	Variolation introduced into Great Britain	Edward Jenner inoculates James Phipps cowpox, and calls the procedure vaccina ("vacca" is Latin for cow)

Table of Contents

Milestones in the History of Vaccination

1870
Pasteur creates the [liv]e attenuated bacterial [vaccin]e (chicken cholera)

1884-85
Pasteur creates the first live attenuated viral vaccine for use in humans

1900
Paul Ehrlich formulates receptor theory of immunity

1901
First Nobel Prize in Medicine to von Behring for diphtheria antitoxin

1909
Theobald Smith discovers a method for inactivating diphtheria toxin

Table of Contents

Milestones in the History of Vaccination

1919
Calmette and Guerin create BCG, the first live attenuated bacterial vaccine for humans

1923
First whole-cell pertussis vaccine tested
Gaston Ramon develops diphtheria toxoid

1926
Ramon and Christian Zoeller develop tetanus toxoid

1931
Goodpasture describes a technique for viral culture in hens' eggs

1936
Thomas Francis and Magill develop the inactivated influenza

Table of Contents

Milestones in the History of Vaccination

1948	1954	1955	1961	1963
...ders and colleagues ...e Lansing Type II ...s in human cell line	Enders and Peebles isolate measles virus Francis Field Trial of inactivated polio vaccine	Inactivated polio vaccine licensed	Human diploid cell line developed	Measles vaccine licensed Trivalent oral polio vaccine licensed

Table of Contents

Milestones in the History of Vaccination

1965
Bifurcated needle for smallpox vaccine licensed

1966
World Health Assembly calls for global smallpox eradication

1967
Maurice Hilleman develops Jeryl Lynn strain of mumps virus

1969
Stanley Plotkin develops RA 27/3 strain of rubella vaccine virus

1971
MMR vaccine lic

14 Meningococcal Disease

15 Mumps

16 Pertussis

lestones in the History of Vaccination

1977
indigenous case
of smallpox
(Somalia)

1979
Last wild poliovirus
transmission in the U.S.

1981
First hepatitis B
vaccine licensed

1983
Smallpox vaccine withdrawn
from civilian market

1986
First recombinant vaccine
licensed (hepatitis B)
National Childhood
Vaccine Injury Act

Table of Contents

Milestones in the History of Vaccination

1989
Two-dose measles vaccine recommendation

1990
First polysaccharide conjugate vaccine licensed (*Haemophilus influenzae* type b)

1994
Polio elimination certified in the Americas
Vaccines for Children program begins

1995
Varicella vaccine licensed
Hepatitis A vaccine licensed
First harmonized childhood immunization schedule published

1996
Acellular pertussis licensed for inf

Milestones in the History of Vaccination

1997	1998	1999	2000	2003
ial polio vaccination ecommended	First rotavirus vaccine licensed	Exclusive use of inactivated polio vaccine recommended Rotavirus vaccine withdrawn	Pneumococcal conjugate vaccine licensed for infants	Live attenuated influenza vaccine licensed

Table of Contents

Milestones in the History of Vaccination

2004 Inactivated influenza vaccine recommended for all children 6–23 months of age

2004 Indigenous transmission of rubella virus interrupted

2005 Acellular pertussis vaccines licensed for adolescents and adults

2005 MMR-varicella (MMRV) licensed

2006 Second generation r vaccine license

B Vaccines

C Vaccine Information Statements

D Vaccine Safety

E Data and Statistics

F Immunization Resources

lestones in the History of Vaccination →

2006
man papillomavirus ccine licensed

2006
First herpes zoster vaccined licensed

2009
H1N1 influenza pandemic declared

2010
Influenza vaccine recommended for all persons 6 months and older

2013
First quadrivalent influenza vaccine licensed

Immunology and Vaccine-Preventable Diseases

Immunology is a complicated subject, and a detailed discussion of it is beyond the scope of this text. However, an understanding of the basic function of the immune system is useful in order to understand both how vaccines work and the basis of recommendations for their use. The description that follows is simplified. Many excellent immunology textbooks are available to provide additional detail.

Immunity is the ability of the human body to tolerate the presence of material indigenous to the body ("self"), and to eliminate foreign ("nonself") material. This discriminatory ability provides protection from infectious disease, since most microbes are identified as foreign by the immune system. Immunity to a microbe is usually indicated by the presence of antibody to that organism. Immunity is generally specific to a single organism or group of closely related organisms. There are two basic mechanisms for acquiring immunity, active and passive.

Active immunity is protection that is produced by the person's own immune system. This type of immunity usually lasts for many years, often during a lifetime.

Passive immunity is protection by products produced by an animal or human and transferred to another human, usually by injection. Passive immunity often provides effective protection, but this protection wanes (disappears) with time, usually within a few weeks or months.

The immune system is a complex system of interacting cells whose primary purpose is to identify foreign ("nonself") substances referred to as antigens. Antigens can be either live (such as viruses and bacteria) or inactivated. The immune system develops a defense against the antigen. This defense is known as the immune response and usually involves the production of protein molecules by B lymphocytes, called antibodies (or immunoglobulins), and of specific cells, including T-lymphocytes (also known as cell-mediated immunity) whose purpose is to facilitate the elimination of foreign substances.

The most effective immune responses are generally produced in response to a live antigen. However, an antigen does not necessarily have to be alive, as occurs with infection with a virus or bacterium, to produce an immune response. Some proteins, such as hepatitis B surface antigen, are easily recognized by the immune system. Other material, such as polysaccharide (long chains of sugar molecules that make up the cell wall of certain bacteria) are less effective antigens, and the immune response may not provide as good protection.

Immunity

- Self vs. nonself
- Protection from infectious disease
- Usually indicated by the presence of antibody
- Generally specific to a single organism

Active Immunity

- Protection produced by the person's own immune system
- Often lifetime

Passive Immunity

- Protection transferred from another animal or human
- Effective protection that wanes with time

Antigen

- A live (e.g., viruses and bacteria) or inactivated substance capable of producing an immune response

Antibody

- Protein molecules (immunoglobulins) produced by B lymphocytes to help eliminate an antigen

Principles of Vaccination

Passive Immunity

Passive immunity is the transfer of antibody produced by one human or other animal to another. Passive immunity provides protection against some infections, but this protection is temporary. The antibodies will degrade during a period of weeks to months, and the recipient will no longer be protected.

The most common form of passive immunity is that which an infant receives from its mother. Antibodies are transported across the placenta during the last 1–2 months of pregnancy. As a result, a full-term infant will have the same antibodies as its mother. These antibodies will protect the infant from certain diseases for up to a year. Protection is better against some diseases (e.g., measles, rubella, tetanus) than others (e.g., polio, pertussis).

Many types of blood products contain antibody. Some products (e.g., washed or reconstituted red blood cells) contain a relatively small amount of antibody, and some (e.g., intravenous immune globulin and plasma products) contain a large amount.

In addition to blood products used for transfusion (e.g., whole blood, red cells, and platelets) there are three major sources of antibody used in human medicine. These are homologous pooled human antibody, homologous human hyperimmune globulin, and heterologous hyperimmune serum.

Homologous pooled human antibody is also known as immune globulin. It is produced by combining (pooling) the IgG antibody fraction from thousands of adult donors in the United States. Because it comes from many different donors, it contains antibody to many different antigens. It is used primarily for postexposure prophylaxis for hepatitis A and measles and treatment of certain congenital immuno-globulin deficiencies.

Homologous human hyperimmune globulins are antibody products that contain high titers of specific antibody. These products are made from the donated plasma of humans with high levels of the antibody of interest. However, since hyperimmune globulins are from humans, they also contain other antibodies in lesser quantities. Hyperimmune globulins are used for postexposure prophylaxis for several diseases, including hepatitis B, rabies, tetanus, and varicella.

Heterologous hyperimmune serum is also known as antitoxin. This product is produced in animals, usually horses (equine), and contains antibodies against only one antigen. In the United States, antitoxin is available for treatment of botulism and diphtheria. A problem with this product is serum sickness, an immune reaction to the horse protein.

Immune globulin from human sources is polyclonal; it contains many different kinds of antibodies. In the 1970s, techniques were developed to isolate and "immortalize" (cause to grow indefinitely) single B cells, which led to the development of monoclonal antibody products. Monoclonal antibody is produced from a single clone of B cells, so these products contain antibody to only one antigen or closely related group of antigens. Monoclonal antibody products have many applications, including the diagnosis of certain types of cancer (colorectal, prostate, ovarian, breast), treatment of cancer (B-cell chronic lymphocytic leukemia, non-Hodgkin lymphoma), prevention of transplant rejection, and treatment of autoimmune diseases (Crohn's disease, rheumatoid arthritis) and infectious diseases.

A monoclonal antibody product is available for the prevention of respiratory syncytial virus (RSV) infection. It is called palivizumab (Synagis). Palivizumab is a humanized monoclonal antibody specific for RSV. While certain antibody products like immune globulins interfere with live-virus vaccines, monoclonal antibody products specific to one, non-vaccine microbe do not interfere with live vaccines. Since palivizumab does not contain any other antibody except RSV antibody, it will not interfere with the response to a live virus vaccine.

Active Immunity

Active immunity is stimulation of the immune system to produce antigen-specific humoral (antibody) and cellular immunity. Unlike passive immunity, which is temporary, active immunity usually lasts for many years, often for a lifetime.

One way to acquire active immunity is to survive infection with the disease-causing form of the organism. While exceptions (like malaria) exist, in general, once persons recover from infectious diseases, they will have lifelong immunity to that disease. The persistence of protection for many years after the infection is known as immunologic memory. Following exposure of the immune system to an antigen, certain cells (memory B cells) continue to circulate in the blood (and also reside in the bone marrow) for many years. Upon reexposure to the antigen, these memory cells begin to replicate and produce antibody very rapidly to reestablish protection.

Another way to produce active immunity is by vaccination. Vaccines interact with the immune system and often produce an immune response similar to that produced by the natural infection, but they do not subject the recipient to the disease and its potential complications. Many vaccines also produce immunologic memory similar to that acquired by having the natural disease.

Monoclonal Antibody

- Derived from a single type, or clone, of antibody-producing cells (B cells)

- Antibody is specific to a single antigen or closely related group of antigens

- Used for diagnosis and therapy of certain cancers and autoimmune and infectious diseases, as well as prevention of transplant rejection

Antibody for Prevention of RSV

- Palivizumab (Synagis)
  - monoclonal
  - contains only RSV antibody
  - will not interfere with the response to a live-virus vaccine

Active Immunity

- Immune system produces antigen-specific humoral and cellular immunity

- Lasts for many years, often lifetime

- Sources
  - infection with disease-causing form of organism
  - vaccination

Vaccination

- Active immunity produced by vaccine

- Immunity and immunologic memory similar to natural infection but without risk of disease

Principles of Vaccination

1

Classification of Vaccines

- Live attenuated
  - viral
  - bacterial
- Inactivated

Inactivated Vaccines

- Whole
  - viruses
  - bacteria
- Fractional
  - protein-based
    - toxoid
    - subunit
  - polysaccharide-based
    - pure
    - conjugate

Live Attenuated Vaccines

- Attenuated (weakened) form of the "wild" virus or bacterium
- Must replicate to produce an immune response
- Immune response virtually identical to natural infection
- Usually produce immunity with one dose*
- Severe reactions possible
- Interference from circulating antibody
- Fragile – must be stored and handled carefully
- Viral: measles, mumps, rubella, vaccinia, varicella, zoster, yellow fever, rotavirus, intranasal influenza, oral polio**
- Bacterial: BCG**, oral typhoid

*except those administered orally
**not available in the United States

Many factors may influence the immune response to vaccination. These include the presence of maternal antibody, nature and dose of antigen, route of administration, and the presence of an adjuvant (e.g., aluminum-containing material added to improve the immunogenicity of the vaccine). Host factors such as age, nutritional factors, genetics, and coexisting disease, may also affect the response.

Classification of Vaccines

There are two basic types of vaccines: live attenuated and inactivated. The characteristics of live and inactivated vaccines are different, and these characteristics determine how the vaccine is used.

Live attenuated vaccines are produced by modifying a disease-producing ("wild") virus or bacterium in a laboratory. The resulting vaccine organism retains the ability to replicate (grow) and produce immunity, but usually does not cause illness. The majority of live attenuated vaccines available in the United States contain live viruses. ~~However, one live attenuated bacterial vaccine is available.~~ *See 9/2015 Errata*

Inactivated vaccines can be composed of either whole viruses or bacteria, or fractions of either. Fractional vaccines are either protein-based or polysaccharide-based. Protein-based vaccines include toxoids (inactivated bacterial toxin) and subunit or subvirion products. Most polysaccharide-based vaccines are composed of pure cell wall polysaccharide from bacteria. Conjugate polysaccharide vaccines contain polysaccharide that is chemically linked to a protein. This linkage makes the polysaccharide a more potent vaccine.

General Rule: The more similar a vaccine is to the disease-causing form of the organism, the better the immune response to the vaccine

Live Attenuated Vaccines

Live vaccines are derived from "wild," or disease-causing, viruses or bacteria. These wild viruses or bacteria are attenuated, or weakened, in a laboratory, usually by repeated culturing. For example, the measles virus used as a vaccine today was isolated from a child with measles disease in 1954. Almost 10 years of serial passage using tissue culture media was required to transform the wild virus into attenuated vaccine virus.

4

To produce an immune response, live attenuated vaccines must replicate (grow) in the vaccinated person. A relatively small dose of virus or bacteria is administered, which replicates in the body and creates enough of the organism to stimulate an immune response. Anything that either damages the live organism in the vial (e.g., heat, light) or interferes with replication of the organism in the body (circulating antibody) can cause the vaccine to be ineffective.

Although live attenuated vaccines replicate, they usually do not cause disease such as may occur with the "wild" form of the organism. When a live attenuated vaccine does cause "disease," it is usually much milder than the natural disease and is referred to as an adverse reaction.

The immune response to a live attenuated vaccine is virtually identical to that produced by a natural infection. The immune system does not differentiate between an infection with a weakened vaccine virus and an infection with a wild virus. Live attenuated vaccines produce immunity in most recipients with one dose, except those administered orally. However, a small percentage of recipients do not respond to the first dose of an injected live vaccine (such as MMR or varicella) and a second dose is recommended to provide a very high level of immunity in the population.

Live attenuated vaccines may cause severe or fatal reactions as a result of uncontrolled replication (growth) of the vaccine virus. This only occurs in persons with immunodeficiency (e.g., from leukemia, treatment with certain drugs, or human immunodeficiency virus [HIV] infection).

A live attenuated vaccine virus could theoretically revert to its original pathogenic (disease-causing) form. This is known to happen only with live (oral) polio vaccine.

Active immunity from a live attenuated vaccine may not develop because of interference from circulating antibody to the vaccine virus. Antibody from any source (e.g., transplacental, transfusion) can interfere with replication of the vaccine organism and lead to poor response or no response to the vaccine (also known as vaccine failure). Live attenuated vaccines are fragile and can be damaged or destroyed by heat and light. They must be handled and stored carefully.

Currently available live attenuated viral vaccines are measles, mumps, rubella, vaccinia, varicella, zoster (which contains the same virus as varicella vaccine but in much higher amount), yellow fever, rotavirus, and influenza (intranasal). Oral polio vaccine is a live viral vaccine but is no longer available in the United States. Live attenuated bacterial vaccines are bacille Calmette-Guérin (BCG—not currently available in the US) and oral typhoid vaccine.

Principles of Vaccination

Inactivated Vaccines

Inactivated vaccines are produced by growing the bacterium or virus in culture media, then inactivating it with heat and/or chemicals (usually formalin). In the case of fractional vaccines, the organism is further treated to purify only those components to be included in the vaccine (e.g., the polysaccharide capsule of pneumococcus).

Inactivated vaccines are not alive and cannot replicate. The entire dose of antigen is administered in the injection. These vaccines cannot cause disease from infection, even in an immunodeficient person. Inactivated antigens are less affected by circulating antibody than are live agents, so they may be given when antibody is present in the blood (e.g., in infancy or following receipt of antibody-containing blood products).

Inactivated vaccines always require multiple doses. In general, the first dose does not produce protective immunity, but "primes" the immune system. A protective immune response develops after the second or third dose. In contrast to live vaccines, in which the immune response closely resembles natural infection, the immune response to an inactivated vaccine is mostly humoral. Little or no cellular immunity results. Antibody titers against inactivated antigens diminish with time. As a result, some inactivated vaccines may require periodic supplemental doses to increase, or "boost," antibody titers.

Currently available whole-cell inactivated vaccines are limited to inactivated whole viral vaccines (polio, hepatitis A, and rabies). Inactivated whole virus influenza vaccine and whole inactivated bacterial vaccines (pertussis, typhoid, cholera, and plague) are no longer available in the United States. Fractional vaccines include subunits (hepatitis B, influenza, acellular pertussis, human papillomavirus, anthrax) and toxoids (diphtheria, tetanus). A subunit vaccine for Lyme disease is no longer available in the United States.

Polysaccharide Vaccines

Polysaccharide vaccines are a unique type of inactivated subunit vaccine composed of long chains of sugar molecules that make up the surface capsule of certain bacteria. Pure polysaccharide vaccines are available for three diseases: pneumococcal disease, meningococcal disease, and *Salmonella* Typhi. A pure polysaccharide vaccine for *Haemophilus influenzae* type b (Hib) is no longer available in the United States.

The immune response to a pure polysaccharide vaccine is typically T-cell independent, which means that these vaccines are able to stimulate B cells without the assistance of T-helper cells. T-cell–independent antigens, including polysaccharide vaccines, are not consistently immunogenic in children younger than 2 years of age. Young children do not respond consistently to polysaccharide antigens, probably because of immaturity of the immune system.

Repeated doses of most inactivated protein vaccines cause the antibody titer to go progressively higher, or "boost." This does not occur with polysaccharide antigens; repeat doses of polysaccharide vaccines usually do not cause a booster response. Antibody induced with polysaccharide vaccines has less functional activity than that induced by protein antigens. This is because the predominant antibody produced in response to most polysaccharide vaccines is IgM, and little IgG is produced.

In the late 1980s, it was discovered that the problems noted above could be overcome through a process called conjugation, in which the polysaccharide is chemically combined with a protein molecule. Conjugation changes the immune response from T-cell independent to T-cell dependent, leading to increased immunogenicity in infants and antibody booster response to multiple doses of vaccine.

The first conjugated polysaccharide vaccine was for Hib. A conjugate vaccine for pneumococcal disease was licensed in 2000. A meningococcal conjugate vaccine was licensed in 2005.

Recombinant Vaccines

Vaccine antigens may also be produced by genetic engineering technology. These products are sometimes referred to as recombinant vaccines. Five genetically engineered vaccines are currently available in the United States. Hepatitis B, human papillomavirus (HPV), and influenza (one brand) vaccines are produced by insertion of a segment of the respective viral gene into the gene of a yeast cell or virus. The modified yeast cell or virus produces pure hepatitis B surface antigen, HPV capsid protein, or influenza hemagglutinin when it grows. Live typhoid vaccine (Ty21a) is *Salmonella* Typhi bacteria that have been genetically modified to not cause illness. Live attenuated influenza vaccine has been engineered to replicate effectively in the mucosa of the nasopharynx but not in the lungs.

Selected References

Siegrist C-A. Vaccine immunology. In Plotkin SA, Orenstein WA, Offit PA. *Vaccines*, 5th ed. China: Saunders, 2008:17–36.

Plotkin S. Vaccines, vaccination, and vaccinology. *J. Infect Dis* 2003; 187:1347–59.

Plotkin S. Correlates of vaccine-induced immunity. *Clin Infect Dis* 2008; 47:401–9.

Polysaccharide Vaccines

Pure polysaccharide

- pneumococcal
- meningococcal
- *Salmonella* Typhi (Vi)

Conjugate polysaccharide

- *Haemophilus influenzae* type b (Hib)
- pneumococcal
- meningococcal

Pure Polysaccharide Vaccines

- Not consistently immunogenic in children younger than 2 years of age
- No booster response
- Antibody with less functional activity
- Immunogenicity improved by conjugation

Recombinant Vaccines

- Genetic engineering technology
- Viral: hepatitis B, human papillomavirus, influenza (one brand), live attenuated influenza
- Bacterial: *Salmonella* Typhi (Vi) (Ty21a)

see Errata 9/2015

Principles of Vaccination

This chapter discusses issues that are commonly encountered in vaccination practice. A more thorough discussion of issues common to more than one vaccine can be found in the *General Recommendations on Immunization: Recommendations of the Advisory Committee on Immunization Practices*. These recommendations are revised every 3 to 5 years as needed; the most current edition was published in January 2011 (MMWR 2011;60 (No. RR-2):1-61). All providers who administer vaccine should have a copy of this report and be familiar with its content. It can be downloaded from the *MMWR* website or ordered in print version from the Centers for Disease Control and Prevention.

Timing and Spacing of Vaccines

The timing and spacing of vaccine doses are two of the most important issues in the appropriate use of vaccines. Specific circumstances that are commonly encountered in immunization practice are the timing of antibody-containing blood products and live vaccines (particularly measles and varicella-containing vaccines), simultaneous and nonsimultaneous administration of different vaccines, and the interval between subsequent doses of the same vaccine.

General Rule: Inactivated vaccines are generally not affected by circulating antibody to the antigen. Live attenuated vaccines may be affected by circulating antibody to the antigen.

Antibody–Vaccine Interactions

The presence of circulating antibody to a vaccine antigen may reduce or completely eliminate the immune response to the vaccine. The amount of interference produced by circulating antibody generally depends on the type of vaccine administered and the amount of antibody.

Inactivated antigens, which include recombinant vaccines, are generally not affected by circulating antibody, so they can be administered before, after, or at the same time as the antibody. Simultaneous administration of antibody (in the form of immune globulin) and vaccine is recommended for postexposure prophylaxis of certain diseases, such as hepatitis B, rabies, and tetanus.

Live Injected Vaccines

Live vaccines must replicate in order to cause an immune response. Antibody against injected live vaccine antigen may interfere with replication. If a live injectable vaccine (measles-mumps-rubella [MMR], varicella, or combination

Antibody and Measles- and Varicella-Containing* Vaccines	
Product Given First	**Action**
Vaccine	Wait 2 weeks before giving antibody
Antibody	Wait 3 months or longer before giving vaccine (See Table, Appendix A)

*except zoster vaccine

measles-mumps-rubella-varicella [MMRV]) must be given around the time that antibody is given, the two must be separated by enough time so that the antibody does not interfere with viral replication. If the live vaccine is given first, it is necessary to wait at least 2 weeks (i.e., an incubation period) before giving the antibody. If the interval between the vaccine and antibody is less than 2 weeks, the recipient should be tested for immunity or the vaccine dose should be repeated.

If the antibody is given before a dose of MMR or varicella-containing vaccine, it is necessary to wait until the antibody has waned (degraded) before giving the vaccine to reduce the chance of interference by the antibody. The necessary interval between an antibody-containing product and MMR or varicella-containing vaccine (except zoster vaccine) depends on the concentration of antibody in the product, but is always 3 months or longer. A table listing the recommended intervals between administration of antibody products and live vaccines (MMR and varicella-containing) is included in Appendix A and in the *General Recommendations on Immunization* (2011). The interval between administration of an antibody product and MMR or varicella vaccination can be as long as 11 months. Zoster vaccine is not known to be affected by circulating antibody so it can be administered at any time before or after receipt of an antibody-containing blood product.

Yellow fever vaccine also is not known to be affected by circulating antibody. Because few North Americans are immune to yellow fever, these products do not contain significant amounts of antibody to yellow fever virus.

Although passively acquired antibodies can interfere with the response to rubella vaccine, the low dose of anti-Rho(D) globulin administered to postpartum women has not been demonstrated to reduce the response to the rubella vaccine. Because of the importance of rubella and varicella immunity among childbearing age women, women without evidence of immunity to rubella or varicella should receive MMR or varicella vaccine (but not MMRV) in the postpartum period. Vaccination should not be delayed because of receipt of anti-Rho(D) globulin or any other blood product during the last trimester of pregnancy or at delivery. These women should be vaccinated immediately after delivery and, if possible, tested 3 months later to ensure immunity to rubella and, if necessary, to measles.

Live Oral and Intranasal Vaccines

Oral typhoid vaccine is not known to be affected by the administration of immune globulin or blood products. Oral typhoid vaccine may be given simultaneously with blood products, or separated by any interval. The replication of live attenuated influenza (LAIV) and rotavirus vaccines are not believed to be affected by antibody-containing blood products. These can be given any time before or after administration of antibody-containing blood products.

Products Containing Type-Specific or Negligible Antibody

Some blood products do not contain antibodies that interfere with vaccine replication. Palivizumab (Synagis), used for the prevention of respiratory syncytial virus (RSV) infection in infants and young children, contains antibody directed only at RSV. Washed red blood cells contain a negligible amount of antibody. These products can be given anytime before or after administration of MMR or varicella-containing vaccines.

Simultaneous and Nonsimultaneous Administration

General Rule: All vaccines can be administered at the same visit as all other vaccines.*

*exception: in children with functional or anatomic asplenia pneumococcal conjugate vaccine (PCV13) and Menactra brand meningococcal conjugate vaccines should not be administered at the same visit; separate these vaccines by at least 4 weeks

Simultaneous administration (that is, administration on the same day) of the most widely used live and inactivated vaccines does not result in decreased antibody responses or increased rates of adverse reaction. Simultaneous administration of all vaccines for which a child is eligible is very important in childhood vaccination programs because it increases the probability that a child will be fully immunized at the appropriate age. A study during a measles outbreak in the early 1990s showed that about one-third of measles cases in unvaccinated but vaccine-eligible preschool children could have been prevented if MMR had been administered at the same visit when another vaccine was given.

All indicated vaccines should be administered at the same visit. In children with functional or anatomic asplenia pneumococcal conjugate vaccine (PCV13) and Menactra brand meningococcal conjugate vaccine should not be administered at the same visit, and should be separated by at least 4 weeks. This is because children with functional or anatomic asplenia are at very high risk of pneumococcal invasive disease and Menactra is thought to interfere with the antibody response to pneumococcal conjugate vaccine. PCV13 should be administered first and then Menactra four weeks later. Individual vaccines should not be mixed

Products Containing Type-Specific or Negligible Antibody

- Palivizumab (Synagis)
  - monoclonal
  - contains only RSV antibody
- Red blood cells (RBCs), washed
  - negligible antibody content

Spacing of Vaccine Combinations Not Given Simultaneously

Combination	Minimum Interval
Two live parenteral, or live intranasal influenza vaccine	4 weeks
All other	None*

*in children with functional or anatomic asplenia pneumococcal conjugate vaccine (PCV13) and Menactra brand meningococcal conjugate vaccines should not be administered at the same visit; separate these vaccines by at least 4 weeks

Spacing of Live Vaccines Not Given Simultaneously

- If two live parenteral vaccines, or live intranasal influenza vaccine, are given less than 4 weeks apart the vaccine given second should be repeated

- Exception is yellow fever vaccine given less than 4 weeks after measles vaccine, mumps vaccine, rubella vaccine, or varicella vaccine

See 9/2015 Errata

in the same syringe unless they are licensed for mixing by the Food and Drug Administration. Only the sanofi-pasteur DTaP-IPV/Hib (Pentacel) vaccine is licensed for mixing in the same syringe. For additional guidelines, see the Vaccine Administration chapter.

Combination vaccines are generally preferred over simultaneous administration of single component vaccines. Considerations should include an assessment of the number of injections, vaccine availability, likelihood of improved coverage, likelihood of patient return, and storage and costs. Considerations should also include patient choice and the potential for adverse events. Because of the increased risk of febrile seizures following the first dose of MMRV vaccine compared to MMR and varicella vaccines, for the first dose of vaccine to prevent measles, mumps, rubella and varicella, unless the parent or caregiver expresses a preference for MMRV vaccine, separate MMR and Varicella vaccines should be administered for children 12 through 47 months of age.

Nonsimultaneous Administration of Different Vaccines

If live parenteral (injected) vaccines (MMR, MMRV, varicella, zoster, and yellow fever) and live intranasal influenza vaccine (LAIV) are not administered at the same visit, they should be separated by at least 4 weeks. This interval is intended to reduce or eliminate interference from the vaccine given first on the vaccine given later. If two live parenteral vaccines or LAIV are administered at an interval of less than 4 weeks, then the vaccine given second should be repeated in 4 weeks or confirmed to have been effective by serologic testing of the recipient (serologic testing is not recommended following LAIV, varicella, or zoster vaccines). An exception to this recommendation is yellow fever vaccine administered less than 4 weeks after single-antigen measles vaccine. A 1999 study demonstrated that yellow fever vaccine is not affected by measles vaccine given 1–27 days earlier. The effect of nonsimultaneously administered yellow fever vaccine with each of the following vaccines: mumps; varicella; zoster; LAIV; and rubella is not known. ~~So doses given nonsimultaneously can be counted.~~ *See 9/2015 Errata*

Live vaccines administered by the oral route (oral polio vaccine [OPV] oral typhoid, and rotavirus) are not believed to interfere with each other if not given simultaneously. These vaccines may be given at any time before or after each other. Rotavirus vaccine is not approved for children older than 32 weeks, oral typhoid is not approved for children younger than 6 years of age, and OPV is no longer available in the United States, so these vaccines are not likely to be given to the same child.

Parenteral live vaccines (MMR, MMRV, varicella, zoster, and yellow fever) and LAIV are not believed to have an effect on live vaccines given by the oral route (OPV, oral typhoid, and rotavirus). Live oral vaccines may be given at any time before or after live parenteral vaccines or LAIV.

All other combinations of two inactivated vaccines, or live and inactivated vaccines, may be given at any time before or after each other. In children with functional or anatomic asplenia PCV13 and Menactra brand meningococcal conjugate vaccine should not be administered at the same visit.

Interval Between Doses of the Same Vaccine

Immunizations are recommended for members of the youngest age group at risk for a disease for whom efficacy and safety of a vaccine have been demonstrated.

General Rule: Increasing the interval between doses of a multidose vaccine does not diminish the effectiveness of the vaccine.*Decreasing the interval between doses of a multidose vaccine may interfere with antibody response and protection.

*after the series has been completed

Most vaccines in the childhood immunization schedule require two or more doses for development of an adequate and persisting antibody response. Studies have demonstrated that recommended ages and intervals between doses of the same antigen(s) provide optimal protection or have the best evidence of efficacy. Table 1 of the *General Recommendations on Immunization* (included in Appendix A) shows the recommended and minimal ages and intervals between doses of vaccines most frequently used in the United States.

Administering doses of a multidose vaccine at shorter than the recommended intervals might be necessary when an infant or child is behind schedule and needs to be brought up-to-date quickly or when international travel is pending. In these cases, an accelerated schedule using the minimum age or minimum interval criteria can be used. Accelerated schedules should not be used routinely.

For routine vaccination, vaccine doses should not be administered at intervals less than the recommended minimal intervals or earlier than the minimal ages. Two exceptions to this may occur. The first is for measles vaccine during a measles outbreak or before travelling abroad. Infants 6

> ### Minimum Intervals and Ages
> Vaccine doses should not be administered at intervals less than the minimum intervals or earlier than the minimum age

2

through 11 months should receive one MMR dose, and this dose should not be counted (should be repeated at 12 months of age or older). The second exception involves administering a dose a few days earlier than the minimum interval or age, which is unlikely to have a substantially negative effect on the immune response to that dose. Although vaccinations should not be scheduled at an interval or age less than the recommended minimums, a child may have erroneously been brought to the office early, or may have come for an appointment not specifically for vaccination. In these situations, the clinician can consider administering the vaccine earlier than the minimum interval or age. If the parent/child is known to the clinician and the physician has confidence that the child will return for a visit, it is preferable to reschedule the child for vaccination closer to the recommended interval. If the parent/child is not known to the clinician or is not reliable (e.g., habitually misses appointments), it may be preferable to administer the vaccine at that visit than to reschedule a later appointment that may not be kept.

Vaccine doses administered up to 4 days before the minimum interval or age can be counted as valid. This 4-day recommendation does not apply to rabies vaccine because of the unique schedule for this vaccine. Doses administered 5 days or earlier than the minimum interval or age should not be counted as valid doses and should be repeated as age appropriate. The repeat dose should generally be spaced after the invalid dose by an interval at least equal to the recommended minimum interval shown in Table 1 of the General Recommendations. In certain situations, local or state requirements might mandate that doses of selected vaccines be administered on or after specific ages, superseding this 4-day "grace period".

In some cases, a scheduled dose of vaccine may not be given on time. If this occurs, the dose should be given at the next visit. Not all permutations of all schedules for all vaccines have been studied. However, available data indicate that intervals between doses longer than those routinely recommended do not affect seroconversion rate or titer when the schedule is completed. Consequently, it is not necessary to restart the series or add doses of any vaccine because of an extended interval between doses. The only exception to this rule is oral typhoid vaccine in some circumstances. Some experts recommend repeating the series of oral typhoid vaccine if the four-dose series is extended to more than 3 weeks.

Violation of Minimum Intervals or Minimum Age

- ACIP recommends that vaccine doses given up to four days before the minimum interval or age be counted as valid

- Immunization programs and/ or school entry requirements may not accept all doses given earlier than the minimum age or interval

Extended Interval Between Doses

- Not all permutations of all schedules for all vaccines have been studied

- Available studies of extended intervals have shown no significant difference in final titer

- It is not necessary to restart the series or add doses because of an extended interval between doses

Number of Doses

For live injected vaccines, the first dose administered at the recommended age usually provides protection. An additional dose is given to provide another opportunity for vaccine response in the small proportion of recipients who do not respond to the first dose. For instance, approximately 95% of recipients will respond to a single dose of measles vaccine. The second dose is given to ensure that nearly 100% of persons are immune (i.e., the second dose is "insurance"). Immunity following live vaccines is long-lasting, and booster doses are not necessary.

For inactivated vaccines, the first dose administered at the recommended age usually does not provide protection (hepatitis A vaccine is an exception). A protective immune response may not develop until the second or third dose. For inactivated vaccines, antibody titers may decrease (wane) below protective levels after a few years. This phenomenon is most notable for pertussis vaccine; tetanus and diphtheria vaccine immunity also wanes. For these vaccines, periodic "boosting" is required. An additional dose is given to raise antibody back to protective levels.

Not all inactivated vaccines require boosting throughout life. For example, additional doses of Hib vaccine are not required after completion of the infant primary series and 12-15 month old booster dose because Hib disease is very rare in children older than 5 years of age. Hepatitis B vaccine does not require boosting because of immunologic memory to the vaccine and the long incubation period of hepatitis B (which can produce an "autoboost").

Adverse Reactions Following Vaccination

Vaccines are intended to produce active immunity to specific antigens. An adverse reaction is an untoward effect caused by a vaccine that is extraneous to the vaccine's primary purpose of producing immunity. Adverse reactions are also called vaccine side effects. A vaccine adverse event refers to any medical event that occurs following vaccination. An adverse event could be a true adverse reaction or just a coincidental event, with further research needed to distinguish between them.

Acute vaccine adverse reactions fall into three general categories: local, systemic, and allergic. The most common type of adverse reactions are local reactions, such as pain, swelling, and redness at the site of injection. Local reactions may occur with up to 80% of vaccine doses, depending on the type of vaccine. Local adverse reactions generally occur within a few hours of the injection and are usually mild and self-limited. On rare occasions, local reactions may be very exaggerated or severe. Some of these reactions, referred to

Vaccine Adverse Reactions

- Adverse reaction
  - extraneous effect caused by vaccine
  - side effect
- Adverse event
  - any medical event following vaccination
  - may be true adverse reaction
  - may be only coincidental
- Local adverse reactions
  - pain, swelling, redness at site of injection
  - occur within a few hours of injection
  - usually mild and self-limited
- Systemic adverse reactions
  - fever, malaise, headache
  - nonspecific
  - may be unrelated to vaccine
- Severe allergic (anaphylaxis)
  - due to vaccine or vaccine component
  - rare
  - risk minimized by screening

2

as Arthus reactions, are most frequently seen with diphtheria and tetanus toxoids. Arthus reactions are not allergic reactions. Arthus reactions are believed to be due to very high titers of antibody, usually caused by too many doses of toxoid.

Systemic adverse reactions are more generalized events and include fever, malaise, myalgias (muscle pain), headache, loss of appetite, and others. These symptoms are nonspecific; they may occur in vaccinated persons because of the vaccine or may be caused by something unrelated to the vaccine.

Systemic adverse reactions were relatively frequent with DTP vaccine, which contained a whole-cell pertussis component. However, comparison of the frequency of systemic adverse events among vaccine and placebo recipients shows they are less common with inactivated vaccines currently in use, including acellular pertussis vaccine.

Systemic adverse reactions may occur following receipt of live attenuated vaccines. Live attenuated vaccines must replicate in order to produce immunity. The adverse reactions that follow live attenuated vaccines, such as fever or rash, represent symptoms produced from viral replication and are similar to a mild form of the natural disease. Systemic adverse reactions following live vaccines are usually mild, and occur 3–21 days after the vaccine was given (i.e., after an incubation period of the vaccine virus). LAIV replicates in the mucous membranes of the nose and throat, not in the lungs. As a result, LAIV may cause upper respiratory symptoms (like a cold) but not influenza-like symptoms.

A third type of acute vaccine adverse reactions are allergic reactions. Allergic reactions may be caused by the vaccine antigen itself or some other component of the vaccine, such as cell culture material, stabilizer, preservative, or antibiotic used to inhibit bacterial growth. Severe allergic reactions (anaphylaxis) may be life-threatening. Fortunately, they are rare. The risk of an allergic reaction can be decreased by good screening prior to vaccination. All providers who administer vaccines must have an emergency protocol and supplies to treat anaphylaxis.

Reporting Vaccine Adverse Events

Providers should report any clinically significant adverse event that occurs after the administration of any vaccine licensed in the United States to the Vaccine Adverse Event Reporting System (VAERS), which includes reporting from both public and private sectors.

Live Attenuated Vaccines

- Must replicate to produce immunity
- Symptoms usually mild
- Occur after an incubation period (usually 3-21 days)

Providers should report a clinically significant adverse event even if they are unsure whether a vaccine caused the event. The telephone number to call for answers to questions and to obtain VAERS forms is (800) 822-7967, or visit the VAERS website at http://vaers.hhs.gov. VAERS accepts reports of adverse reactions through their online system.

Contraindications and Precautions to Vaccination

Contraindications and precautions to vaccination generally dictate circumstances when vaccines will not be given. Many contraindications and precautions are temporary, and the vaccine can be given at a later time.

A contraindication is a condition that increases the likelihood of a serious adverse reaction to a vaccine for a patient with that condition. If the vaccine were given in the presence of that condition, the resulting adverse reaction could seriously harm the recipient. For instance, administering MMR vaccine to a person with a true anaphylactic allergy to gelatin could cause serious illness or death in the recipient. In general, vaccines should not be administered when a contraindication condition is present.

A precaution is a condition in a recipient that *might increase* the chance or severity of a serious adverse reaction, or that might compromise the ability of the vaccine to produce immunity (such as administering measles vaccine to a person with passive immunity to measles from a blood transfusion). Injury could result, but the chance of this happening is less than with a contraindication. In general, vaccines are deferred when a precaution condition is present. However, situations may arise when the benefit of protection from the vaccine outweighs the risk of an adverse reaction, and a provider may decide to give the vaccine.

There are very few true contraindication and precaution conditions. Only four of these conditions are generally considered to be permanent contraindications: severe (anaphylactic) allergic reaction to a vaccine component or following a prior dose of a vaccine; encephalopathy not due to another identifiable cause occurring within 7 days of pertussis vaccination; severe combined immunodeficiency (SCID) and a history of intussusception as contraindications to rotavirus vaccine.

Conditions considered permanent precautions to further doses of pediatric DTaP are temperature of 105°F or higher within 48 hours of a dose, collapse or shock-like state (hypotonic hyporesponsive episode) within 48 hours of a dose, persistent inconsolable crying lasting 3 or more hours occurring within 48 hours of a dose, or a seizure, with

2

Contraindication

- A condition that increases the likelihood of a serious adverse reaction to a vaccine for a patient with that condition

Precaution

- A condition in a recipient that might increase the chance or severity of an adverse reaction, or
- Might compromise the ability of the vaccine to produce immunity

Contraindications and Precautions

Permanent contraindications to vaccination:

- Severe allergic reaction to a vaccine component or following a prior dose
- Encephalopathy not due to another identifiable cause occurring within 7 days of pertussis vaccination
- Severe combined immunodeficiency (rotavirus vaccine)
- History of intussusception (rotavirus vaccine)

Condition	Live	Inactivated
Allergy to component	C	C
Encephalopathy	---	C
Pregnancy	C	V*
Immuno-suppression	C	V
Severe illness	P	P
Recent blood product	P**	V

C=contraindication P=precaution
V=vaccinate if indicated

*except HPV. **MMR and varicella containing (except zoster vaccine) only

2

or without fever, occurring within 3 days of a dose. The occurrence of one of these events in a child following DTaP vaccine is not a precaution to later vaccination with the adolescent/adult formulation of pertussis vaccine (Tdap).

Two conditions are temporary precautions to vaccination: moderate or severe acute illness (all vaccines), and recent receipt of an antibody-containing blood product. The latter precaution applies only to MMR and varicella-containing (except zoster) vaccines. Two conditions are temporary contraindications to vaccination with live vaccines: pregnancy and immunosuppression.

Allergy

A severe (anaphylactic) allergic reaction following a dose of vaccine will almost always contraindicate a subsequent dose of that vaccine. Anaphylactic reactions are those that are mediated by IgE, occur within minutes or hours of receiving the vaccine, and require medical attention. Examples of symptoms and signs typical of anaphylactic reactions are generalized urticaria (hives), swelling of the mouth and throat, difficulty breathing, wheezing, hypotension, or shock. These reactions are very rare following vaccination and can be further minimized with appropriate screening.

A table listing vaccine contents is included in Appendix B. Persons may be allergic to the vaccine antigen or to a vaccine component such as animal protein, antibiotic, preservative, or stabilizer. The most common animal protein allergen is egg protein found in vaccines prepared using embryonated chicken eggs (e.g., yellow fever and influenza vaccines). Ordinarily, a person who can eat eggs or egg products can receive vaccines that contain egg; persons with histories of anaphylactic or anaphylactic-like allergy to eggs or egg proteins should be referred for further evaluation. Asking persons whether they can eat eggs without adverse effects is a reasonable way to screen for those who might be at risk from receiving yellow fever and egg-containing influenza vaccines.

Studies have shown that children who have a history of severe allergy to eggs rarely have reactions to MMR vaccine. This is probably because measles and mumps vaccine viruses are both grown in chick embryo fibroblasts, not actually in eggs. It appears that gelatin, not egg, might be the cause of allergic reactions to MMR. As a result, in 1998, the ACIP removed severe egg allergy as a contraindication to measles and mumps vaccines. Egg-allergic children may be vaccinated with MMR without prior skin testing.

Certain vaccines contain trace amounts of neomycin. Persons who have experienced an anaphylactic reaction to neomycin should not receive these vaccines. Most often,

2

neomycin allergy presents as contact dermatitis, a manifestation of a delayed-type (cell-mediated) immune response, rather than anaphylaxis. A history of delayed-type reactions to neomycin is not a contraindication for administration of vaccines that contain neomycin.

Latex is sap from the commercial rubber tree. Latex contains naturally occurring impurities (e.g., plant proteins and peptides), which are believed to be responsible for allergic reactions. Latex is processed to form natural rubber latex and dry natural rubber. Dry natural rubber and natural rubber latex might contain the same plant impurities as latex but in lesser amounts. Natural rubber latex is used to produce medical gloves, catheters, and other products. Dry natural rubber is used in syringe plungers, vial stoppers, and injection ports on intravascular tubing. Synthetic rubber and synthetic latex also are used in medical gloves, syringe plungers, and vial stoppers. Synthetic rubber and synthetic latex do not contain natural rubber or natural latex, and therefore, do not contain the impurities linked to allergic reactions.

The most common type of latex sensitivity is contact-type (type 4) allergy, usually as a result of prolonged contact with latex-containing gloves. However, injection-procedure-associated latex allergies among diabetic patients have been described. Allergic reactions (including anaphylaxis) after vaccination procedures are rare. Only one report of an allergic reaction after administration of hepatitis B vaccine in a patient with known severe allergy (anaphylaxis) to latex has been published.

If a person reports a severe (anaphylactic) allergy to latex, vaccines supplied in vials or syringes that contain natural rubber should not be administered unless the benefit of vaccination clearly outweighs the risk of an allergic reaction to the vaccine. For latex allergies other than anaphylactic allergies (e.g., a history of contact allergy to latex gloves), vaccines supplied in vials or syringes that contain dry natural rubber or natural rubber latex can be administered.

Pregnancy

The concern with vaccination of a pregnant woman is infection of the fetus and is theoretical. Only smallpox (vaccinia) vaccine has been shown to cause fetal injury. However, since the theoretical possibility exists, live vaccines should not be administered to women known to be pregnant.

Since inactivated vaccines cannot replicate, they cannot cause fetal infection. In general, inactivated vaccines may be administered to pregnant women for whom they are indicated. An exception is human papillomavirus vaccine,

Vaccination of Pregnant Women
- Live vaccines should not be administered to women known to be pregnant
- In general inactivated vaccines may be administered to pregnant women for whom they are indicated
- HPV vaccine should be deferred during pregnancy

General Recommendations on Immunization

which should be deferred during pregnancy because of a lack of safety and efficacy data for this vaccine in pregnant women.

Pregnant women are at increased risk of complications of influenza. Any woman who will be pregnant during influenza season (generally December through March) should receive inactivated influenza vaccine. Pregnant women should not receive live attenuated influenza vaccine.

ACIP recommends that providers of prenatal care implement a Tdap immunization program for all pregnant women. Healthcare personnel should administer a dose of Tdap during each pregnancy, irrespective of the patient's prior history of receiving Tdap. To maximize the maternal antibody response and passive antibody transfer to the infant, optimal timing for Tdap administration is between 27 and 36 weeks gestation although Tdap may be given at any time during pregnancy. For women not previously vaccinated with Tdap, if Tdap is not administered during pregnancy, Tdap should be administered immediately postpartum.

Studies on the persistence of antipertussis antibodies following a dose of Tdap show antibody levels in healthy, nonpregnant adults peak during the first month after vaccination, with subsequent antibody waning after 1 year. Antibody levels in pregnant women likely would be similar. Because antibody levels wane substantially during the first year after vaccination, ACIP concluded a single dose of Tdap at one pregnancy would be insufficient to provide protection for subsequent pregnancies.

Susceptible household contacts of pregnant women should receive MMR and varicella vaccines, and may receive LAIV, zoster and rotavirus vaccines if they are otherwise eligible.

Immunosuppression

Live vaccines can cause severe or fatal reactions in immunosuppressed persons due to uncontrolled replication of the vaccine virus. Live vaccines should not be administered to severely immunosuppressed persons for this reason. Generally the ultimate determination of severe immunosuppression should be made by the provider treating the immunosuppressed patient. Persons with isolated B-cell deficiency may receive varicella vaccine. Inactivated vaccines cannot replicate, so they are safe to use in immunosuppressed persons. However, response to the vaccine may be decreased.

Both diseases and drugs can cause significant immunosuppression. Persons with congenital immunodeficiency, leukemia, lymphoma, or generalized malignancy should not receive live vaccines. However, MMR, varicella, rotavirus, and LAIV vaccines may be given when an immunosuppressed person lives in the same house. Household contacts of immunosuppressed persons may receive zoster vaccine if indicated.

Certain drugs may cause immunosuppression. For instance, persons receiving cancer treatment with alkylating agents or antimetabolites, or radiation therapy should not be given live vaccines. Live vaccines can be given after chemotherapy has been discontinued for at least 3 months. Persons receiving large doses of corticosteroids should not receive live vaccines. For example, this would include persons receiving 20 milligrams or more of prednisone daily or 2 or more milligrams of prednisone per kilogram of body weight per day for 14 days or longer. See Varicella chapter for more information about administration of zoster vaccine to immunosuppressed persons.

Aerosolized steroids, such as inhalers for asthma, are not contraindications to vaccination, nor are alternate-day, rapidly tapering, and short (less than 14 days) high-dose schedules, topical formulations, and physiologic replacement schedules.

The safety and efficacy of live attenuated vaccines administered concurrently with recombinant human immune mediators and immune modulators are not known. There is evidence that use of therapeutic monoclonal antibodies, especially the anti-tumor necrosis factor (TNF) agents adalimumab, infliximab, and etanercept, may lead to reactivation of latent tuberculosis infection and tuberculosis disease and predispose to other opportunistic infections. Because these drugs vary dramatically in the scope and number of immune system targeted components, it is prudent to avoid administration of live attenuated vaccines while patients are taking these drugs. For immunization against seasonal influenza and typhoid, inactivated injectable alternatives are available.

The period of time providers should wait after discontinuation of immune modulator drugs before administering a live-virus vaccine is not specified by ACIP or other authoritative guidelines (except in the case of zoster vaccine). Consultation with the prescribing physician (and possibly a hospital pharmacist) is recommended for management of individual patients and guidance in estimating a particular patient's degree of immunosuppression. No basis exists for interpreting laboratory studies of immune parameters with vaccines' safety or efficacy. Some experts recommend waiting 1 month after discontinuing etanercept and 3 months after discontinuing the other anti-TNF agents. Lymphocyte depleting agents such as alemtuzumab and rituximab may cause prolonged immunosuppression.

Immunosuppression

- Disease
  - congenital immunodeficiency
  - leukemia or lymphoma
  - generalized malignancy
- Chemotherapy
  - alkylating agents
  - antimetabolites
  - radiation
- Corticosteroids
  - 20 mg or more per day of prednisone*
  - 2 mg/kg or more per day of prednisone*
  - NOT aerosols, alternate-day, short courses, topical

*for 14 days or longer

General Recommendations on Immunization

Restarting immunosuppression after live viral vaccination has not been studied, but some experts would recommend at least a 1-month period.

Inactivated vaccines may be administered to immunosuppressed persons. Certain vaccines are recommended or encouraged specifically because immunosuppression is a risk factor for complications from vaccine-preventable diseases (i.e., influenza, invasive pneumococcal disease, invasive meningococcal disease, invasive *Haemophilus influenzae* type b disease, and hepatitis B). However, response to the vaccine may be poor depending on the degree of immunosuppression present. Because a relatively functional immune system is required to develop an immune response to a vaccine, an immunosuppressed person may not be protected even if the vaccine has been given. Additional recommendations for vaccination of immunosuppressed persons are detailed in the *General Recommendations on Immunization*.

HIV Infection

Persons infected with human immunodeficiency virus (HIV) may have no disease manifestations, or they may be severely immunosuppressed. In general, the same vaccination recommendations apply as with other types of immunosuppression. Live-virus vaccines are usually contraindicated in those with severe immunosuppression (defined by the treating provider) but inactivated vaccines may be administered if indicated.

Varicella can be a very severe illness in persons with HIV infection and is often associated with complications. Varicella vaccine can be considered for persons with HIV infection who are not severely immunosuppressed. Zoster vaccine should not be given to persons with AIDS or clinical manifestations of HIV infection. Persons with HIV infection should not receive LAIV; they should receive inactivated influenza vaccine (IIV). Yellow fever vaccine should be considered for persons who do not have AIDS or other symptomatic manifestations of HIV infection, who have established laboratory verification of adequate immune system function, and who cannot avoid potential exposure to yellow fever virus.

Household contacts without evidence of immunity to measles, mumps, rubella, or varicella should receive MMR and varicella vaccines, and may receive rotavirus, zoster and LAIV vaccines if otherwise eligible.

Vaccination of Hematopoietic Cell Transplant Recipients

Hematopoietic cell transplant (HCT) is the infusion of hematopoietic cells from a donor into a patient who has received chemotherapy and often radiation, both of which are usually bone marrow ablative. HCT is used to treat a variety of neoplastic diseases, hematologic disorders, immunodeficiency syndromes, congenital enzyme deficiencies, and autoimmune disorders. HCT recipients can receive either their own cells (i.e., autologous HCT) or cells from a donor other than the transplant recipient (i.e., allogeneic HCT).

Antibody titers to vaccine-preventable diseases (e.g., tetanus, poliovirus, measles, mumps, rubella, and encapsulated bacteria [i.e., *Streptococcus pneumoniae* and *Haemophilus influenzae* type b]) decline during the 1–4 years after allogeneic or autologous HCT if the recipient is not revaccinated. HCT recipients are at increased risk for certain vaccine-preventable diseases. As a result, HCT recipients should be routinely revaccinated after HCT, regardless of the source of the transplanted cells. Revaccination with inactivated vaccines should begin 6 months after HCT. Influenza vaccine also should be administered at 6 months after HCT, but can be given as early as 4 months after HCT. In this circumstance an additional dose should be given. Influenza vaccine should be given annually thereafter for the life of the recipient. Three doses of PCV13 should be given 6 months after HCT, followed by a dose of PPSV23. Revaccination to prevent pertussis should involve a primary series of DTaP followed by a Tdap booster. A dose of MCV4 should be given.

MMR and varicella vaccines should be administered 24 months after transplantation if the HCT recipient is presumed to be immunocompetent.

Household and other close contacts of HCT recipients and healthcare providers who care for HCT recipients should be appropriately vaccinated, particularly against influenza, measles, mumps, rubella, and varicella. Additional details of vaccination of HCT recipients and their contacts can be found in the ACIP statement titled *General Recommendations on Immunization*.

Moderate or Severe Acute Illness

There is no evidence that a concurrent acute illness reduces vaccine efficacy or increases vaccine adverse events. The concern is that an adverse event (particularly fever) following vaccination could complicate the management of a severely ill person. If a person has a moderate or severe acute illness, vaccination with both live and inactivated vaccines should be delayed until the patient has recovered from the illness.

2

Vaccination of Hematopoietic Cell Transplant (HCT) Recipients

- Antibody titers to VPDs decline during the 1-4 years after allogeneic or autologous HCT if the recipient is not revaccinated

- HCT recipients are at increased risk of some VPDs, particularly pneumococcal disease

- Revaccination recommended beginning 6-12 months post-transplant

- Inactivated influenza vaccine at least 6 months following transplant and annual thereafter

- Inactivated vaccines (DTaP/Td, IPV, hepatitis B, Hib, PCV13, PPSV23) at 6 months

- MMR and varicella vaccines at 24 months if immunocompetent

Vaccination of Household Contacts of Hematopoietic Cell Transplant (HCT) Recipients

- Healthy household contacts of HCT recipients should receive MMR and varicella vaccines and annual influenza vaccination

General Recommendations on Immunization

Invalid Contraindications to Vaccination

Some healthcare providers inappropriately consider certain conditions or circumstances to be contraindications or precautions to vaccinations. Such conditions or circumstances are known as invalid contraindications; these misperceptions result in missed opportunities to administer needed vaccines. Some of the most common invalid contraindications are mild illnesses, conditions related to pregnancy and breastfeeding, allergies that are not anaphylactic in nature, and certain aspects of the patient's family history.

Mild Illness

Children with mild acute illnesses, such as low-grade fever, upper respiratory infection (URI), colds, otitis media, and mild diarrhea, should be vaccinated on schedule. Several large studies have shown that young children with URI, otitis media, diarrhea, and/or fever respond to measles vaccine as well as those without these conditions. There is no evidence that mild diarrhea reduces the success of immunization of infants in the United States.

Low-grade fever is not a contraindication to immunization. Temperature measurement is not necessary before immunization if the infant or child does not appear ill and the parent does not say the child is currently ill. ACIP has not defined a body temperature above which vaccines should not be administered. The decision to vaccinate should be based on the overall evaluation of the person rather than an arbitrary body temperature.

Antimicrobial Therapy

Antibiotics do not have an effect on the immune response to most vaccines. The manufacturer advises that Ty21a oral typhoid vaccine should not be administered to persons receiving sulfonamides or other antibiotics; Ty21a should be administered at least 72 hours after a dose of an antibacterial drug.

No commonly used antimicrobial drug will inactivate a live-virus vaccine. However, antiviral drugs may affect vaccine replication in some circumstances. Live attenuated influenza vaccine should not be administered until 48 hours after cessation of therapy using antiviral drugs active against influenza (amantadine, rimantadine, zanamivir, oseltamivir). Antiviral drugs active against herpesviruses (acyclovir, famciclovir) should be discontinued 24 hours before administration of a varicella-containing vaccine, if possible.

Disease Exposure or Convalescence

If a person is not moderately or severely ill, he or she should be vaccinated. There is no evidence that either disease exposure or convalescence will affect the response to a vaccine or increase the likelihood of an adverse event.

Pregnant or Immunosuppressed Person in the Household

It is critical that healthy household contacts of pregnant women and immunosuppressed persons be vaccinated. Vaccination of healthy contacts reduces the chance of exposure of pregnant women and immunosuppressed persons.

Most vaccines, including live vaccines (MMR, varicella, zoster, rotavirus, LAIV, and yellow fever) can be administered to infants or children who are household contacts of pregnant or immunosuppressed persons, as well as to breastfeeding infants (where applicable). Vaccinia (smallpox) vaccine should not be administered to household contacts of a pregnant or immunosuppressed person in a nonemergency situation. Live attenuated influenza vaccine should not be administered to persons who have contact with persons who are hospitalized and require care in a protected environment (i.e., who are in isolation because of immunosuppression). LAIV may be administered to contacts of persons with lesser degrees of immunosuppression.

Transmission of measles and mumps vaccine viruses to household or other contacts has never been documented. Rubella vaccine virus has been shown to be shed in human milk, but transmission to an infant has rarely been documented. Transmission of varicella vaccine virus has been reported very rarely, and most women and older immunosuppressed persons are immune from having had chickenpox as a child. Transmission of zoster vaccine virus to household or other close contacts has not been reported.

Breastfeeding

Breastfeeding does not decrease the response to routine childhood vaccines and is not a contraindication for any vaccine except smallpox. Yellow fever vaccine should be avoided in breastfeeding women. However, when nursing mothers cannot avoid or postpone travel to areas endemic for yellow fever in which risk for acquisition is high, these women should be vaccinated. Breastfeeding also does not extend or improve the passive immunity to vaccine-preventable disease that is provided by maternal antibody except possibly for *Haemophilus influenzae* type b. Breastfed infants should be vaccinated according to recommended schedules.

Although rubella vaccine virus might be shed in human milk, infection of an infant is rare. LAIV may be administered to a woman who is breastfeeding if she is otherwise eligible; the risk of transmission of vaccine virus is unknown but is probably low.

Preterm Birth

Vaccines should be started on schedule on the basis of the child's chronological age. Preterm infants have been shown to respond adequately to vaccines used in infancy.

Studies demonstrate that decreased seroconversion rates might occur among preterm infants with very low birth weight (less than 2,000 grams) after administration of hepatitis B vaccine at birth. However, by 1 month chronological age, all preterm infants, regardless of initial birth weight or gestational age are as likely to respond as adequately as older and larger infants. All preterm infants born to hepatitis B surface antigen (HBsAg)-positive mothers and mothers with unknown HBsAg status must receive immunoprophylaxis with hepatitis B vaccine within 12 hours after birth. Hepatitis B immunoglobulin (HBIG) also must be given to these infants. If the maternal HBsAg status is unknown, and the infant weighs 2,000 grams or more, HBIG must be given within 7 days of birth. If the maternal HBsAg status is positive or the infant weighs less than 2,000 grams, HBIG must be given within 12 hours of birth. Note that if the infant weighs less than 2,000 grams, the initial hepatitis B vaccine dose should not be counted toward completion of the hepatitis B vaccine series, and three additional doses of hepatitis B vaccine should be administered beginning when the infant is 1 month of age.

Preterm infants with a birth weight of less than 2,000 grams who are born to women documented to be HBsAg-negative at the time of birth should receive the first dose of the hepatitis B vaccine series at 1 month of chronological age or at the time of hospital discharge.

Allergy to Products Not Present in Vaccine

Infants and children with nonspecific allergies, duck or feather allergy, or allergy to penicillin, children who have relatives with allergies, and children taking allergy shots can and should be immunized. No vaccine available in the United States contains duck antigen or penicillin.

Allergy That is Not Anaphylactic

Anaphylactic allergy to a vaccine component (such as egg or neomycin) is a true contraindication to vaccination. If an allergy to a vaccine component is not anaphylactic or is not severe, it is not a contraindication to that vaccine.

Family History of Adverse Events

A family history of seizures is a precaution for the use of MMRV vaccine. Immunosuppression may affect the decision for varicella vaccine. A family history of adverse reactions unrelated to immunosuppression or family history of seizures or sudden infant death syndrome (SIDS) is not a contraindication to vaccination. Varicella vaccine should not be administered to persons who have a family history of congenital or hereditary immunodeficiency in first-degree relatives (e.g., parents and siblings) unless the immunocompetence of the potential vaccine recipient has been clinically substantiated or verified by a laboratory.

Tuberculin Skin Test

Infants and children who need a tuberculin skin test (TST) can and should be immunized. All vaccines, including MMR, can be given on the same day as a TST, or any time after a TST is applied. For most vaccines, there are no TST timing restrictions.

MMR vaccine may decrease the response to a TST, potentially causing a false-negative response in someone who actually has an infection with tuberculosis. MMR can be given the same day as a TST, but if MMR has been given and 1 or more days have elapsed, in most situations a wait of at least 4 weeks is recommended before giving a routine TST. No information on the effect of varicella-containing vaccine or LAIV on a TST is available. Until such information is available, it is prudent to apply rules for spacing measles vaccine and TST to varicella vaccine and LAIV.

containing (See 9/2015 Errata)

There is a type of tuberculosis test known as an interferon-gamma release assay (IGRA). Even though this test improves upon the TST because it is less affected by previous doses of BCG vaccine and less affected by previous doses of tuberculosis diagnostic testing, it still may be affected by previous doses of other live vaccines so it is prudent to apply the same spacing rules as for TST.

Multiple Vaccines

As noted earlier in this chapter, administration at the same visit of all vaccines for which a person is eligible is critical to reaching and maintaining high vaccination coverage. Varicella vaccine should not be administered simultaneously with smallpox vaccine; and PCV13 and Menactra should not be administered simultaneously in children with functional or anatomic asplenia.

General Recommendations on Immunization

Screening for Contraindications and Precautions to Vaccination

The key to preventing serious adverse reactions is screening. Every person who administers vaccines should screen every patient for contraindications and precautions before giving the vaccine dose. Effective screening is not difficult or complicated and can be accomplished with just a few questions.

Is the child (or are you) sick today?

There is no evidence that acute illness reduces vaccine efficacy or increases vaccine adverse events. However, as a precaution, with moderate or severe acute illness, all vaccines should be delayed until the illness has improved. Mild illnesses (such as otitis media, upper respiratory infections, and diarrhea) are NOT contraindications to vaccination. Do not withhold vaccination if a person is taking antibiotics.

Does the child have allergies to medications, food, or any vaccine?

A history of anaphylactic reaction such as hives (urticaria), wheezing or difficulty breathing, or circulatory collapse or shock (not fainting) from a previous dose of vaccine or vaccine component is a contraindication for further doses. It may be more efficient to inquire about allergies in a generic way (i.e., any food or medication) rather than to inquire about specific vaccine components. Most parents will not be familiar with minor components of vaccine, but they should know if the child has had an allergic reaction to a food or medication that was severe enough to require medical attention. If a person reports anaphylaxis after eating eggs, a specific protocol should be followed that includes ascertaining the symptoms experienced. For specific information, see Influenza chapter.

Has the child had a serious reaction to a vaccine in the past?

A history of anaphylactic reaction to a previous dose of vaccine or vaccine component is a contraindication for subsequent doses. A history of encephalopathy within 7 days following DTP/DTaP is a contraindication for further doses of pertussis-containing vaccine. Precautions to DTaP (not Tdap) include (a) seizure within 3 days of a dose, (b) pale or limp episode or collapse within 48 hours of a dose, (c) continuous crying for 3 hours within 48 hours of a dose, and (d) fever of 105°F (40°C) or higher within 48 hours of a previous dose. There are other adverse events that might have occurred following vaccination that constitute contraindications or precautions to future doses. Usually vaccines are deferred when a precaution is present. However, situations may arise when the benefit outweighs the risk (e.g., during a community pertussis outbreak). A local reaction (redness or swelling at the site of injection) is not a contraindication to subsequent doses.

Has the child had a seizure, or brain or nerve problem?

DTaP and Tdap are contraindicated for children who have a history of encephalopathy not attributed to an identifiable cause within 7 days following DTP/DTaP. An unstable progressive neurologic problem is a precaution to the use of DTaP and Tdap. Children with stable neurologic disorders (including seizures) unrelated to vaccination may be vaccinated as usual.

A history of Guillain-Barré syndrome is a precaution for tetanus-containing and influenza vaccines.

Patients with a personal or family history of febrile or afebrile seizures have a precaution for MMRV vaccine. Simultaneous MMR and varicella vaccine administration (the single component vaccines) is not associated with an increased risk of fever or seizures and is therefore the acceptable alternative to MMRV.

Has the child had a health problem with asthma, lung disease, heart disease, kidney disease, metabolic disease such as diabetes, or a blood disorder?

Children with any of these conditions should not receive LAIV. Children with these conditions should receive inactivated influenza vaccine only.

Does the child have cancer, leukemia, AIDS, or any other immune system problem?

Live-virus vaccines (e.g., MMR, varicella, rotavirus, and the intranasal live attenuated influenza vaccine [LAIV]) are usually contraindicated in severely immunocompromised children. Persons with severe immunosuppression should not receive MMR, varicella, rotavirus, or LAIV vaccines. However, there are exceptions. For example, MMR and varicella vaccines are recommended for HIV-infected children who do not have evidence of severe immunosuppression. For details, consult the ACIP recommendations for each vaccine.

Has the child taken cortisone, prednisone, other steroids, or anticancer drugs, or had x-ray treatments in the past 3 months?

Live-virus vaccines (e.g., MMR, varicella, zoster, LAIV) should be postponed until after chemotherapy or long-term, high-dose steroid therapy has ended. Details and the length of time to postpone vaccination are described elsewhere in this chapter and in the *General Recommendations on Immunization*.

Has the child received a transfusion of blood or blood products, or been given a medicine called immune (gamma) globulin in the past year?

Certain live virus vaccines (e.g., MMR and varicella) may need to be deferred, depending on the type of blood product and the interval since the blood product was administered. Information on recommended intervals between immune globulin or blood product administration and MMR or varicella vaccination is in Appendix A and in the *General Recommendations on Immunization*.

Is the person pregnant or is there a chance she could become pregnant during the next month?

Live-virus vaccines (e.g., MMR, varicella, zoster, LAIV) are contraindicated during pregnancy because of the theoretical risk of virus transmission to the fetus. Sexually active young women who receive MMR or varicella vaccination should be instructed to practice careful contraception for 1 month following receipt of either vaccine. On theoretical grounds, inactivated poliovirus vaccine should not be given during pregnancy; however, it may be given if the risk of exposure is imminent (e.g., travel to endemic-disease areas) and immediate protection is needed.

Has the child received vaccinations in the past 4 weeks?

If the child was given either live attenuated influenza vaccine or an injectable live-virus vaccine (e.g., MMR. varicella, yellow fever) in the past 4 weeks, he or she should wait 28 days before receiving another live vaccine. Inactivated vaccines may be given at the same time or at any time before or after a live vaccine.

Every person should be screened for contraindications and precautions before vaccination. Standardized screening forms for both children and adults have been developed by the Immunization Action Coalition and are available at http://www.immunize.org.

Selected References

American Academy of Pediatrics. Active and passive immunization. In: Pickering LK, Baker CJ, Kimberlin DW, Long SS, eds. *Red Book: 2012 Report of the Committee on Infectious Diseases*. 29th edition. Elk Grove Village, IL: American Academy of Pediatrics; 2012.

Atkinson WL, Kroger AT, Pickering LK. General immunization practices. In: Plotkin SA, Orentsein WA, Offit PA. eds. *Vaccines*. 5th ed., China: Saunders; 2008.

CDC. General recommendations on immunization: recommendations of the Advisory Committee on Immunization Practices. *MMWR* 2011;60(No. RR-2):1–61.

Dietz VJ, Stevenson J, Zell ER, et al. Potential impact on vaccination coverage levels by administering vaccines simultaneously and reducing dropout rates. *Arch Pediatr Adolesc Med* 1994;148:943–9.

James JM, Burks AW, Roberson RK, Sampson HA. Safe administration of the measles vaccine to children allergic to eggs. *N Engl J Med* 1995;332:1262–9.

King GE, Hadler SC. Simultaneous administration of childhood vaccines: an important public health policy that is safe and efficacious. *Pediatr Infect Dis J* 1994;13:394–407.

Plotkin SA. Vaccines, vaccination and vaccinology. *J. Infect Dis* 2003;187:1349–59.

Tomblyn M, Chiller T, Einsele H, et. al. Guidelines for preventing infectious complications among hematopoietic cell transplant recipients: a global perspective. *Biol Blood Marrow Transplant* 2009;15:1143-1238.

Wood, RA, Berger M, Dreskin M, et. al. An algorithm for treatment of patients with hypersensitivity reactions after vaccines. *Pediatrics* 2008;122 (No. 3) e771-7.

General Recommendations on Immunization

Immunization Strategies for Healthcare Practices and Providers

The Need for Strategies to Increase Immunization Levels

An important component of an immunization provider's practice is ensuring that the vaccines reach all people who need them. While attention to appropriate administration of vaccinations is essential, it cannot be assumed that these vaccinations are being given to every person at the recommended age. Immunization levels in the United States are high, but gaps still exist, and providers can do much to maintain or increase immunization rates among patients in their practice. This chapter describes the need for increasing immunization levels and outlines strategies that providers can adopt to increase coverage in their own practice.

Vaccine-preventable disease rates in the United States are at very low levels. In 2011, only 4 cases of rubella, no cases of diphtheria, 36 cases of tetanus, and no wild-type polio were reported to CDC. Given these immunization successes, one might question the continued interest in strategies to increase immunization levels.

Resurgence of some vaccine-preventable diseases such as pertussis, expanded recommendations for influenza vaccination and HPV vaccination, and gaps in sustainable immunization efforts highlight the need to focus on immunization rates. The viruses and bacteria that cause vaccine-preventable disease and death still exist and can be passed on to unprotected persons or imported from other countries, as demonstrated by pertussis outbreaks that occurred in 2010. Diseases such as measles, mumps, or pertussis can be more severe than often assumed and can result in social and economic as well as physical costs: sick children miss school, parents lose time from work, and illness among healthcare providers can severely disrupt a healthcare system. Although levels of disease are the ultimate outcome of interest, these are a late indicator of the soundness of the immunization system. Immunization levels are a better indicator for determining if there is a problem with immunization delivery, and this chapter will focus on increasing immunization levels and the strategies healthcare providers can use to do this.

Specific concerns about U.S. immunization levels and areas for further study include the following:

Childhood immunization rates are still suboptimal. In 2011, for example, only 84.6% of children 19 to 35 months of age had received four doses of DTaP vaccine.

For other age groups, immunization rates are considerably lower than those for early childhood. According to Behavior Risk Factor Surveillance System (BRFSS) data from 2011, a

3

median of only 64.9% of persons 65 years of age and older received the influenza vaccine in the past 12 months, and 62.3% had ever received pneumococcal vaccine.

Rates of influenza immunization are also unacceptably low among healthcare providers, an important target population for vaccination. Typically, fewer than 70% of healthcare providers receive influenza vaccine.

Sustainable systems for vaccinating children, adolescents, and adults must be developed in the context of a changing healthcare system. High immunization rates cannot rest upon one-time or short-term efforts. Greater understanding of strategies to increase and sustain immunization levels is necessary in order to create lasting, effective immunization delivery systems.

Many strategies have been used to increase immunizations. Some, such as school entry laws, have effectively increased demand for vaccines, but the effectiveness of other strategies (e.g., advertising) is less well documented. Some proven strategies (e.g., reducing costs, linking immunization to Women Infants and Children (WIC) services, home visiting) are well suited to increasing rates among specific populations, such as persons with low access to immunization services.

One key to a successful strategy to increase immunization is matching the proposed solution to the current problem. Although a combination of strategies—directed at both providers and the public—is necessary for increasing and maintaining high immunization rates, this chapter focuses on immunization strategies for healthcare practices and providers.

The AFIX Approach

CDC, through state and other grantees, administers a program designed to move healthcare personnel from a state of unawareness about the problem of low immunization rates in their practice to one in which they are knowledgeable, concerned, motivated to change their immunization practices, and capable of sustaining new behaviors. The acronym used for this approach is AFIX: Assessment of the immunization coverage of public and private providers, Feedback of diagnostic information to improve service delivery, Incentives to motivate providers to change immunization practices or recognition of improved or high performance, and eXchange of information among providers. First conceived by the Georgia Division of Public Health, AFIX is now being used nationwide with both public and private immunization providers and is recommended by governmental and nongovernmental vaccine programs and medical professional societies.

AFIX

Assessment

Feedback

Incentives

e**X**change

Immunization Strategies for Healthcare Practices and Providers

Overview

The AFIX process consists of an assessment of an immunization provider's coverage rates by a trained representative from the state or other immunization grantee program, feedback of the results of the assessment to provider staff, incentives to improve deficiencies and raise immunization rates, and exchange of information and ideas among healthcare providers. Some specific characteristics of this approach have made it one of the most effective for achieving high, sustainable vaccine coverage.

First, AFIX focuses on outcomes. It starts with an assessment, producing an estimate of immunization coverage levels in a provider's office, and these data help to identify specific actions to take in order to remedy deficiencies. Outcomes are easily measurable. Second, AFIX focuses on providers, those who are key to increasing immunization rates. AFIX requires no governmental policy changes, nor does it attempt to persuade clients to be vaccinated, but instead focuses on changing healthcare provider behavior. Third, AFIX, when used successfully, is a unique blend of advanced technology and personal interaction. Much of the AFIX process can be done electronically, increasing speed and accuracy of assessment and feedback and streamlining reporting. However, the personal skills of the assessor and that person's ability to establish rapport with and motivate a provider are critical to achieving lasting results.

Assessment

Assessment refers to the evaluation of medical records to ascertain the immunization rate for a defined group of patients, as well as to provide targeted diagnosis for improvement. This step is essential because several studies have documented that most healthcare providers, while supportive of immunizations, do not have an accurate perception of their own practice's immunization rates. Pediatricians in these studies greatly overestimated the proportion of fully immunized children in their practices. Assessment increases awareness of a provider's actual situation and provides a basis for subsequent actions by provider staff.

CDC has developed a software program, CoCASA, which enables assessment to be done electronically, is flexible enough to accommodate whatever assessment parameters are desired, and provides results that can be printed immediately. This program will be described further in the section titled "AFIX Tools and Resources".

> **Special Characteristics of AFIX**
> - Focuses on outcomes
> - Focuses on providers
> - Blend of advanced technology and personal interaction

3

> **Assessment**
> - Evaluation of medical records to ascertain the immunization rate for a defined group
> - Targeted diagnosis for improvement
> - Assessment increases awareness

Immunization Strategies for Healthcare Practices and Providers

Feedback

- Informing immunization providers about their performance
- Assessment with feedback creates the awareness necessary for behavior change

How to Provide Feedback

- With feeling and precision
- Without judgment
- With confidentiality as appropriate

Incentives

- Something that incites to action or effort
- Vary by provider and stage of progress
- Opportunities for partnership and collaboration

Feedback

Feedback is the process of informing immunization providers about their performance in delivering one or more vaccines to a defined client population. The work of assessment is of no use unless the results are fed back to persons who can make a change. Assessment together with feedback creates the awareness necessary for behavior change.

Feedback generally consists of the immunization program representative meeting with appropriate provider staff and discussing the results of the assessment in order to determine the next steps to be taken. This may be done at a second visit following the assessment of the provider's records, or it may take place the same day. There are advantages and disadvantages to each approach. If CoCASA has been used, the summary report that is generated can identify specific subsets of patients (e.g., those who have not completed the series because of a missed opportunity for immunization) that, if found in substantial numbers, can provide clues to which changes in the provider's practice would be most effective. This can save time and make the feedback session more focused.

The personal element of feedback, as mentioned, is also critical to its success. A reviewer who is involved and committed to the AFIX process, who addresses deficiencies without judgment, and who respects the confidentiality of the data and the efforts of the provider, will be likely to gain the trust of providers and motivate them to increase immunization rates in the practice.

Incentives

An incentive is defined as something that incites one to action or effort. Incentives are built into the AFIX process, recognizing that immunization providers, like everyone else, will accomplish a desired task more successfully if motivated to do so. The assessment and feedback components are not intended to be done in isolation; providers may have sufficient data about their practice's immunization rates, but they must recognize high immunization coverage as a desirable goal and be motivated to achieve it.

Incentives are extremely variable. No one thing will be effective for every provider, and a single provider may need different types of motivation at different stages of progress. Things like small tokens of appreciation and providing resource materials at meetings have helped providers approach their task positively and create an atmosphere of teamwork, but longer-term goals must be considered as well. Since the effort to raise immunization rates may involve an increase in duties for staff, offering assistance in reviewing records or sending reminder notices might more directly address a provider's needs. Incentives pose a challenge to the creativity of the program representative but also offer the opportunity to try new ideas.

Finally, incentives are opportunities for partnerships and collaboration. Professional organizations or businesses have been solicited to publicize the immunization efforts in a newsletter or provide funding for other rewards for provider staff. Many other types of collaboration are possible; these also have the benefit of increasing awareness of immunization among diverse groups.

eXchange of Information

The final AFIX component, eXchange of information, goes hand in hand with incentives. The more information providers have about their own practice's immunization coverage status, how it compares with state norms and with other providers in their community, and what strategies have been successful with other providers, the more knowledgeable and motivated they will be to increase their immunization rates. It is up to the AFIX representative to provide appropriate statistical and educational information and create forums for exchange of information among providers.

Staff members at all levels can benefit from the exchange of ideas about immunization practices and increasing rates of coverage—what has worked or not worked with another provider, streamlining office procedures, or where to obtain educational or other resources. The forums for such exchanges vary widely from informal meetings on the local level to more structured meetings sponsored by government or professional organizations. Immunization training sessions can be combined with sharing of ideas regarding actual situations in which recommendations, such as those from ACIP, are applied.

With the increased use of electronic communication, this method should not be neglected in the information exchange component of AFIX. Although different from face-to-face communication, e-mail exchanges or newsletters sent electronically can be cost-saving and fast means of disseminating information.

VFC/AFIX Initiative

Responsibility for immunization has largely shifted from public health departments to private providers, who now vaccinate nearly 80% of children in the United States. Many of these providers participate in the Vaccines for Children (VFC) program, a federal program whereby funding is provided for state and other immunization programs to purchase vaccines and make them available at no cost to children who meet income eligibility requirements. CDC launched an initiative in 2000 to link some AFIX and VFC

---

eXchange of Information

- Allows access to more experience than an individual can accumulate
- Motivates improvement
- Coordinates resources and efforts

VFC/AFIX

- 2000: Incorporate AFIX activities during VFC site visits
- 2013: VFC visits performed separately from AFIX visits
- VFC/AFIX visits may be combined if state has robust IIS, which assists with AFIX component

3

activities and incorporate AFIX activities during VFC provider site visits in an attempt to avoid duplication of staff time and effort. However, reported concerns with proper storage and handling of vaccine led the federal VFC program to revise this approach. Beginning in 2013, VFC program staff are encouraged to perform VFC compliance visits separate from the AFIX visit to focus on the core components of each program, including the assessment of, and provider training related to, proper vaccine storage practices. VFC programs may choose to continue to combine these program efforts if the state has a robust Immunization Information System (IIS) that assists with performing the AFIX assessment portion of the visits.

VFC serves more than 40,000 private provider sites, and every state participates in the program. VFC provider site visits are conducted to review compliance with federal program requirements, including VFC eligibility screening, and to evaluate vaccine storage and handling procedures. Information about VFC can be found at http://www.cdc.gov/vaccines/programs/vfc/default.htm.

AFIX Tools and Resources

CDC has developed a software program titled Comprehensive Clinic Assessment Software Application (CoCASA) to enable electronic entry of AFIX and VFC site visit data. CoCASA, first released in December 2005, is an update of previous versions of CASA and supersedes previous versions. Using CoCASA, a reviewer enters appropriate basic information about an individual provider and conducts an assessment of patient records. The user also has the option to record AFIX visit outcomes and VFC site visit information.

CoCASA can provide immediate results of the assessment, supplying the reviewer with the information needed for use in the feedback session and noting areas that need further follow-up. CoCASA saves the reviewer time and provides various analysis options. CoCASA reports provide estimates of immunization coverage levels and potential reasons for the coverage level, such as missed opportunities for immunization and patients who did not return to finish the immunization series. The program can generate reports on specific sets of patients. Data from an immunization registry or patient management system can be imported into CoCASA, and data collected during the visit can be exported for further analysis.

Additional resources available for AFIX include the AFIX Guide to the Core Elements for Training and Implementation document. This document generalizes the AFIX process so that it can be applied to any age group and when differences between populations do exist with respect

---

Comprehensive Clinic Assessment Software Application (CoCASA)

- VFC and AFIX results
- Immediate assessment results
- Estimate of coverage levels
- Reasons for deficiencies
- Reports on patient subsets

AFIX Guide to the Core Elements for Training and Implementation

- Generalizes the AFIX process
- Provides strategies for modifying AFIX methodology

---

to the AFIX process, this document clearly identifies the difference and provides helpful strategies for modifying the AFIX methodology.

CoCASA is available on the CDC Vaccines and Immunization website at http://www.cdc.gov/vaccines/programs/cocasa/index.html. Additional information about AFIX, including the Core Elements document, is available on the CDC Vaccines and Immunization website at http://www.cdc.gov/vaccines/programs/afix/index.html.

AFIX Endorsements

AFIX is widely supported as an effective strategy to improve vaccination rates. Many states have shown gradual and consistent improvement in their coverage levels in the public sector, and studies of private pediatricians have also documented substantial improvements in median up-to-date coverage at 24 months. Assessment and feedback of public and private provider sites are recommended by the National Vaccine Advisory Committee (NVAC) in the Standards of Pediatric Immunization Practices, as well as by the Advisory Committee on Immunization Practices (ACIP) in a statement endorsing the AFIX process and recommending its use by all public and private providers. Furthermore, Healthy People 2020 has an objective to increase the proportion of immunization providers who have measured vaccination levels among children in their practice within the past year.

One of the Standards for Adult Immunization Practices issued by NVAC calls upon providers of adult immunization to do annual assessments of coverage levels. Although the use of AFIX among providers who serve adults is not as widespread as among childhood immunization providers, this strategy can be a powerful tool to improve rates in the adult population.

Other Essential Strategies

Although a substantial portion of this chapter is devoted to AFIX, certain other strategies for improvement of immunization levels deserve emphasis. These are complementary to AFIX; their adoption will support the goals of AFIX, i.e., raising immunization coverage levels, and will facilitate the AFIX process and ensure a favorable outcome of an assessment.

Recordkeeping

Patient records are of vital importance in a medical practice, and maintaining these records, whether paper or electronic, is critical to providing optimal healthcare. Immunization records, specifically, should meet all applicable legal requirements as well as requirements of any specific program, such as VFC, in which the provider participates. These

Strategies for High Immunization Levels

- Recordkeeping
- Immunization Information Systems (IIS)
- Recommendations and reinforcement
- Reminder and recall to patients
- Reminder and recall to providers
- Reduction of missed opportunities
- Reduction of barriers to immunization

Records

- Available for inspection
- Easy to interpret
- Accurate, up-to-date, and complete
  - reflect current patient population
  - reflect all vaccines given

3

records should be available for inspection by an AFIX or VFC representative and should be easy to interpret by anyone examining the record.

Immunization records must be accurate. The active medical records must reflect which patients are actually in the practice; charts of persons who have moved or are obtaining services elsewhere should be clearly marked accordingly or removed. Records should be kept up-to-date as new immunizations are administered, and all information regarding the vaccine and its administration should be complete.

Because patients often receive vaccines at more than one provider office, communication between sites is necessary for maintaining complete and accurate immunization records. School-based, public health, and community-based immunization sites should communicate with primary care personnel through quick and reliable methods such as immunization information systems, telephone, fax, or e-mail. This will become increasingly important as venues outside the medical home offer immunizations.

Immunization Information Systems (IIS)

Many recordkeeping tasks, as well as patient reminder/recall activities, can be greatly simplified by participation in a population-based immunization information system (IIS), also known as an immunization registry. An IIS is a computerized information system that contains information about the immunization status of each child in a given geographic area (e.g., a state). In some areas, an IIS is linked to a child's complete medical record. An IIS provides a single data source for all community immunization providers, enabling access to records of children receiving vaccinations at multiple providers. It provides a reliable immunization history for every enrolled child and can also produce accurate immunization records if needed for school or summer camp entry.

The Task Force on Community Preventive Services recommends immunization information systems on the basis of strong evidence of effectiveness in increasing vaccination rates. Specifically, the Task Force concluded that IIS are directly related to increasing vaccination rates through their capabilities to create or support effective interventions such as client reminder/recall systems, provider assessment and feedback, and provider reminders; generate and evaluate public health responses to outbreaks of vaccine-preventable disease; facilitate vaccine management and accountability; determine client vaccination status for decisions made by clinicians, health departments, and schools; and aid surveillance and investigations on vaccination rates, missed vaccination opportunities, invalid dose administration, and disparities in vaccination coverage.

Immunization Information Systems (IIS)

- Single data source for all providers
- Reliable immunization history
- Produce records for patient use
- Increase vaccination rates

Immunization Strategies for Healthcare Practices and Providers

A goal of *Healthy People 2020* is to increase to 95% the proportion of children younger than 6 years of age who participate in fully operational, population-based immunization registries. In 2011, approximately 84% of children in this age group met this participation goal. Federal, state, and local public health agencies are continuing their efforts to improve the registries themselves and to increase participation by immunization providers. IIS are a key to increasing and maintaining immunization levels and provide benefits for providers, patients, and state and federal immunization program personnel. More information about IIS is available on the CDC Vaccines and Immunization website at http://www.cdc.gov/vaccines/programs/iis/index.html.

Recommendations to Parents and Reinforcement of the Need to Return

The recommendation of a healthcare provider is a powerful motivator for patients to comply with vaccination recommendations. Parents of pediatric patients are likely to follow vaccine recommendations of the child's doctor, and even adults who were initially reluctant were likely to receive an influenza vaccination when the healthcare provider's opinion of the vaccine was positive.

Regardless of their child's true immunization status, many parents believe the child is fully vaccinated. Parents may not have been told or may not have understood that return visits are necessary. It is useful for patients to have the next appointment date in hand at the time they leave the provider's office. An additional reminder strategy is to link the timing of the return visit to some calendar event, (e.g., the child's birthday or an upcoming holiday). Even with written schedules or reminders, a verbal encouragement and reminder can be an incentive for a patient's completing the immunization series and can ultimately result in higher coverage levels.

Reminder and Recall Messages to Patients

Patient reminders and recall messages are messages to patients or their parents stating that recommended immunizations are due soon (reminders) or past due (recall messages). The messages vary in their level of personalization and specificity, the mode of communication, (e.g., postcard, letter, telephone), and the degree of automation. Both reminders and recall messages have been found to be effective in increasing attendance at clinics and improving vaccination rates in various settings.

Cost is sometimes thought to be a barrier to the implementation of a reminder/recall system. However, a range of options is available, from computer-generated telephone calls and letters to a card file box with weekly dividers, and

Recommendations and Reinforcement
- Recommend the vaccine
  - powerful motivator
  - patients likely to follow recommendation of the provider
- Reinforce the need to return
  - verbal
  - written
  - link to calendar event

Reminders and Recall to Patients
- Reminder—notification that immunizations are due soon
- Recall—notification that immunizations are past due
- Content of message and technique of delivery vary
- Reminders and recall have been found to be effective

Reminders and Recall to Providers
- Communication to healthcare providers that a patient's immunizations are due soon or past due
- Examples
  - computer-generated list
  - stamped note in the chart
  - "Immunization Due" clip on chart
  - electronic reminder in an electronic medical record

3

these can be adapted to the needs of the provider. The specific type of system is not directly related to its effectiveness, and the benefits of having any system can extend beyond immunizations to other preventive services and increase the use of other recommended screenings.

Both the Standards for Child and Adolescent Immunization Practices and the Standards for Adult Immunization Practices call upon providers to develop and implement aggressive tracking systems that will both remind parents of upcoming immunizations and recall children who are overdue. ACIP supports the use of reminder/recall systems by all providers. The National Center for Immunization and Respiratory Diseases provides state and local health departments with ongoing technical support to assist them in implementing reminder and recall systems in public and private provider sites.

Reminder and Recall Messages to Providers

Providers can create reminder and recall systems that help them remember which patients' routine immunizations are due soon or past due. Provider reminder/recall is different from "feedback," in which the provider receives a message about overall immunization levels for a group of clients. Examples of reminder/recall messages are:

- A computer-generated list that notifies a provider of the children to be seen that clinic session whose vaccinations are past due.

- A stamp with a message such as "No Pneumococcal Vaccine on Record," that a receptionist or nurse can put on the chart of a person age 65 years or older.

- An "Immunization Due" clip that a nurse attaches to the chart of an adolescent who has not had HPV vaccine.

- An electronic reminder which appears when providers access an electronic medical record.

Reminder systems will vary according to the needs of the provider; in addition to raising immunization rates in the practice, they will serve to heighten the awareness of staff members of the continual need to check the immunization status of their patients.

Reduction of Missed Opportunities to Vaccinate

A missed opportunity is a healthcare encounter in which a person is eligible to receive a vaccination but is not vaccinated completely. Missed opportunities occur in all settings in which immunizations are offered, whether routinely or not.

Missed Opportunity

A healthcare encounter in which a person is eligible to receive vaccination but is not vaccinated completely

Immunization Strategies for Healthcare Practices and Providers

Missed opportunities occur for several reasons. At the provider level, many nurses and physicians avoid simultaneous administration of four or even three injectable vaccines. Frequently stated reasons have included concern about reduced immune response or adverse events, and parental objection. These concerns are not supported by scientific data. Providers also may be unaware that a child (or adult) is in need of vaccination (especially if the immunization record is not available at the visit) or may follow invalid contraindications (see Chapter 2 for more information).

Some of the reasons for missed opportunities relate to larger systems; (e.g., a clinic that has a policy of not vaccinating at any visits except well-child care, or not vaccinating siblings). Other reasons relate to large institutional or bureaucratic regulations, such as state insurance laws that deny reimbursement if a vaccine is given during an acute-care visit. The degree of difficulty in eliminating the missed opportunity may vary directly with the size of the system that has to be changed.

Several studies have shown that eliminating missed opportunities could increase vaccination coverage by up to 20 percent. Strategies designed to prevent missed opportunities have taken many different forms, used alone or in combination. Examples include the following:

- **Standing orders.** These are protocols whereby nonphysician immunization personnel may vaccinate clients without direct physician involvement at the time of the immunization. Standing orders are implemented in settings such as clinics, hospitals, and nursing homes. When used alone or in combination with other interventions, standing orders have had positive effects on immunization rates among adults and children.

- **Provider education.** Anyone responsible for administering immunizations should be knowledgeable about principles of vaccination and vaccination scheduling, to the extent required for their position. Providers are largely responsible for educating their patients, so an investment in provider education will result in a higher level of understanding about immunizations among the public in general. Numerous educational materials, in a variety of formats, are available from CDC, the Immunization Action Coalition, and some state health departments, hospitals, or professional organizations. Incorporating some AFIX principles (i.e., assessment, feedback) into a provider education program might have a greater effect on provider behavior than an education effort aimed only at increasing knowledge.

3

Reasons for Missed Opportunities

- Lack of simultaneous administration
- Unaware child (or adult) needs additional vaccines
- Invalid contraindications
- Inappropriate clinic policies
- Reimbursement deficiencies

Strategies for Reducing Missed Opportunities

- Standing orders
- Provider education with feedback
- Provider reminder and recall systems

3

- **Provider reminder and recall systems.** Provider reminder and recall systems are discussed earlier in the chapter. These reminder systems, while effective in increasing immunization levels, can also help avoid missed opportunities if they are a component of other practices directed toward this goal. For example, if a reminder system is used consistently and staff members are knowledgeable about vaccination opportunities and valid contraindications, the system can be an additional aid in promoting appropriate immunization practices.

Reduction of Barriers to Immunization Within the Practice

Despite efforts by providers to adhere to appropriate immunization practices, obstacles to vaccination of patients may exist within the practice setting, sometimes unknown to the provider. Barriers to immunization may be physical or psychological. Physical barriers might be such things as inconvenient clinic hours for working patients or parents, long waits at the clinic, or the distance patients must travel. Providers should be encouraged to determine the needs of their specific patient population and take steps, such as extending clinic hours or providing some immunization clinics, to address obstacles to immunization.

Cost is also a barrier to immunization for many patients. In addition to evaluating their fee schedule for possible adjustments, providers should be knowledgeable about such programs as Vaccines for Children and the State Children's Health Insurance Program and the provisions specific to their state. Enrollment as a VFC provider is recommended for those with eligible children in their practice.

Psychological barriers to healthcare are often more subtle but may be just as important. Unpleasant experiences (e.g., fear of immunizations, being criticized for previously missed appointments, or difficulty leaving work for a clinic appointment) may lead clients to postpone receiving needed vaccinations. Concerns about vaccine safety are also preventing some parents from having their children immunized. Overcoming such barriers calls for both knowledge and interpersonal skills on the part of the provider—knowledge of vaccines and updated recommendations and of reliable sources to direct patients to find accurate information, and skills to deal with fears and misconceptions and to provide a supportive and encouraging environment for patients. For more information on provider resources, see http://www.cdc.gov/vaccines/hcp/patient-ed/conversations/.

Reduction of Barriers to Immunization

- Physical barriers
  - clinic hours
  - waiting time
  - distance
  - cost
- Psychological barriers
  - unpleasant experience
  - vaccine safety concerns

Immunization Strategies for Healthcare Practices and Providers

Acknowledgement

The editors thank Allison Fisher and Maureen Kolasa, CDC, for their assistance in updating this chapter.

Selected References

American Academy of Pediatrics, Committee on Community Health Services and Committee on Practice and Ambulatory Medicine. Increasing Immunization Coverage. *Pediatrics* 2003;112:993–996.

CDC. Noninfluenza Vaccination Coverage Among Adults — United States, 2011. *MMWR* 2013;62:61-76.

CDC. Progress in Immunization Information Systems — United States, 2011. *MMWR* 2013;62:41-60.

CDC. Final State-Level 2011–12 Influenza Vaccination Coverage Estimates. *MMWR* 2012;61:753-776.

CDC. Influenza Vaccination Coverage Among Health-Care Personnel — 2011–12 Influenza Season, United States. *MMWR* 2012;61:753-776.

CDC. Summary of Notifiable Diseases — United States, 2011. *MMWR* 2012;60(No.53):1-118.

CDC. Programmatic strategies to increase vaccination rates —assessment and feedback of provider-based vaccination coverage information. *MMWR* 1996;45:219–220.

CDC. Recommendations of the Advisory Committee on Immunization Practices (ACIP), the American Academy of Pediatrics, and the American Academy of Family Physicians: Use of reminder and recall by vaccination providers to increase vaccination rates. *MMWR* 1998;47:715–717.

Dietz VJ, Baughman AL, Dini EF, Stevenson JM, Pierce BK, Hersey JC. Vaccination practices, policies, and management factors associated with high vaccination coverage levels in Georgia public clinics. *Arch Pediatr Adolesc Med* 2000;154:184–189.

Dini EF, Linkins RW, Sigafoos J. The impact of computer-generated messages on childhood immunization coverage. *Am J Prev Med* 2000;18(2):132–139.

LeBaron CW, Chaney M, Baughman AL, Dini EF, Maes E, Dietz V, et al. Impact of measurement and feedback on vaccination coverage in public clinics, 1988–1994. *JAMA* 1997;277:631–635.

3

3

LeBaron CW, Mercer JT, Massoudi MS, Dini EF, Stevenson JM, Fischer WM, et al. Changes in clinic vaccination coverage after institution of measurement and feedback in 4 states and 2 cities. *Arch Pediatr Adolesc Med* 1999;153:879–886.

Lieu T, Black S, Ray P. Computer-generated recall letters for underimmunized children: how cost-effective? *Pediatr Infect Dis J* 1997;16:28–33.

Lieu T, Capra A, Makol J, Black S, Shinefield H. Effectiveness and cost-effectiveness of letters, automated telephone messages, or both for underimmunized children in a health maintenance organization [Abstract]. *Pediatrics* 1998;101:690–691.

Massoudi MS, Walsh J, Stokley S, Rosenthal J, Stevenson J, Miljanovic B, et al. Assessing immunization performance of private practitioners in Maine: impact of the Assessment, Feedback, Incentives, and eXchange (AFIX) strategy. *Pediatrics* 1999;103:1218–1223.

National Vaccine Advisory Committee. Standards for child and adolescent immunization practices. *Pediatrics* 2003;112:958-63.

National Vaccine Advisory Committee. Recommendations from the National Vaccine Advisory Committee: Standards for Adult Immunization Practice. *Public Health Reports* 2014;129:115-123.

Poland GA, Shefer AM, McCauley M, et al. Standards for adult immunization practices. *Am J Prev Med* 2003;25:144–150.

Szilagyi PG, Rodewald LE, Humiston SG, et al. Immunization practices of pediatricians and family physicians in the United States. *Pediatrics* 1994;94:517–23. Available at http://www.aap.org/research/periodicsurvey/peds10_94b.htm.

Task Force on Community Preventive Services. *Guide to community preventive services*. Atlanta: Centers for Disease Control and Prevention. Available at http://www.thecommunityguide.org.

Yawn BP, Edmonson L, Huber L, Poland GA, Jacobson RM, Jacobsen SJ. The impact of a simulated immunization registry on perceived childhood immunization status. *Am J Managed Care* 1998;4:186–192.

Vaccine safety is a prime concern for the public, manufacturers, immunization providers, and recipients of vaccines. This chapter describes how vaccines licensed for use in the United States are monitored for safety, and presents general information about the provider's role in immunization safety. Further information about contraindications and precautions for individual vaccines, such as pregnancy and immunosuppression, and about potential adverse events associated with the vaccine is contained in the chapter on General Recommendations on Immunization, and in the chapters on specific vaccines.

The Importance of Vaccine Safety Programs

Vaccination is among the most significant public health success stories of all time. However, like any pharmaceutical product, no vaccine is completely safe or completely effective. While almost all known vaccine adverse events are minor and self-limited, some vaccines have been associated with very rare but serious health effects. The following key considerations underscore the need for an active and ongoing vaccine safety program.

Decreases in Disease Risks

Today, vaccine-preventable diseases are at or near record lows. Many people no longer see reminders of the severity and potential life-threatening complications of these diseases. Recent outbreaks of vaccine–preventable diseases show that even vaccinated people are at risk for disease if there is not adequate vaccine coverage in the population. Parents and providers in the United States may be more likely to know someone who has experienced an adverse event following immunization than they are to know someone who has experienced a vaccine-preventable disease. The success of vaccination has led to increased public attention on potential health risks associated with vaccines.

Importance of Vaccine Safety

- Decreases in disease risks and increased attention on vaccine risks
- Public confidence in vaccine safety is critical
  - higher standard of safety is expected of vaccines
  - vaccinees generally healthy (vs. ill for drugs)
  - lower risk tolerance = need to search for rare reactions
  - vaccination universally recommended and mandated

4

Disease	Pre-vaccine Era*	2006§	% decrease
Diphtheria	175,885	0	100
Measles	503,282	55	99.9
Mumps	152,209	6,584	95.7
Pertussis	147,271	15,632	89.4
Polio (paralytic)	16,316	0	100
Rubella	47,745	11	99.9
Congenital Rubella Syndrome	823	1	99.9
Tetanus	1,314	41	99.9
H. influenzae type b and unknown (<5 yrs)	20,000†	208	99.9
Total	1,064,854	22,532	97.9
Vaccine Adverse Events	N/A	15,484	N/A

*Baseline 20th century annual morbidity
§Source: MMWR 2007;56(33):851-64
†Estimated because no national reporting existed in the pre-vaccine era

Vaccination Safety

Public Confidence

Maintaining public confidence in immunizations is critical for preventing a decline in vaccination rates that can result in outbreaks of disease. While the majority of parents understand the benefits of immunization and have their children vaccinated, some have concerns about the safety of vaccines. Public concerns about the safety of whole-cell pertussis vaccine in the 1980s resulted in decreased vaccine coverage and the return of epidemic disease in Japan, Sweden, United Kingdom, and several other countries. Around the same time in the United States, similar concerns led to increases both in the number of lawsuits against manufacturers and the price of vaccines, and to a decrease in the number of manufacturers willing to produce vaccines. This led to the National Childhood Vaccine Injury Act which is discussed in this chapter. Despite high national vaccination coverage rates, there are areas of low coverage that allow outbreaks of vaccine-preventable diseases to occur, many due to concerns about vaccine safety leading parents to refuse or delay their children's immunizations. For example, during 2008, more measles cases were reported than in any year since 1997. More than 90% of those infected had not been vaccinated, or their vaccination status was unknown. In California during January 1- June 30, 2010, 1,337 pertussis cases were reported to the California Department of Public Health, a 418% increase from the 258 cases reported during the same period in 2009. Providing accurate and timely vaccine safety information to healthcare providers, parents, and the general population has a positive effect on vaccine uptake and is a high priority for CDC. Close monitoring and timely assessment of suspected vaccine adverse events can distinguish true vaccine reactions from coincidental unrelated events and help to maintain public confidence in immunizations.

A higher standard of safety is generally expected of vaccines than of other medical interventions because in contrast to most pharmaceutical products, which are administered to ill persons for curative purposes, vaccines are generally given to healthy persons to prevent disease. Public tolerance of adverse reactions related to products given to healthy persons, especially healthy infants and children, is substantially lower than for reactions to products administered to persons who are already sick. This lower tolerance of risk for vaccines translates into a need to investigate the possible causes of very rare adverse events following vaccinations.

Adding to public concern about vaccines is the fact that immunization is mandated by many state and local school entry requirements. Because of this widespread use, safety problems with vaccines can have a potential impact on large numbers of persons. The importance of ensuring the safety of a relatively universal human-directed "exposure" like immunizations is the basis for strict regulatory control of vaccines in the United States by the Food and Drug Administration (FDA).

Sound Immunization Recommendations and Policy

Public health recommendations for vaccine programs and practices represent a dynamic balancing of risks and benefits. Vaccine safety monitoring is necessary to accurately weigh this balance and adjust vaccination policy. This was done in the United States with smallpox and oral polio vaccines as these diseases neared global eradication. Complications associated with each vaccine exceeded the risks of the diseases, leading to discontinuation of routine smallpox vaccination in the United States (prior to global eradication) and a shift to a safer inactivated polio vaccine. Sound immunization policies and recommendations affecting the health of the nation depend upon the ongoing monitoring of vaccines and continuous assessment of immunization benefits and risks.

Adverse Events Following Immunization and Assessment of Causality

Adverse events following immunization can be classified by frequency (common, rare), extent (local, systemic), severity (hospitalization, disability, death), causality, and preventability (intrinsic to vaccine, faulty production, faulty administration). Adverse events following immunizations may be coincidental events or the vaccine may have increased the risk of the adverse event. Some adverse events following immunization may be due to the vaccine preparation itself and the individual response of the vaccinee, and would not have occurred without vaccination. Examples of such events are vaccine-associated paralytic poliomyelitis after oral polio vaccine, or vaccine-strain measles viral infection in an immunodeficient recipient. Other health events may be precipitated by an immunization, such as a vaccine-associated fever precipitating a febrile seizure. Vaccine administration errors may lead to adverse events as well, for example, when administration of a vaccine too high in an adult's arm causes deltoid bursitis. However, many adverse events following immunization are coincidental; they are temporally related to immunization, but occurring by chance without a causal relationship.

To assess causality of an adverse event following immunization, much information is generally needed. A good reference for causality determination is available at www.ncbi.nlm.nih.gov/pubmed/22507656. An adverse health event can be causally attributed to vaccine more readily if: 1) the health problem occurs during a plausible time period

---

4

> **Importance of Vaccine Safety**
> - Ongoing safety monitoring needed for the development of sound policies and recommendations

Vaccination Safety

following vaccination; 2) the adverse event corresponds to those previously associated with a particular vaccine; 3) the event conforms to a specific clinical syndrome whose association with vaccination has strong biologic plausibility (e.g., anaphylaxis) or occurs following the natural disease; 4) a laboratory result confirms the association (e.g., isolation of vaccine strain varicella virus from skin lesions of a patient with rash); 5) the event recurs on re-administration of the vaccine ("positive rechallenge"); 6) a controlled clinical trial or epidemiologic study shows greater risk of a specific adverse event among vaccinated vs. unvaccinated (control) groups; or 7) a finding linking an adverse event to vaccine has been confirmed by other studies.

Assessing and Monitoring Safety of Vaccines
Prelicensure

Vaccines, like other pharmaceutical products, undergo extensive safety and efficacy evaluations in the laboratory, in animals, and in sequentially phased human clinical trials prior to licensure. Phase I human clinical trials usually involve anywhere from 20 to 100 volunteers and focus on detecting serious side effects. Phase II trials generally enroll hundreds of volunteers. These trials might take a few months, or last up to three years. Phase II trials determine the best dose and number of doses for effectiveness and safety. Next, the vaccine moves into Phase III trials, which may last several years. A few hundred to several thousand volunteers may be involved. Some volunteers receive another already-licensed vaccine, allowing researchers to compare one vaccine with another for adverse health effects—anything from a sore arm to a serious reaction. If the vaccine is shown to be safe and effective in Phase III, the manufacturer applies for a license from the FDA. The FDA licenses the vaccine itself (the "product license") and licenses the manufacturing plant where the vaccine will be made (the "establishment license"). During the application, the FDA reviews the clinical trial results, product labeling, the manufacturing plant itself, and the manufacturing protocols.

Fundamental to preventing safety problems is the assurance that any vaccines for public use are made using Good Manufacturing Practices and undergo lot testing for purity and potency. Manufacturers must submit samples of each vaccine lot and results of their own tests for potency and purity to the FDA before releasing them for public use. FDA licensure occurs after a vaccine has met rigorous standards of efficacy and safety, and when its potential benefits in preventing disease clearly outweigh any risks. Phase III trials may be powered sufficiently to identify certain potential adverse reactions prior to licensure. For example, in the pentavalent rotavirus vaccine trials, 70,000 infants received

---

Prelicensure Vaccine Safety Studies

- Laboratory
- Animals
- Humans

Prelicensure Human Studies

- Phases I, II, III trials
- Common reactions are identified
- Vaccines are tested in thousands of persons before being licensed and allowed on the market

---

either vaccine or placebo, so this permitted evaluation of safety with respect to intussusception. However, while rates of common vaccine reactions, such as injection-site reactions and fever, can be estimated before licensure, the comparatively small number of patients enrolled in these trials generally limits detection of rare side effects or side effects that may occur many months after the vaccine is given. Even the largest prelicensure trials (more than 10,000 persons) are inadequate to assess the vaccine's potential to induce rare side effects. Therefore, it is essential to continue to monitor vaccine-associated adverse events once the vaccine has been licensed and recommended for public use.

National Childhood Vaccine Injury Act (NCVIA) of 1986

During the mid-1970s, there were vaccine safety-related lawsuits filed on behalf of those presumably injured by the whole-cell pertussis component of diphtheria-tetanus-pertussis (DTP) vaccine. Legal decisions were reached and damages awarded despite the lack of scientific evidence to support vaccine injury claims. As a result of vaccine manufacturers being held liable, prices soared and many manufacturers halted vaccine production. A vaccine shortage resulted, and public health officials became concerned about the return of epidemic disease. To respond to these concerns, Congress passed the National Childhood Vaccine Injury Act (NCVIA) in 1986. Among the requirements of the NVCIA were the establishment of the Vaccine Adverse Event Reporting System (VAERS) to collect reports of vaccine adverse events, and the National Vaccine Injury Compensation Program to compensate individuals who experience certain health events following immunization. Postlicensure vaccine safety monitoring is now a multi-faceted activity which helps address these concerns as well.

Postlicensure Vaccine Safety Monitoring

Postlicensure evaluation of vaccine safety is critical because rare reactions, delayed reactions, or reactions among subpopulations may not be detected before vaccines are licensed. Several monitoring systems are used in the US to detect and study adverse events that occur after immunizations. In addition to Phase IV trials required of manufacturers, the CDC and FDA use two main systems to monitor the safety of vaccines in use: VAERS and the Vaccine Safety Datalink (VSD). The objectives of postlicensure surveillance are to:

- identify rare adverse reactions after immunization not detected during prelicensure studies;

- monitor increases in known adverse health events after immunization;

Postlicensure Vaccine Safety Systems

- Vaccine Adverse Event Reporting System (VAERS)
- Vaccine Safety Datalink (VSD)

Vaccination Safety

Postlicensure Surveillance

- Identify rare reactions
- Monitor increases in known adverse health events
- Identify risk factors for reactions
- Identify vaccine lots with unusual rates or types of event
- Identify signals

Vaccine Adverse Event Reporting System (VAERS)

- National spontaneous surveillance system
- Jointly administered by CDC and FDA
- Receives about 30,000 reports per year
- Detects
  - new or rare events
  - increases in rates of known side effects
  - patient risk factors
- Additional studies required to confirm VAERS signals
- Not all reports of adverse events are causally related to vaccine

- identify risk factors or preexisting conditions that may be associated with a higher incidence of adverse reactions;

- identify whether there are particular vaccine lots with unusually high rates or certain types of events; and

- identify "signals," possible adverse reactions that may warrant further study to establish the association of an adverse event with vaccination, or affect current immunization recommendations.

The Vaccine Adverse Event Reporting System (VAERS)

The National Childhood Vaccine Injury Act (NCVIA) of 1986 mandated that healthcare providers who administer vaccines and vaccine manufacturers report adverse health events following vaccinations. This act led to the creation of the Vaccine Adverse Event Reporting System (VAERS) in 1990. VAERS is a national spontaneous surveillance system, jointly administered by CDC and FDA, which accepts reports of adverse events after US-licensed vaccinations from health professionals, vaccine manufacturers, and the public. Reports are submitted via the Internet, mail, and fax. All reports are coded using the Medical Dictionary for Regulatory Activities (MedDRA) (http://www.meddramsso.com/) and entered into the VAERS database. VAERS receives about 30,000 US reports per year. Though this may seem like a large number, it is relatively small considering that millions of doses of vaccines are given to adults and children in the US each year.

Healthcare providers are required to report certain adverse health events following specific vaccinations to VAERS (see http://vaers.hhs.gov/resources/VAERS_Table_of_Reportable_Events_Following_Vaccination.pdf) and are encouraged to report any clinically significant adverse event after vaccination even if the reporter is not certain that the incident is vaccine-related. Vaccine manufacturers are required to report all adverse health events that come to their attention (http://www.accessdata.fda.gov/scripts/cdrh/cfdocs/cfcfr/CFRSearch.cfm?fr=600.80). In 2012, US VAERS reports were received from healthcare providers (41%), manufacturers (29%), unknown or other reporters (17 %), and patients or parents (14%).

VAERS collects information about the patient, the vaccination(s) given, the adverse event, and the person reporting the event. Serious adverse event reports as defined in the Federal Register are those involving reported hospitalization or prolongation of hospitalization (if vaccine is given in hospital), death, life threatening illness, or permanent disability. Attempts are made to obtain additional medical information for all reports classified as serious. For these reports, letters to obtain information about recovery status are also sent to the reporters. All patient-identifying information submitted to VAERS, directly or as part of follow-up activities, is protected by strict confidentiality requirements.

Despite limitations inherent to spontaneous reporting systems, VAERS has been able to fulfill its primary purpose of detecting new or rare vaccine adverse events, increases in rates of known side effects, and patient risk factors for particular types of adverse events. Additional studies are required to confirm possible safety signals detected by VAERS because not all reported adverse events are causally related to vaccine. See the section in this chapter titled "Reporting Adverse Events Following Immunization to VAERS" for information on submitting reports. In addition, VAERS often provides early safety data after a vaccine is licensed or during a public health emergency.

VAERS data with personal identifiers removed are available at http://vaers.hhs.gov/index or at http://wonder.cdc.gov/vaers.html.

Vaccine Safety Datalink (VSD)

In 1990, CDC established the Vaccine Safety Datalink to address gaps in the scientific knowledge of rare and serious adverse events following immunizations. This project involves partnerships with large health plans to monitor vaccine safety. A complete list of VSD partners can be found at http://www.cdc.gov/vaccinesafety/Activities/VSD.html. Each participating organization utilizes its electronic health records and immunization registries to contribute to a large linked database. Available information includes data on vaccination (vaccine type, date of vaccination, concurrent vaccinations), health conditions, medical encounters (outpatient visits, inpatient visits, urgent care visits), birth data, and census data.

The VSD allows for planned immunization safety studies, as well as timely investigations of hypotheses that arise from review of medical literature, reports to VAERS, changes in immunization schedules, or the introduction of new vaccines. The Rapid Cycle Analyses (RCA) conducted by the VSD enable CDC and its co-investigators to monitor adverse events following vaccination in near real time, so the public can be informed quickly of possible risks. VSD data come from participating health plans that serve more than 9 million people annually, representing nearly 3% of the United States population, and records for more than 150 million vaccinations, enabling the VSD to study possible rare adverse events after immunization. Data files used in VSD studies remain at each participating site; specific data

---

Vaccine Safety Datalink (VSD)

- Involves partnerships with large health plans

- Links vaccination and health records

- Allows for planned immunization safety studies

- Allows for investigations of hypotheses that arise from review of medical literature, reports to VAERS, changes in immunization schedules, or the introduction of new vaccines

Vaccination Safety

are pulled together for each analysis and do not contain personal identifiers. Further information about VSD is available at http://www.cdc.gov/vaccinesafety/Activities/VSD.html.

Clinical Immunization Safety Assessment (CISA) Project

The CDC supports the Clinical Immunization Safety Assessment (CISA) Project to improve the understanding of adverse events following immunization (AEFI) at the individual-patient level. The CISA Project's goals are to: (1) serve as a vaccine safety resource for consultation on clinical vaccine safety issues, including individual case reviews, and assist with immunization decision-making; (2) assist CDC in developing strategies to assess individuals who may be at increased risk for AEFI; and (3) conduct studies to identify risk factors and preventive strategies for AEFI, particularly in special populations. CISA experts provide advice that has led to a broader understanding of vaccine safety issues and informs clinical or public health practices. A healthcare provider who needs expert opinion on a vaccine safety question about a specific patient can contact CDC at CISAeval@cdc.gov to request a CISA evaluation. Individual case evaluations may lead to development of protocols or guidelines for healthcare providers to help them make the right assessments and manage similar situations. CISA has also contributed to Advisory Committee on Immunization Practices (ACIP) recommendations. Established in 2001, the CISA Project currently consists of seven academic centers of excellence with vaccine safety expertise working in partnership with CDC. A list of these centers, and additional information about the CISA Project, can be found at http://www.cdc.gov/vaccinesafety/Activities/cisa.html.

Vaccine Injury Compensation

A main impact of the National Childhood Vaccine Injury Act (NCVIA) of 1986 was the initiation of the National Vaccine Injury Compensation Program (VICP). This program, administered by the Health Resources and Services Administration (HRSA), compensates individuals who experience certain health events following immunization on a "no fault" basis. "No fault" means that persons filing claims are not required to prove negligence on the part of either the healthcare provider or manufacturer to receive compensation. The program covers all routinely recommended childhood vaccines, although adults who receive a covered vaccine may also file a claim. Claims may be based on a Vaccine Injury Table (available at http://www.hrsa.gov/vaccinecompensation/vaccinetable.html), which lists conditions associated with each vaccine and provides a rebuttable presumption of causation, or by proving by preponderant evidence that the vaccine caused an injury not on the Table.

Clinical Immunization Safety Assessment (CISA) Project

- Improve understanding of vaccine safety issues at individual level
- Review individual cases
- Develop strategies to assess individuals
- Conduct studies to identify risk factors

Vaccine Injury Compensation Program (VICP)

- Established by National Childhood Vaccine Injury Act (1986)
- "No fault" program
- Covers all routinely recommended childhood vaccines
- Vaccine Injury Table

This Table was developed initially by Congress and has been modified by the Secretary of the Department of Health and Human Services (DHHS) to better reflect current science regarding which serious adverse events are reasonably certain to be caused by vaccines. The Table was created to provide swift compensation to those possibly injured by vaccines. As more information becomes available from research on vaccine side effects, the Table will continue to be amended.

VICP has provided compensation to individuals injured by rare vaccine-related adverse events and provided liability protection for vaccine manufacturers and administrators. Further information about the VICP is available at http://www.hrsa.gov/vaccinecompensation/vaccinetable. html.

During the 2009 H1N1 influenza pandemic, the government implemented a new compensation program called Countermeasures Injury Compensation Program (CICP). This program provides compensation for certain individuals who are seriously injured by countermeasures as specified in a declaration by the Secretary of DHHS. Both security (bioterrorism) and pandemic countermeasures are covered. The CICP currently covers serious adverse events caused by pandemic influenza vaccines, including the 2009 monovalent H1N1 influenza vaccine that was widely distributed in the 2009 influenza season and any pandemic influenza vaccines in clinical trials such as H5, H7, H9, etc. The CICP also currently covers serious adverse events caused by anthrax, smallpox, and botulism vaccines, including those used by the Department of Defense. Covered countermeasures within the CICP are not limited to vaccines and may include certain medications or devices used to diagnose, prevent, or treat the covered condition (currently pandemic influenza, smallpox, anthrax, botulism, and acute radiation syndrome). People have one year from receipt of the countermeasure to file with the CICP. More information can be found at http://www.hrsa.gov/countermeasurescomp.

The Immunization Provider's Role

Even though federal regulations require vaccines to undergo years of testing before they can be licensed, and vaccines are monitored continually for safety and effectiveness, immunization providers still play a key role in helping to ensure the safety and efficacy of vaccines. They do this through proper vaccine storage and administration, timing and spacing of vaccine doses, observation of contraindications and precautions, management of vaccine adverse reactions, reporting of adverse events following immunization to VAERS, and educating patients and parents about vaccine benefits and risks. Each of these steps is described

The Provider's Role

- Immunization providers can help to ensure the safety and efficacy of vaccines through proper:

  - vaccine storage and administration

  - timing and spacing of vaccine doses

  - observation of contraindications and precautions

  - management of adverse reactions

  - reporting to VAERS

  - benefit and risk communication

4

only briefly here. Further information is available elsewhere in this book or in resource materials from CDC or other organizations.

Vaccine Storage and Administration

To achieve the best possible results from vaccines, immunization providers should carefully follow the recommendations found in each vaccine's package insert for storage, handling, and administration. Other steps to help ensure vaccine safety include: 1) inspecting vaccines upon delivery and monitoring refrigerator and freezer temperatures to ensure maintenance of the cold chain; 2) rotating vaccine stock so the oldest vaccines are used first; 3) never administering a vaccine later than the expiration date; 4) administering vaccines within the prescribed time periods following reconstitution; 5) waiting to draw vaccines into syringes until immediately prior to administration; 6) never mixing vaccines in the same syringe unless they are specifically approved for mixing by the FDA; and 7) recording vaccine and administration information, including lot numbers and injection sites, in the patient's record. If errors in vaccine storage and administration occur, corrective action should be taken immediately to prevent them from happening again and public health authorities should be notified. More information on vaccine storage and handling is available in the "Vaccine Storage and Handling" chapter and CDC's "Vaccine Storage and Handling Toolkit", available on the CDC Vaccines and Immunizations website at http://www.cdc.gov/vaccines/recs/storage/toolkit/.

Timing and Spacing

Timing and spacing of vaccine doses are two of the most important issues in the appropriate use of vaccines. To ensure optimal results from each immunization, providers should follow the recommended immunization schedules for children, adolescents, and adults. Decreasing the timing intervals between doses of the same vaccine may interfere with the vaccine's antibody response. For more specific information on timing and spacing of vaccines, see Chapter 2, "General Recommendations on Immunization." A table showing recommended minimum ages and intervals between vaccine doses is contained in Appendix A.

Providers should also remember the following:

- Administering all needed vaccines during the same visit is important because it increases the likelihood that children will be fully immunized as recommended. Studies have shown that vaccines are as effective when administered simultaneously as they are individually and carry no greater risk for adverse reactions.

- Some vaccines, such as pediatric diphtheria and tetanus, may cause local reactions when given too frequently. Good recordkeeping, maintaining careful patient histories, and adherence to recommended schedules can decrease the chances that patients receive extra doses of vaccines.

4

Contraindications and Precautions

Certain vaccines should not be given, or should be given only under controlled circumstances, to certain patients. A contraindication is a condition that increases the likelihood of a serious adverse reaction to a vaccine for a recipient with that condition. In general, a vaccine should not be administered when a contraindication is present. A precaution is a condition that might increase the likelihood or severity of an adverse reaction in a recipient, or compromise the ability of the vaccine to produce immunity. Vaccination is generally deferred when a precaution is present. Situations may arise when the benefits of vaccination outweigh the risk of a side effect, and the provider may decide to vaccinate the patient. Many contra-indications and precautions are temporary and the vaccine may be given at a later time. More information about contraindications can be found in the Advisory Committee on Immunization Practices (ACIP) statements for individual vaccines. Recommendations for immunizing persons who are immunocompromised can be found in Appendix A. Information on allergic reactions to vaccines can be found in the American Academy of Pediatrics *Red Book*.

Screening for contraindications and precautions is important for preventing serious adverse outcomes after vaccination. Every provider who administers vaccines should screen every patient before giving a vaccine dose. Sample screening questionnaires can be found in Chapter 2, "General Recommendations on Immunization." Many conditions are often inappropriately regarded as contraindi-cations to vaccination. In most cases, the following are not considered contraindications:

- Minor acute illness (e.g., diarrhea and minor upper respiratory tract illnesses, including otitis media) with or without low-grade fever

- Mild to moderate local reactions and/or low-grade or moderate fever following a prior dose of the vaccine

- Current antimicrobial therapy

- Recent exposure to infectious disease

- Convalescent phase of illness

- Pregnant or immunosuppressed person in the household

Contraindication

A condition that increases the likelihood of a serious adverse reaction to a vaccine for a recipient with that condition

Precaution

A condition in a recipient that might:

- Increase the chance or severity of an adverse reaction, or

- Compromise the ability of the vaccine to produce immunity

Invalid Contraindications to Vaccination

- Minor acute illness

- Mild/moderate local reaction or fever following a prior dose

- Antimicrobial therapy

- Disease exposure or convalescence

- Pregnancy or immunosuppression in the household

- Preterm birth

- Breastfeeding

- Allergies to products not in vaccine

4

- Preterm birth

- Breastfeeding

- Allergies to products not in vaccine

Managing Adverse Reactions after Immunization

Providers should use their best clinical judgment regarding specific management of adverse events after immunization. Allergic reactions to vaccines are estimated to occur after vaccination of children and adolescents at a rate of one for every 1.5 million doses of vaccine. All providers who administer vaccines should have procedures in place and be prepared for emergency care of a person who experiences an anaphylactic reaction. Epinephrine and equipment for maintaining an airway should be available for immediate use. All vaccine providers should be familiar with the office emergency plan and should be certified in cardiopulmonary resuscitation.

Reporting Adverse Events Following Immunization to VAERS

Healthcare providers are required by the National Childhood Vaccine Injury Act of 1986 to report certain adverse events to VAERS and are encouraged to report any adverse event even if they are not sure a vaccine was the cause. A table listing reportable events is available at http://vaers.hhs.gov/reportable.htm. Reporting can be done in one of three ways:

1. Online through a secure website: https://vaers.hhs.gov/esub/step1.

2. If a reporter is unable to report by Internet, they may fax a completed VAERS form* to 877-721-0366.

3. Mail a completed VAERS form* to:

    VAERS
    P.O. Box 1100
    Rockville, MD 20849-1100

*A one-page VAERS form can be downloaded from http://vaers.hhs.gov/resources/vaers_form.pdf or can be requested by telephone at 800-822-7967 or by fax at 877-721-0366.

When providers report suspected vaccine reactions to VAERS, they provide valuable information that is needed for the ongoing evaluation of vaccine safety. CDC and FDA use VAERS information to ensure the safest strategies of vaccine use and to further reduce the rare risks associated with vaccines.

Benefit and Risk Communication

Parents, guardians, legal representatives, and adolescent and adult patients should be informed of the benefits and risks of vaccines in understandable language. Opportunity for questions should be provided before each vaccination. Discussion of the benefits and risks of vaccination is sound medical practice and is required by law.

The National Childhood Vaccine Injury Act requires that vaccine information materials be developed for each vaccine covered by the Act. These materials, known as "Vaccine Information Statements" (VISs), must be provided by all public and private vaccination providers before each dose of vaccine. Copies of VISs are available from state health authorities responsible for immunization, or they can be obtained from CDC's website at http://www.cdc.gov/vaccines/pubs/vis/default.htm or from the Immunization Action Coalition at http://www.immunize.org. Translations of VISs into languages other than English are available from certain state immunization programs and from the Immunization Action Coalition website. Further information about VISs and their use is contained in Appendix C.

Healthcare providers should anticipate questions that parents or patients may have regarding the need for or safety of vaccination. Some individuals may refuse certain vaccines, or even reject all vaccinations. Some might have religious or personal objections to vaccinations. Having a basic understanding of how patients view vaccine risk and developing effective approaches to dealing with vaccine safety concerns when they arise are imperative for vaccination providers. Healthcare providers can accomplish this by assessing patients' specific concerns and information needs, providing them with accurate information, and referring them to credible sources for more information. CDC's website contains extensive and up-to-date information on vaccines and tools for discussing vaccines with patients (see http://www.cdc.gov/vaccines/hcp/patient-ed/conversations/index.html for provider resources).

When a parent or patient initiates discussion regarding a vaccine concern, the healthcare provider should discuss the specific concern and provide factual information, using language that is appropriate. Effective, empathetic vaccine risk communication is essential in responding to misinformation and concerns. The Vaccine Information Statements provide an outline for discussing vaccine benefits and risk. Other vaccine safety informational resources are available at http://www.cdc.gov/vaccinesafety/.

For patients who question or refuse vaccination, identifying common ground and discussing measures for deferring vaccinations is a more effective public health strategy for

Benefit and Risk Communication
- Opportunities for questions should be provided before each vaccination
- Vaccine Information Statements (VISs)
  - must be provided before each dose of vaccine
  - public and private providers
  - available in multiple languages

4

4

providers than excluding these patients from their practice. Healthcare providers can reinforce key points regarding each vaccine, including safety, and emphasize risks encountered by unimmunized children. Parents should be informed about state laws pertaining to school or child care entry, which might require that unimmunized children stay home from school during outbreaks. Documentation of these discussions in the patient's record, including the refusal to receive certain vaccines (i.e., informed refusal), might reduce any potential liability if a vaccine-preventable disease occurs in the unimmunized patient.

Acknowlegement

The editors thank Dr. Cindy M. Weinbaum of the Division of Healthcare Quality Promotion, CDC, for her update and critical review of this chapter.

Selected References

American Academy of Pediatrics. Vaccine Safety and Reporting of Adverse Events. In: Pickering LK, Baker CJ, Kimberlin DW, Long SS, eds. *Red Book: 2012 Report of the Committee on Infectious Diseases*. 29th ed. Elk Grove Village, IL: American Academy of Pediatrics; 2012:41-53.

Berger B, Omer S. Could the United States experience rubella outbreaks as a result of vaccine refusal and disease importation? *Human Vaccines*. 6(12):1016.

Bohlke K, Davis RL, Marcy SM, et al. Risk of anaphylaxis after vaccination of children and adolescents. *Pediatrics* 2003;112(4):815–20.

CDC. Suspension of Rotavirus Vaccine after Reports of Intussusception—United States, 1999. *MMWR* 2004;53(34):786-789.

CDC. Syncope after vaccination—United States, January 2005-July 2007 *MMWR* 2008;57(17);457-460.

CDC. General Recommendations on Immunization: Recommendations of the Advisory Committee on Immunization Practices. *MMWR* 2011;60(No. RR-2):1–60.

CDC. Current Trends National Childhood Vaccine Injury Act: Requirements for permanent vaccination records and for reporting of selected events after vaccination. *MMWR* 1988;37(13):197–200.

CDC. Surveillance for safety after immunization: Vaccine Adverse Event Reporting System (VAERS)—United States 1991-2001. *MMWR* 2003; 52(No.SS-1):1–24.

4

Chen RT, Hibbs B. Vaccine safety: current and future challenges. *Pediatr Ann* 1998;27(7):445–55.

Chen RT, Glasser J, Rhodes P, et al. The Vaccine Safety Datalink (VSD) Project: A new tool for improving vaccine safety monitoring in the United States. *Pediatrics* 1997; 99(6):765–73.

Chen RT, Rastogi SC, Mullen JR, et al. The Vaccine Adverse Event Reporting System (VAERS). *Vaccine* 1994;12(6): 542–50.

Iskander JK, Miller ER, Chen RT. The role of the Vaccine Adverse Event Reporting System (VAERS) in monitoring vaccine safety. *Pediatric Annals* 2004;33(9): 599-606.

Slade BA, Leidel L, Vellozzi C, Woo EJ, Hua W, Sutherland A, Izurieta HS, Ball R, Miller N, Braun MM, Markowitz LE, Iskander J. Postlicensure safety surveillance for quadrivalent human papillomavirus recombinant vaccine. *JAMA* 2009 Aug 19;302(7):750-7.

Varricchio F, Iskander J, Destefano F, Ball R, Pless R, Braun MM, Chen RT. Understanding vaccine safety information from the Vaccine Adverse Event Reporting System. *Pediatr Infect Dis J* 2004 Apr 23 (4): 287-294.

Vellozzi C, Broder KR, Haber P, Guh A, Nguyen M, Cano M, Lewis P, McNeil MM, Bryant M, Singleton J, Martin D, DeStefano F. Adverse events following influenza A (H1N1) 2009 monovalent vaccines reported to the Vaccine Adverse Event Reporting System, United States, October 1, 2009-January 31, 2010. *Vaccine* 2010 Oct 21;28(45):7248-55.

VAERS website available at www.vaers.hhs.gov.

Vaccination Safety

This chapter provides an overview of best practice guidance for storage and handling. CDC's *Vaccine Storage and Handling Toolkit*, http://www.cdc.gov/vaccines/recs/storage/toolkit/storage-handling-toolkit.pdf, contains comprehensive information on best practices and recommendations. Manufacturers' product information and package inserts include the most current information about the storage and handling of specific vaccines. Refer to CDC's *Storage and Handling* webpage for links to these and other resources, http://www.cdc.gov/vaccines/recs/storage/default.htm. Participants in the Vaccines for Children (VFC) program or those who have any vaccines purchased with public funds should consult their state or local immunization program for specifics because some program requirements may differ from the information contained in the *Vaccine Storage and Handling* Toolkit.

Vaccine Storage and Handling

There are few immunization issues more important than the appropriate storage and handling of vaccines. Vaccine-preventable disease rates have decreased in part because of proper storage and handling of vaccines. Exposure of vaccines to temperatures outside the recommended ranges can decrease their potency and reduce the effectiveness and protection they provide. Storage and handling errors can cost thousands of dollars in wasted vaccine and revaccination. Errors can also result in the loss of patient confidence when repeat doses are required. It is better to not vaccinate than to administer a dose of vaccine that has been mishandled. Vaccine management, including proper storage and handling procedures, is the basis on which good immunization practices are built.

Vaccines must be stored properly from the time they are manufactured until they are administered. Assuring vaccine quality and maintaining the cold chain is a shared responsibility among manufacturers, distributors, public health staff, and health-care providers. A proper cold chain is a temperature-controlled supply chain that includes all equipment and procedures used in the transport and storage and handling of vaccines from the time of manufacture to administration of the vaccine. By following a few simple steps and implementing best storage and handling practices, providers can ensure that patients will get the full benefit of vaccines they receive.

Storage and Handling Plans

Every facility should have detailed written protocols for routine and emergency vaccine storage and handling and they should be updated annually. These policies and procedures should be available in writing as a reference for all staff members and easily accessible.

Vaccine Storage and Handling

- Vaccine-preventable disease rates decreased in part because of proper storage and handling

- Storage and handling errors

  - decrease potency and reduce effectiveness and protection

  - cost thousands of dollars in wasted vaccine and revaccination

  - loss of patient confidence

- It is better to not vaccinate than to administer a dose of vaccine that has been mishandled

Cold Chain (a temperature-controlled supply chain)

- Vaccines must be stored properly from the time they are manufactured until they are administered

- Shared responsibility among manufacturers, distributors, public health staff, and healthcare providers

Storage and Handling

5

**Vaccine Storage
and Handling Plans**

- Develop and maintain written ROUTINE plan for:

  - ordering and accepting vaccine deliveries

  - storing and handling vaccines

  - managing inventory

  - managing potentially compromised vaccines

- Develop and maintain written EMERGENCY vaccine retrieval and storage plan

  - back-up storage location with appropriate storage units, temperature monitoring capability, and back-up generator that can maintain power to the vaccine storage units

  - adequate supply of packing materials and portable refrigerators and freezers or qualified containers and packouts, or refrigerated truck

Staff Training and Education

- Assign responsibilities to a primary vaccine coordinator

- Designate at least one alternate (back-up) vaccine coordinator

---

A routine storage and handling plan provides guidelines for daily activities, such as:

- Ordering and accepting vaccine deliveries

- Storing and handling vaccines

- Managing inventory

- Managing potentially compromised vaccines

Every facility should also have an emergency vaccine retrieval and storage plan. The plan should identify a back-up location where the vaccines can be stored. Considerations when choosing this site include appropriate storage units, temperature monitoring capability, and a back-up generator that can maintain power to the vaccine storage units. Potential back-up locations might include a local hospital, pharmacy, long-term care facility, or the Red Cross.

There should be an adequate supply of packing materials and portable refrigerators and freezers or qualified containers and packouts on hand to accommodate the facility's largest annual vaccine inventory (e.g., flu season). A refrigerated truck may be needed to move large inventories of vaccine.

Power outages or natural disasters are not the only events that can compromise vaccine. Forgotten vials of vaccine left out on the counter or doses of vaccine stored at improper temperatures due to a storage unit failure are other examples of how vaccines can be potentially compromised. Protocols after an event will vary depending on individual state or agency policies. Contact the local or state health department immunization program (hereafter referred to as "immunization program"), vaccine manufacturer(s), or both for appropriate actions or guidelines that should be followed for all potentially compromised vaccines. Do not discard vaccines unless directed to by the immunization program and/or the manufacturer.

Staff Training and Education

Assign a primary vaccine coordinator who is responsible for ensuring that vaccines are stored and handled correctly at each facility. Designate at least one alternate (back-up) vaccine coordinator who can perform these responsibilities in the absence of the primary coordinator. These responsibilities include, but are not limited to, the following tasks:

- Ordering vaccines

- Overseeing proper receipt and storage of vaccine deliveries

- Organizing vaccines within the storage unit(s)

- Temperature monitoring of the storage unit(s) (i.e., current temperature at least 2 times each workday).

- Recording temperature readings on a log

- Daily physical inspection of the storage unit(s)

- Rotating stock so that vaccines closest to their expiration dates will be used first

- Monitoring expiration dates and ensuring that expired vaccines and diluents are removed from the storage unit(s) and not administered to patients

- Responding to potential temperature excursions

- Overseeing proper vaccine transport

- Maintaining all appropriate vaccine storage and handling documentation, including temperature-excursion responses

- Maintaining storage equipment and maintenance records

- Maintaining proper documentation for the VFC program in participating facilities

- Ensuring that designated staff is adequately trained

A physician partner or member of management should be directly involved with the clinical staff that is responsible for vaccine storage and handling. Management staff should have a clear understanding of the vaccine replacement costs and clinical implications of mismanaged vaccines.

All personnel who handle or administer vaccines should be familiar with the storage and handling policies and procedures for their facility. This includes not only those who administer vaccines, but also anyone who delivers or accepts vaccine shipments and anyone who has access to the unit(s) where vaccines are stored. Vaccine storage and handling training should be provided to all new personnel who handle or administer vaccines, including temporary staff. Continuing education for staff is essential when new vaccines are stocked and when there are any changes to the storage and handling guidelines for a particular vaccine. CDC has a free web-based storage and handling module as part of the online training tool, "*You Call the Shots*," at http://www.cdc.gov/vaccines/ed/youcalltheshots.htm. Continuing education credit for a variety of healthcare professionals and a certificate of completion are available. Many immunization programs and professional organizations also offer vaccine storage and handling training programs.

Training and Education

- Staff who
  - handle or administer vaccines
  - deliver or accept vaccine shipments
  - have access to vaccine storage unit(s)
- Provide training and continuing education when
  - new or temporary staff are oriented
  - new vaccines are stocked
  - changes to storage and handling guidelines occur

5

Storage and Handling

Receiving and Unpacking Vaccine Deliveries

Proper vaccine storage and handling is important from the moment the vaccine arrives at the facility. All office staff should be trained to notify the vaccine coordinator or the alternate (back-up) coordinator when a vaccine delivery has arrived. This is extremely important for receptionists or other front desk staff since they may be the first to know that vaccines have been delivered. Avoid having other people accept deliveries who may not understand the importance of storage at appropriate temperatures. The vaccine coordinator should request delivery during office hours and update vaccine orders to reflect any period of time the office will be closed, such as holidays or scheduled vacation time.

Examine deliveries right away and store vaccines at the proper temperatures immediately upon arrival. Examine the shipping container and its contents for any evidence of damage during shipment. Cross check the contents with the packing slip to be sure they match. Check heat and cold temperature monitors/indicators if either are included in the shipping container following instructions on the monitors for reading and reporting. If a monitor indicates a possible temperature excursion during shipping, the monitor reading should be documented for future reference. Report the reading to the distributor within the required timeframe if VFC vaccines or other vaccines purchased with public funds are involved. Vaccines sent directly by the manufacturer are in specially designed boxes and may not contain heat or cold temperature monitors.

Allowable shipping time varies among distributors and manufacturers and is dependent on the type of container and packout. Determine if shipping time was within allowable limits noted on shipping insert or container. If the shipping time was more than the allowable limit or there are any discrepancies with the packing slip or concerns about the contents, immediately notify the primary vaccine coordinator (or the alternate [back-up] coordinator). If neither is available, notify a supervisor immediately. Label the vaccines "Do NOT Use" and store the vaccines under appropriate conditions separate from other vaccines. Then, according to your facility's procedures, contact your immunization program, the distributor, and/or vaccine manufacturer(s) for guidance.

Record the contents of each container on an inventory log (stock record). This log should include the name of each vaccine, the number of doses for each vaccine received, the date it was received, the condition of the vaccines upon arrival, the names of the vaccine manufacturers, the lot numbers, the expiration dates for each vaccine, and any action taken regarding questionable vaccines.

Vaccine Storage and Temperature Monitoring Equipment

These items should be selected carefully, used properly, maintained regularly (including professionally serviced when needed), and monitored consistently to ensure the recommended temperatures are maintained. This chapter provides only general guidelines for equipment. Providers should consult their immunization program, particularly providers of VFC vaccines or other vaccines purchased with public funds, for any specific storage equipment requirements.

Keep a logbook for each piece of vaccine storage equipment. The serial number of each piece of equipment, the date each piece of equipment was installed, the dates of any routine maintenance tasks (such as cleaning), the dates of any repairs or service, and the contact information of the service provider should be recorded. A logbook is also an ideal place to keep the instructions that came with the equipment.

Freezers and Refrigerators

Using proper vaccine storage units can help prevent costly vaccine losses and the inadvertent administration of compromised vaccines. CDC recommends stand-alone units, meaning self-contained units that either freeze or refrigerate, and are suitable for vaccine storage. These units can vary in size, from compact, counter-top or under-the-counter style to large, pharmaceutical grade units. Studies demonstrated that stand-alone units maintain the required temperatures better than combination units, particularly the freezer section of household, combination units.

If existing equipment is a household, combination refrigerator/freezer, CDC recommends using only the refrigerator compartment for refrigerated vaccines. Use a separate stand-alone freezer to store frozen vaccines. Research found that freezers in household combination units cannot hold proper storage temperatures for frozen vaccines particularly during defrost cycles. This applies to both temporary and long-term storage.

Any freezer or refrigerator used for vaccine storage must be able to maintain the required temperature range throughout the year. The unit should be dedicated to the storage of biologics and must be large enough to hold inventory a provider might have at the busiest point in the year without crowding (including flu vaccine). There should also be enough room to store water bottles in the refrigerator and frozen water bottles in the freezer to stabilize the temperatures and help maintain temperature longer in a power outage.

5

Freezers and Refrigerators

- Stand-alone units that only freeze or refrigerate

  - can vary in size from compact, counter-top or under-the-counter to large, pharmaceutical grade

  - maintain required temperatures better than combination units, particularly the freezer section of these units

- If existing equipment is a household, combination refrigerator/freezer

  - only use refrigerator for vaccine storage

  - use a stand-alone freezer for frozen vaccines

  - applies to both temporary and long-term storage

- Able to maintain required temperature range throughout year

- Dedicated to storage of biologics

- Large enough to hold year's largest vaccine inventory without crowding (including flu vaccine)

- If stand-alone freezer is manual defrost, must defrost regularly and have another storage unit that maintains appropriate temperatures for temporary storage during defrosting

- Frost-free or automatic defrost cycle may be preferred

Storage and Handling

Storage Unit Placement

- Promote good air circulation around storage unit
  - place in well-ventilated room
  - allow for space on all sides and top
  - allow at least 4 inches between storage unit and a wall
  - do not block motor cover
  - ensure unit stands level with at least 1 to 2 inches between bottom of unit and floor

Dormitory-style Refrigerator

- Small combination freezer/refrigerator unit with one external door and an evaporator plate (cooling coil), which is usually located inside an icemaker compartment (freezer) within the refrigerator
- NOT recommended for vaccine storage under any circumstances, even temporarily
- Prohibited for storage of VFC vaccines or other vaccines purchased with public funds
- NOT recommended for vaccine storage under any circumstances, even temporarily

If your stand-alone freezer is manual defrost, you must defrost regularly and have another storage unit that maintains appropriate temperatures for temporary storage of the vaccine while defrosting. A frost-free unit with an automatic defrost cycle may be preferred if regular manual defrosting cannot be assured.

Good air circulation around a vaccine storage unit is essential for proper cooling functions. A storage unit should be in a well-ventilated room with space around the sides and top and at least 4 inches between the unit and a wall. Nothing should block the cover of the motor compartment and the unit should be level and stand firmly with at least 1 to 2 inches between the bottom of the unit and the floor.

CDC does not recommend storage of any vaccine in a dormitory-style or bar-style, combined refrigerator/freezer unit under any circumstances, even temporarily. A dormitory-style refrigerator is defined as a small combination freezer/refrigerator unit with one exterior door and an evaporator plate (cooling coil), which is usually located inside an icemaker compartment within the refrigerator. These units have exhibited severe temperature control and stability issues throughout the entire storage area. Dormitory-or bar-style units pose a significant risk of freezing vaccines, even when used for temporary storage. The use of this type of unit is prohibited for storage of VFC vaccines or other vaccines purchased with public funds.

Temperature Monitoring Devices

Temperature Monitoring is a critical part of good storage and handling practice. CDC recommends using only a calibrated digital data logger with a current and valid certificate of calibration testing (also known as a Report of Calibration). This certificate informs the user of a temperature monitoring device's level of accuracy compared to a recognized standard. Calibrated temperature monitoring devices are required for providers who receive VFC vaccines or other vaccines purchased with public funds.

All temperature monitoring devices, through normal use, drift over time, which affects their accuracy. Because of this, temperature monitoring devices should undergo periodic calibration testing. Testing should be performed every 1 to 2 years from the last testing date or according to the manufacturer's suggested timeline. CDC recommends that testing meets standards defined in the *Vaccine Storage and Handling Toolkit*. If calibration testing indicates that your temperature monitoring device is no longer accurate, it should be replaced. Immunization programs are often excellent resources for information on temperature monitoring devices.

Several types of temperature monitoring devices are available. CDC recommends digital data loggers with the following characteristics: a digital display easily readable from outside the unit; a detachable probe in a buffered material, which more closely reflects vaccine temperatures rather than air temperature in the unit; an alarm for out-of-range temperatures; current and minimum and maximum temprature accuracy within +/-1°F (+/-.5°C); a low battery indicator; memory that stores at least 4000 readings; and user programmable logging interval. CDC recommends a back-up digital data logger for each vaccine storage unit. Staff should be trained and understand how to set up, read and analyze temperature data provided by the data logger.

Temperature monitoring device placement within the unit is just as important as device selection. Place the buffered probe with the vaccines. This should be in the middle, center of the storage unit away from walls, ceiling, cooling vents, door, floor, and back of the unit. Prior to storing vaccines in a unit, allow the unit temperature to stabilize for a week before placing vaccines in the unit. CDC recommends using a digital data logger to monitor the temperature in the storage unit prior to storage of vaccines.

Temperature Monitoring

Regular temperature monitoring is key to proper cold chain management. Store frozen vaccines (Varicella, MMRV, and Zoster) in a freezer between -58°F and +5°F (-50°C and -15°C). Store all other routinely recommended vaccines in a refrigerator between 35°F and 46°F (2°C and 8°C). The desired average refrigerator vaccine storage temperature is 40°F (5°C). Exposure to temperatures outside these ranges may result in reduced vaccine potency and increased risk of vaccine-preventable diseases.

CDC recommends reviewing and recording temperatures in both the freezer and refrigerator units at least 2 times each workday, in the morning and before leaving at the end of the workday.

This best practice recommendation applies to all vaccine storage units, regardless of whether or not there is a temperature alarm, or a digital data logger that continuously records temperatures in the unit. These readings will provide a better indication of any problems with the storage unit's function.

Reviewing and recording temperatures also provides an opportunity to visually inspect the storage unit, reorganize the vaccines when necessary (e.g., moving vaccine away

Temperature Monitoring Devices

- Use only calibrated temperature monitoring devices with a certificate of calibration testing (Report of Calibration) from an accredited laboratory
  - required for providers who receive VFC vaccines or vaccines purchased with public funds
- Calibration testing every 1 to 2 years from last calibration testing date or according to the manufacturer's suggested timeline

Digital Data Logger Characteristics

- Digital temperature display outside storage unit
- Detachable probe in a buffered material
- Alarm
- Current and minimum and maximum temperatures
- Accuracy within +/-1°F (+/-.5°C)
- Low battery indicator
- Measures current and daily minimum and maximum temperatures in the unit
- Memory for storing at least 4,000 readings
- Uses programmable logging interval

Storage and Handling

Recommended Temperatures

- Freezer
  - between -58°F and +5°F (between -50°C and -15°C)
- Refrigerator
  - between 35°F and 46°F (between 2°C and 8°C)
  - average: 40°F (5°C)

Temperature Monitoring

- Review and record temperatures in both freezer and refrigerator units 2 times each day, once in the morning and once before leaving at the end of the workday
- Post temperature log on the door of each storage unit
- If using a continuous temperature monitor, download temperature data and review weekly
- Keep temperature logs (hard copies and downloaded data) 3 years or according to individual state record retention requirements

Temperature Excursion

- If stored vaccines have been exposed to temperatures outside recommended ranges
  - store the vaccines properly
  - separate from other vaccine supplies
  - mark "Do NOT Use"
  - contact immunization program, vaccine manufacturer(s), or both for guidance

from walls or cold air vents), identify vaccines and diluents with short expiration dates, remove any expired vaccines and diluents, and provide a timely response to temperature excursions.

Post a temperature log on each storage unit door or nearby in a readily accessible and visible location. In addition, if using a device that enables download of temperature data, review and store data at least once every week and reset the device before returning to storage unit monitoring.

CDC recommends maintaining an ongoing file of temperature data, including hard copies and downloaded data for at least 3 years or according to individual state record retention requirements. As the storage unit ages, recurring temperature variances or problems can be tracked and documented. This data can be important when evaluating the need for a new storage unit or if there is a potential need to recall and revaccinate patients because of improperly stored vaccine.

Twice daily temperature monitoring may not be accomplished when a provider's office is closed. A digital data logger that stores data and/or can be accessed remotely can provide information on storage temperatures while the office is closed and help assure that timely corrective action can be taken if temperatures go out of range. Providers should determine how they are to be notified in the event of an emergency (e.g., a power outage) during hours when the facility is not open.

Equally important to temperature monitoring is taking timely corrective action when there is a temperature excursion. If it is discovered that stored vaccines have been exposed to temperatures outside the recommended ranges, these vaccines should remain properly stored, but separated from other vaccine supplies and marked "Do NOT Use" until guidance can be obtained. Protocols after an event will vary depending on individual state or agency policies. Contact your immunization program, vaccine manufacturer(s), or both for guidance.

Vaccine and Diluent Placement and Labeling

Vaccines should be stored in the center of the unit as this is the area where appropriate temperatures are typically most stable. A storage unit should be big enough so that vaccines can be placed in the part of the unit best able to maintain the constant, required temperature away from the walls, coils, cooling vents, ceiling, door, floor and back of the unit. Vaccines and diluents should be kept in their original packaging with the lids on until ready for administration and stacked in rows with vaccine and diluent of the same type. Trays or uncovered containers/bins that allow for air circulation can be used to organize the vaccines and diluents within the storage unit. Do not store vaccines in unit doors or in deli, vegetable, or fruit crisper drawers. Avoid storing vaccines on the refrigerator top shelf. If the top shelf must be used, place water bottles close to the vent and only store vaccines not sensitive to coldest temperatures (e.g., MMR).

Some diluents must be refrigerated and others may be stored in the refrigerator or at room temperature. Always follow the manufacturer's guidance in the product information/package inserts. If possible, store diluent next to the corresponding vaccine. Some of these diluents may contain vaccine antigen. Never store diluents in the freezer.

There should be space between the vaccine and diluent stacks or containers. This will help to avoid confusion between products, provide for air circulation around and through stacks for even cooling, and protect vaccines from unnecessary light exposure. Not only live attenuated vaccines, but also some inactivated vaccines must be protected from light. Information on light sensitivity can be found in the manufacturer's product information/package insert.

Each vaccine and diluent stack or container should be clearly labeled. This can be accomplished by attaching labels directly to the shelves on which vaccines and diluents are stored or by placing labels on the containers. Store pediatric and adult vaccines on different shelves. Use color coded labels that include the vaccine type, as well as age and gender indications, if applicable. Having each vaccine and diluent stack or container labeled helps decrease the chance that someone will inadvertently administer the wrong vaccine or use the wrong diluent to reconstitute a vaccine. Vaccines that sound or look alike should not be stored next to each other, e.g., DTaP and Tdap. VFC vaccines and other vaccines purchased with public funds should be identified and stored separately from vaccines purchased with private funds.

Vaccine Storage Troubleshooting

To maintain the proper temperature ranges, the freezer and refrigerator units must be in good working condition and they must have power at all times. There are several things that can be done to prevent problems.

Plug storage units directly into wall outlets. Do not use power outlets with built-in circuit switches (they have little red reset buttons), outlets that can be activated by a wall switch, or multi-outlet power strips. These can be tripped or switched off, resulting in loss of electricity to the storage

Vaccine and Diluent Placement and Labeling

- Store vaccines away from walls, coils, cooling vents, top shelf, ceiling, door, floor, and back of unit

- Keep vaccines and diluents in original packaging with lids on to protect from light

- Stack in rows with same type of vaccine and diluent

- Use uncovered storage containers to organize vaccines and diluents

- Do not store vaccines in storage unit doors, on the top shelf, on the floor, or in deli, vegetable or fruit crisper drawers

- Store pediatric and adult vaccines on different shelves

- Use labels with vaccine type, age, and gender indications or color coding

- Do not store sound-alike and look-alike vaccines next to each other

- VFC vaccines and other vaccines purchased with public funds should be identified and stored separately from vaccines purchased with private funds

Storage and Handling

Diluent Storage

- Store diluent as directed in manufacturer's product information
- Store refrigerated diluent with corresponding vaccine (these diluents may contain vaccine antigen)
- Never store diluents in the freezer
- Label diluent to avoid inadvertent use of the wrong diluent when reconstituting a vaccine

unit. Plug only one storage unit into an outlet. This will help to prevent a safety switch from being triggered to turn off power and reduce the risk of overloading the outlet which could be a fire hazard.

Use plug guards or safety-lock plugs to prevent someone from inadvertently unplugging the unit. A temperature alarm system that will alert staff to after-hour temperature excursions, particularly if large vaccine inventories are maintained, may be helpful in assuring a timely response to storage problems. Label circuit breakers to alert custodians and electricians not to unplug vaccine storage units or turn off the power. This can be done by posting a warning sign near the electrical outlet, on storage units, and at the circuit breaker box. Warning signs should include emergency contact information.

Place containers of water, labeled "Do NOT Drink," in the refrigerator to help stabilize the temperature in the unit. Place water bottles where vaccines are not stored, such as the door, top shelf, and on the floor of the storage unit. The same principle applies to the freezer. Store frozen water bottles in the freezer and the freezer door. Be careful that the water bottles do not weigh down doors so much that the seals are compromised and the doors do not close properly. These measures will help keep the temperature stable with frequent opening and closing of the storage unit.

In addition to temperature monitoring, a physical inspection of storage units should be performed daily. An inspection should include the following:

- Are the vaccines placed properly in the unit?

- Are the vaccines in their original packaging?

- Are vaccines being stored away from the walls, coils, cooling vents, ceiling, and floor and not in the doors?

During a workday it is easy for vaccines to be shifted into an area of the storage unit where the temperature may not be appropriate or stable, such as against a wall, under a cold air vent, or in the door. CDC recommends that vaccines be kept in storage units dedicated only to vaccines. If other biologic specimens, such as blood or urine, must be stored in the same unit as vaccines, specimens should be stored on a lower shelf. This is to ensure that if a specimen leaks, the vaccines will not be contaminated. Food and beverages should not be stored in a vaccine storage unit because frequent opening of the unit can lead to temperature instability.

While it is important to take measures to prevent problems, equally important is taking immediate corrective action when a problem does exist, for example, when the storage unit temperature falls outside the recommended range. Staff should know who to contact in case of a malfunction or disaster.

If you experience a power outage, immediately begin to implement your emergency plan. Depending on room temperature, storage temperatures may be maintained for only a very short period of time. If there is an extended period of time before the situation can be corrected and there are no other storage units available on site, move the vaccines to the back-up storage facility using the guidelines in the emergency plan.

Vaccine and Diluent Inventory Control

Conduct a vaccine inventory monthly to ensure adequate supplies to meet demand. Include vaccine diluents in the inventory. Determining factors for the amount of vaccine and diluent ordered include: projected demand, storage capacity, and current vaccine supply. Avoid overstocking vaccine supplies, which could lead to vaccine wastage or having outdated vaccine on hand.

Check vaccine and diluent expiration dates a minimum of weekly. Rotate stock so that vaccines and diluents with the soonest expiration dates are used first to avoid waste from expiration. If the date on the label has a specific month, day, and year, the vaccine can be used through the end of that day. If the expiration date on the label is a month and year, the vaccine can be used through the last day of that month. A multidose vial of vaccine that has been stored and handled properly and is normal in appearance can be used through the expiration date printed on the vial unless otherwise stated in the manufacturer's product information. Some vaccines should be used within a certain time frame after the first time a needle is inserted (e.g., multidose vials), after the vaccine is reconstituted (e.g., vaccines requiring reconstitution), or if the manufacturer deems it is necessary to shorten the expiration date. This time frame is called the "beyond use date" or BUD. The BUD is the date or time after which the vaccine should not be used. It may not be the same as the expiration date printed on the vial by the manufacturer. The BUD varies among vaccines and can be found in the package insert. Check the package insert to determine if the vaccine has a BUD, and for the correct time frame (e.g., days, hours) the vaccine can be stored once the vial has been entered or has been reconstituted. Calculate the BUD using the time interval found in the vaccine's package insert. Label the vaccine with the correct beyond use date/time and your initials. Refer to the CDC's *Vaccine Inventory Management* for specific vaccine product information, including the beyond use dates at http://www.cdc.gov/vaccines/recs/storage/toolkit/storage-handling-

Preventive Measures

- Plug unit directly into wall; do NOT use multi-outlet power strip
- Do NOT use power outlets with built-in circuit switchers
- Do NOT use power outlets that can be activated by a wall switch
- Plug only one unit into an outlet
- Use a plug guard or safety-lock plug
- Install a temperature alarm
- Label circuit breakers and electrical outlets
- Post warning signs that include emergency contact information
- Use water bottles in refrigerator and frozen water bottles in freezer to maintain temperature
- Perform daily inspection of storage unit(s)
- If other biologics must be stored in the same unit, store them BELOW the vaccines to avoid contamination
- Never store food and beverages in the same unit with vaccines
- Take immediate corrective action when there is a problem

Vaccine and Diluent Inventory Control

- Conduct a monthly vaccine and diluent inventory
- Order vaccine based on
  - projected demand
  - storage capacity
  - current supply
- Avoid overstocking

5

Storage and Handling

Expiration Dates

- Monitor vaccine and diluent expiration dates at minimum, weekly

- Rotate stock so that vaccine and diluent with soonest expiration dates are used first

- If normal in appearance and stored and handled properly, product can be used

  - through end of day indicated if expiration date is mm/dd/yyyy (e.g., 12/15/2015 – use through 12/15/2015)

  - through end of month indicated if expiration date is mm/yyyy (e.g., 12/2015 – use through 12/31/2015)

- Multidose vials

  - can be used through expiration date on vial unless otherwise stated in manufacturer's product information

- Reconstituted vaccine

  - expiration date/time might change once opened or reconstituted. This is referred to as the Beyond Use Date (BUD) and is provided in the manufacturer's product information

- Note any change in expiration date/time on vial

- Never use expired vaccine or diluent

toolkit.pdf. Note on a vial any change from the original expiration date/time printed on it, along with your initials. Never use expired vaccine or diluent and immediately remove them from the storage unit.

Emergency or Off-Site/ Satellite Facility Transport

General guidance regarding transport is provided here and in CDC's *Vaccine Storage and Handling Toolkit*. Providers should also contact vaccine manufacturers and/or their immunization program for guidance. Some immunization programs may have vaccine packing and transport practices and procedures for maintaining the cold chain in the field that are specific to their area.

Vaccine manufacturers do not generally recommend or provide guidance for transport of vaccines and CDC discourages regular transport. If possible, have vaccines delivered directly to the off-site/satellite facility. Each transport increases the risk that vaccines will be exposed to inappropriate storage conditions.

Plan for emergencies by ensuring that you have proper equipment to maintain the cold chain during transport. CDC recommends that if emergency transport of vaccines is necessary, it should be done using a qualified container and pack-out or portable refrigerator/freezer. Vaccine manufacturers do not recommend re-use of shipping containers and packing material for routine transport.

If vaccines must be transported to an off-site/satellite facility, the amount of vaccines transported should be limited to the amount needed for that workday, including transport and work time (maximum 8 hours). CDC recommends using a digital data logger with a current and valid certificate of calibration testing. CDC does not recommend cold chain monitors (CCMs) since they do not provide adequate data on excursions that may occur during transport.

The facility's standard operating procedure (SOP) should specify that:

- Vaccines are attended at all times during transport to maintain the cold chain

- Vaccines are not placed in the vehicle trunk

- Vaccines are delivered directly to the facility

- Vaccines are promptly unpacked and placed in appropriate storage units on arrival

A digital data logger with a current and valid certificate of calibration testing is placed with the vaccines during transport.

Diluents should be transported with their corresponding vaccines to ensure that there are always equal numbers of vaccine and diluent for reconstitution. Follow manufacturer guidance for specific temperature requirements. Diluents that contain antigen (e.g., DTaP-IPV diluent used with Hib lyophilized vaccine) should be transported with their corresponding vaccines at refrigerator temperature. NEVER transport any diluents at freezer temperature. Refer to CDC's *Vaccine Storage and Handling Toolkit*, or your immunization program for guidance on vaccine and diluent transport.

Transporting Varicella-Containing Vaccines to Off-Site/Satellite Facilities

The vaccine manufacturer does not recommend transporting varicella-containing vaccines to off-site/satellite facilities. Varicella-containing vaccines are fragile. If these vaccines must be transported to an off-site/satellite facility, CDC recommends transport with a portable freezer unit that maintains the temperature between -58°F and +5°F (-50°C and -15°C). Portable freezers may be available for rent in some places. If varicella-containing vaccines must be transported and a portable freezer unit is not available, do not use dry ice.

Varicella-containing vaccines may also be transported at refrigerator temperature between 35°F and 46°F, (2°C and 8°C) for up to 72 continuous hours prior to reconstitution using the guidelines in CDC's *Vaccine Storage and Handling Toolkit*.

Having a patient pick up a dose of vaccine (e.g., zoster vaccine) at a pharmacy and transporting it in a bag to a clinic for administration is not an acceptable transport method for zoster vaccine or any other vaccine.

Monitoring Temperatures at Off-Site/Satellite Facility

Vaccines should be placed in an appropriate storage unit(s) at the recommended temperature range(s) immediately upon arrival at the alternate facility. CDC recommends placing a digital data logger in the storage unit(s) with the vaccines. Read and document temperatures 2 times during the workday. CDC does not recommend keeping vaccines in a transport container unless it is a portable refrigerator or freezer unit. If vaccines must be kept in transport containers during an off-site clinic:

Transport to Off-Site/Satellite Facilities

- Not recommended by vaccine manufacturers

- If possible, have vaccines delivered directly to the off-site/satellite facility

- Plan for emergencies by ensuring you have proper equipment to maintain cold chain during transport

- If transport is necessary, use a qualified container and pack-out or portable refrigerator/freezer

- Vaccine manufacturers do not recommend re-use of shipping containers and packing material for routine transport

Transport of Varicella-containing Vaccines to Off-Site/Satellite Facilities

- The manufacturer does not recommend transporting varicella-containing vaccines to off-site facilities

- If vaccine must be transported, use a portable freezer that maintains the temperature between -58°F and +5°F (-50°C and -15°C)

- Do NOT use dry ice

- Varicella-containing vaccines may be also transported at refrigerator temperature between 35°F and 46°F (2°C and 8°C), for up to 72 continuous hours prior to reconstitution

- Must use the guideline in CDC's *Vaccine Storage and Handling Toolkit*

- Patient transport of vaccine (e.g. zoster) from pharmacy to a clinic for administration is not an acceptable transport method for any vaccine

5

Storage and Handling

- Container(s) should remain closed as much as possible.

- Calibrated temperature monitoring device(s) (preferably with a buffered probe) should be placed as close as possible to vaccines.

- The temperature(s) inside the containers(s) should be read and documented at least hourly.

- Only the amount of vaccine needed at one time (no more than 1 multidose vial or 10 doses) should be removed for preparation and administration by each vaccinator.

Vaccine Preparation

Most vaccines are supplied in single-dose vials or manufacturer-filled syringes. These preparations do not contain a bacteriostatic (preservative) agent. Once a single-dose vial is opened, meaning that the protective cap has been removed, it should be discarded at the end of the workday if not used. The same is true for an activated manufacturer-filled syringe. Removing the needle cap or attaching a needle activates a manufacturer-filled syringe and breaks the sterile seal. Multidose vials contain a bacteriostatic (preservative) agent. Once opened, a multidose vial may be used through the expiration date unless contaminated or the manufacturer's product information specifies a different timeframe (BUD).

CDC recommends that providers draw up vaccine only at the time of administration and not predraw vaccines. Filling a syringe before it is needed increases the risk for administration errors. Once in the syringe, vaccines are difficult to tell apart. Other problems associated with this practice are wasted vaccine, the risk of inappropriate temperature conditions, resulting in potentially reduced vaccine potency, and possible bacterial contamination in vaccines that do not contain a preservative, such as single-dose vials.

Syringes other than those filled by the manufacturer should be used only for immediate administration and not for vaccine storage. If for some reason, like a large flu clinic, more than one dose of a particular vaccine must be predrawn, draw up only a few syringes at one time (no more than 10 doses or the contents of a single multidose vial). In accordance with best practice standards, these syringes should be administered by the person who filled them.

As an alternative to predrawing vaccine, CDC recommends using manufacturer-filled syringes for large immunization events, such as community influenza clinics. These syringes are designed for both storage and administration.

Vaccine Preparation

- Once the protective cap is removed, vaccine in single-dose vial should be used or discarded at end of workday

- Once manufacturer-filled syringe is activated (remove needle cap or attach needle) sterile seal is broken and should be used or discarded at end of workday

- Do not predraw vaccine
  - increases risk for administration errors
  - wasted vaccine
  - possible bacterial growth in vaccines that do not contain a preservative
  - administration syringes not designed for storage

- Consider using manufacturer-filled syringes for large immunization events because they are designed for both storage and administration

Vaccine Disposal

Unused vaccine and diluent doses may be returnable under certain circumstances. Contact the vaccine supplier, which may be the immunization program or the vaccine manufacturer, for specific policies regarding the disposition of returnable vaccine, unopened vials, expired vials, unused doses, and potentially compromised vaccine due to inappropriate storage conditions.

In general, most empty vaccine vials are not considered hazardous or pharmaceutical waste and do not require disposal in a biomedical waste container. However, requirements for medical waste disposal are regulated by state environmental agencies so you should contact your immunization program or state environmental agency to ensure that your disposal procedures are in compliance with state and federal regulations.

Acknowledgement

The editors thank Donna Weaver, Patricia Beckenhaupt, and JoEllen Wolicki, National Center for Immunization and Respiratory Diseases, CDC, for their contribution to this chapter.

Selected References

Centers for Disease Control and Prevention (CDC). General recommendations on immunization: recommendations of the Advisory Committee on Immunization Practices. *MMWR* 2011;60(no. RR-2): 23-27. http://www.cdc.gov/vaccines/pubs/ACIP-list.htm

CDC. Recommendations and Guidelines: Storage and Handling: http://www.cdc.gov/vaccines/recs/storage/default.htm

Food and Drug Administration (FDA): http://www.fda.gov/BiologicsBloodVaccines/Vaccines/ApprovedProducts/ucm093830.htm

Manufacturers' Product Information: http://www.immunize.org/packageinserts/

National Institute of Standards and Technology (NIST). Thermal Analysis of Refrigeration Systems Used for Vaccine Storage, 2009, Household, Dormitory-Style Refrigerators and Data Loggers. http://www.nist.gov/manuscript-publication-search.cfm?pub_id=904574

Immunization Action Coalition Storage and Handling Handouts: http://www.immunize.org/clinic/storage-handling.asp

---

Vaccine Disposal

- Consult immunization program or vaccine manufacturer regarding returnable vaccines

- Refer to CDC's *Vaccine Storage and Handling Toolkit* for comprehensive storage and handling guidance.

5

Storage and Handling

Proper vaccine administration is a critical component of a successful immunization program. It is a key part of ensuring that vaccination is as safe and effective as possible. This chapter provides best practice guidance for vaccine administration. The guidance should be used in conjunction with professional standards for medication administration and guidance from the vaccine manufacturer.

The foundation of medication administration is application of the "Rights of Medication Administration." These rights should be applied to each encounter when vaccines are administered. These rights include the:

- Right patient

- Right vaccine and diluent (when applicable)

- Right time (including the correct age and interval, as well as before the product expiration time/date)

- Right dosage

- Right route (including the correct needle gauge and length and technique)

- Right site

- Right documentation

Vaccine providers should also incorporate the evidence-based safe injection practices, outlined on CDC's Injection Safety Information for Providers webpage, http://www.cdc.gov/injectionsafety/providers.html.

Staff Training and Education

Improper administration of vaccines may result in injuries or prevent the vaccines from providing optimal protection. All personnel who will administer vaccines should receive comprehensive, competency-based training regarding vaccine administration policies and procedures before administering vaccines. Providers need to validate staff's knowledge and skills regarding vaccine administration with a skills checklist. *See the Skills Checklist for Immunization* at http://www.eziz.org/assets/docs/IMM-694.pdf for an example. Competency-based training should be integrated into existing staff education programs such as new staff orientation and annual education requirements. Staff should receive ongoing education, such as whenever vaccine administration recommendations are updated, or when new vaccines are added to the facility's inventory, to maintain staff competency. Accountability checks should be put in place to ensure policies and procedures are followed. Trainings should also be offered to temporary personnel

6

Vaccine Administration

- Key to ensuring vaccination is as safe and effective as possible

- Incorporate

  - professional standards for medication administration

  - manufacturer's vaccine-specific guidelines

  - evidence-based safe injection practices on CDC's Injection Safety Information for Providers webpage

Staff Training and Education

- Before administering vaccines, all personnell who administer vaccines should

  - receive competency-based training

  - validate knowledge and skills

- Integrate training into

  - new staff orientation

  - annual education requirements

  - when vaccine administration recommendations are updated

  - when new vaccines are added to the inventory

Vaccine Administration

who may be filling in on days when the facility is short staffed or helping during peak times such as flu season. Evidence-based injection safety information and educational programs for healthcare personnel are available on the CDC Injection Safety website at http://www.cdc.gov/injection-safety/providers.html. In addition, the Immunization Action Coalition (IAC) offers web-based educational programs and job aids. IAC resources for administering vaccines can be found at http://www.immunize.org/clinic/administering-vaccines.asp.

Patient Care Before Administering Vaccine

All immunization providers should be knowledgeable regarding appropriate strategies to prepare and care for patients whenever vaccines will be administered.

Immunization Assessment

The patient's immunization history should be reviewed at every healthcare visit. When the patient arrives, providers should obtain a complete immunization history, and compare the patient's immunization record to the medical record and immunization information system or registry data, if available. Use the current immunization schedule based on the age of the patient to determine all recommended vaccines that are needed. Assess for all routinely recommended vaccines as well as any vaccines that are indicated based on health status, occupation, or other risk factors. If a documented immunization history is not available, administer the vaccines that are indicated based on the person's age, medical condition and other risk factors. With the exception of influenza and pneumococcal polysaccharide vaccine (PPSV23), providers should only accept written, dated records as evidence of vaccination; self-reported doses of influenza vaccine and PPSV23 are acceptable. This prevents missing an opportunity to vaccinate while the patient or parent searches for the immunization record.

Screening for Contraindications and Precautions

Patients and their family members count on providers and their staff to administer vaccines safely. Screening for contraindications and precautions can prevent adverse events following vaccination. All patients should be screened for contraindications and precautions prior to administering any vaccine, even if the patient has previously received that vaccine. The patient's status may change from one visit to the next or recommendations regarding contraindications and precautions may have changed. Staff should be knowledgeable of all possible contraindications and precautions to vaccination and only valid contraindications should

---

Patient Care Before Administering Vaccines

- Obtain complete immunization history at every healthcare visit
  - accept only written, dated records (exception influenza and PPSV23 self-report)
  - use recommended schedule to determine vaccines needed based on age, medical condition, and risk factors
- Screen for contraindications and precautions prior to administering any vaccine(s)
- Discuss vaccine benefits and risks and vaccine-preventable disease risks using VISs and other reliable resources
- Provide after-care instructions

be followed. Information about contraindications and precautions can be found at http://www.cdc.gov/vaccines/recs/vac-admin/contraindications.htm

Screening for contraindications and precautions should be included in vaccine administration procedures. Using a standardized screening tool helps staff assess patients correctly and consistently. Many state immunization programs and other organizations have developed standardized screening tools. Two examples are Screening Checklist for Contraindications to Vaccines for Children and Teens at http://www.immunize.org/catg.d/p4060.pdf and Screening Checklist for Contraindications to Vaccines for Adults at http://www.immunize.org/catg.d/p4065.pdf. In addition, both screening checklists are available in other languages. To save time, some facilities ask patients to answer screening questions prior to seeing the provider, such as electronically via an electronic healthcare portal or with a paper copy and pen while in the waiting or exam room.

Patient or Parent Education including Vaccine Safety & Risk Communication

Research shows that parents want clear, consistent information from multiple sources they consider credible. Many of today's parents do not know very much about vaccine-preventable diseases, and therefore do not understand vaccines' disease-protection benefits. They often cite the Internet as the source of vaccine information. However, some of the information available online is not accurate and conflicting. It can be difficult for a parent to know which sites to believe. Therefore, parents may turn to their most trusted information source of vaccine information: their child's doctor or nurse. Healthcare professionals need to be ready to provide parents with timely and transparent information about vaccine benefits and risks.

Establishing an open dialogue promotes a safe, trust-building environment in which individuals can freely evaluate information, discuss vaccine concerns and make informed decisions regarding immunizations. Not all parents want the same level of medical or scientific information about vaccines. Healthcare professionals are encouraged to assess the level of information that each parent wants and provide clear and transparent information. Research shows that a provider's recommendation for vaccination is a powerful motivator.

Immunization providers may be asked about many topics, including vaccine-preventable diseases, specific vaccines, the immunization schedule, and vaccine safety issues. Fortunately, there are many resources available to help providers stay up-to-date on all of these vaccine-related issues.

6

Vaccine Administration

Vaccine Information Statements (VISs) are information sheets produced by the Centers for Disease Control and Prevention (CDC) that explain to vaccine recipients, their parents, or their legal representatives both the benefits and risks of a vaccine. Federal law requires that VISs be handed out whenever vaccinations routinely recommended for children are administered, but CDC encourages the use of ALL VISs, whether the vaccine is covered by the law or not. The VIS should be given every time a dose of vaccine is administered, even if the patient has received the vaccine and a VIS in the past. VISs can be provided at the same time as the screening questionnaire, while the patient is waiting to be seen. They include information that may help the patient or parent respond to the screening questions. In addition to traditional paper copies, VISs are increasingly available in electronic formats that can read on smart phones and other devices.

Providers can also use the CDC website titled, *Provider Resources for Vaccine Conversations with Parents*, available at http://www.cdc.gov/vaccines/hcp/patient-ed/conversations/index.html to talk to parents of infants and young children. The materials available on this website are based on formative, mixed methods research, informed by risk communication principles, and reviewed annually by subject matter experts. In addition, all fact sheets are co-branded with the American Academy of Pediatrics and the American Academy of Family Physicians. In addition, healthcare professionals may find the CDC resource, *Tips and Time-savers for Talking with Parents about HPV Vaccine*, available at http://www.cdc.gov/vaccines/who/teens/for-hcp-tipsheet-hpv.pdf, helpful when talking with parents of adolescents.

A best practice strategy is to allow time for questions and discussion of after-care instructions with patients or parents/guardians before the vaccines are administered. This allows the parent to comfort the child immediately after the injection. After-care instructions should include information and strategies for dealing with side effects such as injection site pain, fever, fussiness (infants especially) and for determining when medical attention should be sought. An age-appropriate dose of a non-aspirin-containing pain reliever may be considered to decrease discomfort and fever after vaccination. The prophylactic use of antipyretics before or at the time of vaccination is not recommended. Examples of after-care instructional materials for parents and patients are *After the Shots* at http://www.immunize.org/catg.d/p4014.pdf and *After Receiving Vaccines* at http://www.aimtoolkit.org/adult/After_Receiving_Vaccine_D_112309%20AIM.pdf.

Patient Care During Vaccine Administration

Patients should be prepared for vaccination with consideration for their age and stage of development. Parents/guardians and patients should be encouraged to take an active role before, during and after the administration of vaccines. *Be There for Your Child During Shots* is a handout for parents. It is located at http://www.eziz.org/assets/docs/IMM-686ES.pdf.

Vaccine safety concerns and the need for multiple injections have increased anxiety associated with immunizations for patients, parents and health-care personnel. Health-care providers need to display confidence and establish an environment that promotes a sense of security and trust. Everyone involved should work to provide immunizations in the safest and least stressful way possible. Simple strategies that can be used by both parents and providers to make receiving vaccines easier include:

- Displaying a positive attitude through facial expressions, body language, and comments

- Using a soft and calm tone of voice

- Making eye contact, even with small children

- Explaining why vaccines are needed (e.g., "this medicine will protect you from getting sick" or "this shot is a shield to protect your body against infection")

- Being honest and explaining what to expect (e.g., do not say that "the injection won't hurt")

Positioning & Comforting Restraint

When determining patient positioning and restraint, consider the patient's comfort, safety, age, activity level, and the site of administration. Parent participation has been shown to increase the child's comfort. When vaccines are being administered to infants and small children, the parent/guardian should be encouraged to hold the child during administration. The parent/guardian should be instructed on how to help the child stay still so the vaccine can be administered safely. If the parent is uncomfortable, another person may assist or the patient may be positioned safely. *Comforting Restraint for Immunizations* at http://www.eziz.org/assets/docs/IMM-720ES.pdf outlines positioning techniques.

While definitive guidelines for positioning patients during vaccination have not been established, some recommendations have been suggested. Research supports the belief that children are less fearful and experience less pain when receiving an injection if they are sitting up rather than lying

---

6

Patient Care During Vaccine Administration

- Consider patient's age and stage of development

- Encourage participation of parent/guardian and patient

- Use simple strategies to ease vaccination process
  - positive attitude
  - soft, calm voice
  - eye contact
  - explain why the vaccine is needed
  - honest about what to expect

Positioning and Comforting Restraint

- Encourage parent/guardian to hold child

- Sitting, rather than lying down

- Be aware of syncope (fainting)
  - have patient seated or lying down during vaccination
  - be aware of symptoms that precede syncope
  - if patient faints, provide supportive care and protect patient from injury
  - observe patient (seated or lying down) for at least 15 minutes after vaccination

Vaccine Administration

down. The exact mechanism behind this phenomenon is unknown; it may be that the child's anxiety level is reduced, which in turn reduces the child's perception of pain. Parents should be instructed to hold infants and children in a position comfortable for the child and parent, in which one or more limbs are exposed for injections. All providers who administer vaccines to older children, adolescents, and adults should be aware of the potential for syncope (fainting) after vaccination and the related risk of injury caused by falls. Clinicians should: (1) make sure the person who is being vaccinated is always seated or lying down; (2) be aware of symptoms that precede fainting (e.g. weakness, dizziness, pallor); and (3) provide supportive care and take appropriate measures to prevent injuries if such symptoms occur. The Advisory Committee on Immunization Practices (ACIP) also recommends that providers consider observing the patient (with patient seated or lying down) for 15 minutes after vaccination.

Procedural Pain Management

Concern and anxiety about injections are common for all ages. Fear of injections and needlestick pain are often cited as reasons why children and adults, including health-care personnel, refuse vaccines. Immunizations are the most common source of iatrogenic pain and are administered repeatedly to children throughout infancy, childhood and adolescence. If not addressed, this pain can have long term effects such as pre-procedural anxiety, fear of needles and avoidance of healthcare behaviors through the lifetime. It has been estimated that up to 25% of adults have a fear of needles, with most fears developing in childhood. Decreasing pain associated with immunizations during childhood may help to prevent this distress and future healthcare avoidance behaviors.

Pain is a subjective phenomenon influenced by multiple factors, including an individual's age, anxiety level, previous healthcare experiences, and culture. Although pain from immunizations is, to some extent, unavoidable, there are some things that parents and healthcare providers can do to help when children and adults need vaccines. Evidence-based strategies to ease the pain associated with the injection process include:

Breastfeeding

Breastfeeding has been demonstrated as a soothing measure for infants up to 12 months of age receiving injections. Several aspects of breastfeeding are thought to decrease pain, including holding the child, skin-to-skin contact, sweet-tasting milk and the act of sucking. Potential adverse events such as gagging or spitting up were not reported. Breastfeeding should occur before, during and after the administration of vaccines. Allow adequate time for the infant to latch onto the nipple properly. Bottle feeding with breast milk or formula should not be considered a substitute for breastfeeding for pain management.

Sweet tasting solutions

Sweet tasting liquids are an analgesic for infants up to 12 months of age. Sweetened liquids are recommended for infants who are not breastfed during vaccination. Several studies have demonstrated a reduction in crying after injections when young children (12 months or younger) ingest a small amount (a few drops to half a teaspoon) of a sugary solution prior to administration of the vaccine. Coughing and/or gagging may occur but infrequently (less than 5% of patients). Parents should be counseled that sweet tasting liquids should only be used for the management of pain associated with a procedure such as an injection.

Injection technique

Aspiration prior to injection and slowly injecting medication are practices that have not been evaluated scientifically. Aspiration was originally recommended for safety reasons and injecting medication slowly was thought to decrease pain from sudden distension of muscle tissue. Although aspiration is advocated by some experts, and most nurses are taught to aspirate before injection, there is no evidence that this procedure is necessary. The ACIP's General Recommendations on Immunization document states that aspiration is not required before administering a vaccine. There are no reports of any person being injured because of failure to aspirate. In addition, the veins and arteries within reach of a needle in the anatomic areas recommended for vaccination are too small to allow an intravenous push of vaccine without blowing out the vessel. A 2007 study from Canada compared infants' pain response using slow injection, aspiration, and slow withdrawal with another group using rapid injection, no aspiration, and rapid withdrawal. Based on behavioral and visual pain scales, the group that received the vaccine rapidly without aspiration experienced less pain. No adverse events were reported with either injection technique.

Order of injections

Frequently children and adults receive 2 or more injections at an immunization encounter. Some vaccines are associated with more pain than others. Because procedure pain can increase with each injection, the order the vaccines are administered may effect the overall pain response. Some vaccines cause a painful or stinging sensation when the injecting the vaccine; examples include measles, mumps and rubella (MMR) and human papillomavirus (HPV) vaccines. Injecting the most painful vaccine (e.g., MMR, PCV13, or

---

Procedural Pain Management
- Evidence-based strategies to ease pain
  - breastfeeding
  - sweet tasting solutions
  - injection technique (aspiration may increase pain)
  - order of injections (administer most painful vaccine last)
  - tactile stimulation (rub/ stroke near injection site prior to and during injection)
  - distraction
  - topical anesthetic

6

Vaccine Administration

HPV) last when multiple injections are being administered can decrease the pain associated with the injections.

Tactile Stimulation

Rubbing or stroking the skin near the injection site prior to and during the injection process with moderate intensity may decrease pain in older children (4 years and older) and adults. The mechanism for this is thought to be that the sensation of touch competes with the feeling of pain from the injection, and thereby results in less pain.

Distraction

Psychological interventions such as distraction in children have been demonstrated to be effective at reducing stress and the perception of pain during the injection process. Distraction is defined as using tactics which are intended to take the patient's attention away from the procedure. Distraction can be led by the provider, child or parent. Certain types of parental behaviors (e.g., nonprocedural talk, suggestions on how to cope, humor) have been related to decreases in children's distress and pain, whereas others (e.g., reassurances, apologies) have been related to increases in children's distress and pain. Parents should be encouraged to use distraction methods and instructed in appropriate distraction techniques. Distraction can be accomplished through a variety of techniques (e.g., playing music, books, pretending to blow away the pain, deep breathing techniques).

Topical anesthetics

Topical analgesia may be applied to decrease pain at the injection site. These products (e.g., 5% lidocaine-prilocaine emulsion) should be used only for the ages recommended and as directed by the product manufacturer. Parents should be educated in the appropriate use of topical analgesics including the exact site(s) the medication should be applied. These analgesics often need to be applied before (20 to 60 minutes depending on the product) vaccine administration to be effective.

Following are other techniques used by some providers. There is insufficient evidence to recommend these techniques to relieve the pain associated with vaccine administration.

Dual administrators

Some providers suggest that having two individuals simultaneously administer vaccines at separate sites will decrease anxiety from anticipation of the next injection(s), while others believe this technique actually increases anxiety by making the child feel overpowered and vulnerable. At this time there is insufficient evidence to make a recommendation either for or against this technique.

Physical intervention "The 5 S's"

A 2012 study found an intervention which included swaddling, holding the infant in a side/stomach position, shushing, swinging gently, and sucking provided decreased pain scores on a validated pain scale and decreased crying time for infants 2 and 4 months of age immediately following routine vaccinations.

Route of administration

As of March 2013, there are two FDA licensed vaccines (IPV and PPSV23) that can be administered by either the subcutaneous or intramuscular route. There is insufficient evidence to support one route (subcutaneous or intramuscular) versus the other as a way to reduce injection pain, in vaccines for which either route may be used. When more than one route is an option the number of injections and available sites may influence the vaccinator's choice.

Infection Control

Healthcare providers should follow appropriate precautions to minimize the risks of spreading disease during the administration of vaccines.

Hand hygiene

Hand hygiene is critical to prevent the spread of illness and disease. Hand hygiene should be performed before vaccine preparation, between patients, and any time hands become soiled, e.g., diapering or cleansing excreta. Hands should be cleansed with a waterless alcohol-based hand rub or, when hands are visibly dirty or contaminated with blood or other body fluids, washed thoroughly with soap and water.

Gloves

Occupational Safety and Health Administration (OSHA) regulations do not require gloves to be worn when administering vaccines unless the person administering the vaccine is likely to come into contact with potentially infectious body fluids or has open lesions on the hands. If gloves are worn, they should be changed and hand hygiene performed between patients. Gloves will not prevent needlestick injuries. Any needlestick injury should be reported immediately to the site supervisor, with appropriate care and follow-up given as directed by local/state guidelines.

Equipment Disposal

Immediately after use, all used syringe/needle devices should be placed in biohazard containers that are closable, puncture-resistant, leakproof on sides and bottom and labeled or color-coded. This practice helps prevent accidental needlesticks and reuse. Used needles should not be recapped, cut, or detached from the syringes before

---

Infection Control

- Hand hygiene should be performed
  - before vaccine preparation
  - between patients
  - any time hands become soiled
- Gloves are not required when administering vaccines unless the person administering the vaccine is likely to come into contact with potentially infectious body fluids or has open lesions on hands
  - if gloves are worn, they should be changed and hand hygiene performed between patients
- Equipment disposal
  - place used syringes and needles (do not cut, recap, or detach from syringe) in a puncture-resistant biohazard container
  - dispose of empty or expired vaccine vials as medical waste

Vaccine Administration

disposal. Empty or expired vaccine vials are considered medical waste and should be disposed of according to state regulations. More information can be found at OSHA's website, https://www.osha.gov/pls/oshaweb/owadisp.show_document?p_table=INTERPRETATIONS&p_id=21010&p_text_version=FALSE

Vaccine Preparation

Proper vaccine handling and preparation is critical in maintaining the integrity of the vaccine during transfer from the manufacturer's vial to the syringe and ultimately to the patient. Vaccines should be drawn up in a designated clean medication area that is not adjacent to areas where potentially contaminated items are placed. Multidose vials to be used for more than one patient should not be kept or accessed in the immediate patient treatment area. This is to prevent inadvertent contamination of the vial through direct or indirect contact with potentially contaminated surfaces or equipment that could then lead to infections in subsequent patients. If a multidose vial enters the immediate patient treatment area, it should be discarded after use. See other frequently asked questions on injection safety at http://www.cdc.gov/injectionsafety/providers/provider_faqs_multivials.html

Equipment Selection

Syringe Selection

A separate needle and syringe should be used for each injection. A parenteral vaccine may be delivered in either a 1-mL or 3-mL syringe as long as the prescribed dosage is delivered. OSHA requires that safety-engineered injection devices (e.g., needle-shielding syringes or needle-free injectors) be used for injectable vaccination in all clinical settings to reduce risk for injury and disease transmission. Personnel who will be using these products should be involved in evaluation and selection of these products and should receive training with these devices before using them in the clinical area. Some syringes and needles are packaged with an expiration date. This can be a consideration when ordering injection supplies. Never administer medications from the same syringe to more than one patient, even if the needle is changed.

Needle Selection

Vaccine must reach the desired tissue site for optimal immune response to occur. Use of longer needles has been associated with less redness or swelling than occurs with shorter needles because of the injection into deeper muscle mass. Therefore, needle selection should be based on the prescribed route, size of the individual, and injection technique. A supply of needles in varying lengths appropriate

---

Vaccine Preparation

- Equipment selection

  - use a separate 1-mL or 3-mL sterile syringe for each injection

  - OSHA requires safety-engineered injection devices to reduce risk of injury and disease transmission

  - some syringes and needles are packaged with an expiration date

  - select a separate sterile needle for each injection based on route, size of individual and injection technique

for the facility's patient population should be available to staff. Typically, vaccines are not highly viscous so a fine gauge needle (22- to 25-gauge) can be used. As with syringes, some needles are packaged with an expiration date. Check the expiration date on the needle and syringe packaging, if present. Do not use if the equipment has expired.

Inspecting Vaccine

Each vaccine and diluent vial should be carefully inspected for damage or contamination prior to use. The expiration date printed on the vial or box should be checked. Vaccine can be used through the last day of the month indicated by the expiration date unless otherwise stated on the package labeling. The expiration date or time for some vaccines changes once the vaccine vial is opened or the vaccine is reconstituted. This information is available in the manufacturer's product information. Regardless of expiration date, vaccine and diluent should only be used as long as they are normal in appearance and have been stored and handled properly. Expired vaccine or diluent should never be used.

Reconstitution

Several vaccines are supplied in a lyophilized (freeze-dried) form that requires reconstitution with a liquid diluent. Vaccines should be reconstituted according to manufacturer guidelines using only the specific diluent supplied by the manufacturer for that vaccine. Each diluent is specific to the corresponding vaccine in volume, sterility, pH, and chemical balance. If the wrong diluent is used, the vaccine dose is not valid and will need to be repeated using the correct diluent.

Reconstitute vaccine just before using. Inject all the diluent into the vaccine vial and agitate the vial to ensure thorough mixing (follow the specific instructions provided in the product information). Use all of the diluent supplied for a single dose and then draw up all of the vaccine after it is thoroughly reconstituted. Changing the needle between drawing vaccine from the vial and administering the vaccine is not necessary unless the needle is contaminated or damaged. For additional information on reconstituted vaccines, see *Preparing Reconstituted Vaccine* at http://www.eziz.org/assets/docs/IMM-897.pdf and Vaccine with Diluents: How to use them at http://www.immunize.org/catg.d/p3040.pdf.

Beyond Use Date (BUD)

Some vaccines should be used within a certain time frame after the first time a needle is inserted into a multidose vial (commonly referred to as "entering" the vial.) For other vaccines, this time frame is based on the date/time the vaccine was reconstituted. This time frame is called the

6

Vaccine Preparation

- Inspect vaccine and diluent vial for damage or contamination

- Check the expiration date; never administer expired vaccine or diluent

- Reconstitute vaccine, if applicable, according to manufacturers guidelines just before administration using ONLY the manufacturers supplied diluent for that vaccine.

- Agitate vial to thoroughly mix vaccine

- Inspect vaccine for discoloration, precipitate or if it cannot be re-suspended

Vaccine Administration

"beyond use date" or BUD. The BUD is the date or time after which the vaccine should not be used. It may not be the same as the expiration date printed on the vial by the manufacturer. The BUD varies among vaccines and can be found in the package insert. Check the package insert to determine if the vaccine has a BUD and for the correct time frame (e.g., days, hours) the vaccine can be stored once the vial has been entered or has been reconstituted. Calculate the beyond use date using the time interval found in the vaccine's package insert. Label the vaccine with the correct beyond use date/time and your initials. If the reconstituted vaccine is not used immediately, write the BUD and your initials on the label and store it properly. Refer to the CDC's *Vaccine Inventory Management* for specific vaccine product information, including the beyond use dates at http://www.cdc.gov/vaccines/recs/storage/toolkit/storage-handling-toolkit.pdf

Filling Syringes

Prepare vaccine just prior to administration. Agitate the vial to mix the vaccine thoroughly and obtain a uniform suspension prior to withdrawing each dose. Whenever solution and container permit, inspect the vaccine visually for discoloration, precipitation or if it cannot be re-suspended prior to administration. If problems are noted (e.g., vaccine cannot be re-suspended), the vaccine should not be administered.

Standard medication preparation guidelines should be followed for drawing a dose of vaccine into a syringe. A vaccine dose should not be drawn into the syringe until it is to be administered. The cap on top of a vaccine vial functions as a dust cover. Once removed, cleansing the exposed rubber stopper with a pre-packaged sterile alcohol wipe is recommended. Do not enter a vial with a used syringe or needle. Once the syringe(s) are filled, label the syringe with the type of vaccine. Administer the doses as soon as possible after filling. CDC recommends that providers draw up vaccines only at the time of administration. Do NOT predraw doses before they are needed. (See Vaccine Preparation in the Storage and Handling chapter) Medications packaged as single-use vials or syringes should never be used for more than one patient. Single-dose vials and manufacturer-filled syringes are designed for single-dose administration and should be discarded if vaccine has been withdrawn or reconstituted and subsequently not used within the time frame specified by the manufacturer.

Vaccines should never be combined in a single syringe except when specifically approved by the FDA and packaged for that specific purpose. Most combination vaccines will be

---

Vaccine Preparation

- Filling syringe

  - remove the vial dust cover and withdraw the vaccine according to standard medication preparation guidelines just prior to vaccination

  - single-dose vials should only be used for a single dose

  - once a dose is drawn up, it should be used within the manufacturer specified time or discarded at the end of the workday

  - once a manufacturer-filled syringe is activated (i.e., needle attached or needle covered removed) it should be used or discarded at the end of the workday

combined by the manufacturer. As of March 2013, there are two binary vaccines (i.e. vaccines whose antigens are divided between freeze-dried portion and diluent) that must be combined by the provider at the time of administration, i.e., DTaP-IPV/Hib (Pentacel), and MCV4 (Menveo).

Vaccine should never be transferred from one syringe to another. Partial doses from separate vials should not be combined to obtain a full dose. Both of these practices increase the risk of contamination. Instilling air into a multidose vial prior to withdrawing a vaccine dose may not be necessary. It could cause a "spritz" of vaccine to be lost the next time the vial is entered, which through time can decrease the amount of vaccine in the vial and lead to the loss of a dose (e.g., obtaining only 9 full doses from a 10-dose vial).

Route and Site

The recommended route and site for each vaccine are based on clinical trials, practical experience and theoretical considerations. This information is included in the manufacturer's product information for each vaccine, see manufacturers' package insert at http://www.immunize.org/packageinserts/. There are five routes used to administer vaccines. Deviation from the recommended route may reduce vaccine efficacy or increase local adverse reactions.

Oral (PO) Route

Rotavirus vaccines (RV1 [Rotarix] RV5, [RotaTeq]) and oral typhoid (TY21a [Vivotif]) are the only U.S.-licensed vaccines that are administered by the oral route. RV1 (Rotarix) requires reconstitution prior to oral administration. Oral vaccines should generally be administered prior to administering injections or performing other procedures that might cause discomfort. Administer the liquid slowly down one side of the inside of the cheek (between the cheek and gum) toward the back of the infant's mouth. Care should be taken not to go far enough back to initiate the gag reflex. Never administer or spray (squirt) the vaccine directly into the throat. Detailed information on oral delivery of these vaccines is included in each manufacturer's product information.

ACIP does not recommend readministering a dose of rotavirus vaccine to an infant who regurgitates, spits out, or vomits during or after administration. No data exist on the benefits or risks associated with readministering a dose. The infant should receive the remaining recommended doses of rotavirus vaccine following the routine schedule. There are no restrictions on the infant's consumption of breast milk or any other liquid before or after administration of either of these vaccines.

6

Vaccine Preparation "Nevers"

- Never combine vaccines into a single syringe except when specifically approved by the FDA and packaged for that specific purpose

- Never transfer vaccine from one syringe to another

- Never draw partial doses of vaccine from separate vials to obtain a full dose

Oral (PO) Route Rotavirus Vaccines

- Administer oral vaccines, in general, prior to administering injections or performing other procedures that might cause discomfort

- Administer liquid slowly down one side of the inside cheek (between the cheek and gum) toward the back of infant's mouth

- Take care not to go far enough back to initiate the gag reflex

- Never administer or spray (squirt) vaccine directly into the throat

- Do not readminister a dose of rotavirus vaccine if the infant regurgitates, spits out or vomits during or after administration

Vaccine Administration

6

Intranasal (NAS) Route
Live Attenuated Influenza Vaccine (LAIV)

- Use the special sprayer provided
- Seat the patient with head tilted back with a provider hand supporting the back of the patient's head
- Instruct the patient to breathe normally
- Insert the tip of the sprayer and spray half the dose in one nostril then remove the dose divider clip and administer the other half-dose in the other nostril
- Health-care personnel who are immunosuppressed and require protective isolation should not administer LAIV

Subcutaneous (subcut) Route

- Site
  - thigh for infants younger than 12 months of age
  - upper outer triceps of arm for children older than 12 months and adults (can be used for infants if necessary)
- Needle gauge and length
  - 23- to 25-gauge needle, 5/8- inch
- Technique
  - follow standard medication administration guidelines for site assessment/selection and site preparation
  - pinch up tissue at site
  - insert needle at 45° angle and inject
  - withdraw needle and apply light pressure to injection site for several seconds with gauze pad

Intranasal (NAS) Route

The live attenuated influenza vaccine (LAIV, FluMist) is currently the only vaccine administered by the nasal route. The vaccine dose (0.2 mL) is inside a special sprayer device. A plastic clip on the plunger divides the dose into two equal parts. The patient should be seated in an upright position with head tilted back. Instruct the patient to breathe normally. The provider should gently place a hand behind the patient's head. The tip of the nasal sprayer should be inserted slightly into the nostril. Half of the contents of the sprayer (0.1 mL) are sprayed into the nostril. The dose-divider clip is then removed and the procedure is repeated in the other nostril. Detailed information on the nasal administration of LAIV is included in the manufacturer's product information. The dose does not need to be repeated if the patient coughs, sneezes, or expels the dose in any other way.

It is possible for the LAIV spray to cause low-level contamination of the environment with vaccine virus, but there have been no reports of vaccine virus transmission by this route. No instances of illness or attenuated vaccine virus infections have occured among inadvertently exposed health-care personnel or immunocompromised patients. Health-care personnel at increased risk for influenza complications, including those with underlying medical conditions, pregnant women, persons 50 years of age or older, or with immunosuppressive conditions, may safely administer LAIV. The only exception is personnel with immunosuppression severe enough to require a protective environment (e.g., for hematopoietic cell transplant). However, healthcare personnel with this level of immunosuppression are not likely to be administering any vaccines.

Subcutaneous (subcut) Route

Subcutaneous injections are administered into the fatty tissue found below the dermis and above muscle tissue.

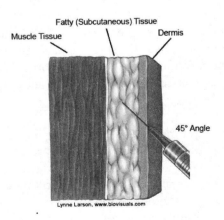

Muscle Tissue — Fatty (Subcutaneous) Tissue — Dermis — 45° Angle

Lynne Larson, www.biovisuals.com

Site

The recommended subcutaneous sites for vaccine administration are the thigh (for infants younger than 12 months of age) and the upper outer triceps of the arm (for persons 1 year of age and older). If necessary, the upper outer triceps area can be used to administer subcutaneous injections to infants.

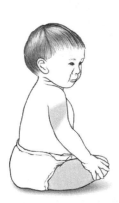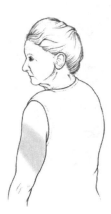

Source: California Department of Public Health

Needle Gauge and Length

5/8-inch, 23- to 25-gauge needle

Technique

- Follow standard medication administration guidelines for site assessment/selection and site preparation.

- To avoid reaching the muscle, pinch up the fatty tissue, insert the needle at a 45° angle and inject the vaccine into the tissue.

- Withdraw the needle and apply light pressure to the injection site for several seconds with a gauze pad.

Subcutaneous Administration Technique

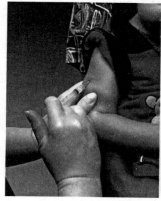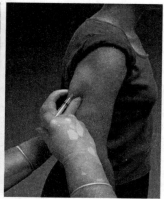

Source: California Department of Public Health

**Intramuscular (IM) Route
Infants 12 Months and Younger**

- Site
  - vastus lateralis muscle (anterolateral thigh)
- Needle gauge and length:
  - 22- to 25-gauge
  - neonates and preterm infants: 5/8-inch
    - 5/8-inch needle is adequate only if the skin is stretched flat between thumb and forefinger
  - 1 month and older: 1-inch

Vaccine Administration

**Intramuscular (IM) Route
Toddlers 1 Year
through 2 Years**

- Site

  - vastus lateralis muscle
    (anterolateral thigh) is
    preferred

  - deltoid muscle (upper arm)
    may be used if the muscle
    mass is adequate

- Needle gauge and length

  - 22- to 25-gauge

  - 5/8 to 1-inch

    – 5/8-inch needle is
    adequate only for the
    deltoid muscle and only
    if the skin is stretched
    flat between thumb and
    forefinger

Intramuscular (IM) Route

Intramuscular injections are administered into muscle tissue below the dermis and subcutaneous tissue.

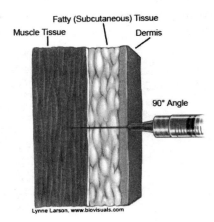

Site

Almost all inactivated vaccines are administered by the intramuscular route. Many inactivated vaccines contain an adjuvant, which is a vaccine component that enhances the immune response to the antigen. Adjuvants can cause an exaggerated local reaction (e.g., pain, swelling, redness) if not injected into the muscle, so proper technique is critical.

There are only two routinely recommended IM sites for administration of vaccines, the vastus lateralis muscle (anterolateral thigh) and the deltoid muscle (upper arm). Injection at these sites reduces the chance of involving neural or vascular structures. The preferred site depends on the age of the individual and the degree of muscle development.

Because there are no large blood vessels in the recommended sites, aspiration before injection of vaccines (i.e., pulling back on the syringe plunger after needle insertion but before injection) is not necessary. Also, some safety-engineered syringes do not allow for aspiration.

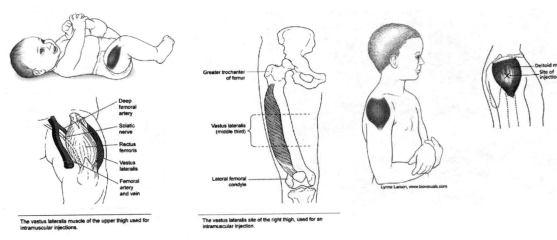

The vastus lateralis muscle of the upper thigh used for intramuscular injections.

The vastus lateralis site of the right thigh, used for an intramuscular injection.

Two left images: Lynne Larson, www.biovisuals.com

Needle Gauge

22- to 25-gauge needle

Needle Length

The needle should be long enough to reach the muscle mass and prevent vaccine from seeping into subcutaneous tissue, but not so long as to involve underlying nerves, blood vessels, or bone. The health-care provider should be familiar with the anatomy of the area into which the vaccine will be injected.

Age-Based Recommendations

Decisions on needle size and site of injection must be made for each person on the basis of the size of the muscle, the thickness of adipose tissue at the injection site, the volume of the material to be administered, and injection technique.

Infants (12 Months and Younger)

For the majority of infants, the anterolateral aspect of the thigh is the recommended site for injection because it provides a large muscle mass. The muscles of the buttock are not used for administration of vaccines in infants and children because of concern about potential injury to the sciatic nerve, which is well documented after injection of antimicrobial agents into the buttock. If the gluteal muscle must be used, care should be taken to define the anatomic landmarks. If the gluteal muscle is chosen, injection should be administered lateral and superior to a line between the posterior superior iliac spine and the greater trochanter or in the ventrogluteal site, the center of a triangle bounded by the anterior superior iliac spine, the tubercle of the iliac crest, and the upper border of the greater trochanter.

Injection technique is the most important parameter to ensure efficient intramuscular vaccine delivery. If the subcutaneous and muscle tissue are bunched to minimize the chance of striking bone, a 1-inch needle is required to ensure intramuscular administration in infants aged 1 month and older. For the majority of infants, a 1-inch, 22- to 25-gauge needle is sufficient to penetrate muscle in an infant's thigh. For neonates (first 28 days of life) and preterm infants, a 5/8-inch needle usually is adequate if the skin is stretched flat between thumb and forefinger and the needle inserted at a 90-degree angle to the skin.

Toddlers (1 Year through 2 Years)

For toddlers, the vastus lateralis muscle in the anterolateral thigh is preferred. The needle should be at least 1-inch long. The deltoid muscle can be used if the muscle mass is adequate. A 5/8-inch needle is adequate only for the deltoid muscle and only if the skin is stretched flat between thumb and forefinger and the needle inserted at a 90° angle to the skin.

Vaccine Administration

Intramuscular (IM) Route Children/Adolescents 3 through 18 Years

- Site
  - deltoid muscle (upper arm) is preferred
  - vastus lateralis muscle (anterolateral thigh) may be used
- Needle gauge and length
  - 22- to 25- gauge
  - 5/8 to 1-inch
    - 5/8-inch needle is adequate only for the deltoid muscle and only if the skin is stretched flat between thumb and forefinger
- Most young children in this age range require a 5/8 or 1-inch needle
- In general, older children and adolescents require a 1-inch needle

Intramuscular (IM) Route Adults 19 Years and Older

- Site:
  - deltoid muscle (upper arm) is preferred
  - vastus lateralis muscle (anterolateral thigh) may be used
- Needle gauge: 23- to 25-gauge

Children/Adolescents (3 through 18 Years)

The deltoid muscle is preferred for children aged 3 through 18 years of age. The needle size for deltoid injections can range from 22- to 25-gauge and from 5/8- to 1-inch, depending on technique. Most young children in this age range require a 5/8- or 1-inch needle. In general, older children and adolescents require a 1-inch needle. One study found that obese adolescents may need a 1½-inch needle in order to reach muscle tissue. If there is any doubt, knowledge of body mass may be helpful in estimating the appropriate needle length. The vastus lateralis muscle in the anterolateral thigh is an alternative site if the deltoid sites cannot be used. A 1- or 1¼-inch needle will be sufficient to reach muscle tissue in most older children and adolescents.

Adults (19 Years and Older)

For adults, the deltoid muscle is recommended for routine intramuscular vaccinations. The anterolateral thigh also can be used. For men and women weighing less than 130 lbs (60 kg) a 5/8 to 1-inch needle is sufficient to ensure intramuscular injection into the deltoid muscle if a 90° angle is used and the tissue is not bunched. For men and women who weigh 130-152 lbs (60-70 kg), a 1-inch needle is sufficient. For women who weigh 152-200 lbs (70-90 kg) and men who weigh 152-260 lbs (70-118 kg), a 1 to 1½-inch needle is recommended. For women who weigh more than 200 lbs (more than 90 kg) or men who weigh more than 260 lbs (more than 118 kg), a 1½-inch needle is recommended. As with adolescents, the vastus lateralis muscle in the anterolateral thigh is an alternative site if the deltoid sites cannot be used.

Gender		Needle Length
Male	Female	
Less than 130 pounds	Less than 130 pounds	5/8 – 1-inch
130 – 152 pounds	130 – 152 pounds	1-inch
153 – 260 pounds	153 – 200 pounds	1 – 1½-inches
260+ pounds	200+ pounds	1½-inches

Technique

- Follow standard medication administration guidelines for site assessment/selection and site preparation.

- To avoid injection into subcutaneous tissue, spread the skin of the selected vaccine administration site taut between the thumb and forefinger, isolating the muscle. Another technique, acceptable mostly for pediatric and geriatric patients, is to grasp the tissue and "bunch up" the muscle.

- Insert the needle fully into the muscle at a 90° angle and inject the vaccine into the tissue.

- Withdraw the needle and apply light pressure to the injection site for several seconds with a gauze pad.

Intramuscular Administration Technique

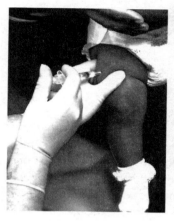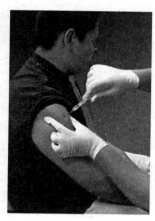

Source: California Department of Public Health

Intradermal (ID) Route

Fluzone Intradermal is the only U.S.-licensed vaccine that is administered by the intradermal route. This Fluzone formulation is not the same as intramuscular formulations of inactivated influenza vaccine (IIV). Other IIV formulations should NOT be administered by the intradermal route.

Site

The site of administration is the deltoid region of the upper arm. The patient should be seated with the arm bent at the elbow and the hand on the hip to ensure that the site of administration is prominent.

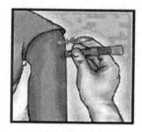

Source: Sanofi Pasteur Inc.

Intramuscular (IM) Injection Technique

- Follow standard medication administration guidelines for site assessment/selection and site preparation

- Spread the skin of the site taut between the thumb and forefinger, isolating the muscle

- Another technique, acceptable mostly for pediatric and geriatric patients, is to grasp the tissue and "bunch up" the muscle

- Insert the needle fully into the muscle at a 90° angle and inject

- Withdraw the needle and apply light pressure to the injection site for several seconds with a gauze pad

Intradermal (ID) Route

- Site
  - deltoid region of the upper arm

- Needle gauge and length
  - manufacturer prefilled microinjection syringe is used to administer a 0.1 mL dose into the dermal layer of the skin
  - syringe contains a 30-gauge, 1.5 mL microneedle

- Technique
  - hold the syringe between the thumb and the middle finger
  - using a short quick motion insert the needle perpendicular to the skin
  - push on the plunger with the index finger without aspirating
  - after the vaccine is delivered, remove the syringe
  - push firmly on the plunger until the needle shield is activated

Vaccine Administration

Needle Gauge and Length

A manufacturer prefilled microinjection syringe is used to administer a 0.1 mL dose into the dermal layer of the skin. The syringe contains a 30-gauge, 1.5 mL microneedle.

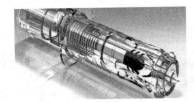

Source: Sanofi Pasteur Inc.

Technique

The syringe should be gently shaken before the needle cap is removed. Hold the syringe between the thumb and the middle finger. Using a short quick motion insert the needle perpendicular to the skin into the deltoid region of the upper arm. Push on the plunger with the index finger without aspirating. Because the needle is very short the vaccine will be delivered just under the skin into the dermal layer. This vaccine should NOT be administered into the volar aspect of the forearm or by the intradermal technique used to administer a tuberculin skin test.

After the vaccine is delivered, remove the syringe and point it away from anyone. Push firmly on the plunger with the thumb until a click is heard. A protective shield will cover the needle and the syringe can be disposed of in a sharps container.

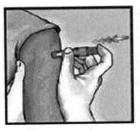 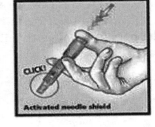

Source: Sanofi Pasteur Inc.

Multiple Vaccinations

If multiple vaccines are administered at a single visit, administration of each preparation at a different anatomic site is desirable. For infants and younger children, if more than two vaccines are injected in a single limb, the thigh is the preferred site because of the greater muscle mass. For older children and adults, the deltoid muscle can be used for more than one intramuscular injection. The injection sites should be separated by 1 inch or more, if possible, so that any local reactions can be differentiated. Vaccines that are the most reactive (e.g., tetanus toxoid-containing and PCV13)

Multiple Vaccinations

- Administer each vaccine at a different anatomic site
- Use anterolateral thigh for infants and young children
- Use deltoid for older children and adults if muscle mass is adequate
- Separate injections by at least 1 inch, or more if possible
- Use a separate limb for most reactive vaccines (e.g., tetanus toxoid-containing and PCV13), if possible
- Use combination vaccines when appropriate to reduce the number of injections

should be administered in different limbs if possible. Use of combination vaccines can reduce the number of injections. A number of job aids are available for immunization providers. See *Giving All the Doses Under 12 Months* (http://www.aimtoolkit.org/docs/Giving_all_doses_under_12mths.pdf), *Giving All the Doses 12 Months and Older* (http://www.aimtoolkit.org/docs/Giving_all_the_doses_12mths.pdf), and *Giving All the Doses for Age 11 Years and Older* (http://www.aimtoolkit.org/docs/7_Givingallthedoses_adolescent_013113.pdf).

If a vaccine and an immune globulin preparation are administered simultaneously (e.g., Td/Tdap and tetanus immune globulin [TIG] or hepatitis B vaccine and hepatitis B immune globulin [HBIG]), separate anatomic sites should be used.

The location of all injection sites should be documented in the patient's medical record. Health-care providers should consider using a vaccination site map so that all persons administering vaccines routinely use the same anatomic site for each different vaccine.

Vaccinating Persons with Bleeding Disorders

Individuals with a bleeding disorder or who are receiving anticoagulant therapy may develop hematomas in IM injection sites. When any intramuscularly administered vaccine is indicated for a patient with a bleeding disorder, the vaccine should be administered intramuscularly if a physician familiar with the patient's bleeding risk determines that the vaccine can be administered by this route with reasonable safety. Prior to administration of IM vaccines the patient or family should be instructed about the risk of hematoma formation from the injection. If the patient periodically receives antihemophilia or similar therapy, IM vaccine administration should be scheduled shortly after such therapy is administered. A 23-gauge or finer needle should be used and firm pressure applied to the site for at least 2 minutes after injection. The site should not be rubbed or massaged. Patients receiving anticoagulation therapy presumably have the same bleeding risk as patients with clotting factor disorders and providers should follow the same guidelines for intramuscular administration.

Nonstandard Administration

CDC discourages deviating from the recommended route, site, dosage, or number of doses for any vaccine. Deviation can result in reduced protection and increase the risk of an exaggerated local reaction. For certain vaccines, the ACIP recommends revaccination if a nonstandard route or site is used. Hepatitis B vaccine administered by any route other than the intramuscular route, or in adults at any

---

Vaccinating Persons with Bleeding Disorders

- Individuals with bleeding disorder or receiving anticoagulant therapy may develop hematomas in IM injection sites

- Administer vaccines by recommended IM route IF physician familiar with patient's bleeding risk determines vaccine can be safely administered

- Prior to vaccination, instruct about risk of hematoma

- Schedule shortly after antihemophelia or similar therapy

- Use 23-gauge or finer needle and apply firm pressure to injection site for at least 2 minutes after injection

- Do NOT rub or massage injection site

Vaccine Administration

Nonstandard Administration

- CDC discourages deviation from recommended route, site, dosage, or number of vaccine doses

- Revaccination is recommended if :

  - hepatitis B vaccine is administered by any route other than IM or in any site of an adult other than deltoid or anterolateral thigh

  - rabies vaccine is administered in gluteal site

  - HPV vaccine is administered by any route other than IM

  - less than the standard dose is administered unless serologic testing indicates an adequate response

  - if a partial dose of a parenteral vaccine is administered because the syringe or needle leaks or the patient jerks away

site other than the deltoid or anterolateral thigh, should not be counted as valid and should be repeated. Doses of rabies vaccine administered in the gluteal site should not be counted as valid doses and should be repeated. Revaccination is recommended when HPV vaccine is administered by any route other than IM. All vaccines should be administered by the manufacturer's recommended route, but there are no ACIP recommendations to repeat doses of other vaccines administered by another route. For additional information, see the ACIP General Recommendations at http://www.cdc.gov/mmwr/pdf/rr/rr6002.pdf.

Larger than recommended dosages can be hazardous because of excessive local or systemic concentrations of antigens or other vaccine constituents deposited into the tissue. Administering volumes smaller than recommended (e.g., inappropriately divided doses) might result in inadequate protection. Using reduced doses administered at multiple vaccination visits that equal a full dose or using smaller divided doses is not recommended. In addition, some vaccines (e.g., IIV, HepB, HepA) require different dosages (amount) based on the patient's age. Any vaccination using less than the standard dose should not be counted, and the person should be revaccinated according to age unless serologic testing indicates that an adequate response has developed. If a partial dose of a parenteral vaccine is administered because the syringe or needle leaks or the patient jerks away, the dose should be repeated.

Managing Acute Vaccine Reactions

Severe, life-threatening anaphylactic reactions following vaccination are rare. Thorough screening for contraindications and precautions prior to vaccination can often prevent reactions. Staff must have in place and be familiar with procedures for managing a reaction. Staff should be familiar with the signs and symptoms of anaphylaxis because they usually begin within minutes of vaccination. These signs and symptoms can include, but are not limited to: flushing, facial edema, urticaria, itching, swelling of the mouth or throat, wheezing, and difficulty breathing. Each staff member should know their role in the event of an emergency and all vaccination providers should be certified in cardiopulmonary resuscitation (CPR). Epinephrine and equipment for maintaining an airway should be available for immediate use. After the patient is stabilized, arrangements should be made for immediate transfer to an emergency facility for additional evaluation and treatment, see *Medical Management of Vaccine Reactions in Children and Teens* at http://www.immunize.org/catg.d/p3082a.pdf and *Medical Management of Vaccine Reactions in Adult Patients* at http://www.immunize.org/catg.d/p3082.pdf.

Documentation

All vaccines administered should be fully documented in the patient's permanent medical record. Healthcare providers who administer vaccines covered by the National Childhood Vaccine Injury Act are required to ensure that the permanent medical record of the recipient indicates:

- Date of administration

- Vaccine manufacturer

- Vaccine lot number

- ~~Expiration date~~ *See 9/2015 Errata*

- Name and title of the person who administered the vaccine and the address of the facility where the permanent record will reside

- Vaccine information statement (VIS)

  - date printed on the VIS

  - date VIS given to patient or parent/guardian

Best practice documentation guidelines for medications also include the vaccine type. The ACIP U.S. Vaccine Abbreviations list can be found at http://www.cdc.gov/vaccines/acip/committee/guidance/vac-abbrev.html), route, dosage (volume), and site. Accurate documentation can help prevent administration errors and curtail the number and costs of excess vaccine doses administered. Providers also should update patients' permanent medical records to reflect any documented episodes of adverse events after vaccination and any serologic test results related to vaccine-preventable diseases (e.g., those for rubella screening and antibody to hepatitis B surface antigen). Participation in immunization information systems is encouraged. Additional documentation resources are located at http://www.immunize.org/handouts/document-vaccines.asp. The patient or parent/guardian should be provided with an immunization record that includes the vaccines administered, including the dates of administration.

Although there is no national law, it is also important to document when parents or adult patients refuse vaccine despite the immunization providers' recommendation. Many professional organizations such as the American Academy of Pediatrics and others have developed forms to document when vaccines are refused. See Decision to Not Vaccinate My Child at http://www.immunize.org/catg.d/p4059.pdf and Refusal to Consent to Vaccination (Adult) at http://www.aimtoolkit.org/adult/vaccine/RefusaltoConsent_Adult%20final_040313.pdf for examples.

Documentation in Permanent Medical Record

- Required for vaccines covered by National Childhood Vaccine Injury Act

  - date of administration

  - vaccine manufacturer

  - vaccine lot number

  - ~~expiration date~~ *See 9/2015 Errata*

  - name and title of person who administered vaccine and address of facility where permanent record will reside

  - vaccine information statement (VIS)

- date on VIS

- date provided to patient or parent/guardian

- Best practice documentation

  - vaccine type (ACIP abbreviation)

  - route

  - dosage (volume)

  - site

- Document vaccine refusal

Immunization Information System (IIS)/ Registry

- Confidential, population-based, computerized database

- All providers are encouraged to use IIS/registry

- Some state IIS utilize barcoding technology

  - 2D barcodes on some vaccine vials and VISs

6

Vaccine Administration

Strategies to Prevent Errors

- Adhere to "Rights of Medication Administration"

- Provide ongoing staff training and education

- Involve staff in selection of products to be used

- Use standardized ACIP vaccine abbreviations

- Keep current reference materials available for staff

- Rotate vaccines so those with shortest expiration dates are in front and check frequently to remove any expired vaccines

- Do not store sound-alike and look-alike vaccines next to each other

- Color code and label vaccines with type, age, and gender, if applicable

- Store pediatric and adult vaccines on separate shelves

- Administer only vaccines that you have prepared

- Triple check your work before administering a vaccine

- Avoid interruptions when selecting and preparing vaccines

- Consider using standing orders

- Counsel parents and patients about vaccines to be administered and about importance of maintaining personal immunization records

Immunization information systems (IIS) or registries are confidential, population-based, computerized databases in which immunization doses administered by participating providers to persons residing within a given geopolitical area can be documented. All immunization providers are encouraged to participate and document administered vaccines in an IIS. For additional information regarding Immunization Information Systems, see http://www.cdc.gov/vaccines/programs/iis/index.html.

Some states' IIS are able to utilize barcoding technology. Implementation of a 2D barcode on vaccine vials and VISs will allow for rapid, accurate, and automatic capture of certain data, including vaccine product identifier, lot number, and expiration date, and VIS edition date using a handheld imaging device, or scanner, which could populate these fields in an electronic health record (EHR) and/or an IIS. For additional information on barcoding and vaccines, see http://www.cdc.gov/vaccines/programs/iis/2d-vaccine-barcodes/index.html.

Strategies to Prevent Administration Errors

Vaccine administration errors can result in a patient receiving an ineffective immunization. This can leave the person vulnerable to infection. Vaccine administration errors may also diminish patient confidence in their healthcare providers. Common vaccine administration errors include:

- Doses administered too early (before the minimum age or interval has been met)

- Wrong vaccine (e.g., Tdap instead of DTaP)

- Wrong dosage (e.g., pediatric formulation of hepatitis B vaccine administered to an adult)

- Wrong route

- Vaccine administered outside the approved age range

- Expired vaccine or diluent administered

- Vaccine which was not stored properly administered

- Vaccine administered to a patient with a contraindication for that vaccine

- Wrong diluent used to reconstitute the vaccine or only the diluent was administered

In addition to strict adherence to the "Rights of Medication Administration" and ongoing training and education of staff, there are other strategies that can be implemented to help prevent administration errors.

When possible, involve staff in the selection of vaccine products to be used in your facility. Different brands of the same vaccine can have different schedules, age indications, or other indications. Stocking multiple brands may lead to staff confusion and vaccine administration errors.

Use standardized abbreviations to avoid confusion about which vaccines have been administered. See ACIP *Abbreviations for Vaccines* at http://www.cdc.gov/vaccines/acip/committee/guidance/vac-abbrev.html.

Keep current reference materials available for staff on each vaccine used in your facility. Keep reference sheets for timing and spacing, recommended sites, routes, and needle lengths posted for easy reference in your medication preparation area. For additional information, see clinic resources for administering vaccines at http://www.immunize.org/handouts/administering-vaccines.asp.

Rotate vaccines so that those with the shortest expiration dates are in the front of the storage unit. Use these first and frequently check the storage unit to remove any expired vaccine.

Consider the potential for product mix-ups when storing vaccines. Do not store sound-alike and look-alike vaccines next to each other (e.g., DTaP and Tdap). Consider color coding labels on vaccine storage containers and/or including the vaccine type, age indications, and gender if applicable. Store the pediatric and adult vaccines on separate shelves in the storage unit. See Vaccine Label Examples at http://www.cdc.gov/vaccines/recs/storage/guide/vaccine-storage-labels.pdf.

Administer only vaccines that you have prepared for administration. Triple check your work before you administer a vaccine and ask other staff to do the same.

Avoid interruptions when selecting and preparing the appropriate vaccine(s) for administration.

Consider using standing orders if appropriate for your facility. Standing orders provide protocols for administering vaccines in a consistent, systematic format. For standing order templates, see Standing Orders for Administering Vaccines at http://www.immunize.org/standing-orders/.

Counsel parents and patients about vaccines to be administered and on how important it is for them to maintain immunization records on all family members. Educated clients may notice a potential error and help prevent it.

Establish an environment that values the reporting and investigation of errors as part of risk management and quality improvement. Promote a "just culture" where staff is

Strategies to Prevent Errors

- Establish an environment that values reporting and investigating errors as part of risk management and quality improvement

- Promote a "just culture" where staff is willing to report errors trusting that the situation and those involved will be treated fairly

- Error reporting should provide opportunities to discover how errors occur and to share ideas to prevent or reduce those errors without fear of punishment and ridicule

6

Vaccine Administration

willing to report errors trusting that the situation and those involved will be treated fairly. Error reporting should provide opportunities to discover how the errors occur and to share ideas to prevent or reduce those errors in the future without fear of punishment and ridicule.

Vaccine Adverse Event Reporting System (VAERS)

The Vaccine Adverse Event Reporting System (VAERS) accepts all reports of adverse events occurring with vaccinations, including reports of vaccination errors. VAERS is primarily concerned with monitoring adverse health events and encourages reporting of clinically significant adverse health events following vaccination. Using clinical judgment, healthcare professionals can decide whether or not to report a medical error at their own discretion. For example, a healthcare professional may elect to report vaccination errors that do not have an associated adverse health event, especially if they think the vaccination error may pose a safety risk (e.g., administering a live vaccine to an immunocompromised patient) or that the error would be preventable with public health action or education.

Acknowledgement

The editors thank JoEllen Wolicki, Dr. Cindy Weinbaum, and Donna Weaver, CDC, for their contribution to this chapter.

Selected References and Resources

Centers for Disease Control and Prevention (CDC). General recommendations on immunization: recommendations of the Advisory Committee on Immunization Practices. *MMWR* 2011;60(no. RR-2): 23-27, http://www.cdc.gov/mmwr/pdf/rr/rr6002.pdf

Centers for Disease Control and Prevention (CDC). Injection Practices: Information for Providers: http://www.cdc.gov/injectionsafety/providers.html

Centers for Disease Control and Prevention (CDC). Recommendations and Guidelines: Vaccine Administration: http://www.cdc.gov/vaccines/recs/vac-admin/default.htm

Cohen, Michael R. *Medication Errors*, 2nd ed. Washington, D.C.: American Pharmacists Assoc.; 2007.

Harrington JW, Logan SJ, Harwell C, et al. Effective analgesia using physical interventions for infant immunizations. *Pediatrics* 2012;129: 815-21.

VAERS

- VAERS accepts all reports, including reports of vaccination errors

- VAERS is primarily concerned with monitoring adverse health events and encourages reporting of clinically significant adverse health events following vaccination

- Healthcare professionals can decide whether or not to report a medical error at their own discretion

  - if they think the vaccination error may pose a safety risk (e.g., administering a live vaccine to an immunocompromised patient)

  - the error would be preventable with public health action or education

Immunization Action Coalition (IAC). Various resources on vaccine administration http://www.immunize.org/clinic/administering-vaccines.asp

Ipp M, Taddio A, Sam J, et al. Vaccine-related pain: randomized controlled trial of two injection techniques. *Arch Dis Child* 2007;92: 1105-08.

Reis EC, Roth EK, Syphan JL, et al. Effective pain reduction for multiple immunization injections in young infants. *Arch Pediatr Adolesc Med* 2003;157: 115-1120.

Smith, SF, Duell DJ, and Martin, BC. *Clinical Nursing Skills: Basic to Advanced Skills*, 8th ed. Saddle River, NJ: Pearson Education, Inc.; 2012.

Taddio A, Appleton M, Bortolussi R, et al. Reducing the pain childhood vaccination: an evidence-based clinical practice guideline. *Can Med Assc Journal* 2010;182:E843-E855.

Taddio A, Ilersich AL, Ipp M, et al. Physical interventions and injection techniques for reducing injection pain during routine childhood immunizations systematic review of randomized controlled trials and quasi-randomized controlled trials. *Clinical Therapeutics* Supplement B 2009;31: S48-S76.

Taddio A, Chambers C, Halperin S, et al. Inadequate pain management during routine childhood immunizations: the nerve of it. *Clinical Therapeutics* Supplement B 2009;31: S152-S167.

6

Vaccine Administration

Diphtheria is an acute, toxin-mediated disease caused by the bacterium *Corynebacterium diphtheriae*. The name of the disease is derived from the Greek diphthera, meaning leather hide. The disease was described in the 5th century BCE by Hippocrates, and epidemics were described in the 6th century AD by Aetius. The bacterium was first observed in diphtheritic membranes by Klebs in 1883 and cultivated by Löffler in 1884. Antitoxin was invented in the late 19th century, and toxoid was developed in the 1920s.

Corynebacterium diphtheriae

C. diphtheriae is an aerobic gram-positive bacillus. Toxin production (toxigenicity) occurs only when the bacillus is itself infected (lysogenized) by a specific virus (bacteriophage) carrying the genetic information for the toxin (tox gene). Only toxigenic strains can cause severe disease.

Culture of the organism requires selective media containing tellurite. If isolated, the organism must be distinguished in the laboratory from other *Corynebacterium* species that normally inhabit the nasopharynx and skin (e.g., diphtheroids).

C. diphtheriae has four biotypes—gravis, intermedius, mitis and belfanti. All strains may produce toxin and can cause severe disease. All isolates of *C. diphtheriae* should be tested for toxigenicity.

Pathogenesis

Susceptible persons may acquire toxigenic diphtheria bacilli in the nasopharynx. The organism produces a toxin that inhibits cellular protein synthesis and is responsible for local tissue destruction and pseudomembrane formation. The toxin produced at the site of the membrane is absorbed into the bloodstream and then distributed to the tissues of the body. The toxin is responsible for the major complications of myocarditis and neuritis and can also cause low platelet counts (thrombocytopenia) and protein in the urine (proteinuria).

Non-toxin producing strains may cause mild to moderate pharyngitis but are not associated with formation of a pseudomembrane. While rare severe cases have been reported, these may actually have been caused by toxigenic strains that were not detected because of inadequate culture sampling.

7

Diphtheria

- Greek *diphthera* (leather hide)
- Recognized by Hippocrates in 5th century BCE
- Epidemics described in 6th century
- *C. diphtheriae* described by Klebs in 1883
- Toxoid developed in 1920s

Corynebacterium diphtheria

- Aerobic gram-positive bacillus
- Toxin production occurs only when *C. diphtheriae* infected by virus (phage) carrying tox gene
- If isolated, must be distinguished from normal diphtheroid

Diphtheria

Clinical Features

The incubation period of diphtheria is 2–5 days (range, 1–10 days).

Disease can involve almost any mucous membrane. For clinical purposes, it is convenient to classify diphtheria into a number of manifestations, depending on the anatomic site of disease.

Anterior Nasal Diphtheria

The onset of anterior nasal diphtheria is indistinguishable from that of the common cold and is usually characterized by a mucopurulent nasal discharge (containing both mucus and pus) which may become blood-tinged. A white membrane usually forms on the nasal septum. The disease is usually fairly mild because of apparent poor systemic absorption of toxin in this location, and it can be terminated rapidly by diphtheria antitoxin and antibiotic therapy.

Pharyngeal and Tonsillar Diphtheria

The most common sites of diphtheria infection are the pharynx and the tonsils. Infection at these sites is usually associated with substantial systemic absorption of toxin. The onset of pharyngitis is insidious. Early symptoms include malaise, sore throat, anorexia, and low-grade fever (<101°F). Within 2–3 days, a bluish-white membrane forms and extends, varying in size from covering a small patch on the tonsils to covering most of the soft palate. Often by the time a physician is contacted, the membrane is greyish-green, or black if bleeding has occurred. There is a minimal amount of mucosal erythema surrounding the membrane. The pseudomembrane is firmly adherent to the tissue, and forcible attempts to remove it cause bleeding. Extensive pseudomembrane formation may result in respiratory obstruction.

While some patients may recover at this point without treatment, others may develop severe disease. Fever is usually not high, even though the patient may appear quite toxic. Patients with severe disease may develop marked edema of the submandibular areas and the anterior neck along with lymphadenopathy, giving a characteristic "bullneck" appearance. If enough toxin is absorbed, the patient may develop severe prostration, striking pallor, rapid pulse, stupor, and coma, and may even die within 6 to 10 days.

Laryngeal Diphtheria

Laryngeal diphtheria can be either an extension of the pharyngeal form or can involve only this site. Symptoms include fever, hoarseness, and a barking cough. The membrane can lead to airway obstruction, coma, and death.

Cutaneous (Skin) Diphtheria

In the United States, cutaneous diphtheria has been most often associated with homeless persons. Skin infections are quite common in the tropics and are probably responsible for the high levels of natural immunity found in these populations. Skin infections may be manifested by a scaling rash or by ulcers with clearly demarcated edges and membrane, but any chronic skin lesion may harbor *C. diphtheriae* along with other organisms. Generally, the organisms isolated from cases in the United States were nontoxigenic. The severity of the skin disease with toxigenic strains appears to be less than from other sites. Cutaneous diphtheria is no longer reported to the National Notifiable Diseases Surveillance System in the United States.

Rarely, other sites of involvement include the mucous membranes of the conjunctiva and vulvovaginal area, as well as the external auditory canal.

Complications

Most complications of diphtheria, including death, are attributable to effects of the toxin. The severity of the disease and complications are generally related to the extent of local disease. The toxin, when absorbed, affects organs and tissues distant from the site of invasion. The most frequent complications of diphtheria are myocarditis and neuritis.

Myocarditis may present as abnormal cardiac rhythms and can occur early in the course of the illness or weeks later, and can lead to heart failure. If myocarditis occurs early, it is often fatal.

Neuritis most often affects motor nerves and usually resolves completely. Paralysis of the soft palate is most frequent during the third week of illness. Paralysis of eye muscles, limbs, and diaphragm can occur after the fifth week. Secondary pneumonia and respiratory failure may result from diaphragmatic paralysis.

Other complications include otitis media and respiratory insufficiency due to airway obstruction, especially in infants.

Death

The overall case-fatality rate for diphtheria is 5%–10%, with higher death rates (up to 20%) among persons younger than 5 and older than 40 years of age. The case-fatality rate for diphtheria has changed very little during the last 50 years.

Diphtheria Complications
- Most attributable to toxin
- Severity generally related to extent of local disease
- Most frequent complications are myocarditis and neuritis
- Death occurs in 5%-10%

Diphtheria

Laboratory Diagnosis

Diagnosis of diphtheria is usually made on the basis of clinical presentation since it is imperative to begin presumptive therapy quickly.

Culture of the lesion is done to confirm the diagnosis. It is critical to take a swab of the pharyngeal area, especially any discolored areas, ulcerations, and tonsillar crypts. Culture medium containing tellurite is preferred because it provides a selective advantage for the growth of this organism. If diphtheria bacilli are isolated, they must be tested for toxin production.

A blood agar plate is also inoculated for detection of hemolytic streptococcus. Gram stain and Kenyon stain of material from the membrane itself can be helpful when trying to confirm the clinical diagnosis. The Gram stain may show multiple club-shaped forms that look like Chinese characters. Other *Corynebacterium* species (diphtheroids) that can normally inhabit the throat may confuse the interpretation of direct stain. However, treatment should be started if clinical diphtheria is suggested, even in the absence of a Gram stain.

In the event that prior antibiotic therapy may have impeded a positive culture in a suspect diphtheria case, three sources of evidence can aid in presumptive diagnosis: 1) a positive polymerase chain reaction test for diphtheria tox genes, or 2) isolation of *C. diphtheriae* from cultures of specimens from close contacts, or 3) a low nonprotective diphtheria antibody titer (less than 0.1 IU) in serum obtained prior to antitoxin administration. This is done by commercial laboratories and requires several days. To isolate *C. diphtheriae* from carriers, it is best to inoculate a Löffler or Pai slant with the throat swab. After an incubation period of 18–24 hours, growth from the slant is used to inoculate a medium containing tellurite.

Medical Management
Diphtheria Antitoxin

Diphtheria antitoxin, produced in horses, was used for treatment of diphtheria in the United States since the 1890s. It is not indicated for prophylaxis of contacts of diphtheria patients. Since 1997, diphtheria antitoxin has been available only from CDC, through an Investigational New Drug (IND) protocol. Diphtheria antitoxin does not neutralize toxin that is already fixed to tissues, but it will neutralize circulating (unbound) toxin and prevent progression of disease. The patient must be tested for sensitivity before antitoxin is given. Consultation on the use of diphtheria antitoxin is available through the duty officer at the CDC through CDC's Emergency Operations Center at 770-488-7100.

Diphtheria Antitoxin

- Produced in horses
- First used in the U.S. in the 1890s
- Used only for treatment of diphtheria
- Neutralizes only unbound toxin

After a provisional clinical diagnosis is made, appropriate specimens should be obtained for culture and the patient placed in isolation. Persons with suspected diphtheria should be given diphtheria antitoxin and antibiotics in adequate dosage. Respiratory support and airway maintenance should also be administered as needed.

Antibiotics

Treatment with erythromycin orally or by injection (40 mg/kg/day; maximum, 2 gm/day) for 14 days, or procaine penicillin G daily, intramuscularly (300,000 U/day for those weighing 10 kg or less, and 600,000 U/day for those weighing more than 10 kg) for 14 days. The disease is usually not contagious 48 hours after antibiotics are instituted. Elimination of the organism should be documented by two consecutive negative cultures after therapy is completed.

Preventive Measures

For close contacts, especially household contacts, a diphtheria booster, appropriate for age, should be given. Contacts should also receive antibiotics—benzathine penicillin G (600,000 units for persons younger than 6 years old and 1,200,000 units for those 6 years old and older) or a 7- to 10-day course of oral erythromycin (40 mg/kg/day for children and 1 g/day for adults). For compliance reasons, if surveillance of contacts cannot be maintained, they should receive benzathine penicillin G. Identified carriers in the community should also receive antibiotics. Maintain close surveillance and begin antitoxin at the first signs of illness.

Contacts of cutaneous diphtheria should be treated as described above; however, if the strain is shown to be nontoxigenic, investigation of contacts should be discontinued.

Epidemiology
Occurrence

Diphtheria occurs worldwide, particularly in tropical countries. Diphtheria is a rare disease in industrialized countries including the United States. In the United States during the pre-vaccine era, the highest incidence was in the Southeast during the winter.

Reservoir

Human carriers are the reservoir for C. *diphtheriae* and are usually asymptomatic. In outbreaks, high percentages of children are found to be transient carriers.

Diphtheria Epidemiology
- Reservoir
  - human carriers
  - usually asymptomatic
- Transmission
  - respiratory
  - skin and fomites rarely
- Temporal pattern
  - winter and spring
- Communicability
  - without antibiotics, seldom more than 4 weeks

Diphtheria

Transmission

Transmission is most often person-to-person spread from the respiratory tract. Rarely, transmission may occur from skin lesions or articles soiled with discharges from lesions of infected persons (fomites).

Temporal Pattern

In temperate areas, diphtheria most frequently occurs during winter and spring.

Communicability

Transmission may occur as long as virulent bacilli are present in discharges and lesions. The time is variable, but without antibiotics, organisms usually persist 2 weeks or less and seldom more than 4 weeks. Chronic carriers may shed organisms for 6 months or more. Effective antibiotic therapy promptly terminates shedding.

Secular Trends in the United States

Globally, diphtheria was once a major cause of morbidity and mortality among children. In England and Wales during the 1930s, diphtheria was among the top three causes of death for children younger than 15 years of age. During the 1920s in the United States, 100,000–200,000 cases of diphtheria (140–150 cases per 100,000 population) and 13,000–15,000 deaths were reported each year. In 1921, a total of 206,000 cases and 15,520 deaths were reported. The number of cases gradually declined to about 19,000 in 1945 (15 per 100,000 population). A more rapid decrease began with the widespread use of diphtheria toxoid in the late 1940s.

From 1970 through 1979, an average of 196 cases per year were reported. This included a high proportion of cutaneous cases from an outbreak in Washington State. Beginning in 1980, all cutaneous cases were excluded from reporting. Diphtheria was seen most frequently in Native Americans and persons in lower socioeconomic strata.

From 1980 through 2011, 55 cases of diphtheria were reported in the United States, an average of 1 or 2 per year (range, 0–5 cases per year). Only 5 cases have been reported since 2000.

Of 53 reported cases with known patient age since 1980, 34 (64%) were in persons 20 years of age or older; 41% of cases were among persons 40 years of age or older. Most cases have occurred in unimmunized or inadequately immunized persons. The current age distribution of cases corroborates the finding of inadequate levels of circulating antitoxin in many adults (up to 60% with less than protective levels).

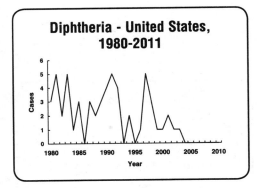

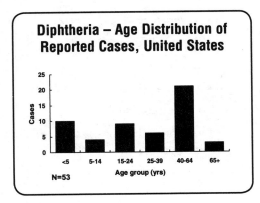

Although diphtheria disease is rare in the United States, it appears that toxigenic *Corynebacterium diphtheriae* continues to circulate in areas of the country with previously endemic diphtheria. In 1996, 8 isolates of toxigenic *C. diphtheriae* were obtained from persons in a Native American community in South Dakota. None of the infected persons had classic diphtheria disease, although five had either pharyngitis or tonsillitis. The presence of toxigenic *C. diphtheriae* in this community is a good reminder for providers not to let down their guard against this organism.

Diphtheria continues to occur in other parts of the world. A major epidemic of diphtheria occurred in countries of the former Soviet Union beginning in 1990. By 1994, the epidemic had affected all 15 Newly Independent States (NIS). More than 157,000 cases and more than 5,000 deaths were reported. In the 6 years from 1990 through 1995, the NIS accounted for more than 90% of all diphtheria cases reported to the World Health Organization (WHO) from the entire world. In some NIS countries, up to 80% of the epidemic diphtheria cases have been among adults. The outbreak and the age distribution of cases are believed to be due to several factors, including a lack of routine immunization of adults in these countries. Globally, reported cases of diphtheria have declined from 11,625 in 2000 to 4,880 cases in 2011.

Diphtheria Toxoid
Characteristics

Beginning in the early 1900s, prophylaxis was attempted with toxin–antitoxin mixtures. Toxoid was developed around 1921 but was not widely used until the early 1930s. It was incorporated with tetanus toxoid and pertussis vaccine and became routinely used in the 1940s.

Diphtheria toxoid is produced by growing toxigenic *C. diphtheriae* in liquid medium. The filtrate is incubated with formaldehyde to convert toxin to toxoid and is then adsorbed onto an aluminum salt.

Single-antigen diphtheria toxoid is not available. Diphtheria toxoid is combined with tetanus toxoid as pediatric diphtheria-tetanus toxoid (DT) or adult tetanus-diphtheria (Td), and with both tetanus toxoid and acellular pertussis vaccine as DTaP and Tdap. Diphtheria toxoid is also available as combined DTaP-HepB-IPV (Pediarix) and DTaP-IPV/Hib (Pentacel)—see Pertussis chapter for more information. Pediatric formulations (DT and DTaP) contain a similar amount of tetanus toxoid as adult Td, but contain 3 to 4 times as much diphtheria toxoid. Children younger than 7 years of age should receive either DTaP or pediatric DT. Persons 7 years of age or older should receive the adult

7

Diphtheria Toxoid

- Converted from toxin to toxoid
- Schedule
  - 3 or 4 doses plus booster
  - booster every 10 years
- Efficacy
  - approximately 95%
- Duration
  - approximately 10 years
- Should be administered with tetanus toxoid as DTaP, DT, Td, or Tdap

Diphtheria

Routine DTaP Primary Vaccination Schedule

Dose	Age	Interval
Primary 1	2 months	---
Primary 2	4 months	4 weeks
Primary 3	6 months	4 weeks
Primary 4	15-18 months	6 months

Children Who Receive DT

- The number of doses of DT needed to complete the series depends on the child's age at the first dose:

  - if first dose given at younger than 12 months of age, 4 doses are recommended

  - if first dose given at 12 months or older, 3 doses complete the primary series

Tetanus, Diphtheria and Pertussis Booster Doses

- 4 through 6 years of age, before entering school (DTaP)

- 11 or 12 years of age (Tdap)

- Every 10 years thereafter (Td)

Routine Td Schedule for Unvaccinated Persons 7 Years of Age and Older

Dose*	Interval
Primary 1	---
Primary 2	4 weeks
Primary 3	6 to 12 months

Booster dose every 10 years

*ACIP recommends that one of these doses (preferably the first) be administered as Tdap

formulation (adult Td), even if they have not completed a series of DTaP or pediatric DT. Two brands of Tdap are available—Boostrix (approved for persons 10 years of age or older) and Adacel (approved for persons 10 through 64 years of age). DTaP and Tdap vaccines do not contain thimerosal as a preservative.

Immunogenicity and Vaccine Efficacy

After a primary series of three properly spaced diphtheria toxoid doses in adults or four doses in infants, a protective level of antitoxin (defined as greater than 0.1 IU of antitoxin/mL) is reached in more than 95%. Diphtheria toxoid has been estimated to have a clinical efficacy of 97%.

Vaccination Schedule and Use

DTaP (diphtheria and tetanus toxoids and acellular pertussis vaccine) is the vaccine of choice for children 6 weeks through 6 years of age. The usual schedule is a primary series of 4 doses at 2, 4, 6, and 15–18 months of age. The first, second, and third doses of DTaP should be separated by a minimum of 4 weeks. The fourth dose should follow the third dose by no less than 6 months, and should not be administered before 12 months of age.

If a child has a valid contraindication to pertussis vaccine, pediatric DT should be used to complete the vaccination series. If the child was younger than 12 months old when the first dose of DT was administered (as DTP, DTaP, or DT), the child should receive a total of four primary DT doses. If the child was 12 months of age or older at the time the first dose of DT was administered, three doses (third dose 6–12 months after the second) complete the primary DT series.

If the fourth dose of DT, DTP or DTaP is administered before the fourth birthday, a booster (fifth) dose is recommended at 4 through 6 years of age. The fifth dose is not required if the fourth dose was given on or after the fourth birthday.

Vaccines containing reduced diphtheria (i.e., Td and Tdap) are indicated for children 7 years and older and for adults. A primary series is three or four doses, depending on whether the person has received prior doses of diphtheria-containing vaccine, and the age these doses were administered. The number of doses recommended for children who received one or more doses of DTP, DTaP, or DT before age 7 years is discussed above. For unvaccinated persons 7 years and older (including persons who cannot document prior vaccination), the primary series is three doses. The first two doses should be separated by at least 4 weeks, and the third dose given 6 to 12 months after the second. ACIP recommends that one of these doses (preferably the first) be administered as Tdap.

A booster dose of Td should be given every 10 years. Persons who have never received Tdap should be given a dose of Tdap as one of these boosters. Refer to the pertussis chapter for more information about Tdap.

Interruption of the recommended schedule or delay of subsequent doses does not reduce the response to the vaccine when the series is finally completed. There is no need to restart a series regardless of the time elapsed between doses.

Diphtheria disease might not confer immunity. Persons recovering from diphtheria should begin or complete active immunization with diphtheria toxoid during convalescence.

Contraindications and Precautions to Vaccination

Persons with a history of a severe allergic reaction (anaphylaxis) to a vaccine component or following a prior dose should not receive additional doses of diphtheria toxoid. Diphtheria toxoid should be deferred for those persons who have moderate or severe acute illness, but persons with minor illness may be vaccinated. Immunosuppression and pregnancy are not contraindications to receiving diphtheria toxoid. See pertussis chapter for additional information on contraindications and precautions to Tdap.

Adverse Events Following Vaccination

Rarely, severe systemic adverse events, such as generalized urticaria, anaphylaxis, or neurologic complications have been reported following administration of diphtheria toxoid.

Adverse Reactions Following Vaccination

Local reactions, generally erythema and induration with or without tenderness, are common after the administration of vaccines containing diphtheria toxoid. Local reactions are usually self-limited and require no therapy. A nodule may be palpable at the injection site for several weeks. Abscess at the site of injection has been reported. Fever and other systemic symptoms are not common.

Exaggerated local (Arthus-type) reactions are occasionally reported following receipt of a diphtheria- or tetanus-containing vaccine. These reactions present as extensive painful swelling, often from shoulder to elbow. They generally begin 2–8 hours after injections and are reported most often in adults, particularly those who have received frequent doses of diphtheria or tetanus toxoid. Persons experiencing these severe reactions usually have very high

Diphtheria and Tetanus Toxoids Contraindications and Precautions

- Severe allergic reaction to vaccine component or following a prior dose

- Moderate or severe acute illness

Diphtheria and Tetanus Toxoids Adverse Events

- Reports of severe systemic adverse events (urticaria, anophylaxis, neurologic complications) are rare

Diphtheria and Tetanus Toxoids Adverse Reactions

- Local reactions (erythema, induration) are common

- Fever and systemic symptoms not common

- Exaggerated local reactions (Arthus-type) occasionally reported

7

serum antitoxin levels; they should not be given further routine or emergency booster doses of Td more frequently than every 10 years. Less severe local reactions may occur in persons who have multiple prior boosters.

Vaccine Storage and Handling

All diptheria-toxoid containing vaccines should be maintained at refrigerator temperature between 35°F and 46°F (2°C and 8°C). Manufacturer package inserts contain additional information and can be found at http://www.fda.gov/BiologicsBloodVaccines/Vaccines/ApprovedProducts/ucm093830.htm. For complete information on best practices and recommendations please refer to CDC's Vaccine Storage and Handling Toolkit, http://www.cdc.gov/vaccines/recs/storage/toolkit/storage-handling-toolkit.pdf.

Suspect Case Investigation and Control

Immediate action on all highly suspect cases is warranted until they are shown not to be caused by toxigenic C. diphtheriae. The following action should also be taken for any toxigenic C. diphtheriae carriers who are detected.

1. Contact state health department or CDC.

2. Obtain appropriate cultures and preliminary clinical and epidemiologic information (including vaccine history).

3. Begin early presumptive treatment with antitoxin and antibiotics. Impose strict isolation until at least two cultures are negative 24 hours after antibiotics were discontinued.

4. Identify close contacts, especially household members and other persons directly exposed to oral secretions of the patient. Culture all close contacts, regardless of their immunization status. Ideally, culture should be from both throat and nasal swabs. After culture, all contacts should receive antibiotic prophylaxis. Inadequately immunized contacts should receive DTaP/DT/Td/Tdap boosters. If fewer than three doses of diphtheria toxoid have been given, or vaccination history is unknown, an immediate dose of diphtheria toxoid should be given and the primary series completed according to the current schedule. If more than 5 years have elapsed since administration of diphtheria toxoid-containing vaccine, a booster dose should be given. If the most recent dose was within 5 years, no booster is required (see the ACIP's 1991 Diphtheria, Tetanus, and Pertussis: Recommendations for Vaccine Use and Other Preventive Measures for

schedule for children younger than 7 years of age). Unimmunized contacts should start a course of DTaP/DT/Td vaccine and be monitored closely for symptoms of diphtheria for 7 days.

5. Treat any confirmed carrier with an adequate course of antibiotic, and repeat cultures at a minimum of 2 weeks to ensure eradication of the organism. Persons who continue to harbor the organism after treatment with either penicillin or erythromycin should receive an additional 10-day course of erythromycin and should submit samples for follow-up cultures.

6. Treat any contact with antitoxin at the first sign of illness.

Acknowledgment

The editors thank Dr. Cindy Weinbaum, CDC for her assistance in updating this chapter.

Selected References

CDC. Diphtheria, tetanus, and pertussis: Recommendations for vaccine use and other preventive measures: recommendations of the Immunization Practices Advisory Committee (ACIP). MMWR 1991;40(No. RR-10):1-28.

CDC. Pertussis vaccination: use of acellular pertussis vaccines among infants and young children. Recommendations of the Advisory Committee on Immunization Practices (ACIP). *MMWR* 1997;46 (No. RR-7):1–25.

CDC. Preventing tetanus, diphtheria, and pertussis among adolescents: use of tetanus toxoid, reduced diphtheria toxoid and acellular pertussis vaccines. Recommendations of the Advisory Committee on Immunization Practices (ACIP). *MMWR* 2006;55(No. RR-3):1–34.

CDC. Preventing tetanus, diphtheria, and pertussis among adults: use of tetanus toxoid, reduced diphtheria toxoid and acellular pertussis vaccines. Recommendations of the Advisory Committee on Immunization Practices (ACIP) and Recommendation of ACIP, supported by the Healthcare Infection Control Practices Advisory Committee (HICPAC), for Use of Tdap Among Health-Care Personnel. *MMWR* 2006;55(No. RR-17):1–33.

Farizo KM, Strebel PM, Chen RT, Kimbler A, Cleary TJ, Cochi SL. Fatal respiratory disease due to *Corynebacterium diphtheriae*: case report and review of guidelines for management, investigation, and control. *Clin Infect Dis* 1993;16:59–68.

7

Diphtheria

Vitek CR, Wharton M. Diphtheria in the former Soviet Union: reemergence of a pandemic disease. *Emerg Infect Dis* 1998;4:539–50.

Vitek CR, Wharton M, Diphtheria toxoid. In Plotkin SA, Orenstein WA, Offit, PA, eds. Vaccines. 5th ed. China: Saunders, 2008:139-56.

7

Haemophilus influenzae is a cause of bacterial infections that are often severe, particularly among infants. It was first described by Pfeiffer in 1892. During an outbreak of influenza he found the bacteria in sputum of patients and proposed a causal association between this bacterium and the clinical syndrome known as influenza. The organism was given the name *Haemophilus* by Winslow, et al. in 1920. It was not until 1933 that Smith, et al. established that influenza was caused by a virus and that *H. influenzae* was a cause of secondary infection.

In the 1930s, Margaret Pittman demonstrated that *H. influenzae* could be isolated in encapsulated and unencapsulated forms. She identified six capsular types (a–f), and observed that virtually all isolates from cerebrospinal fluid (CSF) and blood were of the capsular type b.

Before the introduction of effective vaccines, *H. influenzae* type b (Hib) was the leading cause of bacterial meningitis and other invasive bacterial disease among children younger than 5 years of age; approximately one in 200 children in this age group developed invasive Hib disease. Nearly all Hib infections occurred among children younger than 5 years of age, and approximately two-thirds of all cases occurred among children younger than 18 months of age.

Haemophilus influenzae

Haemophilus influenzae is a gram-negative coccobacillus. It is generally aerobic but can grow as a facultative anaerobe. In vitro growth requires accessory growth factors, including "X" factor (hemin) and "V" factor (nicotinamide adenine dinucleotide [NAD]).

Chocolate agar media are used for isolation. *H. influenzae* will generally not grow on blood agar, which lacks NAD.

H. influenzae has encapsulated (typeable) and unencapsulated nontypeable strains. The outermost structure of encapsulated *H. influenzae* is composed of polyribosyl-ribitol-phosphate (PRP), a polysaccharide that is responsible for virulence and immunity. Six antigenically and biochemically distinct capsular polysaccharide serotypes have been described; these are designated types a through f. There are currently no vaccines to prevent disease caused by non-b encapsulated or nontypeable strains. In the prevaccine era, type b organisms accounted for 95% of all strains that caused invasive disease.

8

> ### *Haemophilus influenzae* type b
> - Severe bacterial infection, particularly among infants
> - During late 19th century believed to cause influenza
> - Immunology and microbiology clarified in 1930s

> ### *Haemophilus influenzae*
> - Aerobic gram-negative bacteria
> - Polysaccharide capsule
> - Six different serotypes (a-f) of polysaccharide capsule
> - 95% of invasive disease caused by type b (prevaccine)

Haemophilus influenzae type B

Haemophilus influenzae type b Pathogenesis

- Organism colonizes nasopharynx

- In some persons organism invades bloodstream and causes infection at distant site

- Antecedent upper respiratory tract infection may be a contributing factor

Haemophilus influenzae type b 1986 Incidence* by Age Group

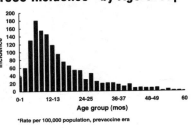

*Rate per 100,000 population, prevaccine era

Pathogenesis

The organism enters the body through the nasopharynx. Organisms colonize the nasopharynx and may remain only transiently or for several months in the absence of symptoms (asymptomatic carrier). In the prevaccine era, Hib could be isolated from the nasopharynx of 0.5%–3% of normal infants and children but was not common in adults. Nontypeable (unencapsulated) strains are also frequent inhabitants of the human respiratory tract.

In some persons, the organism causes an invasive infection. The exact mode of invasion to the bloodstream is unknown. Antecedent viral or mycoplasma infection of the upper respiratory tract may be a contributing factor. The bacteria spread in the bloodstream to distant sites in the body. Meninges are especially likely to be affected.

Incidence is strikingly age-dependent. In the prevaccine era, up to 60% of invasive disease occurred before age 12 months, with a peak occurrence among children 6–11 months of age. Passive protection of some infants is provided by transplacentally acquired maternal IgG antibodies and breastfeeding during the first 6 months of life. Children 60 months of age and older account for less than 10% of invasive disease. The presumed reason for this age distribution is the acquisition of immunity to Hib with increasing age.

Antibodies to Hib capsular polysaccharide are protective. The precise level of antibody required for protection against invasive disease is not clearly established. However, a titer of 1 µg/mL 3 weeks postvaccination correlated with protection in studies following vaccination with unconjugated purified polyribosyl-ribitol-phosphate (PRP) vaccine and suggested long-term protection from invasive disease.

Acquisition of both anticapsular and serum bactericidal antibody is inversely related to the age-specific incidence of Hib disease.

In the prevaccine era, most children acquired immunity by 5–6 years of age through asymptomatic infection by Hib bacteria. Since only a relatively small proportion of children carry Hib at any time, it has been postulated that exposure to organisms that share common antigenic structures with the capsule of Hib (so-called "cross-reacting organisms") may also stimulate the development of anticapsular antibodies against Hib. Natural exposure to Hib also induces antibodies to outer membrane proteins, lipopolysaccharides, and other antigens on the surface of the bacterium.

The genetic constitution of the host may also be important in susceptibility to infection with Hib. Risk for Hib disease has been associated with a number of genetic markers, but the mechanism of these associations is unknown. No single genetic relationship regulating susceptibility or immune responses to polysaccharide antigens has yet been convincingly demonstrated.

Clinical Features

Invasive disease caused by *H. influenzae* type b can affect many organ systems. The most common types of invasive disease are meningitis, epiglottitis, pneumonia, arthritis, and cellulitis.

Meningitis is infection of the membranes covering the brain and spinal cord and is the most common clinical manifestation of invasive Hib disease, accounting for 50%–65% of cases in the prevaccine era. Hallmarks of Hib meningitis are fever, decreased mental status, and stiff neck (these symptoms also occur with meningitis caused by other bacteria). Hearing impairment or other neurologic sequelae occur in 15%–30% of survivors. The case-fatality rate is 3%–6%, despite appropriate antimicrobial therapy.

Epiglottitis is an infection and swelling of the epiglottis, the tissue in the throat that covers and protects the larynx during swallowing. Epiglottitis may cause life-threatening airway obstruction.

Septic arthritis (joint infection), cellulitis (rapidly progressing skin infection which usually involves face, head, or neck), and pneumonia (which can be mild focal or severe empyema) are common manifestations of invasive disease. Osteomyelitis (bone infection) and pericarditis (infection of the sac covering the heart) are less common forms of invasive disease.

Otitis media and acute bronchitis due to *H. influenzae* are generally caused by nontypeable strains. Hib strains account for only 5%–10% of *H. influenzae* causing otitis media.

Non-type b encapsulated strains can cause invasive disease similar to type b infections. Nontypeable (unencapsulated) strains may cause invasive disease but are generally less virulent than encapsulated strains. Nontypeable strains are rare causes of serious infection among children but are a common cause of ear infections in children and bronchitis in adults.

Laboratory Diagnosis

A Gram stain of an infected body fluid may demonstrate small gram-negative coccobacilli suggestive of invasive *Haemophilus* disease. CSF, blood, pleural fluid, joint fluid,

Haemophilus influenzae type b Clinical Features*

- Epiglottitis 17%
- Meningitis 50%
- Pneumonia 15%
- Osteomyelitis 2%
- Arthritis 8%
- Cellulitis 6%
- Bacteremia 2%

*prevaccine era

Haemophilus influenzae type b Meningitis

- Accounted for approximately 50%-65% of cases in the prevaccine era
- Hearing impairment or neurologic sequelae in 15%-30%
- Case-fatality rate 3%-6% despite appropriate antimicrobial therapy

Haemophilus influenzae type B

and middle ear aspirates should be cultured on appropriate media. A positive culture for *H. influenzae* (Hi) establishes the diagnosis.

All isolates of *H. influenzae* should be serotyped. This is an extremely important laboratory procedure that should be performed on every isolate of *H. influenzae*, especially those obtained from children younger than 15 years of age. Two tests are available for serotyping Hi isolates: slide agglutination and serotype-specific real-time PCR. These tests determine whether an isolate is type b, which is the only type that is potentially vaccine preventable. Serotyping is usually done by either a state health department laboratory or a reference laboratory. State health departments with questions about serotyping should contact the CDC Meningitis and Vaccine-Preventable Diseases Branch Laboratory at 404-639-3158.

Detection of antigen or DNA may be used as an adjunct to culture, particularly in diagnosing *H. influenzae* infection in patients who have been partially treated with antimicrobial agents, in which case the organism may not be viable on culture. Slide agglutination is used to detect Hib capsular polysaccharide antigen in CSF, but a negative test does not exclude the diagnosis, and false-positive tests have been reported. Antigen testing of serum and urine is not recommended because of false positives. Furthermore, no slide agglutination assay is available to identify non-b Hi serotypes. Serotype-specific real-time PCR is currently available to detect the specific target gene of each *H. influenzae* serotype and can be used for detection of *H. influenzae* in blood, CSF, or other clinical specimens.

Medical Management

Hospitalization is generally required for invasive Hib disease. Antimicrobial therapy with an effective third-generation cephalosporin (cefotaxime or ceftriaxone), or chloramphenicol in combination with ampicillin should be begun immediately. The treatment course is usually 10 days. Ampicillin-resistant strains of Hib are now common throughout the United States. Children with life-threatening illness in which Hib may be the etiologic agent should not receive ampicillin alone as initial empiric therapy.

Haemophilus influenzae type b
Medical Management

- Hospitalization required
- Treatment with an effective 3rd generation cephalosporin, or chloramphenicol plus ampicillin
- Ampicillin-resistant strains now common throughout the United States

Epidemiology

Occurrence

Hib disease occurs worldwide.

Reservoir

Humans (asymptomatic carriers) are the only known reservoir. Hib does not survive in the environment on inanimate surfaces.

Transmission

The primary mode of Hib transmission is presumably by respiratory droplet spread, although firm evidence for this mechanism is lacking. Neonates can acquire infection by aspiration of amniotic fluid or contact with genital tract secretions during delivery.

Temporal Pattern

Several studies in the prevaccine era described a bimodal seasonal pattern in the United States, with one peak during September through December and a second peak during March through May. The reason for this bimodal pattern is not known.

Communicability

The contagious potential of invasive Hib disease is considered to be limited. However, certain circumstances, particularly close contact with a case-patient (e.g., household, child care, or institutional setting) can lead to outbreaks or direct secondary transmission of the disease.

Secular Trends in the United States

H. influenzae infections became nationally reportable in 1991. Serotype-specific reporting continues to be incomplete.

Before the availability of national reporting data, several areas conducted active surveillance for *H. influenzae* disease, which allowed estimates of disease nationwide. In the early 1980s, it was estimated that about 20,000 cases occurred annually in the United States, primarily among children younger than 5 years of age (40–50 cases per 100,000 population). The incidence of invasive Hib disease began to decline dramatically in the late 1980s, coincident with licensure of conjugate Hib vaccines, and has declined by more than 99% compared with the prevaccine era.

From 2003 through 2010, an average of 2,562 invasive *H. influenzae* infections per year were reported to CDC in all age groups (range 2,013–3,151 per year). Of these, an average of 398 (approximately 16%) per year were among children younger than 5 years of age. Serotype was known for 52%

Haemophilus influenzae type b Epidemiology

- Reservoir
  - human
    - asymptomatic carriers
- Transmission
  - neonates
    - aspiration of amniotic fluid
    - genital track secretions during delivery
    - respiratory droplets
- Temporal pattern
  - peaks in Sept-Dec and March-May
- Communicability
  - generally limited but higher in some circumstances

8

Incidence*of Invasive Hib Disease, 1990-2010

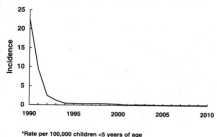

*Rate per 100,000 children <5 years of age

Haemophilus influenzae - United States, 2003-2010

- Average of 2,562 infections per year reported to CDC in all age groups
  - of these, 398 (16%) were children younger than 5 years

of the invasive cases in this age group. Two-hundred-two (average of 25 cases per year) were due to type b. In 2011, among children younger than 5 years of age, 14 cases of invasive disease due to Hib were reported in the United States. An additional 13 cases of Hib are estimated to have occurred among the 226 reports of invasive *H. influenzae* infections with an unknown serotype.

During 2010-2011, 33% of children younger than 5 years of age with confirmed invasive Hib disease were younger than 6 months of age and too young to have completed a three-dose primary vaccination series. Sixty-seven percent were age 6 months or older and were eligible to have completed the primary vaccination series. Of these age-eligible children, 64% were either unvaccinated, incompletely vaccinated (fewer than 3 doses), or their vaccination status was unknown. Thirty-six percent of children aged 6–59 months with confirmed type b disease had received three or more doses of Hib vaccine, including 5 who had received a booster dose 14 or more days before onset of their illness. The cause of Hib vaccine failure in these children is not known.

Risk factors for Hib disease include exposure factors and host factors that increase the likelihood of exposure to Hib. Exposure factors include household crowding, large household size, child care attendance, low socioeconomic status, low parental education levels, and school-aged siblings. Host factors include race/ethnicity (elevated risk among Hispanics and Native Americans—possibly confounded by socioeconomic variables that are associated with both race/ethnicity and Hib disease), chronic disease (e.g., sickle cell anemia, antibody deficiency syndromes, malignancies – especially during chemotherapy), and possibly gender (risk is higher for males).

Protective factors (effect limited to infants younger than 6 months of age) include breastfeeding and passively acquired maternal antibody.

Secondary Hib disease is defined as illness occurring 1–60 days following contact with an ill child, and accounts for less than 5% of all invasive Hib disease. Among household contacts, six studies have found a secondary attack rate of 0.3% in the month following onset of the index case, which is about 600-fold higher than the risk for the general population. Attack rates varied substantially with age, from 3.7% among children 2 years of age and younger to 0% among contacts 6 years of age and older. In these household contacts, 64% of secondary cases occurred within the first

8

Haemophilus influenzae type b
Risk Factors for Invasive Disease

- Exposure factors
  - household crowding
  - large household size
  - child care attendance
  - low socioeconomic status
  - low parental education
  - school-aged siblings
- Host factors
  - race/ethnicity
  - chronic disease
  - possibly gender (risk higher for males)

week (excluding the first 24 hours) of disease onset in the index patient, 20% during the second week, and 16% during the third and fourth weeks.

Data are conflicting regarding the risk of secondary transmission among child care contacts. Secondary attack rates have varied from 0% to as high as 2.7%. Most studies seem to suggest that child care contacts are at relatively low risk for secondary transmission of Hib disease particularly if contacts are age-appropriately vaccinated.

Haemophilus influenzae type b Vaccines
Characteristics

A pure polysaccharide vaccine (HbPV) was licensed in the United States in 1985. The vaccine was not effective in children younger than 18 months of age. Estimates of efficacy in older children varied widely, from 88% to -69% (a negative efficacy implies greater disease risk for vaccinees than nonvaccinees). HbPV was used until 1988 but is no longer available in the United States.

The characteristics of the Hib polysaccharide were similar to other polysaccharide vaccines (e.g., pneumococcal, meningococcal). The response to the vaccine was typical of a T-independent antigen, most notably an age-dependent immune response, and poor immunogenicity in children 2 years of age and younger. In addition, no boost in antibody titer was observed with repeated doses, the antibody that was produced was relatively low-affinity IgM, and switching to IgG production was minimal.

Haemophilus influenzae type b Polysaccharide-Protein Conjugate Vaccines

Conjugation is the process of chemically bonding a polysaccharide (a somewhat ineffective antigen) to a protein "carrier," which is a more effective antigen. This process changes the polysaccharide from a T-independent to a T-dependent antigen and greatly improves immunogenicity, particularly in young children. In addition, repeat doses of conjugate vaccines elicit booster responses and allow maturation of class-specific immunity with predominance of IgG antibody. The conjugates also cause carrier priming and elicit antibody to "useful" carrier protein.

The first Hib conjugate vaccine (PRP-D, ProHIBIT) was licensed in December 1987. PRP-D is no longer available in the United States.

Three monovalent conjugate Hib vaccines are currently licensed and available for use. Two (ActHIB and PedvaxHIB) are licensed for use in infants as young as 6 weeks of age.

Haemophilus influenzae type b Polysaccharide Vaccine
- Available 1985-1988
- Not effective in children younger than 18 months of age
- Efficacy in older children varied

Polysaccharide Vaccines
- Age-dependent immune response
- Not consistently immunogenic in children 2 years of age and younger
- No booster response

Polysaccharide Conjugate Vaccines
- Stimulates T-dependent immunity
- Enhanced antibody production, especially in young children
- Repeat doses elicit booster response

Haemophilus influenzae type B

A third Hib vaccine (Hiberix) is approved only for the booster dose of the Hib schedule among children 12 months and older. The vaccines utilize different carrier proteins. Three combination vaccines that contain Hib conjugate vaccine are also available.

Hib Conjugate Vaccines

PRP-T	ActHIB, Pentacel Hiberix (booster dose only) MenHibrix
PRP-OMP	PedvaxHIB, COMVAX

HbOC (HibTiter) no longer available in the United States

Immunogenicity and Vaccine Efficacy

Hib conjugate vaccines licensed for use in infants are highly immunogenic. More than 95% of infants will develop protective antibody levels after a primary series. Clinical efficacy has been estimated at 95% to 100%. Invasive Hib disease in a completely vaccinated infant is not common.

Hib vaccine is immunogenic in patients with increased risk for invasive disease, such as those with sickle-cell disease, leukemia, or human immunodeficiency virus (HIV) infection, and those who have had a splenectomy. However, in persons with HIV infection, immunogenicity varies with stage of infection and degree of immunocompromise. Efficacy studies have not been performed in populations with increased risk of invasive disease.

Vaccination Schedule and Use

All infants, including those born preterm, should receive a primary series of conjugate Hib vaccine (separate or in combination), beginning at 2 months of age. The number of doses in the primary series depends on the type of vaccine used. A primary series of PRP-OMP (PedvaxHIB or COMVAX) vaccine is two doses; PRP-T (ActHIB, Pentacel, or MenHibrix) requires a three-dose primary series (see table below). A booster is recommended at 12–15 months regardless of which vaccine is used for the primary series.

ACIP-Recommended *Haemophilus influenzae* type b (Hib) Routine Vaccine Schedule

Type	Vaccine	2 months	4 months	6 months	12-15 months
PRP-T	ActHIB	X (1st)	X (2nd)	X (3rd)	X
	Pentacel*	X (1st)	X (2nd)	X (3rd)	X
	Hiberix†	—	—	—	X
	MenHibrix§	X (1st)	X (2nd)	X (3rd)	X
PRP-OMP	PedvaxHIB	X (1st)	X (2nd)	—	X
	COMVAX	X (1st)	X (2nd)	—	X

* The recommended age for the 4th dose of Pentacel is 15-18 months, but it can be given as early as 12 months, provided at least 6 months have elapsed since the 3rd dose.

† Hiberix is approved only for the last dose of the Hib series among children 12 months of age and older. The recommended age is 15 months, but to facilitate timely booster vaccination it may be given as early as 12 months.

§ The recommended age for the 4th dose of MenHibrix is 12-18 months.

> ### *Haemophilus influenzae* type b (Hib) Vaccine
>
> - Recommended interval 8 weeks for primary series doses
> - Minimum interval 4 weeks for primary series doses
> - Vaccination at younger than 6 weeks of age may induce immunologic tolerance to subsequent doses of Hib vaccine
> - Minimum age 6 weeks

The recommended interval between primary series doses is 8 weeks, with a minimum interval of 4 weeks. At least 8 weeks should separate the booster dose from the previous (second or third) dose. Hib vaccines may be given simultaneously with all other vaccines.

Limited data suggest that Hib conjugate vaccines given before 6 weeks of age may induce immunologic tolerance to subsequent doses of Hib vaccine. A dose given before 6 weeks of age may reduce the response to subsequent doses. As a result, Hib vaccines, including combination vaccines that contain Hib conjugate, should never be given to a child younger than 6 weeks of age.

With the exception of Hiberix, the monovalent conjugate Hib vaccines licensed for use in infants are interchangeable. A series that includes vaccine of more than one type will induce a protective antibody level. If a child receives different brands of Hib vaccine at 2 and 4 months of age, a third dose of either brand should be administered at 6 months of age to complete the primary series. Either vaccine may be used for the booster dose, regardless of what was administered in the primary series.

Unvaccinated children 7 months of age and older may not require a full series of three or four doses. The number of doses a child needs to complete the series depends on the child's current age.

8

Haemophilus influenzae type B

Hib Vaccine Interchangeability

- Conjugate Hib vaccines licensed for the primary series* are interchangeable for primary series and booster dose

- 3 dose primary series if more than one brand of vaccine used

*ActHIB, Pedvax HIB, COMVAX, Pentacel, and MenHibrix

Unvaccinated Children 7 months of Age and Older

- Children starting late may not need entire 3 or 4 dose series

- Number of doses child requires depends on current age

Haemophilus influenzae type b Vaccine Detailed Schedule for Unvaccinated Children

Vaccine	Age at 1st Dose (months)	Primary series	Booster
PRP-T*	2-6	3 doses, 8 weeks apart	12-15 months
	7-11	2 doses, 4 weeks apart	12-15 months
	12-14	1 dose	2 months later
	15-59†	1 dose	--
PRP-OMP	2-6	2 doses, 8 weeks apart	12-15 months
	7-11	2 doses, 4 weeks apart	12-15 months
	12-14	1 dose	2 months later
	15-59	1 dose	--

*Hiberix brand PRP-T vaccine is approved only for the last dose of the Hib series among children 12 months of age and older.
† MenHibrix brand PRP-T vaccine is not recommended for children 19 months of age or older.

Monovalent Vaccines
PRP-T (ActHIB)

Previously unvaccinated infants aged 2 through 6 months should receive three doses of vaccine administered 2 months apart, followed by a booster dose at age 12–15 months, administered at least 2 months after the last dose. A booster dose at 12-15 months of age is only needed if 2 or 3 primary doses were administered before age 12 months. Unvaccinated children aged 7 through 11 months should receive two doses of vaccine 2 months apart, followed by a booster dose at age 12–15 months, administered at least 2 months after the last dose. Unvaccinated children aged 12 through 14 months should receive one dose of vaccine followed by a booster at least 2 months later. Any previously unvaccinated child aged 15 through 59 months should receive a single dose of vaccine. PRP-T (ActHIB) must be reconstituted only with the 0.4% sodium chloride ActHIB diluent. If ActHIB diluent is not available then the provider must contact the manufacturer (Sanofi Pasteur) to obtain it. Any dose of ActHIB reconstituted with a diluent other than specific ActHIB diluent should not be counted as valid and must be repeated.

PRP-OMP (PedvaxHIB)

Unvaccinated children aged 2 through 11 months should receive two doses of vaccine 2 months apart, followed by a booster dose at 12–15 months of age, at least 2 months after the last dose. Unvaccinated children aged 7 through 11 months should receive two doses of vaccine 2 months apart, followed by a booster dose at age 12–15 months, administered at least 2 months after the last dose. Unvaccinated children aged 12 through 14 months should receive one dose of vaccine followed by a booster at least 2 months later. Any previously unvaccinated child 15 through 59 months of age should receive a single dose of vaccine.

Vaccination of Older Children and Adults and Special Populations

Children with a lapsed Hib immunization series (i.e., children who have received one or more doses of Hib-containing vaccine but are not up-to-date for their age) may not need all the remaining doses of a three- or four-dose series. Vaccination of children with a lapsed schedule is addressed in the catch-up schedule, published annually with the childhood vaccination schedule.

Hib invasive disease does not always result in development of protective anti-PRP antibody levels. Children younger than 24 months of age who develop invasive Hib disease should be considered susceptible and should receive Hib vaccine. Vaccination of these children should start as soon as possible during the convalescent phase of the illness. A complete series as recommended for the child's age should be administered.

In general, Hib vaccination of persons older than 59 months of age is not recommended. The majority of older children are immune to Hib, probably from asymptomatic infection as infants. However, some older children and adults are at increased risk for invasive Hib disease and may be vaccinated if they were not vaccinated in childhood. These include those with functional or anatomic asplenia (e.g., sickle cell disease, postsplenectomy), immunodeficiency (in particular, persons with IgG2 subclass deficiency), early component complement deficiency, infection with HIV, and receipt of chemotherapy or radiation therapy for a malignant neoplasm. Patients undergoing elective splenectomy should receive one dose of Hib vaccine if unimmunized. Persons 15 months of age or older with functional or anatomic asplenia and HIV-infected children should receive at least one dose of Hib vaccine if unimmunized. Adults with HIV do not need a dose of Hib vaccine. Patients receiving hematopoietic cell transplants should receive 3 doses of Hib vaccine 1 month apart beginning 6-12 months post-transplant regardless of

---

Hib Vaccine Following Invasive Disease

- Children younger than 24 months may not develop protective antibody after invasive disease

- Vaccinate during convalescence

- Administer a complete series for age

8

Hib Vaccine Use in Older Children and Adults

- Generally not recommended for persons older than 59 months of age

- 3 doses recommended for all persons who have received a hematopoietic cell transplant

- See the ACIP Hib vaccine statement for further details about vaccination in high-risk groups older than 59 months of age

*MMWR 2014; 63(No. RR-1):8

prior Hib vaccine history. Readers should review the ACIP Hib vaccine statement for further details about vaccination in high-risk groups.

For American Indian/Alaska Natives (AI/AN), PRP-OMP is the preferred vaccine for the primary series doses. Hib meningitis incidence peaks at a younger age among AI/AN infants, and PRP-OMP vaccines produce a protective antibody response after the first dose and provide early protection that AI/AN infants particularly need.

Combination Vaccines

Three combination vaccines that contain *H. influenzae* type b are licensed and available in the United States–DTaP-IPV/Hib (Pentacel, Sanofi Pasteur), Hepatitis B–Hib (COMVAX, Merck), and Hib-MenCY (MenHibrix, GlaxoSmithKline). A fourth combination, TriHiBit, is no longer available in the U.S.

HepB-Hib-PRP-OMP (COMVAX)

COMVAX (Merck) is a combination hepatitis B–Hib vaccine. COMVAX is licensed for use when either or both antigens are indicated. However, because of the potential of immune tolerance to the Hib antigen, COMVAX should not be used in infants younger than 6 weeks of age (i.e., the birth dose of hepatitis B, or a dose at 1 month of age, if the infant is on a 0-1-6-month schedule). Although COMVAX is not licensed for infants whose mothers are known to be hepatitis B surface antigen positive (i.e., acute or chronic infection with hepatitis B virus), the Advisory Committee on Immunization Practices (ACIP) has approved off-label use of COMVAX for these infants (see http://www.cdc.gov/vaccines/programs/vfc/dowloads/resolutions/1003hepb.pdf). COMVAX contains the same dose of Merck's hepatitis B vaccine recommended for these infants, so response to the hepatitis B component of COMVAX should be adequate.

Recommendations for spacing and timing of COMVAX are the same as those for the individual antigens. In particular, the third dose must be given at 12 months of age or older and at least 2 months after the second dose, as recommended for PRP-OMP. Comvax will be removed from existing contracts and pricing programs in early 2015.

DTaP-IPV-Hib-PRP-T (Pentacel)

Pentacel (Sanofi Pasteur) is a combination vaccine that contains lyophilized Hib (ActHIB) vaccine that is reconstituted with a liquid DTaP-IPV solution. Pentacel is licensed by FDA for doses 1 through 4 of the DTaP series among children 6 weeks through 4 years of age. Pentacel should not

---

8

Combination Vaccines Containing Hib

- DTaP-IPV/Hib
  - Pentacel
- Hepatitis B-Hib
  - COMVAX
- Hib-MenCY
  - MenHibrix

COMVAX

- Hepatitis B-Hib combination
- Use when either antigen is indicated
- Cannot use before 6 weeks of age
- May be used in infants whose mothers are HBsAg positive or status is not known

Pentacel

- Contains lyophilized Hib (ActHIB) vaccine that is reconstituted with a liquid DTaP-IPV solution
- Approved for doses 1 through 4 among children 6 weeks through 4 years of age
- The DTaP-IPV solution should not be used separately (i.e., only use to reconstitute the Hib component)

be used for the fifth dose of the DTaP series, or for children 5 years or older regardless of the number of prior doses of the component vaccines.

The DTaP-IPV solution is licensed only for use as the diluent for the lyophilized Hib component and should not be used separately. If the DTaP-IPV solution is inadvertently administered without being used to reconstitute the Hib component the DTaP and IPV doses can be counted as valid. However, PRP-T (ActHIB) must be reconstituted only with the DTaP-IPV diluent supplied in the Pentacel package, or with a specific 0.4% sodium chloride ActHIB diluent. If DTaP-IPV diluent is not available then the provider must contact the manufacturer (Sanofi Pasteur) to obtain the ActHIB diluent. Any dose of ActHIB reconstituted with a diluent other than DTaP-IPV or specific ActHIB diluent should not be counted as valid and must be repeated.

Hib-MenCY (MenHibrix)

MenHibrix is lyophilized and should be reconstituted with a 0.9% saline diluent. MenHibrix is approved as a four dose series for children at 2, 4, 6, and 12 through 18 months. MenHibrix may be used in any infant for routine vaccination against Hib. Infants at increased risk for meningococcal disease should be vaccinated with a 4-dose series of MenHibrix. MenHibrix is not recommended for routine meningococcal vaccination for infants who are not at increased risk for meningococcal disease. Further recommendations for the MenCY component of MenHibrix can be found at http://www.cdc.gov/mmwr/preview/mmwrhtml/mm6203a3.htm?s_cid=mm6203a3_w.

> **MenHibrix**
> - Approved as a 4-dose series
> - Infants at increased risk for meningoccal disease should be vaccinated with a 4-dose series

Contraindications and Precautions to Vaccination

Vaccination with Hib conjugate vaccine is contraindicated for persons known to have experienced a severe allergic reaction (anaphylaxis) to a vaccine component or following a prior dose. Vaccination should be delayed for children with moderate or severe acute illnesses. Minor illnesses (e.g., mild upper respiratory infection) are not contraindications to vaccination. Hib conjugate vaccines are contraindicated for children younger than 6 weeks of age because of the potential for development of immunologic tolerance.

Contraindications and precautions for the use of Pentacel and COMVAX are the same as those for its individual component vaccines (i.e., DTaP, Hib, IPV, and hepatitis B).

> ***Haemophilus influenzae* type b Vaccine Contraindications and Precautions**
> - Severe allergic reaction to vaccine component or following a prior dose
> - Moderate or severe acute illness
> - Age younger than 6 weeks

Haemophilus influenzae type B

> **Haemophilus influenzae type b Vaccine Adverse Reactions**
> - Swelling, redness, or pain in 5%-30% of recipients
> - Systemic reactions infrequent
> - Serious adverse reactions rare

Adverse Reactions Following Vaccination

Adverse reactions following Hib conjugate vaccines are not common. Swelling, redness, or pain have been reported in 5%–30% of recipients and usually resolve within 12–24 hours. Systemic reactions such as fever and irritability are infrequent. Serious reactions are rare.

All serious adverse events that occur after receipt of any vaccine should be reported to the Vaccine Adverse Event Reporting System (VAERS) (http://vaers.hhs.gov/).

Vaccine Storage and Handling

Hib vaccine should be maintained at refrigerator temperature between 35°F and 46°F (2°C and 8°C). Manufacturer package inserts contain additional information and can be found at http://www.fda.gov/BiologicsBloodVaccines/Vaccines/ApprovedProducts/ucm093830.htm. For complete information on best practices and recommendations please refer to CDC's Vaccine Storage and Handling Toolkit, http://www.cdc.gov/vaccines/recs/storage/toolkit/storage-handling-toolkit.pdf.

Surveillance and Reporting of Hib Disease

Invasive Hib disease is a reportable condition in most states. All healthcare personnel should report any case of invasive Hib disease to local and state health departments.

Acknowledgement

The editors thank Dr. Elizabeth Briere, CDC, for her assistance in updating this chapter.

Selected References

MacNeil JR et al; Current Epidemiology and Trends in Invasive *Haemophilus influenzae* Disease – United States, 1989-2008. *Clinical Infectious Diseases*; 2011;53(12): 1230-6.

Briere E., Jackson, ML, Shah S., et al. *Haemophilus influenzae* Type b Disease and Vaccine Booster Dose Deferral, United States, 1998-2009. *Pediatrics* 2012;130:414-20

Livorsi DJ, Macneil JR, Cohn AC, et al. Invasive *Haemophilus influenzae* in the United States, 1999-2008: Epidemiology and outcomes. *J Infect*. 2012 Aug 15. [Epub ahead of print]

American Academy of Pediatrics. *Haemophilus influenzae* infections. In: Pickering L, Baker C, Kimberlin D, Long S, eds. Red Book: 2012 Report of the Committee on Infectious Diseases. 29th ed. Elk Grove Village, IL: *American Academy of Pediatrics*, 2012345-352.

Bisgard KM, Kao A, Leake J, et al. *Haemophilus influenzae* invasive disease in the United States, 1994–1995: near disappearance of a vaccine-preventable childhood disease. *Emerg Infect Dis* 1998;4:229–37.

CDC. *Haemophilus* b conjugate vaccines for prevention of *Haemophilus influenzae* type b disease among infants and children two months of age and older: recommendations of the Advisory Committee on Immunization Practices (ACIP). *MMWR* 1991;40(No. RR-1):1–7.

CDC. Progress toward elimination of *Haemophilus influenzae* type b disease among infants and children—United States, 1998–2000. *MMWR* 2002;51:234–37.

CDC. *Haemophilus influenzae* invasive disease among children aged <5 years—California, 1990–1996. *MMWR* 1998;47:737–40.

CDC. Licensure of a *Haemophilus influenzae* Type b (Hib) Vaccine (Hiberix) and Updated Recommendations for Use of Hib Vaccine. *MMWR* 2009;58:1008-9.

Decker MD, Edwards KM. *Haemophilus influenzae* type b vaccines: history, choice and comparisons. *Pediatr Infect Dis J* 1998;17:S113–16.

Orenstein WA, Hadler S, Wharton M. Trends in vaccine-preventable diseases. *Semin Pediatr Infect Dis* 1997;8:23–33.

8

Haemophilus influenzae type B

8

The first descriptions of hepatitis (epidemic jaundice) are generally attributed to Hippocrates. Outbreaks of jaundice, probably hepatitis A, were reported in the 17th and 18th centuries, particularly in association with military campaigns. Hepatitis A (formerly called infectious hepatitis) was first differentiated epidemiologically from hepatitis B, which has a longer incubation period, in the 1940s. Development of serologic tests allowed definitive diagnosis of hepatitis B. In the 1970s, identification of the virus, and development of serologic tests helped differentiate hepatitis A from other types of non-B hepatitis.

Until 2004, hepatitis A was the most frequently reported type of hepatitis in the United States. In the prevaccine era, the primary methods used for preventing hepatitis A were hygienic measures and passive protection with immune globulin (IG). Hepatitis A vaccines were licensed in 1995 and 1996. These vaccines provide long-term protection against hepatitis A virus (HAV) infection. The similarities between the epidemiology of hepatitis A and poliomyelitis suggest that widespread vaccination of appropriate susceptible populations can substantially lower disease incidence, eliminate virus transmission, and ultimately, eliminate HAV infection.

> **Hepatitis A**
> - Epidemic jaundice attributed to Hippocrates
> - Differentiated from hepatitis B in 1940s
> - Serologic tests developed in 1970s
> - Vaccines licensed in 1995 and 1996

9

Hepatitis A Virus

Hepatitis A is caused by infection with HAV, a nonenveloped RNA virus that is classified as a picornavirus. It was first isolated in 1979. Humans are the only natural host, although several nonhuman primates have been infected in laboratory conditions. Depending on conditions, HAV can be stable in the environment for months. The virus is relatively stable at low pH levels and moderate temperatures but can be inactivated by high temperature (185°F [85°C] or higher), formalin, and chlorine.

> **Hepatitis A Virus**
> - Picornavirus (RNA)
> - Humans are only natural host
> - Stable at low pH
> - Inactivated by temperature of 185°F or higher, formalin, chlorine

Pathogenesis

HAV is acquired by mouth (through fecal-oral transmission) and replicates in the liver. After 10–12 days, virus is present in blood and is excreted via the biliary system into the feces. Peak titers occur during the 2 weeks before onset of illness. Although virus is present in serum, its concentration is several orders of magnitude less than in feces. Virus excretion begins to decline at the onset of clinical illness, and has decreased significantly by 7–10 days after onset of symptoms. Most infected persons no longer excrete virus in the feces by the third week of illness. Children may excrete virus longer than adults.

> **Hepatitis A Pathogenesis**
> - Entry into mouth
> - Viral replication in the liver
> - Virus present in blood and feces 10-12 days after infection
> - Virus excretion may continue for up to 3 weeks after onset of symptoms

Hepatitis A

9

Clinical Features

The incubation period of hepatitis A is approximately 28 days (range 15–50 days). The clinical course of acute hepatitis A is indistinguishable from that of other types of acute viral hepatitis. The illness typically has an abrupt onset of fever, malaise, anorexia, nausea, abdominal discomfort, dark urine and jaundice. Clinical illness usually does not last longer than 2 months, although 10%–15% of persons have prolonged or relapsing signs and symptoms for up to 6 months. Virus may be excreted during a relapse.

The likelihood of symptomatic illness from HAV infection is directly related to age. In children younger than 6 years of age, most (70%) infections are asymptomatic. In older children and adults, infection is usually symptomatic, with jaundice occurring in more than 70% of patients.

Complications

Severe clinical manifestations of hepatitis A infection are rare, however atypical complications may occur, including immunologic, neurologic, hematologic, pancreatic, and renal extrahepatic manifestations. Relapsing hepatitis, cholestatic hepatitis A, hepatitis A triggering autoimmune hepatitis, subfulminant hepatitis, and fulminant hepatitis have also been reported. Fulminant hepatitis is the most severe rare complication, with mortality estimates up to 80%. In the prevaccine era, fulminant hepatitis A caused about 100 deaths per year in the United States. The hepatitis A case-fatality rate among persons of all ages with reported cases was approximately 0.3% but may have been higher among older persons (approximately 2% among persons 40 years of age and older) More recent case-fatality estimates range from 0.3%–0.6% for all ages and up to 1.8% among adults aged >50 years. Vaccination of high risk groups and public health measures have significantly reduced the number of overall hepatitis A cases and fulminant HAV cases. Nonetheless, hepatitis A results in substantial morbidity, with associated costs caused by medical care and work loss.

Laboratory Diagnosis

Hepatitis A cannot be distinguished from other types of viral hepatitis on the basis of clinical or epidemiologic features alone. Serologic testing is required to confirm the diagnosis. Virtually all patients with acute hepatitis A have detectable IgM anti-HAV. Acute HAV infection is confirmed during the acute or early convalescent phase of infection by the presence of IgM anti-HAV in serum. IgM generally becomes detectable 5–10 days before the onset of symptoms and can persist for up to 6 months.

IgG anti-HAV appears in the convalescent phase of infection, remains present in serum for the lifetime of the person, and confers enduring protection against disease. The antibody test for total anti-HAV measures both IgG anti-HAV and IgM anti-HAV. Persons who are total anti-HAV positive and IgM anti-HAV negative have serologic markers indicating immunity consistent with either past infection or vaccination.

Molecular virology methods such as polymerase chain reaction (PCR)-based assays can be used to amplify and sequence viral genomes. These assays are helpful to investigate common-source outbreaks of hepatitis A. Providers with questions about molecular virology methods should consult with their state health department or the CDC Division of Viral Hepatitis.

Medical Management

There is no specific treatment for hepatitis A virus infection. Treatment and management of HAV infection are supportive.

Epidemiology

Occurrence

Hepatitis A occurs throughout the world. It is highly endemic in some areas, particularly Central and South America, Africa, the Middle East, Asia, and the Western Pacific.

Reservoir

Humans are the only natural reservoir of the virus. There are no insect or animal vectors. A chronic HAV state has not been reported.

Transmission

HAV infection is acquired primarily by the fecal-oral route by either person-to-person contact or ingestion of contaminated food or water. Since the virus is present in blood during the illness prodrome, HAV has been transmitted on rare occasions by transfusion. Although HAV may be present in saliva, transmission by saliva has not been demonstrated. Waterborne outbreaks are infrequent and are usually associated with sewage-contaminated or inadequately treated water.

Temporal Pattern

There is no appreciable seasonal variation in hepatitis A incidence. In the prevaccine era, cyclic increases in reported acute cases were observed every 5- 10 years, and were

Hepatitis A Epidemiology
- Reservoir
  - human
- Transmission
  - fecal-oral
- Temporal pattern
  - none
- Communicability
  - 2 weeks before illness to 1 week after onset of jaundice

9

characterized by large community outbreaks of disease. Since introduction of vaccination in the United States, these increases no longer occur.

Communicability

Viral shedding persists for 1 to 3 weeks. Infected persons are most likely to transmit HAV 1 to 2 weeks before the onset of illness, when HAV concentration in stool is highest. The risk then decreases and is minimal the week after the onset of jaundice.

Risk Factors

Groups at increased risk for hepatitis A or its complications include international travelers (particularly high-risk itineraries like travel to rural areas in high-risk countries), contacts of recent international adoptees from HAV endemic countries, men who have sex with men, and users of illegal drugs. Outbreaks of hepatitis A have also been reported among persons working with hepatitis A–infected primates. This is the only occupational group known to be at increased risk for hepatitis A.

Persons with chronic liver disease are not at increased risk of infection but are at increased risk of acquiring fulminant hepatitis A. Persons with clotting factor disorders may be at increased risk of HAV because of administration of solvent/detergent-treated factor VIII and IX concentrates.

Foodhandlers are not at increased risk for hepatitis A because of their occupation, but are noteworthy because of their critical role in common-source foodborne HAV transmission. Health-care personnel do not have an increased prevalence of HAV infections, and nosocomial HAV transmission is rare. Nonetheless, outbreaks have been observed in neonatal intensive care units and in association with adult fecal incontinence. Institutions for persons with developmental disabilities previously were sites of high HAV endemicity. However, as fewer children have been institutionalized, conditions within these institutions have improved, and more children have been vaccinated. HAV incidence and prevalence have decreased, but sporadic outbreaks can occur. Schools are not common sites for HAV transmission. Multiple cases among children at a school require investigation of a common source and efforts to improve vaccination coverage. No worker related HAV infection have been reported in the United States. Consistently, serologic studies in the US have shown no or mildly increased risk of HAV infection in wastewater workers.

Children play an important role in HAV transmission. Children generally have asymptomatic or unrecognized illnesses, so they may serve as a source of infection, particularly for household or other close contacts.

In 2010, 75% of hepatitis A cases (who responded to any question about risk behaviors and exposures) indicated no risk factors for their infection. Of cases indicating at least one risk factor 2-6 weeks prior to the onset of illness, the most frequently reported source of infection was personal contact (sexual or household) with an infected person (7.3%). Employment or attendance at a nursery, day-care center, or preschool involved 3.1% of cases; 4% involved contact with a child or employee in child care; 14.1% occurred among persons reporting recent international travel; and 10.4% occurred in the context of a recognized foodborne or waterborne outbreak. Injection-drug use was a reported risk factor in 2% of cases; men who have sex with men represented 4.9% of cases.

Of the 1,398 case reports of acute hepatitis A received by CDC during 2011, a total of 571 (41%) cases did not include a response (i.e. a "yes" or "no" response to any of the questions about risk behaviors and exposures) to enable assessment of risk behaviors or exposures. Of the 827 case reports that had a response, 646 (78%) indicated no risk behaviors/exposures for acute hepatitis A, and 181 (22%) indicated at least one risk behavior/exposure for acute hepatitis A during the 2-6 weeks prior to onset of illness.

Secular Trends in the United States

Hepatitis A became nationally reportable as a distinct entity in 1966. During the prevaccine era in the United States, hepatitis A occurred in large nationwide epidemics. The largest number of cases reported in one year was in 1971 (59,606) and the last increase in cases occurred from 1994 to 1995. Prior to 2000, the incidence of reported hepatitis A was substantially higher in the western United States than in other parts of the country. From 1987 to 1997, 11 mostly western states (Arizona, Alaska, Oregon, New Mexico, Utah, Washington, Oklahoma, South Dakota, Idaho, Nevada, California) accounted for 50% of all reported cases but only 22% of the U.S. population. Historically, children 2 through 18 years of age have had the highest rates of hepatitis A (15 to 20 cases per 100,000 population in the early to mid-1990s).

In 1996, CDC's Advisory Committee on Immunization Practices (ACIP) recommended administration of hepatitis A vaccine to persons at increased risk for the disease, including international travelers, men who have sex with men, non-injection and injection-drug users, and children living in communities with high rates of disease. In 1999, ACIP also recommended routine vaccination for children living in 11 Western states with average hepatitis A rates of >20 cases per 100,000 population and recommended that vaccination be considered for children in an additional six

9

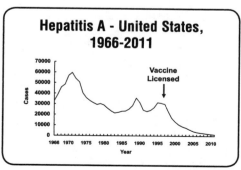

Hepatitis A – United States, 2011

Risk identified 13% (181)

No risk identified 46% (646)

Risk data missing 41% (571)

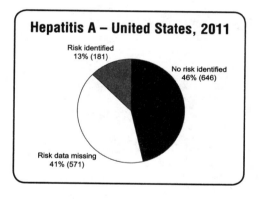

Hepatitis A - United States, 1966-2011

Vaccine Licensed

Hepatitis A

states with rates of 10–20 cases per 100,000 population. ACIP expanded these recommendations in 2006 to include routine vaccination of children in all 50 states.

Hepatitis A rates have been declining since vaccination initiation in 1996, and since 1998 have been at historically low levels. The number of reported acute hepatitis A cases decreased 93.7% overall from 1990 to 2009, and the last increase in cases occurred from 1994 to 1995. Many of the high-incidence states began routine hepatitis A vaccination programs for children in the late 1990s and since 2002, rates have been similar in all parts of the country, ranging from 0.1 case per 100,000 population in Arkansas, Mississippi, and South Dakota to 1.0 case per 100,000 population in Arizona. Since 2002, rates among children have declined and are now similar to other age groups. The wider use of vaccine is largely responsible for the marked decrease in hepatitis A rates in the United States and similar rates of infection throughout the country, and decreased infection rates in children. Beginning in the late 1990s, national age-specific rates declined more rapidly among children than adults; as a result, in recent years, rates have been similar among all age groups. Historic differences in rates among racial/ethnic populations also have narrowed in the vaccine era.

In 2010, a total of 1,670 cases of acute hepatitis A were reported nationwide to CDC. The overall incidence rate for 2010 was 0.5 cases per 100,000 population. The rate was similar among all age groups and gender. However, beginning in 2008, rates among Asian Pacific Islanders were higher than those among all other racial/ethnic populations. Based on data from the National Health and Nutrition Examination Survey (NHANES) conducted from 1999 through 2006, the overall seroprevalence of total antibody to HAV (anti-HAV) among the general U.S. population was 34.9% and 28.1% among U.S.-born individuals alone. Seroprevalence of HAV antibody increases with age, from 22.9% among 6- to 11-year-olds to 59.7% among persons 60 years of age and older. In this survey, anti-HAV seroprevalence was highest among Mexican Americans not born in the U.S. regardless of age, and seroprevalence was higher among U.S.-born Mexican Americans compared with U.S-born non-Hispanic white and non-Hispanic black persons for all age groups. Asian Pacific Islanders were not included as a race/ethnic category in this survey. The 1988 to 1994 NHANES total population age-adjusted seroprevalence of anti-HAV was not significantly different from the 1999-2006 age-adjusted seroprevalence. However, the overall age-adjusted seroprevalence increased among U.S. born children (6-19 years) during 1999-2006 compared to 1988-2004 from 8% to 20.2%. In addition, for individuals younger than 40 years, seroprevalence was higher in vaccinating states compared to non-vaccinating states for all age groups. This suggests increased hepatitis A vaccination rates following the 1999 ACIP recommendations.

The rate of hospitalization for hepatitis A in the United States declined more than 68% from the pre- to post-vaccine era (1996-2004) for all age groups. Similarly the rate of ambulatory care visits declined more than 40%. Medical expenditures for both hospitalizations and ambulatory care visits were estimated to have declined by approximately 68% ($29.1 to $9.3 million).

Case Definition

The 2012 case definition for hepatitis A was approved by the Council of State and Territorial Epidemiologists (CSTE) and published in a 2011 position statement. The clinical description for acute hepatitis A is an acute illness with a discrete onset of any sign or symptom consistent with acute viral hepatitis (e.g., fever, headache, malaise, anorexia, nausea, vomiting, diarrhea, and abdominal pain), and either a) jaundice, or b) elevated serum alanine aminotransferase (ALT) or aspartate aminotransferase (AST) levels. Since HAV cannot be differentiated from other types of viral hepatitis on clinical or epidemiologic features alone, serologic evidence of HAV-specific antibody is necessary. The diagnosis of acute hepatitis A requires the presence of HAV-specific IgM antibody.

Hepatitis A Vaccine
Characteristics

Two inactivated whole-virus hepatitis A vaccines are available: HAVRIX (GlaxoSmithKline) and VAQTA (Merck). To produce each vaccine, cell culture–adapted virus is propagated in human fibroblasts, purified from cell lysates, inactivated with formalin, and adsorbed to an aluminum hydroxide adjuvant. HAVRIX is prepared with a preservative (2-phenoxyethanol); VAQTA does not contain a preservative. HAVRIX is available in two formulations: pediatric (720 ELISA units [EL.U.] per 0.5-mL dose) and adult (1,440 EL.U. per 1.0-mL dose). VAQTA is also available in two formulations: pediatric 0.5ml (25U of antigen) and adult 1.0ml (50U of antigen) formulations. The pediatric formulations of both vaccines are approved for persons 12 months through 18 years. The adult formulations are approved for persons 19 years and older. Both vaccines are approved for 2-dose schedules. The second dose of VAQTA is administered 6-18 months after the first dose, and the second dose of HAVRIX is administered 6-12 months after the first dose.

9

Hepatitis A Vaccines
- Inactivated whole-virus vaccines
- Pediatric and adult formulations
  - pediatric formulations approved for persons 12 months through 18 years
  - adult formulations approved for persons 19 years and older

Hepatitis A

9

Immunogenicity and Vaccine Efficacy

Both monovalent hepatitis A vaccines are highly immunogenic. More than 95% of adults will develop protective antibody within 4 weeks of a single dose of either vaccine, and nearly 100% will seroconvert after receiving two doses. Among children and adolescents, more than 97% will be seropositive within a month of the first dose. In clinical trials, all recipients had protective levels of antibody after two doses.

Both vaccines are effective in preventing clinical hepatitis A. The efficacy of HAVRIX in protecting against clinical hepatitis A was 94% among 40,000 Thai children 1 to 16 years of age who received two doses 1 month apart while living in villages with high HAV disease rates. The efficacy of VAQTA in protecting against clinical hepatitis A was 100% among 1,000 New York children 2 to 16 years of age who received one dose while living in a community with a high HAV disease rate.

Ten year follow-up data of serial anti-HAV levels after two doses of inactivated hepatitis A vaccine is available. A study in Alaska Native/American Indian individuals has shown that seropositivity for hepatitis A persists for at least 10 years after completing the two-dose vaccination at age 12 to 21 months, regardless of maternal anti-HAV status. Data from two other studies using the same population showed that protective anti-HAV levels persist 15 and 17 years after receiving three doses of a lower antigen content, inactivated hepatitis A vaccine starting at ages 3-6 years. Sustained protection will continue to be assessed by persistence of anti-HAV.

Vaccination Schedule and Use

Following its introduction in 1996, hepatitis A vaccine was initially recommended for children and adolescents in communities with high or intermediate HAV endemicity. While this strategy prevented infection in high risk areas of the United States, it had little or no impact on the incidence of HAV infection in the United States.

All children should receive hepatitis A vaccine at age 1 year (i.e., 12 through 23 months). Vaccination should be completed according to the licensed schedules and integrated into the routine childhood vaccination schedule. Children who are not vaccinated by age 2 years can be vaccinated at subsequent visits. States, counties, and communities with existing hepatitis A vaccination programs for children aged 2 through18 years are encouraged to maintain these programs. In these areas, efforts should focus on routine vaccination of children 12 months of age and should enhance, not replace, ongoing programs directed at a broader population of children. In areas without existing hepatitis A vaccination programs, catch-up vaccination of unvaccinated children aged 2 through 18 years can be considered. Such programs might especially be warranted in the context of increasing incidence or ongoing outbreaks among children or adolescents.

Adults 19 years of age and older receive the adult formulation of hepatitis A vaccine according to licensed schedules. Persons at increased risk for HAV infection, or who are at increased risk for complications of HAV infection, should be routinely vaccinated.

For children less than 2 years of age, the vaccine should be administered intramuscularly into the anterolateral area of the thigh. For adults, the vaccine should be administered intramuscularly into the deltoid muscle. A needle length appropriate for the person's age and size (minimum of 1 inch) should be used.

Limited data indicate that vaccines from different manufacturers are interchangeable. Completion of the series with the same product is preferable. However, if the originally used product is not available or not known, vaccination with either product is acceptable.

For both vaccines, the dosage of the 2nd dose should be based on the person's age at the time of the dose, not the age when the first dose was given. For example, if a person received the first dose of the pediatric formulation of VAQTA at 18 years of age, and returns for the second dose at age 19 years, the second dose should be the adult formulation, not the pediatric formulation.

ACIP Recommendation for Routine Hepatitis A Vaccination of Children

- All children should receive hepatitis A vaccine at 12 through 23 months of age

- Vaccination should be integrated into the routine childhood vaccination schedule

- Children who are not vaccinated by 2 years of age can be vaccinated at subsequent visits

- States, counties, and communities with existing hepatitis A vaccination programs for children 2 through 18 years of age should maintain these programs

- New efforts focused on routine vaccination of children 12 months of age should enhance, not replace ongoing vaccination programs for older children

- In areas with without an existing hepatitis A vaccination program catch-up vaccination of unvaccinated children 2 through 18 years of age can be considered

9

Hepatitis A Vaccines

Formulation	HAVRIX	VAQTA
Pediatric		
Age	1 through 18 years	1 through 18 years
Volume	0.5 mL	0.5 mL
Dose	720 (EL.U)	25 U
Schedule*	0, 6-12	0, 6-18
Number of Doses	2	2
Adult		
Age	19 years and older	19 years and older
Volume	1.0 mL	1.0 mL
Dose	1,440 (EL.U)	50 U
Schedule*	0, 6-12	0, 6-18
Number of Doses	2	2

*Months: 0 months represents timing of the initial dose; subsequent number(s) represent months after the initial dose.

Hepatitis A

The minimum interval between the first and second doses of hepatitis A vaccine is 6 calendar months. If the interval between the first and second doses of hepatitis A vaccine extends beyond 18 months, it is not necessary to repeat a dose.

Combination Hepatitis A and Hepatitis B Vaccine

In 2001, the Food and Drug Administration (FDA) approved a combination hepatitis A and hepatitis B vaccine (Twinrix, GlaxoSmithKline). Each dose of Twinrix contains 720 EL.U. of hepatitis A vaccine (equivalent to a pediatric dose of HAVRIX), and 20 mcg of hepatitis B surface antigen protein (equivalent to an adult dose of Engerix-B). The vaccine is administered in a three-dose series at 0, 1, and 6 months. Appropriate spacing of the doses must be maintained to assure long-term protection from both vaccines. The first and second doses should be separated by at least 4 weeks, and the second and third doses should be separated by at least 5 months. Twinrix is approved for persons aged 18 years and older and can be used in persons in this age group with indications for both hepatitis A and hepatitis B vaccines.

In 2007, FDA approved an alternative schedule for Twinrix with doses at 0, 7, and 21 through 30 days and a booster dose 12 months after the first dose.

Because the hepatitis B component of Twinrix is equivalent to a standard dose of hepatitis B vaccine, the schedule is the same whether Twinrix or single-antigen hepatitis B vaccine is used.

Single-antigen hepatitis A vaccine may be used to complete a series begun with Twinrix and vice versa. A person 19 years of age or older who receives one dose of Twinrix may complete the hepatitis A series with two doses of adult formulation hepatitis A vaccine separated by at least 5 months. A person who receives two doses of Twinrix may complete the hepatitis A series with one dose of adult formulation hepatitis A vaccine or Twinrix 5 months after the second dose. A person who begins the hepatitis A series with single-antigen hepatitis A vaccine may complete the series with two doses of Twinrix or one dose of adult formulation hepatitis A vaccine. An 18-year-old should follow the same schedule using the pediatric formulation.

Persons at Increased Risk for Hepatitis A or Severe Outcomes of Infection

Persons at increased risk for hepatitis A should be identified and vaccinated. Hepatitis A vaccine should be strongly considered for persons 1 year of age and older traveling to or working in countries where they would have a high or intermediate risk of hepatitis A virus infection. These

---

Twinrix

- Combination hepatitis A vaccine (pediatric dose) and hepatitis B (adult dose)
- Schedules
  - 0, 1, 6 months, or
  - 0, 7, 21to 30 days and a booster dose 12 months after first dose
- Approved for persons 18 years of age and older

Persons at Increased Risk for Hepatitis A or Severe Outcomes of Infection

- International travelers
- Close contact with an international adoptee from a country of high or intermediate endemicity
- Men who have sex with men
- Persons who use illegal drugs
- Persons who have a clotting factor disorder
- Persons with occupational risk
- Persons with chronic liver disease
- Healthcare workers: not routinely recommended
- Child care centers: not routinely recommended
- Sewer workers or plumbers: not routinely recommended
- Food handlers: may be considered based on local epidemiology

areas include all areas of the world except Canada, Western Europe and Scandinavia, Japan, New Zealand, and Australia.

The first dose of hepatitis A vaccine should be administered as soon as travel is considered. For healthy persons 40 years of age or younger, 1 dose of single antigen vaccine administered at any time before departure can provide adequate protection.

Unvaccinated adults older than 40 years of age, immunocompromised persons, and persons with chronic liver disease planning to travel in 2 weeks or sooner should receive the first dose of vaccine and also can receive immune globulin at the same visit. Vaccine and IG should be administered with separate syringes at different anatomic sites.

Travelers who choose not to receive vaccine should receive a single dose of IG (0.02 mL/kg), which provides protection against HAV infection for up to 3 months. Persons whose travel period is more than 2 months should be administered IG at 0.06 mL/kg. IG should be repeated in 5 months for prolonged travel.

In 2009 ACIP recommended hepatitis A vaccination for all previously unvaccinated persons who anticipate close personal contact (e.g., household contact or regular babysitting) with an international adoptee from a country of high or intermediate endemicity during the first 60 days following arrival of the adoptee in the United States. The first dose of the 2-dose hepatitis A vaccine series should be administered as soon as adoption is planned, ideally 2 or more weeks before the arrival of the adoptee.

Other groups that should be offered vaccine include men who have sex with other men, persons who use illegal drugs, persons who have clotting factor disorders, and persons with occupational risk of infection. Persons with occupational risk include only those who work with hepatitis A-infected primates or with hepatitis A virus in a laboratory setting. No other groups have been shown to be at increased risk of hepatitis A infection due to occupational exposure.

Persons with chronic liver disease are not at increased risk for HAV infection because of their liver disease alone. However, these persons are at increased risk for fulminant hepatitis A should they become infected. Susceptible persons who have chronic liver disease should be vaccinated. Susceptible persons who either are awaiting or have received liver transplants should be vaccinated.

Hepatitis A vaccination is not routinely recommended for healthcare personnel, persons attending or working in child care centers, or persons who work in liquid or solid waste management (e.g., sewer workers or plumbers).

Hepatitis A

These groups have not been shown to be at increased risk for hepatitis A infection. ACIP does not recommend routine hepatitis A vaccination for food service workers, but vaccination may be considered based on local epidemiology.

Prevaccination Serologic Testing

HAV infection produces lifelong immunity to hepatitis A, so there is no benefit of vaccinating someone with serologic evidence of past HAV infection. The risk for adverse events following vaccination of such persons is not higher than the risk for serologically negative persons. As a result, the decision to conduct prevaccination testing should be based chiefly on the prevalence of immunity, the cost of testing and vaccinating (including office visit costs), and the likelihood that testing will interfere with initiating vaccination.

Testing of children is not indicated because of their expected low prevalence of infection. Persons for whom prevaccination serologic testing will likely be most cost-effective include adults who were either born in or lived for extensive periods in geographic areas that have a high endemicity of HAV infection (e.g., Central and South America, Africa, Asia); older adolescents and adults in certain populations (i.e., American Indian/Alaska Native and Hispanic); adults in certain groups that have a high prevalence of infection, and adults 40 years of age and older.

Commercially available tests for total anti-HAV should be used for prevaccination testing.

Postvaccination Serologic Testing

Postvaccination testing is not indicated because of the high rate of vaccine response among adults and children. Testing methods sufficiently sensitive to detect low anti-HAV concentrations after vaccination are not approved for routine diagnostic use in the United States.

Contraindications and Precautions to Vaccination

Hepatitis A vaccine should not be administered to persons with a history of a severe allergic reaction (e.g. anaphylaxis) to a vaccine component or following a prior dose of hepatitis A vaccine, hypersensitivity to alum or, in the case of HAVRIX, to the preservative 2-phenoxyethanol. Vaccination of persons with moderate or severe acute illnesses should be deferred until the person's condition has improved.

The safety of hepatitis A vaccination during pregnancy has not been determined. However, because it is an inactivated vaccine, the theoretical risk to the fetus is low. The risk

---

Hepatitis A Serologic Testing

- Prevaccination
  - not indicated for children
  - may be considered for some adults and older adolescent
- Postvaccination
  - not indicated

Hepatitis A Vaccine Contraindications and Precautions

- Severe allergic reaction to a vaccine component or following a prior dose
- Moderate or severe acute illness

associated with vaccination should be weighed against the risk for HAV infection. Because hepatitis A vaccine is inactivated, no special precautions are needed when vaccinating immunocompromised persons, although response to the vaccine may be suboptimal.

Adverse Reactions Following Vaccination

For both vaccines, the most commonly reported adverse reaction following vaccination is a local reaction at the site of injection. Injection site pain, erythema, or swelling is reported by 20% to 50% of recipients. These symptoms are generally mild and self-limited. Mild systemic complaints (e.g., malaise, fatigue, low-grade fever) are reported by fewer than 10% of recipients. No serious adverse reactions have been reported.

> **Hepatitis A Vaccine Adverse Reactions**
> - Local reaction
>   - 20%-50%
> - Systemic reactions (malaise, fatigue)
>   - <10%
> - No serious adverse reactions reported

9

Vaccine Storage and Handling

Hepatitis A vaccine should be maintained at refrigerator temperature between 35°F and 46°F (2°C and 8°C). Manufacturer package inserts contain additional information and can be found at http://www.fda.gov/BiologicsBloodVaccines/Vaccines/ApprovedProducts/ucm093830.htm. For complete information on best practices and recommendations please refer to CDC's Vaccine Storage and Handling Toolkit, http://www.cdc.gov/vaccines/recs/storage/toolkit/storage-handling-toolkit.pdf.

Postexposure Prophylaxis

Immune globulin (IG) is typically used for postexposure prophylaxis of hepatitis A in susceptible persons. Hepatitis A vaccine may be used for postexposure prophylaxis in healthy persons 12 months through 40 years of age. Immune globulin is preferred for persons older than 40 years of age, children younger than 12 months of age, immunocompromised persons, and persons with chronic liver disease. See *MMWR* 2007;56(No.41):1080-84 (October 19, 2007) for details.

Acknowledgement

The editors thank Drs. Trudy Murphy, Noelle Nelson, and Clive Brown, CDC for their assistance in updating this chapter.

Selected References

Byrd KK, Bruden DL, Bruce MG, Bulkow LR, Zanis CL, Snowball MM, Homan CE, Hennessy TW, Williams JL, Dunaway E, Chaves SS, McMahon BJ. Long term immunogenicity of inactivated hepatitis A vaccine: Follow-up at 15 years.

Pediatric Infectious Disease Journal 2010;5:321–6.

CDC. Update: prevention of hepatitis A virus after exposure to hepatitis A virus in international travelers. Updated recommendations of the Advisory Committee on Immunization Practices (ACIP). *MMWR* 2007;56:1080–84.

CDC. Prevention of hepatitis A through active or passive immunization: recommendations of the Advisory Committee on Immunization Practices (ACIP). *MMWR* 2006;55(No. RR-7):1–23.

CDC. Updated Recommendations from the Advisory Committee on Immunization Practices (ACIP) for Use of Hepatitis A Vaccine in Close Contacts of Newly Arriving International Adoptees. *MMWR* 2009;58;1006–7.

CDC. Viral Hepatitis Surveillance United States 2010. http://www.cdc.gov/hepatitis/Statistics/2010Surveillance/PDFs/2010HepSurveillanceRpt.pdf. Accessed March 19, 2013.

CDC. Hepatitis A outbreak associated with green onions at a restaurant—Monaca, Pennsylvania, 2003. *MMWR* 2003;52:1155–7.

Council of State and Territorial Epidemiologists Position Statement, Infectious Disease, Public Health Reporting and National Notification for Hepatitis A, 11-ID-02. http://c.ymcdn.com/sites/www.cste.org/resource/resmgr/PS/11-ID-02.pdf

Klevens RM, Kruszon-Moran D, Wasley A, Gallagher K, McQuillan GM, Kuhnert W, Teshale EH, Drobeniuc J, Bell BP. Seroprevalence of hepatitis A virus antibodies in the U.S.: results from the National Health and Nutrition Examination Survey. Public Health Rep. 2011 Jul-Aug;126(4):522-32.

Murphy TV, Feinstone SM, and Bell BP. Hepatitis A Vaccine. In: Plotkin SA, Orenstein, WA, and Offit PA, eds. *Vaccines*. 6th ed. China: Saunders; 2013.

Raczniak, Gregory A ; Bulkow, Lisa R ; Bruce, Michael G ; Zanis, Carolyn L ; Baum, Richard L ; Snowball, Mary M ; Byrd, Kathy K ; Sharapov, Umid M ; Hennessy, Thomas W ; McMahon, Brian J. Long-term immunogenicity of hepatitis A virus vaccine in Alaska 17 years after initial childhood series The Journal of infectious diseases, 2013, Vol.207(3), pp.493-6

Sharapov UM, Bulkow LR, Negus SE, Spradling PR, Homan C, Drobeniuc J, Bruce M, Kamili S, Hu DJ, McMahon BJ. Persistence of hepatitis A vaccine induced seropositivity in infants and young children by maternal antibody status: 10-year follow-up. Hepatology. 2012 Aug;56(2):516-22. doi: 10.1002/hep.25687. Epub 2012 Jun 11.

Taylor RM, Davern T, Munoz S, Han SH, McGuire B, Larson AM, Hynan L, Lee WM, Fontana RJ; US Acute Liver Failure Study Group. Fulminant hepatitis A virus infection in the United States: Incidence, prognosis, and outcomes. Hepatology. 2006 Dec;44(6):1589-97.

Zhou F, Shefer A, Weinbaum C, McCauley M, Kong Y. Impact of hepatitis A vaccination on health care utilization in the United States, 1996-2004. Vaccine. 2007 May 4;25(18):3581-7. Epub 2007 Jan 25.

9

Viral hepatitis is a term commonly used for several clinically similar yet etiologically and epidemiologically distinct diseases. Hepatitis A (formerly called infectious hepatitis) and hepatitis B (formerly called serum hepatitis) have been recognized as separate entities since the early 1940s and can be diagnosed with specific serologic tests. Delta hepatitis is an infection dependent on the hepatitis B virus (HBV). It may occur as a coinfection with acute HBV infection or as superinfection of an HBV carrier.

Epidemic jaundice was described by Hippocrates in the 5th century BCE. The first recorded cases of "serum hepatitis," or hepatitis B, are thought to be those that followed the administration of smallpox vaccine containing human lymph to shipyard workers in Germany in 1883. In the early and middle parts of the 20th century, serum hepatitis was repeatedly observed following the use of contaminated needles and syringes. The role of blood as a vehicle for virus transmission was further emphasized in 1943, when Beeson described jaundice that had occurred in seven recipients of blood transfusions. Australia antigen, later called hepatitis B surface antigen (HBsAg), was first described in 1965, and the Dane particle (complete hepatitis B virion) was identified in 1970. Identification of serologic markers for HBV infection followed, which helped clarify the natural history of the disease. Ultimately, HBsAg was prepared in quantity and now comprises the immunogen in highly effective vaccines for prevention of HBV infection.

Hepatitis B Virus

HBV is a small, double-shelled virus in the family Hepadnaviridae. Other Hepadnaviridae include duck hepatitis virus, ground squirrel hepatitis virus, and woodchuck hepatitis virus. The virus has a small circular DNA genome that is partially double-stranded. HBV contains numerous antigenic components, including HBsAg, hepatitis B core antigen (HBcAg), and hepatitis B e antigen (HBeAg). Humans are the only known host for HBV, although some nonhuman primates have been infected in laboratory conditions. HBV is relatively resilient and, in some instances, has been shown to remain infectious on environmental surfaces for more than 7 days at room temperature.

An estimated 2 billion persons worldwide have been infected with HBV, and more than 350 million persons have chronic, lifelong infections. HBV infection is an established cause of acute and chronic hepatitis and cirrhosis. It is the cause of up to 50% of hepatocellular carcinomas (HCC). The World Health Organization estimated that more than 600,000 persons died worldwide in 2002 of hepatitis B-associated acute and chronic liver disease.

Hepatitis B
- Epidemic jaundice described by Hippocrates in 5th century BCE
- Jaundice reported among recipients of human serum and yellow fever vaccines in 1930s and 1940s
- Australia antigen described in 1965
- Serologic tests developed in 1970s

10

Hepatitis B Virus
- Hepadnaviridae family (DNA)
- Numerous antigenic components
- Humans are only known host
- May retain infectivity for more than 7 days at room temperature

Hepatitis B Virus Infection
- More than 350 million chronically infected worldwide
- Established cause of chronic hepatitis and cirrhosis
- Human carcinogen—cause of up to 50% of hepatocellular carcinomas
- More than 600,000 deaths worldwide in 2002

Hepatitis B

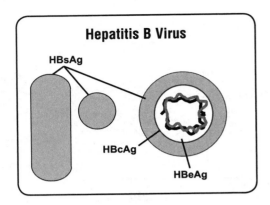

Hepatitis B Virus

HBsAg

HBcAg

HBeAg

Several well-defined antigen–antibody systems are associated with HBV infection. HBsAg, formerly called Australia antigen or hepatitis-associated antigen, is an antigenic determinant found on the surface of the virus. It also makes up subviral 22-nm spherical and tubular particles. HBsAg can be identified in serum 30 to 60 days after exposure to HBV and persists for variable periods. HBsAg is not infectious. Only the complete virus (Dane particle) is infectious. During replication, HBV produces HBsAg in excess of that needed for production of Dane particles. HBsAg is antigenically heterogeneous, with a common antigen (designated a) and 2 pairs of mutually exclusive antigens (d, y, w [including several subdeterminants] and r), resulting in 4 major subtypes: adw, ayw, adr and ayr. The distribution of subtypes varies geographically; because of the common "a" determinant, protection against one subtype appears to confer protection against the other subtypes, and no differences in clinical features have been related to subtype.

HBcAg is the nucleocapsid protein core of HBV. HBcAg is not detectable in serum by conventional techniques, but it can be detected in liver tissue of persons with acute or chronic HBV infection. HBeAg, a soluble protein, is also contained in the core of HBV. HBeAg is detected in the serum of persons with high virus titers and indicates high infectivity. Antibody to HBsAg (anti-HBs) develops during convalescence after acute HBV infection or following hepatitis B vaccination. The presence of anti-HBs indicates immunity to HBV. (Anti-HBs is sometimes referred to as HBsAb, but use of this term is discouraged because of potential confusion with HBsAg.) Antibody to HBcAg (anti-HBc) indicates infection with HBV at an undefined time in the past. IgM class antibody to HBcAg (IgM anti-HBc) indicates recent infection with HBV. Antibody to HBeAg (anti-HBe) becomes detectable when HBeAg is lost and is associated with low infectivity of serum.

Genotype classification based on sequencing of genetic material has been introduced and is becoming the standard: HBV is currently classified into 8 main genotypes (A–H). HBV genotypes are associated with the modes of HBV transmission (vertical vs. horizontal) and with the risk of certain outcomes of chronic infection, such as cirrhosis and HCC. In Alaska, HBV genotype F is associated with HCC in young children as well as adults younger than 30 years of age. In Asia as well as Alaska, HBV genotype C has been associated with a significantly higher risk of HCC than other genotypes.

Clinical Features

The clinical course of acute hepatitis B is indistinguishable from that of other types of acute viral hepatitis. The incubation period ranges from 45 to 160 days (average, 120 days). Clinical signs and symptoms occur more often in adults than in infants or children, who usually have an asymptomatic acute course. However, approximately 50% of adults who have acute infections are asymptomatic.

The preicteric, or prodromal phase from initial symptoms to onset of jaundice usually lasts from 3 to 10 days. It is nonspecific and is characterized by insidious onset of malaise, anorexia, nausea, vomiting, right upper quadrant abdominal pain, fever, headache, myalgia, skin rashes, arthralgia and arthritis, and dark urine, beginning 1 to 2 days before the onset of jaundice. The icteric phase is variable but usually lasts from 1 to 3 weeks and is characterized by jaundice, light or gray stools, hepatic tenderness and hepatomegaly (splenomegaly is less common). During convalescence, malaise and fatigue may persist for weeks or months, while jaundice, anorexia, and other symptoms disappear.

Most acute HBV infections in adults result in complete recovery with elimination of HBsAg from the blood and the production of anti-HBs, creating immunity to future infection.

> ## Hepatitis B Clinical Features
> - Incubation period 45-160 days (average 120 days)
> - Nonspecific prodrome of malaise, fever, headache, myalgia
> - Illness not specific for hepatitis B
> - At least 50% of infections asymptomatic

10

Complications

While most acute HBV infections in adults result in complete recovery, fulminant hepatitis occurs in about 1% to 2% of acutely infected persons. About 200 to 300 Americans die of fulminant disease each year (case-fatality rate 63% to 93%). Although the consequences of acute HBV infection can be severe, most of the serious complications associated with HBV infection are due to chronic infection.

Chronic HBV Infection

The proportion of patients with acute HBV Infection who progress to chronic infection varies with age and immune status. As many as 90% of infants who acquire HBV infection from their mothers at birth or in infancy become chronically infected. Of children who become infected with HBV between 1 year and 5 years of age, 30% to 50% become chronically infected. By adulthood, the risk of acquiring chronic HBV infection is approximately 5%. Acute HBV progresses to chronic HBV in approximately 40% of hemodialysis patients and up to 20% of patients with immune deficiencies.

Persons with chronic infection are often asymptomatic and may not be aware that they are infected; however, they are capable of infecting others and have been referred to as carriers. Chronic infection is responsible for most

> ## Hepatitis B Complications
> - Fulminant hepatitis
> - Hospitalization
> - Cirrhosis
> - Hepatocellular carcinoma
> - Death
>
> ## Chronic Hepatitis B Virus Infection
> - Responsible for most mortality
> - Overall risk 5% among adults
> - Higher risk with early infection
> - Often asymptomatic

Hepatitis B

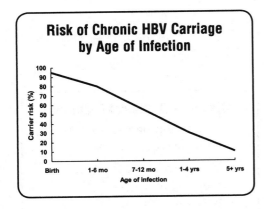

Risk of Chronic HBV Carriage by Age of Infection

Carrier risk (%) — Birth, 1-6 mo, 7-12 mo, 1-4 yrs, 5+ yrs — Age of infection

HBV-related morbidity and mortality, including chronic hepatitis, cirrhosis, liver failure, and hepatocellular carcinoma. Approximately 25% of persons with chronic HBV infection die prematurely from cirrhosis or liver cancer. Chronic active hepatitis develops in more than 25% of carriers and often results in cirrhosis. An estimated 3,000 to 4,000 persons die of hepatitis B-related cirrhosis each year in the United States. Persons with chronic HBV infection are at 12 to 300 times higher risk of hepatocellular carcinoma than noncarriers. An estimated 1,000 to 1,500 persons die each year in the United States of hepatitis B-related liver cancer.

Laboratory Diagnosis

Diagnosis is based on clinical, laboratory, and epidemiologic findings. HBV infection cannot be differentiated on the basis of clinical symptoms alone, and definitive diagnosis depends on the results of serologic testing. Serologic markers of HBV infection vary depending on whether the infection is acute or chronic.

HBsAg is the most commonly used test for diagnosing acute HBV infections or detecting carriers. HBsAg can be detected as early as 1 or 2 weeks and as late as 11 or 12 weeks after exposure to HBV when sensitive assays are used. The presence of HBsAg indicates that a person is infectious, regardless of whether the infection is acute or chronic.

Anti-HBc (core antibody) develops in all HBV infections, appears shortly after HBsAg in acute disease, and indicates HBV infection at some undefined time in the past. Anti-HBc only occurs after HBV infection and does not develop in persons whose immunity to HBV is from vaccine. Anti-HBc generally persists for life and is not a serologic marker for acute infection.

IgM anti-HBc appears in persons with acute disease about the time of illness onset and indicates recent infection with HBV. IgM anti-HBc is generally detectable 4 to 6 months after onset of illness and is the best serologic marker of acute HBV infection. A negative test for IgM-anti-HBc together with a positive test for HBsAg in a single blood sample identifies a chronic HBV infection. HBV DNA assays are used to monitor response to treatment, assess the likelihood of maternal-to-child transmission of HBV, and to detect the presence of occult HBV infection (i.e. infection in someone who tests HBsAg negative).

HBeAg is a useful marker associated strongly with the number of infective HBV particles in the serum and a higher risk of infectivity.

Interpretation of Hepatitis B Serologic Tests

Tests	Results	Interpretation
HBsAg .... Negative anti-HBc .... Negative anti-HBs .... Negative		Susceptible
HBsAg .... Negative anti-HBc .... Negative anti-HBs .... Positive with ≥10mIU/mL*		Immune due to vaccination
HBsAg .... Negative anti-HBc .... Positive anti-HBs .... Positive		Immune due to natural infection
HBsAg .... Positive anti-HBc .... Positive IgM anti-HBc .... Positive anti-HBs .... Negative		Acutely infected
HBsAg .... Positive anti-HBc .... Positive IgM anti-HBc .... Negative anti-HBs .... Negative		Chronically infected
HBsAg .... Negative anti-HBc .... Positive anti-HBs .... Negative		Four interpretations possible[†]

*Postvaccination testing, when it is recommended, should be performed 1-2 months following dose #3.

[†] 1. May be recovering from acute HBV infection.
   2. May be distantly immune and the test is not sensitive enough to detect a very low level of anti-HBs in serum.
   3. May be susceptible with a false positive anti-HBc.
   4. May be chronically infected and have an undetectable level of HBsAg present in the serum.

10

Anti-HBs (surface antibody) is a protective, neutralizing antibody. The presence of anti-HBs following acute HBV infection generally indicates recovery and immunity against reinfection. Anti-HBs can also be acquired as an immune response to hepatitis B vaccine or passively transferred by administration of hepatitis B immune globulin (HBIG). With enzyme immunoassay (EIA), the manufacturer's recommended positive should be considered an appropriate measure of immunity. The level of anti-HBs may also be expressed in milli-international units/mL (mIU/mL). Ten mIU/mL is considered to indicate a protective level of immunity.

Hepatitis B

Medical Management

There is no specific therapy for acute HBV infection. Treatment is supportive.

Two major groups of antiviral treatment have been licensed for the treatment of chronic HBV infection in many countries. These include interferon alpha (IFNa, or PEG-IFNa) and nucleoside or nucleotide analogues such as lamivudine, adefovir, entecavir telbivudine, and tenofovir. Many other drugs are being evaluated. Although the decision to treat and choosing the appropriate therapy remain challenging, considerable progress has been made in the treatment of persons with chronic HBV infection. Patients generally are considered for treatment when they have HBV DNA levels above 2000 IU/ml, serum alanine aminotransferase levels above the upper limit of normal, and severity of liver disease assessed by liver biopsy (or non-invasive markers once validated in HBV-infected patients) showing moderate to severe active necroinflammation and/or at least moderate fibrosis using a standardized scoring system. The majority of patients will require prolonged treatment in order to maintain suppression of viral replication. Consequently, treatment costs in both developing and developed countries are currently prohibitively high. The efficacy of combination therapy will have to be studied further, but it is likely to diminish the occurrence of virus mutants resistant to treatment. Medications have significant side effects that require careful monitoring.

Persons with acute or chronic HBV infections should prevent their blood and other potentially infective body fluids from contacting other persons. They should not donate blood or share toothbrushes or razors with household members.

In the hospital setting, patients with HBV infection should be managed with standard precautions.

Epidemiology
Reservoir

Although other primates have been infected in laboratory conditions, HBV infection affects only humans. No animal or insect hosts or vectors are known to exist.

Transmission

The virus is transmitted by parenteral or mucosal exposure to HBsAg-positive body fluids from persons who have acute or chronic HBV infection. The highest concentrations of virus are in blood and serous fluids; lower titers are found in other fluids, such as saliva, tears, urine, and semen. Semen is a vehicle for sexual transmission and saliva can be a vehicle of transmission through bites; other types of

---

Hepatitis B Epidemiology
- Reservoir
  - human
- Transmission
  - bloodborne
  - subclinical cases transmit
- Communicability
  - 1-2 months before and after onset of symptoms
  - persons with either acute or chronic HBV infection with HBsAg present in blood

exposure, e.g., to saliva through kissing, are unlikely modes of transmission. Transmission of HBV via tears, sweat, urine, stool, or droplet nuclei has not been clearly documented.

In the United States, the most important routes of transmission are perinatal and sexual contact, either heterosexual or homosexual, with an infected person. Fecal-oral transmission does not appear to occur. However, transmission occurs among men who have sex with men, possibly via contamination from asymptomatic rectal mucosal lesions. In the past two decades, outbreaks of hepatitis B have occurred in long-term care facilities (e.g., assisted living facilities and nursing homes) as the result of lack of infection control practices related to blood glucose monitoring.

Hepatitis B virus remains infectious for at least 7 days on environmental surfaces and is transmissible in the absence of visible blood. Direct percutaneous inoculation of HBV by needles during injection-drug use is an important mode of transmission. Breaks in the skin without overt needle puncture, such as fresh cutaneous scratches, abrasions, burns, or other lesions, may also serve as routes for entry. Nosocomial exposures such as transfusion of blood or blood products, hemodialysis, use of meters and lancets for glucose monitoring, insulin pens, and needle-stick or other "sharps" injuries sustained by hospital personnel have all resulted in HBV transmission. Rare transmission to patients from HBsAg-positive health care personnel has been documented. Outbreaks have been reported among patients in dialysis centers in many countries through failure to adhere to recommended infection control practices against transmission of HBV and other blood-borne pathogens in these settings. IG, heat-treated plasma protein fraction and albumin are considered safe. In the past, outbreaks have been traced to tattoo parlors, acupuncturists, and barbers.

Contamination of mucosal surfaces with infective serum or plasma may occur during mouth pipetting, eye splashes, or other direct contact with mucous membranes of the eyes or mouth, such as hand-to-mouth or hand-to-eye contact when hands are contaminated with infective blood or serum. Transfer of infective material to skin lesions or mucous membranes via inanimate environmental surfaces may occur by touching surfaces of various types of hospital equipment. Contamination of mucosal surfaces with infective secretions other than serum or plasma could occur with contact involving semen.

Perinatal transmission from mother to infant at birth is very efficient. If the mother is positive for both HBsAg and HBeAg, 70%–90% of infants will become infected in the absence of postexposure prophylaxis. The risk of perinatal

---

Hepatitis B Perinatal Transmission*

- If mother positive for HBsAg and HBeAg
  - 70%-90% of infants infected
  - 90% of infected infants become chronically infected
- If positive for HBsAg only
  - 10% of infants infected
  - 90% of infected infants become chronically infected

*in the absence of postexposure prophylaxis

10

Hepatitis B

Global Patterns of Chronic HBV Infection

- High (>8%): 45% of global population
  - lifetime risk of infection >60%
  - early childhood infections common
- Intermediate (2%-7%): 43% of global population
  - lifetime risk of infection 20%-60%
  - infections occur in all age groups
- Low (<2%): 12% of global population
  - lifetime risk of infection <20%
  - most infections occur in adult risk groups

transmission is about 10% if the mother is positive only for HBsAg. As many as 90% of infant HBV infections will progress to chronic infection.

The frequency of infection and patterns of transmission vary in different parts of the world. Approximately 45% of the global population live in areas with a high prevalence of chronic HBV infection (8% or more of the population is HBsAg positive), 43% in areas with a moderate prevalence (2% to 7% of the population is HBsAg positive), and 12% in areas with a low prevalence (less than 2% of the population is HBsAg positive).

In China, Southeast Asia, most of Africa, most Pacific Islands, parts of the Middle East, and the Amazon Basin, 8% to 15% of the population carry the virus. The lifetime risk of HBV infection is greater than 60%, and most infections are acquired at birth or during early childhood, when the risk of developing chronic infections is greatest. In these areas, because most infections are asymptomatic, very little acute disease related to HBV occurs, but rates of chronic liver disease and liver cancer among adults are very high. In the United States, Western Europe, and Australia, HBV infection is a disease of low endemicity. Infection occurs primarily during adulthood, and only 0.1% to 0.5% of the population are chronic carriers. Lifetime risk of HBV infection is less than 20% in low prevalence areas.

Communicability

Persons with either acute or chronic HBV infection should be considered infectious any time that HBsAg is present in the blood. When symptoms are present in persons with acute HBV infection, HBsAg can be found in blood and body fluids for 1–2 months before and after the onset of symptoms.

Secular Trends in the United States

Hepatitis has been reportable in the United States for many years. Hepatitis B became reportable as a distinct entity during the 1970s, after serologic tests to differentiate different types of hepatitis became widely available.

The incidence of reported hepatitis B peaked in the mid-1980s, with about 26,000 cases reported each year. Reported cases have declined since that time, and fell below 10,000 cases for the first time in 1996. The decline in cases during the 1980s and early 1990s is generally attributed to reduction of transmission among men who have sex with men and injection-drug users, as a result of HIV prevention efforts.

During 1990–2004, incidence of acute hepatitis B in the United States declined 75%. The greatest decline (94%) occurred among children and adolescents, coincident with an increase in hepatitis B vaccine coverage. A total of 2,895 cases of hepatitis B were reported in 2012.

An estimated 800,000 to 1.4 million persons in the United States are chronically infected with HBV, and an additional 5,000–8,000 persons become chronically infected each year.

Before routine childhood hepatitis B vaccination was recommended, more than 80% of acute HBV infections occurred among adults. Adolescents accounted for approximately 8% of infections, and children and infants infected through perinatal transmission accounted for approximately 4% each. Perinatal transmission accounted for a disproportionate 24% of chronic infections.

In the United States in 2005, the highest incidence of acute hepatitis B was among adults aged 25–45 years. Approximately 79% of persons with newly acquired hepatitis B infection are known to engage in high-risk sexual activity or injection-drug use. Other known exposures (e.g., occupational, household, travel, and healthcare-related) together account for 5% of new infections. Approximately 16% of persons deny a specific risk factor for infection.

Although HBV infection is uncommon among adults in the general population (the lifetime risk of infection is less than 20%), it is highly prevalent in certain groups. Risk for infection varies with occupation, lifestyle, or environment. Generally, the highest risk for HBV infection is associated with lifestyles, occupations, or environments in which contact with blood from infected persons is frequent. In addition, the prevalence of HBV markers for acute or chronic infection increases with increasing number of years of high-risk behavior. For instance, an estimated 40% of injection-drug users become infected with HBV after 1 year of drug use, while more than 80% are infected after 10 years.

Hepatitis B Prevention Strategies

Hepatitis B vaccines have been available in the United States since 1981. Vaccines have had a large impact on acute Hepatitis B disease. However, the impact of vaccine on chronic HBV disease has been less than optimal. However there are examples of positive effects, such as dramatic reductions in complications of hepatocellular carcinoma observed in Alaska Natives.

The three major risk groups (heterosexuals with multiple partners or contact with infected persons, injection-drug users, and men who have sex with men) are not reached

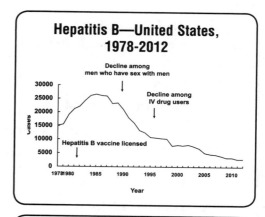

Hepatitis B—United States, 1978-2012

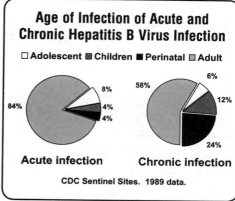

Age of Infection of Acute and Chronic Hepatitis B Virus Infection

☐ Adolescent ■ Children ■ Perinatal ▨ Adult

Acute infection

Chronic infection

CDC Sentinel Sites. 1989 data.

10

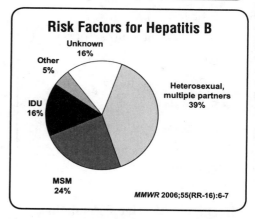

Risk Factors for Hepatitis B

Unknown 16%

Other 5%

IDU 16%

MSM 24%

Heterosexual, multiple partners 39%

MMWR 2006;55(RR-16):6-7

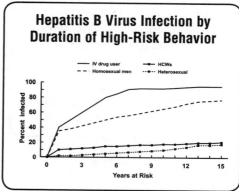

Hepatitis B Virus Infection by Duration of High-Risk Behavior

Hepatitis B

10

effectively by targeted programs. Deterrents to immunization of these groups include lack of awareness of the risk of disease and its consequences, lack of effective public or private sector programs, and vaccine cost. Difficulty in gaining access to these populations is also a problem.

A comprehensive strategy to eliminate hepatitis B virus transmission was recommended in 1991; it includes prenatal testing of pregnant women for HBsAg to identify newborns who require immunoprophylaxis for prevention of perinatal infection and to identify household contacts who should be vaccinated, routine vaccination of infants, vaccination of adolescents, and vaccination of adults at high risk for infection. Recommendations to further enhance vaccination of adults at increased risk of HBV infection were published in 2011.

Hepatitis B Vaccine
Characteristics

A plasma-derived vaccine was licensed in the United States in 1981. It was produced from 22-nm HBsAg particles purified from the plasma of chronically infected humans. The vaccine was safe and effective but was not well accepted, possibly because of unsubstantiated fears of transmission of live HBV and other bloodborne pathogens (e.g., human immunodeficiency virus). This vaccine was removed from the U.S. market in 1992.

The first recombinant hepatitis B vaccine was licensed in the United States in July 1986. A second, similar vaccine was licensed in August 1989.

Recombinant vaccine is produced by inserting a plasmid containing the gene for HBsAg into common baker's yeast (*Saccharomyces cerevisiae*). Yeast cells then produce HBsAg, which is harvested and purified. The recombinant vaccine contains more than 95% HBsAg protein (5 to 40 mcg/mL); yeast-derived proteins may constitute up to 5% of the final product, but no yeast DNA is detectable in the vaccine. HBV infection cannot result from use of the recombinant vaccine, since no potentially infectious viral DNA or complete viral particles are produced in the recombinant system. Vaccine HBsAg is adsorbed to aluminum hydroxide or aluminum hydroxyphosphate sulfate.

Hepatitis B vaccine is produced by two manufacturers in the United States, Merck (Recombivax HB) and GlaxoSmithKline Pharmaceuticals (Engerix-B). Both vaccines are available in both pediatric and adult formulations. Although their antigen content differs, the two vaccines are interchangeable, except for the two-dose schedule for adolescents aged

11 through 15 years. Only Merck vaccine is approved for this schedule. Providers must always follow the manufacturer's dosage recommendations, which may vary by product.

Both the pediatric and adult formulations of Recombivax HB are approved for use in any age group. For example, the adult formulation of Recombivax HB may be used in children (0.5 mL) and adolescents (0.5 mL). However, pediatric Engerix-B is approved for use only in children and adolescents younger than 20 years of age. The adult formulation of Engerix-B is not approved for use in infants and children but may be used in both adolescents (11 through 19 years of age) and adults.

Engerix-B contains aluminum hydroxide as an adjuvant, and Recombivax HB contains aluminum hydroxyphosphate sulfate as an adjuvant. Both vaccines are supplied in single-dose vials and syringes, and no formulation of either vaccine contains thimerosal or any other preservative.

Immunogenicity and Vaccine Efficacy

After three intramuscular doses of hepatitis B vaccine, more than 90% of healthy adults and more than 95% of infants, children, and adolescents (from birth to 19 years of age) develop adequate antibody responses. However, there is an age-specific decline in immunogenicity. After age 40 years, approximately 90% of recipients respond to a three-dose series, and by 60 years, only 75% of vaccinees develop protective antibody titers. The proportion of recipients who respond to each dose varies by age.

The vaccine is 80% to 100% effective in preventing infection or clinical hepatitis in those who receive the complete vaccine series. Larger vaccine doses (2 to 4 times the normal adult dose), or an increased number of doses, are required to induce protective antibody in most hemodialysis patients and may also be necessary for other immunocompromised persons.

The recommended dosage of vaccine differs depending on the age of the recipient and type of vaccine (see table). Hemodialysis patients should receive a 40-mcg dose in a series of three or four doses. Recombivax HB has a special dialysis patient formulation that contains 40 mcg/mL.

The deltoid muscle is the recommended site for hepatitis B vaccination in adults and children, while the antero-lateral thigh is recommended for infants and neonates. Immunogenicity of vaccine in adults is lower when injections are given in the gluteus. Hepatitis B vaccine should be administered to newborns using a needle of at least 5/8 inch length and to older children and adults of at least 1 inch length. Hepatitis B vaccine administered by any route

Hepatitis B

Recommended doses of currently licensed formulations of hepatitis B vaccine, by age group and vaccine type

Age Group	Single-Antigen Vaccine				Combination Vaccine			
	Recombivax HB		Engerix-B		Pediarix		Twinrix	
	Dose (mcg)*	Volume (mL)	Dose (mcg)*	Volume (mL)	Dose (mcg)*	Volume (mL)	Dose (mcg)*	Volume (mL)
Infants (<1 year)	5	0.5	10	0.5	10	0.5	N/A	N/A
Children (1-10 years)	5	0.5	10	0.5	10	0.5	N/A	N/A
Adolescents 11-15 yrs	10†	1.0	N/A	N/A	N/A	N/A	N/A	N/A
11-19 yrs	5	0.5	10	0.5	N/A	N/A	N/A	N/A
Adults (>20 years)	10	1.0	20	1.0	N/A	N/A	20	1.0
Hemodialysis patients and other immunocompromised persons <20 yrs§	5	0.5	10	N/A	N/A	N/A	N/A	N/A
>20 yrs	40¶	1.0	40‡	N/A	N/A	N/A	N/A	N/A

* Recombinant hepatitis B surface antigen protein dose.
† Adult formulation administered on a 2-dose schedule.
§ Higher doses might be more immunogenic, but no specific recommendations have been made.
¶ Dialysis formulation administered on a 3-dose schedule at 0, 1, and 6 months.
‡ Two 1.0 mL doses administered at one site, on a 4-dose schedule at 0, 1, 2, and 6 months.
** Not applicable.

or site other than intramuscularly in the anterolateral thigh or deltoid muscle should not be counted as valid and should be repeated unless serologic testing indicates that an adequate response has been achieved.

Available data show that vaccine-induced antibody levels decline with time. However, immune memory remains intact for more than 20 years following immunization, and both adults and children with declining antibody levels are still protected against significant HBV infection (i.e., clinical disease, HBsAg antigenemia, or significant elevation of liver enzymes). Exposure to HBV results in an anamnestic anti-HBs response that prevents clinically significant HBV infection. Chronic HBV infection has only rarely been documented among vaccine responders.

For adults and children with normal immune status, booster doses of vaccine are not recommended. Routine serologic testing to assess immune status of vaccinees is not recommended. The need for booster doses after longer intervals will continue to be assessed as additional information becomes available.

For hemodialysis patients, the need for booster doses should be assessed by annual testing of vaccinees for antibody levels, and booster doses should be provided when antibody levels decline below 10 mIU/mL.

Hepatitis B Vaccine Long-term Efficacy

- Immunologic memory established following vaccination
- Exposure to HBV results in anamnestic anti-HBs response
- Chronic infection rarely documented among vaccine responders

Hepatitis B Vaccine

- Routine booster doses are NOT routinely recommended for any group

Vaccination Schedule and Use
Infants and Children

Hepatitis B vaccination is recommended for all infants soon after birth and before hospital discharge. Infants and children younger than 11 years of age should receive 0.5 mL (5 mcg) of pediatric or adult formulation Recombivax HB (Merck) or 0.5 mL (10 mcg) of pediatric Engerix-B (GlaxoSmithKline). Primary vaccination consists of three intramuscular doses of vaccine. The usual schedule is 0, 1 to 2, and 6 to 18 months. Infants whose mothers are HBsAg positive or whose HBsAg status is unknown should receive the last dose by 6 months of age (12 to 15 months if Comvax is used).

Because the highest titers of anti-HBs are achieved when the last two doses of vaccine are spaced at least 4 months apart, schedules that achieve this spacing are preferable. However, schedules with 2-month intervals between doses, which conform to schedules for other childhood vaccines, have been shown to produce good antibody responses and may be appropriate in populations in which it is difficult to ensure that infants will be brought back for all their vaccinations. However, the third dose must be administered at least 8 weeks after the second dose, and at least 16 weeks after the first dose. For infants, the third dose should not be given earlier than 24 weeks of age. It is not necessary to add doses or restart the series if the interval between doses is longer than recommended.

Preterm infants born to HBsAg-positive women and women with unknown HBsAg status must receive immunoprophylaxis with hepatitis B vaccine and hepatitis B immune globulin (HBIG) within 12 hours of birth. See the section on Postexposure Management for additional information. Preterm infants weighing less than 2,000 grams have a decreased response to hepatitis B vaccine administered before 1 month of age. However, by chronologic age 1 month, preterm infants, regardless of initial birthweight or gestational age, are as likely to respond as adequately as full-term infants. Preterm infants of low birthweight whose mothers are HBsAg negative can receive the first dose of the hepatitis B vaccine series at chronologic age 1 month. Preterm infants discharged from the hospital before chronologic age 1 month can receive hepatitis B vaccine at discharge if they are medically stable and have gained weight consistently. The full recommended dose should be used. Divided or reduced doses are not recommended.

Comvax

Hepatitis B vaccine is available in combination with *Haemophilus influenzae* type b (Hib) vaccine as Comvax (Merck). Each dose of Comvax contains 7.5 mcg of

Hepatitis B Vaccine Routine Infant Schedule

Dose	Usual Age	Minimum Interval
Primary 1	Birth	---
Primary 2	1-2 months	4 weeks
Primary 3	6-18 months*	8 weeks**

* infants who mothers are HBsAg+ or whose HBsAg status is unknown should receive the third dose at 6 months of age

** at least 16 weeks after the first dose

Third Dose of Hepatitis B Vaccine

- Minimum of 8 weeks after second dose, and
- At least 16 weeks after first dose, and
- For infants, at least 24 weeks of age

Preterm Infants

- Birth dose and HBIG if mother HBsAg positive (within 12 hours of birth)
- Preterm infants who weigh less than 2,000 grams have a decreased response to vaccine administered before 1 month of age
- Delay first dose until chronologic age 1 month if mother documented to be HBsAg negative at the time of birth

Hepatitis B

10

COMVAX

- Hepatitis B-Hib combination
- Use when either antigen is indicated
- Cannot use at younger than 6 weeks of age
- May be used in infants whose mother is HBsAg positive or status is unknown

Pediarix

- DTaP – Hep B – IPV combination
- Approved for 3 doses at 2, 4 and 6 months
- Not approved for booster doses
- Approved for children 6 weeks to 7 years of age
- May be used interchangeably with other pertussis-containing vaccines if necessary
- Can be given at 2, 4, and 6 months to infants who received a birth dose of hepatitis B vaccine (total of 4 doses)
- May be used in infants whose mothers are HBsAg positive or status unknown

PRP-OMP Hib vaccine (PedvaxHIB), and 5 mcg of hepatitis B surface antigen. The dose of hepatitis B surface antigen is the same as that contained in Merck's pediatric formulation. The immunogenicity of the combination vaccine is equivalent to that of the individual antigens administered at separate sites.

Comvax is licensed for use at 2, 4, and 12 through 15 months of age. It may be used whenever either antigen is indicated and the other antigen is not contraindicated. However, the vaccine must not be administered to infants younger than 6 weeks of age because of potential suppression of the immune response to the Hib component (see Chapter 7, *Haemophilus influenzae* type b, for more details). Although it is not labeled for this indication by FDA, ACIP recommends that Comvax may be used in infants whose mothers are HBsAg positive or whose HBsAg status is unknown. Comvax will be removed from existing contracts and pricing programs in early 2015.

Pediarix

In 2002, the Food and Drug Administration approved Pediarix (GlaxoSmithKline), the first pentavalent (5-component) combination vaccine licensed in the United States. Pediarix contains DTaP (Infanrix), hepatitis B (Engerix-B), and inactivated polio vaccines. In prelicensure studies, children who received these vaccine antigens together as Pediarix were at least as likely to develop a protective level of antibody as those who received the vaccines separately; and their antibody titers were also at least as high.

The minimum age for the first dose of Pediarix is 6 weeks, so it cannot be used for the birth dose of the hepatitis B series. Pediarix is approved for the first three doses of the DTaP and IPV series, which are usually given at about 2, 4, and 6 months of age; it is not approved for fourth or fifth (booster) doses of the DTaP or IPV series. However, Pediarix is approved for use through 6 years of age. A child who is behind schedule can still receive Pediarix as long as it is given for doses 1, 2, or 3 of the series, and the child is younger than 7 years of age.

A dose of Pediarix inadvertently administered as the fourth or fifth dose of the DTaP or IPV series does not need to be repeated.

Pediarix may be used interchangeably with other pertussis-containing vaccines if necessary (although ACIP prefers the use of the same brand of DTaP for all doses of the series, if possible). It can be given at 2, 4, and 6 months to infants who received a birth dose of hepatitis B vaccine (total of 4 doses of hepatitis B vaccine). Although not labeled for this indication by FDA, Pediarix may be used in infants whose mothers are HBsAg positive or whose HBsAg status is unknown.

Adolescents

Routine hepatitis B vaccination is recommended for all children and adolescents through age 18 years. All children not previously vaccinated with hepatitis B vaccine should be vaccinated at 11 or 12 years of age with the age-appropriate dose of vaccine. When adolescent vaccination programs are being considered, local data should be considered to determine the ideal age group (e.g., preadolescents, young adolescents) to vaccinate to achieve the highest vaccination rates. The vaccination schedule should be flexible and should take into account the feasibility of delivering three doses of vaccine to this age group. Unvaccinated older adolescents should be vaccinated whenever possible. Those in groups at risk for HBV infection (e.g., Asian and Pacific Islanders, sexually active) should be identified and vaccinated in settings serving this age group (i.e., schools, sexually transmitted disease clinics, detention facilities, drug treatment centers).

Persons younger than 20 years of age should receive 0.5 mL (5 mcg) of pediatric or adult formulation Recombivax HB (Merck) or 0.5 mL (10 mcg) of pediatric formulation Engerix-B (GlaxoSmithKline). The adult formulation of Engerix-B may be used in adolescents, but the approved dose is 1 mL (20 mcg).

The usual schedule for adolescents is two doses separated by no less than 4 weeks, and a third dose 4 to 6 months after the second dose. If an accelerated schedule is needed, the minimum interval between the first two doses is 4 weeks, and the minimum interval between the second and third doses is 8 weeks. However, the first and third doses should be separated by no less than 16 weeks. Doses given at less than these minimum intervals should not be counted and should be repeated.

In 1999, the Food and Drug Administration approved an alternative hepatitis B vaccination schedule for adolescents 11 through 15 years of age. This alternative schedule is for two 1.0-mL (10 mcg) doses of Recombivax HB separated by 4 to 6 months. Seroconversion rates and postvaccination anti-HBs antibody titers were similar using this schedule or the standard schedule of three 5-mcg doses of Recombivax HB. This alternative schedule is approved only for adolescents 11 through 15 years of age, and for Merck's hepatitis B vaccine. The 2-dose schedule should be completed by the 16th birthday.

10

Hepatitis B Vaccine Adolescent Vaccination

- Routine vaccination recommended through age 18 years
- Integrate into routine adolescent immunization visit
- Flexible schedules

Hepatitis B Vaccine Adolescent and Adult Schedule

Dose	Usual Interval	Minimum Interval
Primary 1	---	---
Primary 2	1 month	4 weeks
Primary 3	5 months	8 weeks*

*third dose must be separated from first dose by at least 16 weeks

Alternative Adolescent Vaccination Schedule

- Two 1.0 mL (10 mcg) doses of Recombivax HB separated by 4-6 months
- Approved only for adolescents 11-15 years of age
- Only applies to Merck hepatitis B vaccine

Hepatitis B

Adults at Risk for HBV Infection

- Sexual exposure
  - sex partners of HBsAg-positive persons
  - sexually active persons not in a long-term, mutually monogamous relationship*
  - persons seeking evaluation or treatment for a sexually transmitted disease
  - men who have sex with men
- Percutaneous or mucosal exposure to blood
  - current or recent IDU
  - household contacts of HBsAg-positive persons
  - residents and staff of facilities for developmentally disabled persons
  - healthcare and public safety workers with risk for exposure to blood or blood-contaminated body fluids
  - persons with end-stage renal disease
  - persons with diabetes mellitus
- Other groups
  - international travelers to regions with high or intermediate levels (HBsAg prevalence of 2% or higher) of endemic HBV infection
  - persons with HIV infection

*persons with more than one sex partner during the previous 6 months

Adults (20 Years of Age and Older)

Routine preexposure vaccination should be considered for adults who are at increased risk of HBV infection. Adults 20 years of age and older should receive 1 mL (10 mcg) of pediatric or adult formulation Recombivax HB (Merck) or 1 mL (20 mcg) of adult formulation Engerix-B (GlaxoSmithKline). The pediatric formulation of Engerix-B is not approved for use in adults.

The usual schedule for adults is two doses separated by no less than 4 weeks, and a third dose 4 to 6 months after the second dose. If an accelerated schedule is needed, the minimum interval between the first two doses is 4 weeks, and the minimum interval between the second and third doses is 8 weeks. However, the first and third doses should be separated by no less than 16 weeks. Doses given at less than these minimum intervals should not be counted and should be repeated. It is not necessary to restart the series or add doses because of an extended interval between doses.

Hepatitis B vaccination is recommended for all unvaccinated adults at risk for HBV infection and for all adults requesting protection from HBV infection. Acknowledgment of a specific risk factor should not be a requirement for vaccination.

Persons at risk for infection by sexual exposure include sex partners of HBsAg-positive persons, sexually active persons who are not in a long-term, mutually monogamous relationship (e.g., persons with more than one sex partner during the previous 6 months), persons seeking evaluation or treatment for a sexually transmitted disease, and men who have sex with men.

Persons at risk for infection by percutaneous or mucosal exposure to blood include current or recent injection-drug users (IDU), household contacts of HBsAg-positive persons, residents and staff of facilities for developmentally disabled persons, healthcare and public safety workers with risk for exposure to blood or blood-contaminated body fluids, and persons with end-stage renal disease, including predialysis, hemodialysis, peritoneal dialysis, and home dialysis patients.

Adults with diabetes mellitus (type 1 or type 2) are at increased risk of HBV infection, probably because of breaches in infection control during assisted blood glucose monitoring (e.g., reuse of single patient finger stick devices). In October 2011, ACIP recommended that all previously unvaccinated adults 19 through 59 years of age with diabetes mellitus type 1 and type 2 be vaccinated against hepatitis B as soon as possible after a diagnosis of diabetes is made. ACIP also recommends that unvaccinated adults 60 years of age or older with diabetes may be vaccinated at the discretion of the treating clinician after assessing their risk and the likelihood of an adequate immune response to vaccination.

Other groups at risk include international travelers to regions with high or intermediate levels (HBsAg prevalence of 2% or higher) of endemic HBV infection, long term travelers, and those who may engage in high-risk behaviors or provide health-care while traveling. Persons with HIV infection are also at increased risk.

In settings in which a high proportion of adults have risks for HBV infection (e.g., sexually transmitted disease/human immunodeficiency virus testing and treatment facilities, drug-abuse treatment and prevention settings, healthcare settings targeting services to IDUs, healthcare settings targeting services to MSM, and correctional facilities), ACIP recommends hepatitis B vaccination for all unvaccinated adults. In other primary care and specialty medical settings in which adults at risk for HBV infection receive care, healthcare providers should inform all patients about the health benefits of vaccination, risks for HBV infection, and persons for whom vaccination is recommended; and should vaccinate any adults who report risks for HBV infection or request protection from HBV infection.

Twinrix

In 2001, the Food and Drug Administration approved a combination hepatitis A and hepatitis B vaccine (Twinrix, GlaxoSmithKline). Each dose of Twinrix contains 720 ELISA units of hepatitis A vaccine (equivalent to a pediatric dose of Havrix), and 20 mcg of hepatitis B surface antigen protein (equivalent to an adult dose of Engerix-B). The vaccine is administered in a three-dose series at 0, 1, and 6 months. Appropriate spacing of the doses must be maintained to assure long-term protection from both vaccines. The first and third doses of Twinrix should be separated by at least 6 months. The first and second doses should be separated by at least 4 weeks, and the second and third doses should be separated by at least 5 months. In 2007, the FDA approved an alternative Twinrix schedule of doses at 0, 7, and 21–31 days and a booster dose 12 months after the first dose. It is not necessary to restart the series or add doses if the interval between doses is longer than the recommended interval.

Twinrix is approved for persons 18 years of age and older, and can be administered to persons in this age group for whom either hepatitis A and hepatitis B vaccines is recommended. Because the hepatitis B component of Twinrix is equivalent to a standard adult dose of hepatitis B vaccine, the schedule is the same whether Twinrix or single-antigen hepatitis B vaccine is used. Single-antigen hepatitis A vaccine can be used to complete a series begun with Twinrix or vice versa. See the Hepatitis A chapter for details.

Hepatitis B

Prevaccination Serologic Testing

- Not indicated before routine vaccination of infants or children
- Recommended for
  - all persons born in Africa, Asia, the Pacific Islands, and other regions with HBsAg prevalence of 2% or higher
  - household, sex, and needle-sharing contacts of HBsAg-positive persons
  - men who have sex with men
  - injection drug users
  - certain persons receiving cytotoxic or immunosuppressive therapy

Postvaccination Serologic Testing

- Not routinely recommended following vaccination of infants, children, adolescents, or most adults
- Recommended for:
  - chronic hemodialysis patients
  - other immunocompromised persons
  - persons with HIV infection
  - sex partners of HBsAg+ persons
  - infants born to HBsAg+ women
  - certain healthcare personnel
    - healthcare personnel who have contact with patients or blood should be tested for anti-HBs (antibody to hepatitis B surface antigen) 1 to 2 months after completion of the 3-dose series

Serologic Testing of Vaccine Recipients
Prevaccination Serologic Testing

The decision to screen potential vaccine recipients for prior infection depends on the cost of vaccination, the cost of testing for susceptibility, and the expected prevalence of immune persons in the population being screened. Prevaccination testing is recommended for all foreign-born persons (including immigrants, refugees, asylum seekers, and internationally adopted children) born in Africa, Asia, the Pacific Islands, and other regions with endemicity of HBV infection; household, sex, and needle-sharing contacts of HBsAg-positive persons; men who have sex with men; injection drug users; and certain persons receiving cytotoxic or immunosuppressive therapy. Screening is usually cost-effective, and should be considered for groups with a high risk of HBV infection (prevalence of HBV markers 20% or higher), such as men who have sex with men, injection-drug users, and incarcerated persons. Screening is usually not cost-effective for groups with a low expected prevalence of HBV serologic markers, such as health professionals in their training years.

Serologic testing is not recommended before routine vaccination of infants, children, or adolescents.

Postvaccination Serologic Testing

Testing for immunity following vaccination is not recommended routinely but should be considered for persons whose subsequent management depends on knowledge of their immune status, such as chronic hemo-dialysis patients, other immunocompromised persons, and persons with HIV infection. Testing is also recommended for sex partners of HBsAg-positive persons. Postvaccination testing should be performed 1 to 2 months after completion of the vaccine series.

Infants born to HBsAg-positive women should be tested for HBsAg and antibody to HBsAg (anti-HBs) 1 to 2 months after completion of the final dose of the hepatitis B vaccine series, and at least age 9 months (generally at the next well-child visit). If HBsAg is not present and anti-HBs antibody is present, children can be considered to be protected.

Healthcare personnel who have contact with blood and body fluids of patients who might be infected with HBV, or who are at ongoing risk for injuries with sharp instruments or needlesticks should be routinely tested for antibody 1 to 2 months after completion of the 3-dose hepatitis B vaccine series, assuming they are not previously vaccinated. Data since 2002 indicate the rates of reported exposures are highest among healthcare trainees, and vary by occupation and job duties among non-trainee healthcare personnel (e.g., low for office-based counseling, higher for healthcare personnel performing procedures). All health-care institutions should ensure healthcare personnel receive training to recognize and report exposures, have systems in place to facilitate reporting and postexposure assessment, and have prophylaxis readily accessible for timely administration.

Increasingly, healthcare personnel with documentation of routine hepatitis B vaccination received the series in infancy or as catch-up vaccination in adolescence without postvaccination testing. Antibody to vaccine antigen wanes over time, although protection persists in vaccine recipients who responded initially. A negative anti-HBs serologic response in healthcare personnel who received hepatitis B vaccine in the distant past will not distinguish between failure to respond to the initial vaccination series (lack of protection) and response to the initial vaccination series with subsequent waning of antibody (protected).

CDC recommends evaluating healthcare personnel for hepatitis B virus protection either at matriculation or hire (preexposure) or with post-exposure management, depending on the occupational risk for exposure to potentially contaminated blood or body fluids, and the prevalence of hepatitis B infection in the patient population. Booster doses of hepatitis B vaccine are not recommended for persons with normal immune systems. However, previously vaccinated healthcare personnel for whom preexposure evaluation fails to detect protective anti-HBs should receive a "challenge dose" of hepatitis B vaccine to assess protection, which will be indicated by a rise in anti-HBs, or "memory" response to vaccine antigen.

Healthcare personnel who respond to the challenge dose do not require additional management, even if exposed. Healthcare personnel who do not respond to a challenge dose should complete revaccination and retesting for anti-HBs. Postexposure management of healthcare personnel ensures hepatitis B prophylaxis and assesses vaccine response as dictated by the HBsAg status of the source patient. Detailed guidance for pre- or postexposure evaluation and management of healthcare personnel for hepatitis B protection was published in 2013.

Vaccine Nonresponse

Several factors have been associated with nonresponse to hepatitis B vaccine. These include vaccine factors (e.g., dose, schedule, injection site) and host factors. Older age (40 years and older), male sex, obesity, smoking, and chronic illness have been independently associated with nonresponse to hepatitis B vaccine. Additional vaccine doses for persons who receive post-vaccination testing and who fail to respond to a primary vaccination series administered in the deltoid muscle produce adequate response in 15% to 25% of vaccinees after one additional dose and in 30% to 50% after three additional doses.

Persons who do not respond to the first series of hepatitis B vaccine should complete a second three-dose vaccine series. The second vaccine series should be given on the usual 0, 1, 6-month schedule. Healthcare personnel and others for whom postvaccination serologic testing is recommended should be retested 1 to 2 months after completion of the second vaccine series.

Fewer than 5% of persons receiving six doses of hepatitis B vaccine administered by the appropriate schedule in the deltoid muscle fail to develop detectable anti-HBs antibody. One reason for persistent nonresponse to hepatitis B vaccine is chronic infection with HBV. Persons who fail to develop detectable anti-HBs after six doses should be tested for HBsAg. Persons who are found to be HBsAg positive should be counseled accordingly. Persons who fail to respond to two appropriately administered three-dose series, and who are HBsAg negative should be considered susceptible to HBV infection and should be counseled regarding precautions to prevent HBV infection and the need to obtain HBIG prophylaxis for any known or probable parenteral exposure to HBsAg-positive blood (see the postexposure prophylaxis table in this chapter).

It is difficult to interpret a negative anti-HBs serologic response in a person who received hepatitis B vaccine in the past and was not tested after vaccination. Without postvaccination testing 1 to 2 months after completion of the series, it is not possible to determine if persons testing negative years after vaccination represent true vaccine failure (i.e., no initial response), or have anti-HBs antibody that has waned to below a level detectable by the test. The latter is the most likely explanation, because up to 60% of vaccinated people lose detectable antibody (but not protection) 9 to 15 years after vaccination.

Postexposure Management

After a percutaneous (needle stick, laceration, bite) or permucosal exposure that contains or might contain HBV, blood should be obtained from the person who was the source of the exposure to determine their HBsAg status. Management of the exposed person depends on the HBsAg status of the source and the vaccination and anti-HBs response status of the exposed person. Recommended postexposure prophylaxis is described in the following table.

Management of Nonresponse to Hepatitis B Vaccine

- Complete a second series of three doses
- Should be given on the usual schedule of 0, 1 and 6 months (may be given on a 0, 1, and 4 month or a 0, 2 and 4 month schedule)
- Retest 1-2 months after completing the second series

Persistent Nonresponse to Hepatitis B Vaccine

- Less than 5% of vaccinees do not develop anti-HBs after 6 valid doses
- May be nonresponder or "hyporesponder"
- Check HBsAg status
- If exposed, treat as nonresponder with postexposure prophylaxis

10

Recommended postexposure prophylaxis
for percutaneous or permucosal exposure to hepatitis B virus –
Advisory Committee on Immunization Practices, United States

Vaccination and antibody response status of exposed person	Treatment		
	Source HBsAg-positive	Source HBsAg-negative	Source not tested or status unknown
Unvaccinated	HBIG x 1; Initiate HB vaccine series	Initiate HB vaccine series	Initiate HB vaccine series
Previously vaccinated:			
· Known responder	No treatment	No treatment	No treatment
· Known nonresponder: - After 3 doses	HBIG x 1 and initiate revaccination	No treatment	- If known high-risk source, treat as if source were HBsAg-positive.
- After 6 doses	HBIG x 2 (separated by 1 month)	No treatment	- If known high-risk source, treat as if source were HBsAg-positive.
· Antibody response unknown	Test exposed person for anti-HBs - If adequate,* no treatment - If inadequate,* HBIG x 1 and vaccine booster	No treatment	Test exposed person for anti-HBs - If adequate,* no treatment - If inadequate,* HBIG x 1 and vaccine booster

Abbreviations: HbsAg = hepatitis B surface antigen; HBIG = hepatitis B immune globulin; anti-HBs = antibody to hepatitis B surface antigen; HB = hepatitis B.

Source: Adapted from CDC. A comprehensive immunization strategy to eliminate transmission of hepatitis B virus infection in the United States: recommendations of the Advisory Committee on Immunization Practices (ACIP). Part II: Immunization of adults. *MMWR* 2006;55(No. RR-16).
* A seroprotective (adequate) level of anti-HBs after completion of a vaccination series is defined as anti-HBs $\geq$10 mIU/mL; a response <10 mIU/mL is inadequate and is not a reliable indicator of protection.
Source: *MMWR* 2011:60(RR-7)42.

Hepatitis B vaccine is recommended as part of the therapy used to prevent hepatitis B infection following exposure to HBV. Depending on the exposure circumstance, the hepatitis B vaccine series may be started at the same time as treatment with hepatitis B immune globulin (HBIG).

HBIG is prepared by cold ethanol fraction of plasma from selected donors with high anti-HBs titers; it contains an anti-HBs titer of at least 1:100,000, by RIA. It is used for passive immunization for accidental (percutaneous, mucous membrane) exposure, sexual exposure to an HBsAg-positive person, perinatal exposure of an infant, or household

Hepatitis B

Prevention of Perinatal Hepatitis B Virus Infection

- Begin treatment within 12 hours of birth
- Hepatitis B vaccine (first dose) and HBIG at different sites
- Complete vaccination series at 6 months of age
- Test for response after completion of at least 3 doses of the HepB series at 9 through 18 months of age (generally at the next well-child visit)

exposure of an infant younger than 12 months old to a primary caregiver with acute hepatitis B. Most candidates for HBIG are, by definition, in a high-risk category and should therefore also receive hepatitis B vaccine.

Immune globulin (IG) is prepared by cold ethanol fractionation of pooled plasma and contains low titers of anti-HBs. Because titers are relatively low, IG has no valid current use for HBV disease unless hepatitis B immune globulin is unavailable.

Infants born to women who are HBsAg-positive (i.e., acutely or chronically infected with HBV) are at extremely high risk of HBV transmission and chronic HBV infection. Hepatitis B vaccination and one dose of HBIG administered within 24 hours after birth are 85%–95% effective in preventing chronic HBV infection. Hepatitis B vaccine administered alone beginning within 24 hours after birth is 70%–95% effective in preventing perinatal HBV infection.

The first dose of hepatitis B vaccine and HBIG (0.5 mL) should be given intramuscularly (IM), and are recommended for administration within 12 hours of birth. The hepatitis B vaccine dose is given at the same time as HBIG, but at a different site. The second and third vaccine doses should be given 1 to 2 months and 6 months, respectively, after the first dose. To monitor the success of therapy, testing for HBsAg and anti-HBs is recommended 1-2 months after the final vaccine dose but not before 9 months of age. If the mother's HBsAg status is not known at the time of birth, the hepatitis B vaccination of the infant should be initiated within 12 hours of birth.

HBIG given at birth does not interfere with the immune response to hepatitis B vaccine or other vaccines administered at 2 months of age.

Infants born to HBsAg-positive women and who weigh less than 2,000 grams at birth should receive postexposure prophylaxis as described above. However, the initial vaccine dose (at birth) should not be counted. The next dose in the series should be administered when the infant is chronologic age 1 month, followed by a third dose 1 to 2 months after the second , and the fourth dose at 6 months of age. To monitor the success of postexposure prophylaxis, testing for HBsAg and anti-HBs is recommended 1-2 months after the final vaccine dose, but not before 9 months of age.

Women admitted for delivery whose HBsAg status is unknown should have blood drawn for testing. While test results are pending, the infant should receive the first dose of hepatitis B vaccine (without HBIG) within 12 hours of birth. If the mother is found to be HBsAg positive, the infant should receive HBIG as soon as possible but not later than 7 days of age. If the infant does not receive HBIG, it is important that the second dose of vaccine be administered at 1 or 2 months of age.

Infants with birth weight less than 2,000 grams whose mother's HBsAg status is unknown should receive hepatitis B vaccine within 12 hours of birth. If the maternal HBsAg status cannot be determined within 12 hours of birth HBIG should also be administered. The immune response to hepatitis B vaccine is less reliable in infants weighing less than 2,000 grams. The vaccine dose administered at birth should not be counted as part of the series, and the infant should receive three additional doses beginning at age 1 month (total number of doses should be at least 4). The vaccine series should be completed by 6 months of age.

Non-Occupational Exposure to an HBsAg-Positive Source

Persons who have written documentation of a complete hepatitis B vaccine series and who did not receive postvaccination testing should receive a single vaccine booster dose. Persons who are in the process of being vaccinated but who have not completed the vaccine series should receive the appropriate dose of HBIG and should complete the vaccine series. Unvaccinated persons should receive both HBIG and a dose of hepatitis B vaccine as soon as possible after exposure (preferably within 24 hours) and complete the 3-dose hepatitis B vaccine series according to the appropriate schedule. Hepatitis B vaccine may be administered simultaneously with HBIG in a separate injection site.

Household, sex, and needle-sharing contacts of HBsAg-positive persons should be identified. Unvaccinated sex partners and household and needle-sharing contacts should be tested for susceptibility to HBV infection and should receive the first dose of hepatitis B vaccine immediately after collection of blood for serologic testing. Susceptible persons should complete the vaccine series using an age-appropriate vaccine dose and schedule. Persons who are not fully vaccinated should complete the vaccine series.

Non-Occupational Exposure to a Source with Unknown HBsAg Status

Persons with written documentation of a complete hepatitis B vaccine series require no further treatment. Persons who are not fully vaccinated should complete the vaccine series. Unvaccinated persons should receive the hepatitis B vaccine series with the first dose administered as soon as possible after exposure, preferably within 24 hours.

Hepatitis B

10

**Hepatitis B Vaccine
Contraindications and Precautions**

- Severe allergic reaction to a vaccine component or following a prior dose

- Moderate or severe acute illness

**Hepatitis B Vaccine
Adverse Reactions**

- Anaphylaxis – one case per 1.1 million doses

Contraindications and Precautions to Vaccination

Hepatitis B vaccination is contraindicated for persons with a history of hypersensitivity to yeast or any other vaccine component. Despite a theoretic risk for allergic reaction to vaccination in persons with allergy to *Saccharomyces cerevisiae* (baker's yeast), no evidence exists to document adverse reactions after vaccination of persons with a history of yeast allergy.

Persons with a history of serious adverse events (e.g. anaphylaxis) after receipt of hepatitis B vaccine should not receive additional doses. As with other vaccines, vaccination of persons with moderate or severe acute illness, with or without fever, should be deferred until illness resolves. Vaccination is not contraindicated in persons with a history of multiple sclerosis (MS), Guillain-Barré syndrome (GBS), autoimmune disease (e.g. systemic lupus erythematosis or rheumatoid arthritis) or other chronic diseases.

Pregnancy is not a contraindication to vaccination. Limited data suggest that developing fetuses are not at risk for adverse events when hepatitis B vaccine is administered to pregnant women. Available vaccines contain non-infectious HBsAg and should cause no risk of infection to the fetus.

Adverse Events Following Vaccination

Reported episodes of alopecia (hair loss) after rechallenge with hepatitis B vaccine suggest that vaccination might very rarely trigger episodes of alopecia. However, a population-based study found no statistically significant association between alopecia and hepatitis B vaccination.

In rare instances, other illnesses have been reported after hepatitis B vaccination, including GBS, chronic fatigue syndrome, neurologic disorders (e.g. leukoencephalitis, optic neuritis, and transverse myelitis), rheumatoid arthritis, type 1 diabetes, and autoimmune disease. However, no causal association between those conditions or any chronic illness and hepatitis B vaccine has been demonstrated. Reviews by scientific panels have also found no causal association between hepatitis B vaccination and MS.

Adverse Reactions Following Vaccination

Anaphylaxis has occurred after hepatitis B vaccination, with an estimated incidence of one case per 1.1 million vaccine doses distributed (95% confidence interval = 0.1 - 3.9) among children and adolescents.

Vaccine Storage and Handling

HepB vaccine should be maintained at refrigerator temperature between 35°F and 46°F (2°C and 8°C). Manufacturer package inserts contain additional information and can be found at http://www.fda.gov/BiologicsBloodVaccines/Vaccines/ApprovedProducts/ucm093830.htm. For complete information on best practices and recommendations please refer to CDC's Vaccine Storage and Handling Toolkit, http://www.cdc.gov/vaccines/recs/storage/toolkit/storage-handling-toolkit.pdf.

Acknowledgment

The editors thank Drs. Trudy Murphy, Phyllis Kozarsky, and Philip Spradling, CDC, for their assistance in updating this chapter.

Selected References

Ascherio A, Zhang SM, Hernan MA, et al. Hepatitis B vaccination and the risk of multiple sclerosis. *N Engl J Med* 2001;344:327–32.

CDC. A comprehensive immunization strategy to eliminate transmission of hepatitis B virus infection in the United States: recommendations of the Advisory Committee on Immunization Practices (ACIP). Part 1: Immunization of infants, children, and adolescents. *MMWR* 2005;54(No. RR-16):1–32.

CDC. A comprehensive immunization strategy to eliminate transmission of hepatitis B virus infection in the United States. Recommendations of the Advisory Committee on Immunization Practices (ACIP) Part II: Immunization of Adults. *MMWR* 2006;55(No. RR-16):1–33.

CDC. Recommendations for identification and public health management of persons with chronic hepatitis B virus infection. *MMWR* 2008;57(RR-8);9-11.

CDC. CDC guidance for evaluating health-care personnel for hepatitis B virus protection and for administering posexposure management. *MMWR* 2013;62(RR-10): 1-19.

CDC. Immunization of health-care personnel. Recommendations of the Advisory Committee on Immunization Practices (ACIP). *MMWR* 2011;60(RR-7):1-45.

CDC. Use of hepatitis B vaccination for adults with diabetes mellitus. Recommendations of the Advisory Committee on Immunization Practices (ACIP). *MMWR* 2011;60(No. 50):1709-11.

10

Institute of Medicine. 2012. Adverse effects of vaccines: Evidence and causality. Washington D.C. The National Academies Press.

Institute of Medicine. 2002. Immunization Safety Review: Hepatitis B Vaccine and Demyelinating Neurological Disorders. Washington D.C. The National Academy Press.

Lewis E, Shinefield HR, Woodruff BA, et al. Safety of neonatal hepatitis B vaccine administration. *Pediatr Infect Dis J* 2001;20:1049–54.

Van Damme P, Ward J, Shouval D, Wiersma S, Zanetti A. Hepatitis B vaccine. In: Plotkin SA, Orenstein WA, Offit P, eds. *Vaccines*. 6th edition. China: Saunders; 2013.

Poland GA, Jacobson RM. Clinical practice: prevention of hepatitis B with the hepatitis B vaccine. *N Engl J Med* 2004;351:2832–8.

10

Human papillomavirus (HPV) is the most common sexually transmitted infection in the United States. The relationship of cervical cancer and sexual behavior was suspected for more than 100 years and was established by epidemiologic studies in the 1960s. In the early 1980s, cervical cancer cells were demonstrated to contain HPV DNA. Epidemiologic studies showing a consistent association between HPV and cervical cancer were published in the 1990s. The first vaccine to prevent infection with four types of HPV was licensed in 2006.

Human Papillomaviruses

Human papillomaviruses are small, double-stranded DNA viruses that infect the epithelium. More than 120 HPV types have been identified; they are differentiated by the genetic sequence of the outer capsid protein L1. Most HPV types infect the cutaneous epithelium and can cause common skin warts. About 40 types infect the mucosal epithelium; these are categorized according to their epidemiologic association with cervical cancer. Infection with low-risk, or nononcogenic types, such as types 6 and 11, can cause benign or low-grade cervical cell abnormalities, genital warts and laryngeal papillomas. High-risk, or oncogenic, HPV types act as carcinogens in the development of cervical cancer and other anogenital cancers. High-risk types (currently including types 16 and 18, among others) can cause low-grade cervical cell abnormalities, high-grade cervical cell abnormalities that are precursors to cancer, and anogenital cancers. High-risk HPV types are detected in 99% of cervical cancers. Type 16 is the cause of approximately 50% of cervical cancers worldwide, and types 16 and 18 together account for about 70% of cervical cancers. Infection with a high-risk HPV type is considered necessary for the development of cervical cancer, but by itself it is not sufficient to cause cancer because the vast majority of women with HPV infection do not develop cancer.

In addition to cervical cancer, HPV infection is also associated with anogenital cancers less common than cervical cancer, such as cancer of the vulva, vagina, penis and anus. The association of genital types of HPV with non-genital cancers is less well established, but studies support a role for these HPV types in some oropharyngeal cancers.

Pathogenesis

HPV infection occurs at the basal epithelium. Although the incidence of infection is high, most infections resolve spontaneously. A small proportion of infected persons become persistently infected; persistent infection is the most important risk factor for the development of cervical cancer.

11

Human Papillomaviruses (HPV)

- Small DNA virus
- More than 120 types identified based on the genetic sequence of the outer capsid protein L1
- About 40 types infect the mucosal epithelium

Human Papillomavirus Types and Disease Association

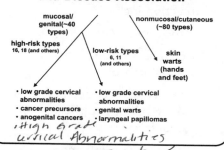

High grade cervical Abnormalities

see 9/2015 Errata

Human Papillomavirus

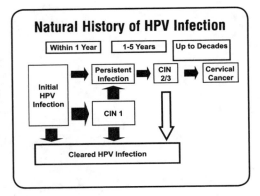

Natural History of HPV Infection

Within 1 Year | 1-5 Years | Up to Decades

Initial HPV Infection → Persistent Infection → CIN 2/3 → Cervical Cancer

Initial HPV Infection → CIN 1

Cleared HPV Infection

The most common clinically significant manifestation of persistent genital HPV infection is cervical intraepithelial neoplasia, or CIN. Within a few years of infection, low-grade CIN—called CIN 1—may develop, which may spontaneously resolve and the infection clear.

Persistent HPV infection, however, may progress directly to higher-grade CIN, called CIN2 or CIN3. High-grade abnormalities are at risk of progression to cancer and so are considered cancer precursors. Some high-grade abnormalities spontaneously regress. If left undetected and untreated, years or decades later CIN2 or 3 can progress to cervical cancer.

Infection with one type of HPV does not prevent infection with another type. Of persons infected with mucosal HPV, 5% to 30% are infected with multiple types of the virus.

11

HPV Clinical Features

- Most HPV infections are asymptomatic and result in no clinical disease
- Clinical manifestations of HPV infection include:
  - anogenital warts
  - recurrent respiratory papillomatosis
  - cervical cancer precursors (cervical intraepithelial neoplasia)
  - cancer (cervical, anal, vaginal, vulvar, penile, and oropharyngeal cancer)

Clinical Features

Most HPV infections are asymptomatic and result in no clinical disease. Clinical manifestations of HPV infection include anogenital warts, recurrent respiratory papillomatosis, cervical cancer precursors (cervical intraepithelial neoplasia), and cancers, including cervical, anal, vaginal, vulvar, penile, and oropharyngeal cancer.

Laboratory Diagnosis

HPV has not been cultured by conventional methods. Infection is identified by detection of HPV DNA from clinical samples. Assays for HPV detection differ considerably in their sensitivity and type specificity, and detection is also affected by the anatomic region sampled as well as the method of specimen collection.

Several HPV tests have been approved by the Food and Drug Administration (FDA) and detect 13-14 high-risk types (HPV 16, 18, 31, 33, 35, 39, 45, 51, 52, 56, 58, 59, 66, 68). Test results are reported as positive or negative for any of the types; some tests specifically identify HPV 16 and 18. These tests are approved for triage of Papanicolaou (Pap) test results (ASC-US, atypical cells of undetermined significance) and in combination with the Pap test for cervical cancer screening in women 30 years of age and older. The tests are not clinically indicated nor approved for use in men.

Epidemiologic and basic research studies of HPV generally use nucleic acid amplification methods that generate type-specific results. The polymerase chain reaction (PCR) assays used most commonly in epidemiologic studies target genetically conserved regions in the L1 gene.

The most frequently used HPV serologic assays are virus-like particle (VLP)-based enzyme immunoassays. However, laboratory reagents used for these assays are not standardized and there are no standards for setting a threshold for a positive result.

Medical Management

There is no specific treatment for HPV infection. Medical management depends on treatment of the specific clinical manifestation of the infection (such as genital warts or abnormal cervical cell cytology).

Epidemiology

Occurrence

HPV infection occurs throughout the world.

Reservoir

Viruses in the papillomavirus family affect other species. Humans are the only natural reservoir of HPV.

Transmission

HPV is transmitted by direct contact, usually sexual, with an infected person. Transmission occurs most frequently with sexual intercourse but can occur following nonpenetrative sexual activity.

Studies of newly acquired HPV infection demonstrate that infection occurs soon after onset of sexual activity. In a prospective study of college women, the cumulative incidence of infection was 40% by 24 months after first sexual intercourse. HPV 16 accounted for 10.4% of infections.

Genital HPV infection also may be transmitted by nonsexual routes, but this appears to be uncommon. Nonsexual routes of genital HPV transmission include transmission from a woman to a newborn infant at the time of birth.

Temporal Pattern

There is no known seasonal variation in HPV infection.

Communicability

HPV is presumably communicable during the acute infection and during persistent infection. This issue is difficult to study because of the inability to culture the virus. Communicability can be presumed to be high because of the large number of new infections estimated to occur each year.

HPV Epidemiology
- Reservoir
  - Human
- Transmission
  - Direct contact, usually sexual
- Temporal pattern
  - None
- Communicability
  - Presumed to be high

11

Human Papillomavirus

Risk Factors

Risk factors for HPV infection are primarily related to sexual behavior, including lifetime and recent sex partners. Results of epidemiologic studies are less consistent for other risk factors, including young age at sexual initiation, number of pregnancies, genetic factors, smoking, and lack of circumcision of male partner.

Disease Burden in the United States

Anogenital HPV infection is believed to be the most common sexually transmitted infection in the United States. An estimated 79 million persons are infected, and an estimated 14 million new HPV infections occur annually with half of these in persons 15-24 years.

The two most common types of cervical cancer worldwide, squamous cell carcinoma followed by adenocarcinoma, are both caused by HPV. The CDC and National Cancer Institute's United States Cancer Statistics Working Group reports that from 2005 through 2009 there were annual averages of 12,595 cases and 3,968 deaths due to cervical cancer. HPV is believed to be responsible for nearly all of these cases of cervical cancer. HPV types 16 and 18 are associated with 70% of these cancers.

In addition to cervical cancer, HPV is believed to be responsible for 90% of anal cancers, 71% of vulvar, vaginal, or penile cancers, and 72% of oropharyngeal cancers.

Population-based estimates, primarily from clinics treating persons with sexually transmitted infections, indicate that about 1% of the sexually active adolescent and adult population in the United States have clinically apparent genital warts. More than 90% of cases of anogenital warts are associated with the low-risk HPV types 6 and 11.

About 8 billion dollars are spent annually on management of sequelae of HPV infections, primarily for the management of abnormal cervical cytology and treatment of cervical neoplasia. This exceeds the economic burden of any other sexually transmitted infection except human immunodeficiency virus.

Prevention
HPV Infection

HPV transmission can be reduced but not eliminated with the use of physical barriers such as condoms. Recent studies demonstrated a significant reduction in HPV infection among young women after initiation of sexual activity when their partners used condoms consistently and correctly.

HPV Disease Burden in the United States

- Anogenital HPV is the most common sexually transmitted infection in the US
  - estimated 79 million infected
  - 14 million new infections/year
- Common among adolescents and young adults

Abstaining from sexual activity (i.e., refraining from any genital contact with another individual) is the surest way to prevent genital HPV infection. For those who choose to be sexually active, a monogamous relationship with an uninfected partner is the strategy most likely to prevent future genital HPV infections.

Cervical Cancer Screening

Most cases and deaths from cervical cancer can be prevented through detection of precancerous changes within the cervix by cervical cytology using the Pap test. Currently available Pap test screening can be done by a conventional Pap or a liquid-based cytology. CDC does not issue recommendations for cervical cancer screening, but various professional groups have published recommendations. Cervical cancer screening recommendations were revised in 2012 after the U.S. Preventive Services Task Force (USPSTF) and a multidisciplinary group, including the American Cancer Society (ASC), American Society for Colposcopy and Cervical Pathology (ASCCP), and the American Society for Clinical Pathology (ASCP) reviewed new evidence. Previously, recommendations varied by organization. Since 2012, all organizations have recommended that screening should begin at age 21 years. While there are slight differences in other aspects of the recommendations, all groups recommend screening in women aged 21 to 65 years with cytology (Pap test) every 3 years. For women aged 30 to 65 years who want to lengthen the screening interval, screening can be done with a combination of cytology and HPV testing ("co-testing") every 5 years.

The use of HPV vaccine does not eliminate the need for continued Pap test screening, since 30% of cervical cancers are caused by HPV types not included in the vaccine.

Human Papillomavirus Vaccine
Characteristics

Three HPV vaccines are licensed in the United States. The vaccines are non-infectious subunit vaccines. The antigen for the vaccines is the L1 major capsid protein of HPV, produced by using recombinant DNA technology. L1 proteins self-assemble into noninfectious, nononcogenic units called virus-like particles (VLP).

Quadrivalent HPV (HPV4) vaccine (Gardasil, Merck) was approved by the FDA in June 2006. The vaccine is approved for females and males 9 through 26 years of age. Each 0.5-mL dose of HPV4 contains 20 micrograms HPV 6 L1 protein, 40 micrograms HPV 11 L1 protein, 40 micrograms HPV 16 L1 protein, and 20 micrograms HPV 18 L1 protein. The vaccine antigen is adsorbed on alum adjuvant.

Cervical Cancer Screening

- Revised in 2012

- Screening should begin at age 21 years

- Screen women 21 to 65 years of age with Pap test every 3 years

- Co-testing (Pap and HPV testing) every 5 years in women 30 to 65 years of age

11

Human Papillomavirus Vaccine

- HPV L1 major capsid protein of the virus is antigen used for immunization

- L1 protein produced using recombinant technology

- L1 proteins self-assemble into virus-like particles (VLP)

- VLPs are noninfectious and nononcogenic

Human Papillomavirus

The vaccine also includes sodium chloride, L-histidine, polysorbate 80, and sodium borate. HPV4 does not contain a preservative or antibiotic. The vaccine is supplied in single-dose vials and syringes. A 9-valent vaccine (Merck) was approved by the FDA in December 2014.

Bivalent HPV (HPV2) vaccine (Cervarix, GlaxoSmithKline) was approved by the FDA in October 2009. The vaccine is approved for females 9 through 25 years of age. HPV2 is not approved for males. The L1 antigen is adsorbed onto aluminum hydroxide. The unique adjuvant system, AS04, is composed of 3-O-desacyl-4'-monophosphoryl lipid A (MPL) adsorbed onto aluminum hydroxide. Each 0.5-mL dose contains 20 micrograms of HPV type 16 L1 protein and 20 micrograms of HPV type 18 L1 protein. HPV2 does not contain a preservative or antibiotic. It is available in 2 types of prefilled syringes.

Immunogenicity and Vaccine Efficacy

HPV vaccines are highly immunogenic. More than 99% of recipients develop an antibody response to HPV types included in the respective vaccines 1 month after completing the three-dose series. However, there is no known serologic correlate of immunity and no known minimal titer determined to be protective. The high efficacy found in the clinical trials to date has precluded identification of a minimum protective antibody titer. Further follow-up of vaccinated cohorts may allow determination of serologic correlates of immunity in the future.

Both HPV vaccines have been found to have high efficacy for prevention of HPV vaccine type–related persistent infection, CIN 2/3 and adenocarcinoma in-situ (AIS). Clinical efficacy for HPV4 against cervical disease was determined in two double-blind, placebo-controlled trials. In women 16 through 26 years of age vaccine efficacy for HPV 16 or 18–related CIN 2/3 or AIS was 97%. HPV4 efficacy against HPV 6, 11, 16 or 18–related genital warts was 99%.

HPV2 efficacy was evaluated in two randomized, double-blind, controlled clinical trials in females aged 15 through 25 years. In the phase III trial, efficacy against HPV 16 or 18-related CIN 2/3 or AIS was 93%.

HPV4 was evaluated in men 16 through 26 years and found to have 88% efficacy against vaccine type genital warts. Among men who have sex with men (MSM), efficacy against anal intraepithelial neoplasia grade 2 or 3 (AIN2/3) was 75%.

Although high efficacy among persons without evidence of infection with vaccine HPV types was demonstrated in clinical trials of both HPV vaccines, there is no evidence of

---

HPV Vaccines

- HPV4 (Gardasil, Merck)
  - approved for females and males 9 through 26 years of age
  - contains types 16 and 18 (high risk) and types 6 and 11 (low risk)
- a 9-valent vaccine licensed in December 2014
- HPV2 (Cervarix, GlaxoSmithKline)
  - approved for females 9 through 25 years of age
  - contains types 16 and 18 (high risk)

11

efficacy against disease caused by vaccine types with which participants were infected at the time of vaccination (i.e., the vaccines had no therapeutic effect on existing infection or disease). Participants infected with one or more vaccine HPV types prior to vaccination were protected against disease caused by the other vaccine types. Prior infection with one HPV type did not diminish efficacy of the vaccine against other vaccine HPV types.

The duration of protection following HPV vaccine is not known. For both vaccines a subset of participants have been followed for more than 60 months with no evidence of waning protection. Study populations will continue to be followed for any evidence of waning immunity.

Vaccination Schedule and Use

ACIP recommends vaccination of females with HPV2 or HPV4 for prevention of cervical cancers and precancers. HPV4 is recommended also for prevention of genital warts. ACIP recommends routine vaccination at age 11 or 12 years with HPV4 or HPV2 for females and with HPV4 for males. The vaccination series can be started beginning at age 9 years.

HPV4 and HPV2 are each administered in a 3-dose series. The second dose should be administered 1 to 2 months after the first dose and the third dose 6 months after the first dose. Vaccination also is recommended for females aged 13 through 26 years and for males aged 13 through 21 years, who have not been previously vaccinated or who have not completed the 3-dose series. For immunocompromised males (including HIV infection) and men who have sex with men, ACIP recommends routine vaccination with HPV4, as for all males, through 26 years of age for those who have not been vaccinated previously or who have not completed the 3-dose series. Males aged 22 through 26 years without these risk factors may be vaccinated as well. HPV2 is neither licensed nor recommended for males.

If females or males reach age 27 years before the vaccination series is complete, the second and/or third doses of vaccine can be administered after age 26 to complete the vaccination series.

Prevaccination assessments (e.g., Pap testing or screening for high-risk HPV DNA, type-specific HPV tests, or HPV antibody) to establish the appropriateness of HPV vaccination are not recommended.

Ideally, vaccine should be administered before potential exposure to HPV through sexual contact; however, persons who may have already been exposed to HPV should be

---

HPV Vaccine Efficacy

- High efficacy among females without evidence of infection with vaccine HPV types

- No evidence of efficacy against disease caused by vaccine types with which participants were infected at the time of vaccination

- Prior infection with one HPV type did not diminish efficacy of the vaccine against other vaccine HPV types

11

HPV Vaccination Recommendations

- ACIP recommends routine vaccination at age 11 or 12 years with HPV4 or HPV2 for females and HPV 4 for males

- The vaccination series can be started as young as 9 years of age

- Vaccination also recommended for females 13 through 26 years of age

- Vaccination also recommended for males 13 through 21 years of age

- All immunocompromised males (including HIV infection) and MSM through 26 years of age should be vaccinated

- Males aged 22 through 26 years may be vaccinated

Human Papillomavirus

vaccinated. Sexually active persons who have not been infected with any of the HPV vaccine types will receive full benefit from vaccination. Vaccination will provide less benefit to persons if they have already been infected with one or more of the HPV vaccine types. However, it is not possible for a clinician to assess the extent to which sexually active persons would benefit from vaccination, and the risk of HPV infection may continue as long as persons are sexually active. Pap testing or screening for HPV DNA or HPV antibody is not recommended prior to vaccination at any age.

Both HPV vaccines are administered in a three-dose series of intramuscular injections. The second and third doses should be administered 1 to 2 and 6 months after the first dose. The third dose should follow the first dose by at least 24 weeks. The third dose need not be repeated as long as it was administered at least 16 weeks after the first dose and at least 12 weeks after the second dose. An accelerated schedule for HPV vaccine is not recommended.

There is no maximum interval between doses. If the HPV vaccine schedule is interrupted, the vaccine series does not need to be restarted. If the series is interrupted after the first dose, the second dose should be given as soon as possible, and the second and third doses should be separated by an interval of at least 12 weeks. If only the third dose is delayed, it should be administered as soon as possible.

Whenever feasible, the same HPV vaccine should be used for the entire vaccination series. No studies address interchangeability of HPV vaccines. However, if the vaccine provider does not know or have available the HPV vaccine product previously administered, either HPV vaccine can be used to complete the series to provide protection against HPV 16 and 18. For protection against HPV 6 or 11-related genital warts, a vaccination series with fewer than 3 doses of HPV4 might provide less protection than a complete 3-dose HPV4 series.

HPV vaccine should be administered at the same visit as other age-appropriate vaccines, such as Tdap and quadrivalent meningococcal conjugate (MCV4) vaccines. Administering all indicated vaccines at a single visit increases the likelihood that adolescents and young adults will receive each of the vaccines on schedule. Each vaccine should be administered using a separate syringe at a different anatomic site.

As mentioned, prevaccination assessments (e.g. Pap testing or screening for high-risk HPV DNA, type-specific HPV tests, or HPV antibody) to establish the appropriateness

> **HPV Vaccination Schedule**
> - Routine schedule is 0, 1 to 2, 6 months
> - An accelerated schedule using minimum intervals is not recommended
> - Series does not need to be restarted if the schedule is interrupted
> - Prevaccination assessments not recommended
> - No therapeutic effect on HPV infection, genital warts, cervical lesions

of HPV vaccination are not recommended at any age. HPV vaccination can provide protection against infection with HPV vaccine types not already acquired. Therefore, vaccination is recommended through the recommended age for females regardless of whether they have an abnormal pap test result, and for females or males regardless of known HPV infection.

Women should be advised that the vaccine will not have a therapeutic effect on existing HPV infection, genital warts or cervical lesions.

A history of genital warts or clinically evident genital warts indicates infection with HPV, most often type 6 or 11. However, these persons may be infected with HPV types other than the HPV4 vaccine types, and therefore they may receive HPV4 vaccine if they are in the recommended age group. Persons with a history of genital warts should be advised that data do not indicate HPV4 vaccine will have any therapeutic effect on existing HPV infection or genital warts.

Because HPV vaccines are subunit vaccines, they can be administered to persons who are immunosuppressed because of disease or medications. However, the immune response and vaccine efficacy might be less than that in persons who are immunocompetent. Women who are breastfeeding may receive HPV vaccine.

Contraindications and Precautions to Vaccination

A severe allergic reaction (e.g., anaphylaxis) to a vaccine component or following a prior dose of HPV vaccine is a contraindication to receipt of HPV vaccine. Anaphylactic allergy to latex is a contraindication to bivalent HPV vaccine in a prefilled syringe since the tip cap contains natural rubber latex. A moderate or severe acute illness is a precaution to vaccination, and vaccination should be deferred until symptoms of the acute illness improve. A minor acute illness (e.g., diarrhea or mild upper respiratory tract infection, with or without fever) is not a reason to defer vaccination.

HPV vaccine is not recommended for use during pregnancy. The vaccine has not been causally associated with adverse pregnancy outcomes or with adverse effects on the developing fetus, but data on vaccination during pregnancy are limited. Pregnancy testing before vaccination is not needed. However, if a woman is found to be pregnant after initiation of the vaccination series, the remainder of the series should be delayed until after completion of the

11

> **HPV Vaccine Contraindications and Precautions**
> - Contraindication
>   - severe allergic reaction to a vaccine component or following a prior dose
> - Precaution
>   - moderate or severe acute illnesses (defer until symptoms improve)

Human Papillomavirus

pregnancy. No intervention is indicated. Women known to be pregnant should delay initiation of the vaccine series until after delivery.

Pregnancy registries for both HPV2 and HPV4 have been terminated. However, vaccination with either vaccine during pregnancy may still be reported to VAERS or to the manufacturer: GlaxoSmithKline at 1-888-825-5249 (for HPV2), or Merck at 1-877-888-4231 (for HPV4).

Adverse Reactions Following Vaccination

The most common adverse reactions reported during clinical trials of HPV vaccines were local reactions at the site of injection. In prelicensure clinical trials, local reactions, such as pain, redness or swelling were reported by 20% to 90% of recipients. A temperature of 100°F during the 15 days after vaccination was reported in 10% to 13% of recipients of either vaccine. A similar proportion of placebo recipients reported an elevated temperature. Local reactions generally increased in frequency with increasing doses. However, reports of fever did not increase significantly with increasing doses. No serious adverse events have been associated with either HPV vaccine based on monitoring by CDC and the Food and Drug Administration.

A variety of systemic adverse reactions were reported by vaccine recipients, including nausea, dizziness, myalgia and malaise. However, these symptoms occurred with equal frequency among both vaccine and placebo recipients.

Syncope has been reported among adolescents who received HPV and other vaccines recommended for this age group (Tdap, MCV4). Recipients should always be seated during vaccine administration. Clinicians should consider observing recipient for 15 minutes after vaccination.

Vaccine Storage and Handling

HPV vaccines should be maintained at refrigerator temperature between 35°F and 46°F (2°C and 8°C). Manufacturer package inserts contain additional information and can be found at http://www.fda.gov/BiologicsBloodVaccines/Vaccines/ApprovedProducts/ucm093830.htm. For complete information on best practices and recommendations please refer to CDC's Vaccine Storage and Handling Toolkit, http://www.cdc.gov/vaccines/recs/storage/toolkit/storage-handling-toolkit.pdf.

Acknowledgment

The editors thank Drs. Lauri Markowitz and Elizabeth Unger for their assistance in updating this chapter.

Selected References

American College of Obstetricians and Gynecologists. Human papillomavirus vaccination. ACOG committee opinion No. 467. *Obstet Gynecol* 2010;116:800–803.

CDC. Human papillomavirus vaccination. Recommendations of the Advisory Committee on Immunization Practices (ACIP). *MMWR* 2014;63(No. 5):1-30.

CDC. Quadrivalent human papillomavirus vaccine. Recommendations of the Advisory Committee on Immunization Practices (ACIP). *MMWR* 2007;56 (No.RR-2):1–24.

CDC. FDA licensure of bivalent human papillomavirus vaccine (HPV2, Cervarix) for use in females and updated HPV vaccination recommendations from the Advisory Committee on Immunization Practices (ACIP). *MMWR* 2010;59(No. 20):626-9.

CDC. Recommendations on the use of quadrivalent human papillomavirus vaccine in males – Advisory Committee on Immunization Practices (ACIP), 2011. *MMWR* 2011;60 (No. 50):1705-8.

Dunne E, Markowitz L. Genital human papillomavirus infection. *Clin Infect Dis* 2006;43:624–9.

Koutsky LA, Kiviat NB. Genital human papillomavirus. In: Holmes KK, Sparling PF, Mårdh PA, et al, eds. *Sexually Transmitted Diseases*. 3rd ed. New York: McGraw-Hill;1999:347-59.

Moyer VA. Screening for cervical cancer: U.S. Preventive Services Task Force recommendation statement. *Ann Intern Med* 2012;156:880-91, W312.

Saslow D, Solomon D, Lawson HW, et al. American Cancer Society, American Society for Colposcopy and Cervical Pathology, and American Society for Clinical Pathology screening guidelines for the prevention and early detection of cervical cancer. *American Journal of Clinical pathology* 2012; 137:516-42.

Satterwhite CL, Torrone E, Meites E, et al. Sexually Transmitted Infections Among US Women and Men: Prevalence and Incidence Estimates, 2008. *Sex Transm Dis.* 2013;40:187-93

Schiller JT, Lowy DR, Markowitz LE. Human papillomavirus vaccines. In: Plotkin SA, Orenstein WA, Offit PA, eds. *Vaccines*. 6th ed. China: Saunders 2012:235-256.

11

Trottier H, Franco E. The epidemiology of genital human papillomavirus infection. *Vaccine 2006*;24(suppl1):51–15.

U.S. Cancer Statistics Working Group. United States Cancer Statistics; 1999-2009 Incidence and Mortality Web-based Report. Atlanta: U.S. Department of Health and Human Services, Centers for Disease Control and Prevention and National Cancer Institute; 2013. Available at: www.cdc.gov/uscs.

Winer R, Hughes J, Feng Q, et al. Condom use and the risk of genital human papillomavirus infection in young women. *N Engl J Med* 2006;354:2645–54.

Winer R, Lee S, Hughes J, et al. Genital human papillomavirus infection incidence and risk factors in a cohort of female university students. *Am J Epidemiol* 2003;157: 218-26.

11

Influenza is a highly infectious viral illness. The name "influenza" originated in 15th century Italy, from an epidemic attributed to "influence of the stars." The first pandemic, or worldwide epidemic, that clearly fits the description of influenza was in 1580. At least four pandemics of influenza occurred in the 19th century, and three occurred in the 20th century. The pandemic of "Spanish" influenza in 1918–1919 caused an estimated 21 million deaths worldwide. The first pandemic of the 21st century occurred in 2009–2010.

Smith, Andrewes, and Laidlaw isolated influenza A virus in ferrets in 1933, and Francis isolated influenza B virus in 1936. In 1936, Burnet discovered that influenza virus could be grown in embryonated hens' eggs. This led to the study of the characteristics of the virus and the development of inactivated vaccines. The protective efficacy of these inactivated vaccines was determined in the 1950s. The first live attenuated influenza vaccine was licensed in 2003.

Influenza Virus

Influenza is a single-stranded, helically shaped, RNA virus of the orthomyxovirus family. Basic antigen types A, B, and C are determined by the nuclear material. Type A influenza has subtypes that are determined by the surface antigens hemagglutinin (H) and neuraminidase (N). Three types of hemagglutinin in humans (H1, H2, and H3) have a role in virus attachment to cells. Two types of neuraminidase (N1 and N2) have a role in virus penetration into cells.

Influenza A causes moderate to severe illness and affects all age groups. The virus infects humans and other animals. Influenza A viruses are perpetuated in nature by wild birds, predominantly waterfowl. Most of these viruses are not pathogenic to their natural hosts and do not change or evolve. Influenza B generally causes milder disease than type A and primarily affects children. Influenza B is more stable than influenza A, with less antigenic drift and consequent immunologic stability. It affects only humans. Influenza C is rarely reported as a cause of human illness, probably because most cases are subclinical. It has not been associated with epidemic disease.

The nomenclature to describe the type of influenza virus is expressed in this order: 1) virus type, 2) geographic origin where it was first isolated, 3) strain number, 4) year of isolation, and 5) virus subtype.

Influenza

- Highly infectious viral illness
- First pandemic in 1580
- At least 4 pandemics in 19th century
- Estimated 21 million deaths worldwide in pandemic of 1918-1919
- Virus first isolated in 1933

Influenza Virus

- Single-stranded RNA virus
- Orthomyxoviridae family
- 3 types: A, B, C
- Subtypes of type A determined by hemagglutinin and neuraminidase

Influenza Virus Strains

- Type A-moderate to severe illness
  - all age groups
  - humans and other animals
- Type B-milder disease
  - primarily affects children
  - humans only
- Type C-rarely reported in humans
  - no epidemics

Influenza Virus

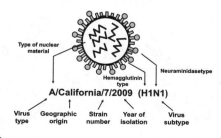

12

Influenza

12

Antigenic Changes

Hemagglutinin and neuraminidase periodically change, apparently due to sequential evolution within immune or partially immune populations. These changes may take the form of antigenic drift or antigenic shift, the latter associated with pandemics.

In antigenic drift, antigenic mutants emerge and are selected as the predominant virus to the extent that they differ from the antecedent virus, which is suppressed by specific antibody arising in the population as a result of infection. This cycle repeats continuously. In interpandemic periods, mutants arise by serial point mutations in the RNA coding for hemagglutinin.

Antigenic drift is a minor change in surface antigens that results from point mutations in a gene segment. Antigenic drift may result in an epidemic, since the protection that remains from past exposures to similar viruses is incomplete. Drift occurs in all three types of influenza virus (A,B,C). For instance, during most of the 1997–1998 influenza season, A/Wuhan/359/95 (H3N2) was the predominant influenza strain isolated in the United States. A/Wuhan was a drifted distant relative of the 1968 Hong Kong H3N2 strain. In the last half of the 1997–1998 influenza season, a drifted variant of A/Wuhan appeared. This virus, named A/Sydney/5/97, was different enough from A/Wuhan (which had been included in the 1997–1998 vaccine) that the vaccine did not provide much protection. Both A/Wuhan and A/Sydney circulated late in the 1997–1998 influenza season. A/Sydney became the predominant strain during the 1998–1999 influenza season and was included in the 1998–1999 vaccine. In antigenic shift, at irregular intervals of 10 to >40 years, viruses showing major antigenic differences from prevalent subtypes appear and, because the population does not have protective antibody against these new antigens, cause pandemic disease. Antigenic shift involves a major change in one or both surface antigens (H or N). Antigenic shifts are probably due to genetic recombination (an exchange of a gene segment) between influenza A viruses that affect humans and/or animals. An antigenic shift may result in a worldwide pandemic if the virus is efficiently transmitted from person to person. An antigenic shift occurred in 1968 when H3N2 (Hong Kong) influenza appeared. It completely replaced the type A strain (H2N2, or Asian influenza) that had circulated throughout the world for the prior 10 years.

Since the late 19th century, five occurrences of antigenic shifts have led to pandemics (1889–1891, 1918–1920, 1957–1958, 1968–1969, and 2009-2010). A pandemic may start from a single focus and spread along routes of travel. Typically, there are high attack rates involving all age groups, and mortality is usually markedly increased. Severity is generally not greater in the individual patient (except for the 1918–1919 strain), but because large numbers of persons are infected, the number, if not the proportion, of severe and fatal cases will be large. Onset may occur in any season of the year. Secondary and tertiary waves may occur up to 2 years later, usually in the winter.

In April 2009, a novel influenza A(H1N1) virus appeared and quickly spread across North America. By May 2009 the virus had spread to many areas of the world. Influenza morbidity caused by 2009 pandemic H1N1 virus remained above seasonal baselines throughout spring and summer 2009 and was the cause of the first influenza pandemic since 1968.

In the United States, the 2009 pandemic was characterized by a substantial increase in influenza activity in Spring 2009 that was well beyond seasonal norms. Influenza activity peaked in late October 2009, and returned to the seasonal baseline by January 2010. During this time, more than 99 percent of viruses characterized were the 2009 pandemic influenza A(H1N1) virus.

In January 2011, CDC estimated that pandemic H1N1 influenza virus caused more than 60 million Americans to become ill, and led to more than 270,000 hospitalizations and 12,500 deaths. Ninety percent of hospitalizations and deaths occurred in persons younger than 65 years of age. With typical seasonal influenza approximately 90% of deaths occur in persons older than 65 years.

In response to the pandemic a monovalent influenza vaccine was produced and deployed in a nationwide vaccination campaign.

Typically in an epidemic, influenza attack rates are lower than in pandemics. The major impact is observed in morbidity, with high attack rates and excess rates of hospitalization, especially for adults with respiratory disease. Absenteeism from work and school is high, and visits to healthcare providers increase. In the Northern Hemisphere, epidemics usually occur in late fall and continue through early spring. In the Southern Hemisphere, epidemics usually occur 6 months before or after those in the Northern Hemisphere.

Sporadic outbreaks can occasionally be localized to families, schools, and isolated communities.

2009 Influenza A(H1N1)

- In April 2009 a novel influenza A(H1N1) virus appeared and quickly spread across North America
- By May 2009 the virus had spread to many areas of the world
- Cause of the first influenza pandemic since 1968
- Pandemic monovalent influenza vaccine produced and deployed in nationwide vaccination campaign

12

Influenza

Influenza Pathogenesis

- Respiratory transmission of virus
- Replication in respiratory epithelium with subsequent destruction of cells
- Viremia rarely documented
- Virus shed in respiratory secretions for 5-10 days

Influenza Clinical Features

- Incubation period 2 days (range 1-4 days)
- 50% of infected persons develop classic symptoms
- Abrupt onset of fever, myalgia, sore throat, nonproductive cough, headache

12

Pathogenesis

Following respiratory transmission, the virus attaches to and penetrates respiratory epithelial cells in the trachea and bronchi. Viral replication occurs, which results in the destruction of the host cell. Viremia has rarely been documented. Virus is shed in respiratory secretions for 5–10 days.

Clinical Features

The incubation period for influenza is usually 2 days, but can vary from 1 to 4 days. Influenza illness can vary from asymptomatic infection to severe. In general, only about 50% of infected persons will develop the classic clinical symptoms of influenza.

"Classic" influenza disease is characterized by the abrupt onset of fever, myalgia, sore throat, nonproductive cough, and headache. The fever is usually 101°–102°F, and accompanied by prostration (bedridden). The onset of fever is often so abrupt that the exact hour is recalled by the patient. Myalgias mainly affect the back muscles. Cough is believed to be a result of tracheal epithelial destruction. Additional symptoms may include rhinorrhea (runny nose), headache, substernal chest burning and ocular symptoms (e.g., eye pain and sensitivity to light).

Systemic symptoms and fever usually last from 2 to 3 days, rarely more than 5 days. They may be decreased by such medications as aspirin or acetaminophen. Aspirin should not be used for infants, children, or teenagers because they may be at risk for contracting Reye syndrome following an influenza infection. Recovery is usually rapid, but some patients may have lingering asthenia (lack of strength or energy) for several weeks.

Influenza Complications

- Pneumonia
  - secondary bacterial
  - primary influenza viral
- Reye syndrome
- Myocarditis
- Death is reported than less than 1 per 1,000 cases

Complications

The most frequent complication of influenza is pneumonia, most commonly secondary bacterial pneumonia (e.g., *Streptococcus pneumoniae*, *Haemophilus influenzae*, or *Staphylococcus aureus*). Primary influenza viral pneumonia is an uncommon complication with a high fatality rate. Reye syndrome is a complication that occurs almost exclusively in children taking aspirin, primarily in association with influenza B (or varicella zoster), and presents with severe vomiting and confusion, which may progress to coma due to swelling of the brain.

Other complications include myocarditis (inflammation of the heart) and worsening of chronic bronchitis and other chronic pulmonary diseases. Death is reported in less than 1 per 1,000 cases. The majority of deaths typically occur among persons 65 years of age and older.

Impact of Influenza

An increase in mortality typically accompanies an influenza epidemic. Increased mortality results not only from influenza and pneumonia but also from cardiopulmonary and other chronic diseases that can be exacerbated by influenza.

The number of influenza-associated deaths varies substantially by year, influenza virus type and subtype, and age group. In a study of influenza seasons from 1976-77 through 2006-07, the estimated number of annual influenza-associated deaths from respiratory and circulatory causes ranged from a low of 3,349 (1985-86 season) to a high of 48,614 (2003-04 season), with an average of 23,607 annual influenza-associated deaths. Persons 65 years of age and older account for approximately 90% of deaths attributed to pneumonia and influenza. During seasons with prominent circulation of influenza A(H3N2) viruses, 2.7 times more deaths occurred than during seasons when A(H3N2) viruses were not prominent.

The risk for complications and hospitalizations from influenza are higher among persons 65 years of age and older, young children, and persons of any age with certain underlying medical conditions. An average of more than 200,000 hospitalizations per year are related to influenza, with about 37% occurring in persons younger than 65 years. A greater number of hospitalizations occur during years that influenza A(H3N2) is predominant. In nursing homes, attack rates may be as high as 60%, with fatality rates as high as 30%. The cost of a severe epidemic has been estimated to be $12 billion.

Among children 0–4 years of age, hospitalization rates have varied from 100 per 100,000 healthy children to as high as 500 per 100,000 for children with underlying medical conditions. Hospitalization rates for children 24 months of age and younger are comparable to rates for persons 65 and older. Children 24-59 months of age are at less risk of hospitalization from influenza than are younger children, but are at increased risk for influenza-associated clinic and emergency department visits.

Healthy children 5 through 18 years of age are not at increased risk of complications of influenza. However, children typically have the highest attack rates during community outbreaks of influenza. They also serve as a major source of transmission of influenza within communities. Influenza has a substantial impact among school-aged children and their contacts. These impacts include school absenteeism, medical care visits, and parental work loss. Studies have documented 5 to 7 influenza-related outpatient visits per 100 children annually, and these children frequently receive antibiotics.

Impact of Influenza-United States, 1976-2007

- The number of influenza-associated deaths varies substantially by year, influenza virus type and subtype, and age group

- Annual influenza-associated deaths ranged from 3,349 (1985-86 season) to 48,614 (2003-04 season), with an average of 23,607 annual deaths

- Persons 65 years of age and older account for approximately 90% of deaths

- 2.7 times more deaths occurred during seasons when A(H3N2) viruses were prominent

Impact of Influenza-United States

- Highest rates of complications and hospitalization among persons 65 years and older, young children, and persons of any age with certain underlying medical conditions

- Average of more than 200,000 influenza-related excess hospitalizations

- 37% of hospitalizations among persons younger than 65 years of age

- Greater number of hospitalizations during years that A(H3N2) is predominant

12

Influenza

Laboratory Diagnosis

The diagnosis of influenza is usually suspected on the basis of characteristic clinical findings, particularly if influenza has been reported in the community.

Virus can be isolated from throat and nasopharyngeal swabs obtained within 3 days of onset of illness. Culture is performed by inoculation of the amniotic or allantoic sac of chick embryos or certain cell cultures that support viral replication. A minimum of 48 hours is required to demonstrate virus, and 1 to 2 additional days to identify the virus type. As a result, culture is helpful in defining the etiology of local epidemics, but not in individual case management.

Serologic confirmation of influenza requires demonstration of a significant rise in influenza IgG. The acute-phase specimen should be taken less than 5 days from onset, and a convalescent specimen taken 10–21 days (preferably 21 days) following onset. Complement fixation (CF) and hemagglutination inhibition (HI) are the serologic tests most commonly used. The key test is HI, which depends on the ability of the virus to agglutinate erythrocytes and inhibition of this process by specific antibody. Diagnosis requires at least a fourfold rise in antibody titer. Rapid diagnostic testing for influenza antigen is available, but because these tests fail to detect many patients with influenza, CDC recommends antiviral treatment with oseltamivir or zanamivir as early as possible for patients with confirmed or suspected influenza who have severe, complicated, or progressive illness; who require hospitalization; or who are at greater risk for serious influenza-related complications.

Details about the laboratory diagnosis of influenza are available on the CDC influenza website at http://www.cdc.gov/flu/professionals/diagnosis/index.htm

Epidemiology

Occurrence

Influenza occurs throughout the world.

Reservoir

Humans are the only known reservoir of influenza types B and C. Influenza A viruses may infect both humans and animals. There is no chronic carrier state.

Transmission

Influenza is primarily transmitted from person to person via large virus-laden droplets (particles more than 5 microns in diameter) that are generated when infected persons cough or sneeze. These large droplets can then settle on

12

the mucosal surfaces of the upper respiratory tracts of susceptible persons who are near (within 3 feet) infected persons. Transmission may also occur through direct contact or indirect contact with respiratory secretions such as when touching surfaces contaminated with influenza virus and then touching the eyes, nose or mouth.

Temporal Pattern

Influenza activity peaks from December to March in temperate climates, but may occur earlier or later. During 1982–2012, peak influenza activity in the United States occurred most frequently in January (17% of seasons), and February (47% of seasons). However, peak influenza activity occurred in March, April, or May in 17% of seasons. Influenza occurs throughout the year in tropical areas.

Communicability

Adults can transmit influenza from the day before symptom onset to approximately 5 days after symptoms begin. Children can transmit influenza to others for 10 or more days.

12

Secular Trends in the United States

There is a documented association between influenza and increased morbidity in high-risk adult populations. Hospitalization for adults with high-risk medical conditions increases two- to fivefold during major epidemics.

The impact of influenza in the United States is quantified by measuring pneumonia and influenza (P and I) deaths. Death certificate data are collected from 122 U.S. cities with populations of more than 100,000 (total of approximately 70,000,000). P and I deaths include all deaths for which pneumonia is listed as a primary or underlying cause or for which influenza is listed on the death certificate.

An expected ratio of deaths due to P and I compared with all deaths for a given period of time is determined. The epidemic threshold for influenza seasons is generally estimated at 1.645 standard deviations above observed P and I deaths for the previous 5-year period excluding periods during influenza outbreaks. Influenza epidemic activity is signaled when the ratio of deaths due to P and I exceeds the threshold ratio for 2 consecutive weeks.

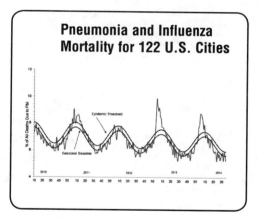

Pneumonia and Influenza Mortality for 122 U.S. Cities

Influenza Vaccines
Characteristics

Two types of influenza vaccine are available in the United States, inactivated influenza vaccine (IIV) and live attenuated influenza vaccine (LAIV). IIV has been

Influenza Vaccines
- Inactivated subunit (IIV)
  - intramuscular or intradermal
- Live attenuated vaccine (LAIV)
  - intranasal

12

available since the 1940s. IIV is administered by the intra-muscular or intradermal route. Trivalent vaccine contains three inactivated viruses: type A(H1N1), type A(H3N2), and type B. Quadrivalent influenza vaccines were introduced for the 2013-2014 season. They contain the same antigens as trivalent vaccines, with the exception that quadrivalent vaccines contain two type B strains. Only split-virus and subunit inactivated vaccines are available in the United States. Vaccine viruses are grown in chicken eggs, and the final product contains residual egg protein. The vaccine is available in both pediatric (0.25-mL dose) and adult (0.5-mL dose) formulations.

Multiple manufacturers produce inactivated influenza vaccine each year for the U.S. market. Vaccines are available in multiple presentations (single dose syringes and vials, multi-dose vials) and in preservative-free formulations. Approved age indications vary by manufacturer and product. Clinicians should obtain inactivated influenza vaccine appropriate for the age groups they plan to vaccinate. ACIP does not recommend use of influenza vaccine outside the vaccine's FDA-approved age indication. Tables listing each year's influenza vaccines are available in the annual ACIP influenza statement, and on the CDC influenza website at http://www.cdc.gov/flu/.

Flucelvax was approved by the FDA in November 2012. It is a trivalent subunit IIV prepared from virus propagated in Madin Darby Canine Kidney (MDCK) cells. It is a cell-culture inactivated influenza vaccine (ccIIV). It is approved for persons 18 years old or older.

One inactivated influenza vaccine product, FluBlok, is a recombinant influenza vaccine (RIV). It is trivalent, administered by intramuscular injection, and is indicated for persons aged 18 through 49 years. RIV is manufactured without the use of influenza viruses; therefore, similarly to IIVs, no shedding of vaccine virus will occur. No preference is expressed for RIV vs. IIV within specified indications.

In 2009 the Food and Drug Administration (FDA) approved a new formulation of inactivated influenza vaccine produced by sanofi pasteur, brand name Fluzone High-Dose. This vaccine is approved only for persons 65 years of age or older. Each dose of this vaccine contains 4 times as much hemagglutinin as the regular formulation of Fluzone for adults. ACIP has not expressed a preference for the high dose Fluzone formulation or any other inactivated vaccine for use in persons 65 years and older.

In 2011 the FDA approved a IIV formulation administered by the intradermal route. The product is Fluzone Intradermal produced by sanofi pasteur. It is approved for persons 18 through 64 years of age. This vaccine formulation is not the same as intramuscular IIV preparations. Each 0.1 mL dose contains 27 micrograms of hemagglutinin. The vaccine is administered with a specially designed prefilled syringe with a 30 gauge 1.5 millimeter microneedle.

In 2014, the FDA approved Alfuria influenza vaccine to be administered by the Stratis® Jet Injector. FDA approved this method of administration for adults 18 through 64 years of age.

Live attenuated influenza vaccine (LAIV) was approved for use in the United States in 2003. It contains the same influenza viruses as IIV. The viruses are cold-adapted, and replicate effectively in the mucosa of the nasopharynx. The vaccine viruses are grown in chicken eggs, and the final product contains residual egg protein. The vaccine is provided in a single-dose sprayer unit; half of the dose is sprayed into each nostril. LAIV does not contain thimerosal or any other preservative. LAIV is approved for use only in healthy, nonpregnant persons 2 through 49 years of age.

Vaccinated children can shed vaccine viruses in nasopharyngeal secretions for up to 3 weeks. One instance of transmission of vaccine virus to a contact has been documented.

Immunogenicity and Vaccine Efficacy

IIV

For practical purposes, the duration of immunity following inactivated influenza vaccination is less than 1 year because of waning of vaccine-induced antibody and antigenic drift of circulating influenza viruses. Influenza vaccine efficacy varies by the similarity of the vaccine strain(s) to the circulating strain and the age and health status of the recipient. Vaccines are effective in protecting about 60% of healthy vaccinees younger than 65 years of age from illness when the vaccine strain is similar to the circulating strain. However, the vaccine is less effective in preventing illness among persons 65 years of age and older.

Although the vaccine is not highly effective in preventing clinical illness among the elderly, it is effective in preventing complications and death. Some studies show that, among elderly persons, the vaccine is 50%–60% effective in preventing hospitalization and 80% effective in preventing death. During a 1982–1983 influenza outbreak in Genesee County, Michigan, unvaccinated nursing home residents were four times more likely to die than were vaccinated residents.

LAIV

LAIV has been tested in groups of both healthy children and healthy adults. A randomized, double-blind, placebo-controlled trial among healthy children 60–84 months

Transmission of LAIV Virus

- LAIV replicates in the nasopharyngeal mucosa
- Vaccinated children can shed vaccine viruses in nasopharyngeal secretions for up to 3 weeks
- One instance of transmission of vaccine virus to a contact has been documented

Inactivated Influenza Vaccine Efficacy

- About 60% effective among healthy persons younger than 65 years of age
- 50-60% effective in preventing hospitalization among elderly persons
- 80% effective in preventing death among elderly persons

Influenza and Complications Among Nursing Home Residents

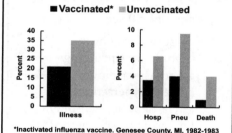

*Inactivated influenza vaccine. Genesee County, MI, 1982-1983

LAIV Efficacy in Healthy Children

- 87% effective against culture-confirmed influenza in children 60 – 84 months old
- 27% reduction in febrile otitis media (OM)
- 28% reduction in OM with accompanying antibiotic use
- Decreased fever and OM in vaccine recipients who developed influenza

12

Influenza

Inactivated Influenza Vaccine Recommendations

- Advisory Committee on Immunization Practices recommends annual influenza vaccination for all persons 6 months of age and older

- Protection of persons at higher risk for influenza-related complications should continue to be a focus of vaccination efforts as providers and programs transition to routine vaccination of all persons aged 6 months and older

Inactivated Influenza Vaccine Recommendations

- When vaccine supply is limited, vaccination efforts should focus on delivering vaccination to the following groups of persons:

    - children 6 months through 4 years (59 months) of age

    - persons 50 years and older

    - persons with chronic pulmonary (including asthma), cardiovascular (except hypertension), renal, hepatic, neurologic, hematologic, or metabolic disorders (including diabetes mellitus)

    - persons who are immunosuppressed (including immunosuppression caused by medications or by human immunodeficiency virus)

    - women who are or will be pregnant during the influenza season

of age assessed the efficacy of the trivalent LAIV against culture-confirmed influenza during two influenza seasons. In year 1, when vaccine and circulating virus strains were well matched, efficacy was 87% against culture-confirmed influenza. In year 2, when the type A component was not well matched between vaccine and circulating virus strains, efficacy was also 87%. Other results from this trial included a 27% reduction in febrile otitis media and a 28% reduction in otitis media with concomitant antibiotic use. Receipt of LAIV also resulted in decreased fever and otitis media in vaccine recipients who developed influenza.

A randomized, double-blind, placebo-controlled trial among 3,920 healthy working adults aged 18–49 years assessed several endpoints and documented reductions in illness, absenteeism, healthcare visits, and medication use during influenza outbreak periods. This study was conducted during the 1997–98 influenza season, when the vaccine and circulating type A strains were not well matched. This study did not include laboratory virus testing of cases. Some studies among children have demonstrated greater efficacy for LAIV compared to IIV. There is no evidence in adults that efficacy of LAIV is greater than that of IIV.

Vaccination Schedule and Use
IIV

Influenza activity peaks in temperate areas between late December and early March. IIV should be offered as soon as it becomes available.

Organized vaccination campaigns generally should be scheduled no earlier than mid-October. Although most influenza vaccination activities should be completed by December (particularly for high-risk groups), providers should continue to provide vaccine throughout influenza season.

One dose of IIV may be administered annually for persons 9 years of age or older. Children 6 months through 8 years of age receiving influenza vaccine for the first time should receive two doses administered at least 28 days apart.

In addition, certain children 6 months through 8 years of age who previously received influenza vaccine may be recommended to receive a second dose. Refer to the current ACIP influenza recommendations for guidance on this issue.

Inactivated influenza vaccine should be given by the intra-muscular (IM) or intradermal route (Fluzone Intradermal only). Other methods, such as subcutaneous, topical, or mucosal should not be used unless approved by the Food and Drug Administration or recommended by ACIP.

Beginning in the 2010-2011 influenza season the Advisory Committee on Immunization Practices recommended annual influenza vaccination for all persons 6 months of age and older. Protection of persons at higher risk for influenza-related complications should continue to be a focus of vaccination efforts as providers and programs transition to routine vaccination of all persons aged 6 months and older.

When vaccine supply is limited, vaccination efforts should focus on delivering vaccination to the following groups of persons: children 6 months–4 years (59 months) of age; persons 50 years and older; persons with chronic pulmonary (including asthma), cardiovascular (except hypertension), renal, hepatic, neurologic, hematologic, or metabolic disorders (including diabetes mellitus); persons who are immunosuppressed (including immunosuppression caused by medications or by human immunodeficiency virus); women who are or will be pregnant during the influenza season; children 6 months through 18 years of age and receiving long-term aspirin therapy and who therefore might be at risk for experiencing Reye syndrome after influenza virus infection; residents of nursing homes and other chronic-care facilities; American Indians/Alaska Natives; persons who are morbidly obese (body-mass index is 40 or greater); healthcare personnel; household contacts and caregivers of children younger than 5 years of age and adults 50 years of age and older, with particular emphasis on vaccinating contacts of children aged younger than 6 months; and household contacts and caregivers of persons with medical conditions that put them at higher risk for severe complications from influenza.

Case reports and limited studies suggest that pregnant women may be at increased risk for serious medical complications of influenza as a result of increases in heart rate, stroke volume and oxygen consumption; decreases in lung capacity; and changes in immunologic function. A study found that the risk of hospitalization for influenza-related complications was more than four times higher for women in the second or third trimester of pregnancy than for nonpregnant women. The risk of complications for these pregnant women was comparable to that for nonpregnant women with high-risk medical conditions, for whom influenza vaccine has been traditionally recommended.

ACIP recommends vaccination of women who will be pregnant during influenza season. Vaccination can occur during any trimester. Influenza season in the United States generally occurs in December through March. Only IIV should be administered to pregnant women.

Available data suggest that persons with HIV infection may have prolonged influenza illnesses and are at increased

- children 6 months through 18 years of age and receiving long-term aspirin therapy and who therefore might be at risk for experiencing Reye syndrome after influenza virus infection
- residents of nursing homes and other chronic-care facilities
- American Indians/Alaska Natives
- persons who are morbidly obese (body-mass index is 40 or greater)
- healthcare personnel
- household contacts and caregivers of children younger than 5 years of age and adults 50 years of age or older, with particular emphasis on vaccinating contacts of children aged younger than 6 months
- household contacts and caregivers of persons with medical conditions that put them at higher risk for severe complications from influenza

Pregnancy and Inactivated Influenza Vaccine

- Risk of hospitalization 4 times higher than nonpregnant women
- Risk of complications comparable to nonpregnant women with high-risk medical conditions
- Vaccination (with IIV) recommended if pregnant during influenza season
- Vaccination can occur during any trimester

12

Influenza

HIV Infection and Inactivated Influenza Vaccine

- Persons with HIV at increased risk of complications of influenza
- IIV induces protective antibody titers in many HIV-infected persons
- IIV will benefit many HIV-infected person

Simultaneous Administration of LAIV and Other Vaccines

- Inactivated vaccines can be administered either simultaneously or at any time before or after LAIV
- Other live vaccines can be administered on the same day as LAIV
- Live vaccines not administered on the same day should be administered at least 4 weeks apart

---

risk of complications of influenza. Many persons with HIV infection will develop protective antibody titers following inactivated influenza vaccine. In persons who have advanced HIV disease and low CD4+ T-lymphocyte cell counts, IIV vaccine may not induce protective antibody titers. A second dose of vaccine does not improve the immune response in these persons.

Efforts should be made to vaccinate household and other close contacts of high-risk persons. These include healthcare personnel, employees of long-term care facilities, and household contacts of high-risk persons. These individuals may be younger and healthier and more likely to be protected from illness than are elderly persons. All healthcare providers should receive annual inactivated influenza vaccine. Groups that should be targeted include physicians, nurses, and other personnel in hospitals and outpatient settings who have contact with high-risk patients in all age groups, and providers of home care to high-risk persons (e.g., visiting nurses, volunteers). LAIV may be administered to healthy healthcare personnel 49 years of age or younger, except those who have contact with severely immunosuppressed persons who require hospitalization and care in a protective environment (i.e., in isolation because of severe immunosuppression).

LAIV

LAIV is approved for healthy, nonpregnant persons 2 through 49 years of age. The vaccine can be administered to eligible persons as soon as it becomes available in the late summer or fall. Vaccination can continue throughout influenza season. One dose of LAIV may be administered by the intranasal route to persons 9 through 49 years of age. Children 2 through 8 years of age receiving influenza vaccine for the first time should receive two doses administered at least 4 weeks apart.

In addition, certain children 6 months through 8 years of age who previously received influenza vaccine may be recommended to receive a second dose. Refer to the current ACIP influenza recommendations for guidance on this issue.

Close contacts of persons at high risk for complications from influenza should receive influenza vaccine. Contacts of persons at high risk of complications of influenza may receive LAIV if they are otherwise eligible (i.e., 2 through 49 years of age, healthy and not pregnant). Persons in close contact with severely immunosuppressed persons who are hospitalized and receiving care in a protected environment should not receive LAIV.

Inactivated vaccines do not interfere with the immune response to live vaccines. Inactivated vaccines, such as tetanus and diphtheria toxoids, can be administered either simultaneously or at any time before or after LAIV. Other live vaccines can be administered on the same day as LAIV. Live vaccines not administered on the same day should be administered at least 4 weeks apart.

Contraindications and Precautions to Vaccination

IIV

Persons with a severe allergic reaction (anaphylaxis) to a vaccine component or following a prior dose of inactivated influenza vaccine should not receive IIV. In 2011, ACIP revised its recommendation for influenza vaccination of persons with egg allergy. Persons whose allergy involves only urticaria without other symptoms may receive IIV. See the ACIP influenza vaccine recommendations for further information. Persons with a moderate or severe acute illness normally should not be vaccinated until their symptoms have decreased. A history of Guillian Barre' syndrome (GBS) within 6 weeks following a previous dose of influenza vaccine is a precaution for IIV. Pregnancy, breastfeeding, and immunosuppression are not contraindications to inactivated influenza vaccination.

LAIV

Persons who should not receive LAIV include children younger than 2 years of age; persons 50 years of age and older; persons with chronic medical conditions, including asthma, a recent wheezing episode, reactive airways disease or other chronic pulmonary or cardiovascular conditions, metabolic disease such as diabetes, renal disease, or hemoglobinopathy, such as sickle cell disease; and children or adolescents receiving long-term therapy with aspirin or aspirin-containing therapy, because of the association of Reye syndrome with wild-type influenza infection. Persons in these groups should receive inactivated influenza vaccine.

As with other live-virus vaccines, LAIV should not be given to persons who are immunosuppressed because of disease, including HIV, or who are receiving immunosuppressive therapy. Pregnant women should not receive LAIV. Immunosuppressed persons and pregnant women should receive inactivated influenza vaccine. Since LAIV contains residual egg protein, it should not be administered to persons with a history of severe allergy to egg or any other vaccine component. A history of Guillian Barre' syndrome (GBS) within 6 weeks following a previous dose of influenza vaccine is a precaution for LAIV.

Inactivated Influenza Vaccine Contraindications and Precautions

- Severe allergic reaction (e.g., anaphylaxis) to a vaccine component or following a prior dose of inactivated influenza
- Moderate or severe acute illness
- History of Guillian-Barré syndrome (GBS) within 6 weeks following a previous dose of influenza vaccine

Live Attenuated Influenza Vaccine Contraindications and Precautions

- Children younger than 2 years of age*
- Persons 50 years of age or older*
- Persons with chronic medical conditions*
- Children and adolescents receiving long-term aspirin or aspirin-containing therapy*
- Immunosuppression from any cause*
- Pregnant women*
- Severe allergy to egg or other vaccine components
- History of Guillian Barré syndrome (GBS) within 6 weeks following a previous dose of influenza vaccine
- Children younger than 5 years with recurrent wheezing*
- Recent wheezing
- Moderate or severe acute illness

*These persons should receive inactivated influenza vaccine

12

Influenza

As with all vaccines, LAIV should be deferred for persons with a moderate or severe acute illness. If clinical judgment indicates that nasal congestion might impede delivery of the vaccine to the nasopharyngeal mucosa, deferral of administration should be considered until the condition has improved.

The effect on safety and efficacy of LAIV coadministration with influenza antiviral medications has not been studied. However, because influenza antiviral agents reduce replication of influenza viruses, LAIV should not be administered until 48 hours after cessation of influenza antiviral therapy, and influenza antiviral medications should not be administered for 2 weeks after receipt of LAIV.

Adverse Events Following Vaccination
IIV

Local reactions are the most common adverse events following vaccination with IIV.

Although the incidence of Guillain-Barré syndrome (GBS) in the general population is very low, persons with a history of GBS have a substantially greater likelihood of subsequently developing GBS than do persons without such a history, irrespective of vaccination. As a result, the likelihood of coincidentally developing GBS after influenza vaccination is expected to be greater among persons with a history of GBS than among persons with no history of GBS. Whether influenza vaccination might be causally associated with this risk for recurrence is not known. It seems prudent for persons known to have developed GBS within 6 weeks of a previous influenza vaccination to avoid subsequent influenza vaccination. For most persons with a history of GBS who are at high risk for severe complications from influenza, the established benefits of influenza vaccination justify yearly vaccination. Unlike the 1976 swine influenza vaccine, subsequent inactivated vaccines prepared from other virus strains have not been clearly associated with an increased frequency of Guillain-Barré syndrome (GBS). However, obtaining a precise estimate of a small increase in risk is difficult for a rare condition such as GBS, which has an annual background incidence of only one to two cases per year per 100,000 adult population.

LAIV

Among children the most common adverse events are nonspecific systemic symptoms (e.g. runny nose and headaches). However, there have been no significant differences between LAIV and placebo recipients in the proportion with these symptoms. Guillain-Barré syndrome has not been associated with LAIV in post-licensure safety monitoring.

Influenza Vaccine Adverse Events

- IIV
  - local reactions – common
  - Guillain-Barré syndrome – expected to be greater among persons with a history of GBS than among persons with no history of GBS
- LAIV
  - nonspecific systemic symptoms – common

Inactivated Influenza Vaccine Adverse Reactions

- Local reactions (soreness, redness)
  - 15% - 20%
- Fever, malaise, myalgia
  - less than 1%
- Allergic reactions (hives, angioedema, anaphylaxis)
  - rare

Adverse Reactions Following Vaccination
IIV

Local reactions include soreness, erythema, and induration at the site of injection. These reactions are transient, generally lasting 1 to 2 days. Local reactions are reported in 15%–20% of vaccinees.

Nonspecific systemic symptoms, including fever, chills, malaise, and myalgia, are reported in fewer than 1% of IIV recipients. These symptoms usually occur in those with no previous exposure to the viral antigens in the vaccine. They usually occur within 6–12 hours of IIV vaccination and last 1–2 days. Recent reports indicate that these systemic symptoms are no more common than in persons given a placebo injection.

Rarely, immediate hypersensitivity, presumably allergic, reactions (such as hives, angioedema, allergic asthma, or systemic anaphylaxis) occur after vaccination with IIV. These reactions probably result from hypersensitivity to a vaccine component. Severe allergic and anaphylactic reactions can occur in response to a number of influenza vaccine components, but such reactions are rare. Most currently available influenza vaccines are prepared by means of inoculation of virus into chicken eggs.

ACIP recommends that persons with egg allergy who report only hives after egg exposure should receive IIV, with several additional safety measures, as summarized below:

1. Persons with a history of egg allergy who have experienced only hives after exposure to egg should receive influenza vaccine, with the following additional safety measures

    a. Because studies published to date involved use of IIV, IIV rather than LAIV should be used;

    b. Vaccine should be administered by a healthcare provider who is familiar with the potential manifestations of egg allergy; and

    c. Vaccine recipients should be observed for at least 30 minutes for signs of a reaction after administration of each vaccine dose.

2. Persons who report having had reactions to egg involving such symptoms as angioedema, respiratory distress, lightheadedness, or recurrent emesis; or who required epinephrine or another emergency medical intervention, particularly those that occurred immediately or within a short time (minutes to hours) after egg exposure, are more likely to have a serious

12

12

systemic or anaphylactic reaction upon reexposure to egg proteins. Before receipt of vaccine, such persons should be referred to a physician with expertise in the management of allergic conditions for further risk assessment.

The potential exists for hypersensitivity reactions to any vaccine component. Although exposure to vaccines containing thimerosal can lead to induction of hypersensitivity, most patients do not develop reactions to thimerosal administered as a component of vaccines, even when patch or intradermal tests for thimerosal indicate hypersensitivity. When it has been reported, hypersensitivity to thimerosal has usually consisted of local delayed-type hypersensitivity reactions.

In 1976 there was a small increased risk of GBS following vaccination with an influenza vaccine made to protect against a swine flu virus. The increased risk was approximately 1 additional case of GBS per 100,000 people who received swine flu vaccine. The Institute of Medicine (IOM) conducted a thorough scientific review of this issue in 2003 and concluded that people who received the 1976 swine influenza vaccine had an increased risk for developing GBS. The exact reason for this association is unknown.

Several studies assessing the risk of GBS after seasonal flu vaccines in the years following the 1976 swine influenza vaccination campaign either have not been associated with an increased risk of GBS or have been associated with a small increase in risk of 1 to 2 cases per million people vaccinated. Studies assessing GBS following the 2009 (H1N1) swine-origin flu vaccine also showed that there is a small increased risk of GBS of about 1-3 cases per million people vaccinated. It is important to keep in mind that severe illness and death can result from influenza, and vaccination is the best way to prevent influenza disease and its complications.

LAIV

In a clinical trial, children 6 through 23 months of age had an increased risk of wheezing. An increased risk of wheezing was not reported in older children.

In other clinical trials, among healthy adults, a significantly increased rate of cough, runny nose, nasal congestion, sore throat, and chills was reported among vaccine recipients. These symptoms were reported in 10%–40% of vaccine recipients, a rate 3%–10% higher than reported for placebo recipients. There was no increase in the occurrence of fever among vaccine recipients. No serious adverse reactions have been identified in LAIV recipients, either children or adults.

Live Attenuated Influenza Vaccine Adverse Reactions

- Children
  - no significant increase in URI symptoms, fever, or other systemic symptoms
  - increased risk of wheezing in children 6-23 months of age
- Adults
  - significantly increased rate of cough, runny nose, nasal congestion, sore throat, and chills reported among vaccine recipients
  - no increase in the occurrence of fever
- No serious adverse reactions identified

Few data are available concerning the safety of LAIV among persons at high risk for development of complications of influenza, such as immunosuppressed persons or those with chronic pulmonary or cardiac disease. Therefore, persons at high risk of complications of influenza should not receive LAIV. These persons should continue to receive inactivated influenza vaccine.

Vaccine Storage and Handling

Inactivated influenza vaccines should be maintained at refrigerator temperature between 35°F and 46°F (2°C and 8°C). Manufacturer package inserts contain additional information and can be found at http://www.fda.gov/BiologicsBloodVaccines/Vaccines/ApprovedProducts/ucm093830.htm. For complete information on best practices and recommendations please refer to CDC's Vaccine Storage and Handling Toolkit, http://www.cdc.gov/vaccines/recs/storage/toolkit/storage-handling-toolkit.pdf.

LAIV is intended for intranasal administration only and should never be administered by injection. LAIV is supplied in a prefilled single-use sprayer containing 0.2 mL of vaccine. Approximately 0.1 mL (i.e., half of the total sprayer contents) is sprayed into the first nostril while the recipient is in the upright position. An attached dose-divider clip is removed from the sprayer to administer the second half of the dose into the other nostril. If the vaccine recipient sneezes after administration, the dose should not be repeated.

Strategies for Improving Influenza Vaccine Coverage

On average, fewer than 50% of persons in high-risk groups receive influenza vaccine each year. By November 2012 only 47.3 percent of pregnant women had received influenza vaccine for the 2012-2013 season. This points to the need for more effective strategies for delivering vaccine to high-risk persons, their healthcare providers, and household contacts. Persons for whom the vaccine is recommended can be identified and immunized in a variety of settings.

In physicians' offices and outpatient clinics, persons who should receive inactivated influenza vaccine should be identified and their charts marked. IIV use should be promoted, encouraged and recommended beginning in October and continuing through the influenza season. Those without regularly scheduled visits should receive reminders.

In nursing homes and other residential long-term care facilities, immunization with IIV should be routinely provided

12

Influenza

to all residents at one period of time immediately preceding the influenza season; consent should be obtained at the time of admission.

In acute care hospitals and continuing care centers, persons for whom vaccine is recommended who are hospitalized from October through March should be vaccinated prior to discharge. In outpatient facilities providing continuing care to high-risk patients (e.g., hemodialysis centers, hospital specialty-care clinics, outpatient rehabilitation programs), all patients should be offered IIV shortly before the onset of the influenza season.

Visiting nurses and others providing home care to high-risk persons should identify high-risk patients and administer IIV in the home, if necessary.

In facilities providing services to persons 50 years of age and older (e.g., retirement communities, recreation centers), inactivated influenza vaccine should be offered to all unvaccinated residents or attendees on site. Education and publicity programs should also be conducted in conjunction with other interventions.

For travelers, indications for influenza vaccine should be reviewed prior to travel and vaccine offered, if appropriate.

Administrators of all of the above facilities and organizations should arrange for influenza vaccine to be offered to all personnel before the influenza season. Additionally, household members of high-risk persons and others with whom they will be in contact should receive written information about why they should receive the vaccine and where to obtain it.

Antiviral Agents for Influenza

In the United States, four antiviral agents are approved for preventing or treating influenza: amantadine, rimantadine, zanamivir, and oseltamivir.

Testing of influenza A isolates from the United States and Canada has demonstrated that most of these viruses are resistant to amantadine and rimantadine. The ACIP recommends that neither amantadine nor rimantadine be used for the treatment or chemoprophylaxis of influenza A in the United States.

Zanamivir and oseltamivir are members of a class of drugs called neuraminidase inhibitors and are active against both influenza type A and type B. Zanamivir is provided as a dry powder that is administered by inhalation. It is approved for treatment of uncomplicated acute influenza A or B in persons 7 years of age and older who have been

---

Influenza Antiviral Agents*

- Amantadine and rimantadine
  - not recommended because of documented resistance in U.S. influenza isolates
- Zanamivir and oseltamivir
  - neuraminidase inhibitors
  - effective against influenza A and B
  - oseltamavir and zanamavir approved for prophylaxis

*see influenza ACIP statement or CDC influenza website for details

symptomatic for no more than 48 hours. Oseltamivir is provided as an oral capsule. It is approved for the treatment of uncomplicated influenza A or B in persons 2 weeks of age and older who have been symptomatic for no more than 48 hours. Zanamivir is approved for prophylaxis of influenza in persons 5 years and older. Oseltamivir is approved for prophylaxis of influenza infection among persons 1 year of age and older.

In 2007-08, a significant increase in the prevalence of oseltamivir resistance was reported among influenza A(H1N1) viruses worldwide. During the 2007-08 influenza season, 10.9% of H1N1 viruses tested in the U.S. were resistant to oseltamivir. During 2008 more than 90% of H1N1 viruses were resistant to oseltamivir. For the 2008-09 influenza season CDC recommends that persons who test positive for influenza A should receive only zanamivir if treatment is indicated. Oseltamivir should be used alone only if recent local surveillance data indicate that circulating viruses are likely to be influenza A(H3N2) or influenza B viruses, which have not been found to be resistant to oseltamivir. As of 2013 seasonal viruses are almost 100% susceptible to oseltamivir as well as zanamivir.

Antiviral agents for influenza are an adjunct to vaccine and are not a substitute for vaccine. Vaccination remains the principal means for preventing influenza-related morbidity and mortality. Additional information on the use of influenza antiviral drugs can be found in the current ACIP statement on influenza vaccine and on the CDC influenza website at http://www.cdc.gov/flu.

Nosocomial Influenza Control

Many patients in general hospitals, and especially in referral centers, are likely to be at high risk for complications of influenza. Hospitalized susceptible patients may acquire influenza from other patients, hospital employees, or visitors. The preferred method of control is to administer inactivated influenza vaccine to high-risk patients and medical personnel.

During community influenza A activity, the use of antiviral prophylaxis may be considered for high-risk patients who were not immunized or were immunized too recently to have protective antibody levels. Antiviral agents may also be considered for unimmunized hospital personnel. Other measures include restricting visitors with respiratory illness, cohorting patients with influenza for 5 days following onset of illness, and postponing elective admission of patients with uncomplicated illness.

12

Influenza Surveillance

- Monitor prevalence of circulating strains and detect new strains

- Estimate influenza-related morbidity, mortality and economic loss

- Rapidly detect outbreaks

- Assist disease control through rapid preventive action

Influenza

Influenza Surveillance

Influenza surveillance is intended to monitor the prevalence of circulating strains and detect new strains necessary for vaccine formulation; estimate influenza-related impact on morbidity, mortality, and economic loss; rapidly detect outbreaks; and assist disease control through rapid preventive action (e.g., chemoprophylaxis of unvaccinated high-risk patients).

CDC receives weekly surveillance reports from the states showing the extent of influenza activity. Reports are classified into four categories: no cases, sporadic, regional (cases occurring in counties collectively contributing less than 50% of a state's population), widespread (cases occurring in counties collectively contributing 50% or more of a state's population).

Weekly surveillance reports are available at http://www.cdc.gov/flu/weekly/fluactivity.htm

Acknowledgement

The editors thank Drs. Lisa Grohskopf, Jerome Tokars, Tom Shimabukuro, and Scott Epperson, CDC for their assistance in updating this chapter.

Selected References

A special issue of *Clinical Infectious Diseases* (January 2011) focused on the 2009 H1N1 influenza pandemic.

Bhat N, Wright JG, Broder KR, et al. Influenza-associated deaths among children in the United States, 2003–2004. *N Engl J Med.* 2005;353:2559–67.

CDC. Estimates of deaths associated with seasonal influenza – United States, 1976-2007. *MMWR* 2010;59(No. 33): 1057-62.

Centers for Disease Control and Prevention. [Prevention and Control of Seasonal Influenza with Vaccines Recommendations of the Advisory Committee on Immunization Practices — United States, 2013–2014]. MMWR 2013;62(No. RR-7):[1-46].

CDC. Influenza vaccination of healthcare personnel. Recommendations of the Healthcare Infection Control Practices Advisory Committee (HICPAC) and the Advisory Committee on Immunization Practices (ACIP). *MMWR* 2006; 55(No. RR-2):1–16.

Fedson DS, Houck P, Bratzler D. Hospital-based influenza and pneumococcal vaccination: Sutton's law applied to prevention. *Infect Control Hosp Epidemiol* 2000;21:692–9.

12

Glezen WP, Couch RB. Influenza viruses. In: Evans AS, Kaslow RA, eds. Viral Infections of Humans. *Epidemiology and Control*. 4th edition. New York, NY: Plenum Medical Book Company;1997:473–505.

Monto AS, Ohmit SE, Petrie JG, et al. Comparative efficacy of inactivated and live attenuated influenza vaccines. *N Engl J Med* 2009;361:1260-7.

Murphy KR, Strunk RC. Safe administration of influenza vaccine in asthmatic children hypersensitive to egg protein. *J Pediatr* 1985;106:931–3.

Neuzil KM, Zhu Y, Griffin MR, et al. Burden of interpandemic influenza in children younger than 5 years: a 25 year prospective study. *J Infect Dis* 2002;185:147–52.

Nichol KL, Lind A, Margolis KL, et al. The effectiveness of vaccination against influenza in healthy, working adults. *N Engl J Med* 1995;333:889–93.

Saxen H, Virtanen M. Randomized, placebo-controlled double blind study on the efficacy of influenza immunization on absenteeism of healthcare workers. *Pediatr Infect Dis J* 1999;18:779–83.

12

Influenza

Measles is an acute viral infectious disease. References to measles can be found from as early as the 7th century. The disease was described by the Persian physician Rhazes in the 10th century as "more to be dreaded than smallpox."

In 1846, Peter Panum described the incubation period of measles and lifelong immunity after recovery from the disease. Enders and Peebles isolated the virus in human and monkey kidney tissue culture in 1954. The first live attenuated vaccine was licensed for use in the United States in 1963 (Edmonston B strain).

Before a vaccine was available, infection with measles virus was nearly universal during childhood, and more than 90% of persons were immune by age 15 years. Measles is still a common and often fatal disease in developing countries. The World Health Organization estimates there were 145,700 deaths globally from measles in 2013.

Measles Virus

The measles virus is a paramyxovirus, genus *Morbillivirus*. It is 120–250 nm in diameter, with a core of single-stranded RNA, and is closely related to the rinderpest and canine distemper viruses. Two membrane envelope proteins are important in pathogenesis. They are the F (fusion) protein, which is responsible for fusion of virus and host cell membranes, viral penetration, and hemolysis, and the H (hemagglutinin) protein, which is responsible for adsorption of virus to cells.

There is only one antigenic type of measles virus. Although studies have documented changes in the H glycoprotein, these changes do not appear to be epidemiologically important (i.e., no change in vaccine efficacy has been observed).

Measles virus is rapidly inactivated by heat, sunlight, acidic pH, ether, and trypsin. It has a short survival time (less than 2 hours) in the air or on objects and surfaces.

Pathogenesis

Measles is a systemic infection. The primary site of infection is the respiratory epithelium of the nasopharynx. Two to three days after invasion and replication in the respiratory epithelium and regional lymph nodes, a primary viremia occurs with subsequent infection of the reticuloendothelial system. Following further viral replication in regional and distal reticuloendothelial sites, a second viremia occurs 5–7 days after initial infection. During this viremia, there may be infection of the respiratory tract and other organs. Measles virus is shed from the nasopharynx beginning with the prodrome until 3–4 days after rash onset.

Measles
- Highly contagious viral illness
- First described in 7th century
- Near universal infection of childhood in prevaccination era
- Common and often fatal in developing countries

Measles Virus
- Paramyxovirus (RNA)
- Hemagglutinin important surface antigen
- One antigenic type
- Rapidly inactivated by heat, sunlight, acidic pH, ether and trypsin

13

Measles Pathogenesis
- Respiratory transmission of virus
- Replication in nasopharynx and regional lymph nodes
- Primary viremia 2-3 days after exposure
- Secondary viremia 5-7 days after exposure with spread to tissues

Measles

Measles Clinical Features

- Incubation period 10-12 days
- Prodrome 2-4 days
  - stepwise increase in fever to 103°F–105°F
  - cough, coryza, conjunctivitis
  - Koplik spots (rash on mucous membranes)
- Rash
  - 2-4 days after prodrome, 14 days after exposure
  - persists 5-6 days
  - begins on face and upper neck
  - maculopapular, becomes confluent
  - fades in order of appearance

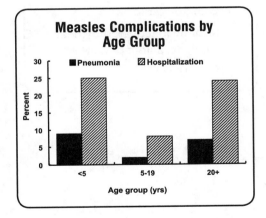

Measles Complications by Age Group

Measles Complications

Diarrhea	8%
Otitis media	7%
Pneumonia	6%
Encephalitis	0.1%
Seizures	0.6-0.7%
Death	0.2%

Based on 1985-1992 surveillance data

Clinical Features

The incubation period of measles, from exposure to prodrome, averages 10–12 days. From exposure to rash onset averages 14 days (range, 7–21 days).

The prodrome lasts 2–4 days (range 1–7 days). It is characterized by fever, which increases in stepwise fashion, often peaking as high as 103°F –105°F. This is followed by the onset of cough, coryza (runny nose), or conjunctivitis.

Koplik spots, a rash present on mucous membranes, is considered to be pathognomonic for measles. It occurs 1–2 days before the rash to 1–2 days after the rash, and appears as punctate blue-white spots on the bright red background of the buccal mucosa.

The measles rash is a maculopapular eruption that usually lasts 5–6 days. It begins at the hairline, then involves the face and upper neck. During the next 3 days, the rash gradually proceeds downward and outward, reaching the hands and feet. The maculopapular lesions are generally discrete, but may become confluent, particularly on the upper body. Initially, lesions blanch with fingertip pressure. By 3–4 days, most do not blanch with pressure. Fine desquamation occurs over more severely involved areas. The rash fades in the same order that it appears, from head to extremities.

Other symptoms of measles include anorexia; diarrhea, especially in infants; and generalized lymphadenopathy.

Complications

Approximately 30% of reported measles cases have one or more complications. Complications of measles are most common among children younger than 5 years of age and adults 20 years of age and older.

From 1985 through 1992, diarrhea was reported in 8% of measles cases, making this the most commonly reported complication of measles. Otitis media was reported in 7% of cases and occurs almost exclusively in children. Pneumonia (in 6% of reported cases) may be viral or superimposed bacterial, and is the most common cause of measles-related death.

Acute encephalitis occurs in approximately 0.1% of reported cases. Onset generally occurs 6 days after rash onset (range 1–15 days) and is characterized by fever, headache, vomiting, stiff neck, meningeal irritation, drowsiness, convulsions, and coma. Cerebrospinal fluid shows pleocytosis and elevated protein. The case-fatality rate is approximately 15%. Some form of residual neurologic damage occurs in as many as 25% of cases. Seizures (with or without fever) are reported in 0.6%–0.7% of cases.

Death from measles was reported in approximately 0.2% of the cases in the United States from 1985 through 1992. As with other complications of measles, the risk of death is highest among young children and adults. Pneumonia accounts for about 60% of deaths. The most common causes of death are pneumonia in children and acute encephalitis in adults.

Subacute sclerosing panencephalitis (SSPE) is a rare degenerative central nervous system disease believed to be due to persistent measles virus infection of the brain. Onset occurs an average of 7 years after measles (range 1 month–27 years), and occurs in five to ten cases per million reported measles cases. The onset is insidious, with progressive deterioration of behavior and intellect, followed by ataxia (awkwardness), myoclonic seizures, and eventually death. SSPE has been extremely rare since the early 1980s.

Measles illness during pregnancy results in a higher risk of premature labor, spontaneous abortion, and low-birth-weight infants. Birth defects (with no definable pattern of malformation) have been reported rarely, without confirmation that measles was the cause.

"Atypical measles" occurs only in persons who received inactivated (killed) measles vaccine (KMV) and are subsequently exposed to wild-type measles virus. An estimated 600,000 to 900,000 persons received KMV in the United States from 1963 to 1967. KMV sensitizes the recipient to measles virus antigens without providing protection. Subsequent infection with measles virus leads to signs of hypersensitivity polyserositis. The illness is characterized by fever, pneumonia, pleural effusions, and edema. The rash is usually maculopapular or petechial, but may have urticarial, purpuric, or vesicular components. It appears first on the wrists or ankles. Atypical measles may be prevented by revaccinating with live measles vaccine. Moderate to severe local reactions with or without fever may follow vaccination; these reactions are less severe than with wild measles virus infection.

Modified measles occurs primarily in patients who received immune globulin (IG) as postexposure prophylaxis and in young infants who have some residual maternal antibody. It is usually characterized by a prolonged incubation period, mild prodrome, and sparse, discrete rash of short duration. Similar mild illness has been reported among previously vaccinated persons.

Rarely reported in the United States, hemorrhagic measles is characterized by high fever (105°F–106°F), seizures, delirium, respiratory distress, and hemorrhage into the skin and mucous membranes.

13

Measles

Measles in an immunocompromised person can be severe with a prolonged course. It is reported almost exclusively in persons with T-cell deficiencies (certain leukemias, lymphomas, and acquired immunodeficiency syndrome [AIDS]). It may occur without the typical rash, and a patient may shed virus for several weeks after the acute illness.

Measles in developing countries has resulted in high attack rates among children younger than 12 months of age. Measles is more severe in malnourished children, particularly those with vitamin A deficiency. Complications include diarrhea, dehydration, stomatitis, inability to feed, and bacterial infections (skin and elsewhere). The case-fatality rate may be as high as 25%. Measles is also a leading cause of blindness in African children.

Laboratory Diagnosis

Isolation of measles virus is not recommended as a routine method to diagnose measles. However, virus isolates are extremely important for molecular epidemiologic surveillance to help determine the geographic origin of the virus and the viral strains circulating in the United States.

Measles virus can be isolated from urine, nasopharyngeal aspirates, heparinized blood, or throat swabs. Specimens for virus culture should be obtained from every person with a clinically suspected case of measles and should be shipped to the state public health laboratory or CDC, at the direction of the state health department. Clinical specimens for viral isolation should be collected at the same time as samples taken for serologic testing. Because the virus is more likely to be isolated when specimens are collected within 3 days of rash onset, collection of specimens for virus isolation should not be delayed until serologic confirmation is obtained. Clinical specimens should be obtained within 7 days, and not more than 10 days, after rash onset. A detailed protocol for collection of specimens for viral isolation is available on the CDC website at http://www.cdc.gov/measles/lab-tools/rt-pcr.html.

Serologic testing, most commonly by enzyme-linked immunoassay (EIA), is widely available and may be diagnostic if done at the appropriate time. Generally, a previously susceptible person exposed to either vaccine or wild-type measles virus will first mount an IgM response and then an IgG response. The IgM response will be transient (1–2 months), and the IgG response should persist for many years. Uninfected persons should be IgM negative and will be either IgG negative or IgG positive, depending upon their previous infection or vaccination history.

Measles Laboratory Diagnosis

- Isolation of measles virus from urine, nasopharynx, blood, throat
- Significant rise in measles IgG by any standard serologic assay (e.g., EIA, HI)
- Positive serologic test for measles IgM antibody

EIA for IgM antibody requires only a single serum specimen and is diagnostic if positive. The preferred reference test is a capture IgM test developed by CDC. This test should be used to confirm every case of measles that is reported to have some other type of laboratory confirmation. IgM capture tests for measles are often positive on the day of rash onset. However, in the first 72 hours after rash onset, up to 20% of tests for IgM may give false-negative results. Tests that are negative in the first 72 hours after rash onset should be repeated. IgM is detectable for at least 30 days after rash onset and frequently longer.

A variety of tests for IgG antibodies to measles are available and include EIA, hemagglutination inhibition (HI), indirect fluorescent antibody tests, microneutralization, and plaque reduction neutralization. Complement fixation, while widely used in the past, is no longer recommended.

IgG testing for acute measles requires demonstration of a four-fold rise in titer of antibody against measles virus, so two serum specimens are always required. The first specimen should be drawn as soon after rash onset as possible. The second specimen should be drawn 10–30 days later. The tests for IgG antibody should be conducted on both specimens at the same time. The same type of test should be used on both specimens. The specific criteria for documenting an increase in titer depend on the test.

Tests for IgG antibody require two serum specimens, and a confirmed diagnosis cannot be made until the second specimen is obtained. As a result, IgM tests are generally preferred to confirm the diagnosis of measles.

Epidemiology
Occurrence

Measles occurs throughout the world. However, interruption of indigenous transmission of measles has been achieved in the United States and other parts of the Western Hemisphere.

Reservoir

Measles is a human disease. There is no known animal reservoir, and an asymptomatic carrier state has not been documented.

Transmission

Measles transmission is primarily person to person via large respiratory droplets. Airborne transmission via aerosolized droplet nuclei has been documented in closed areas (e.g., office examination room) for up to 2 hours after a person with measles occupied the area.

13

Measles Epidemiology
- Reservoir
  - human
- Transmission
  - respiratory Airborne
- Temporal pattern
  - peak in late winter–spring
- Communicability
  - 4 days before to 4 days after rash onset

Measles

Measles - United States, 1950-2011

Measles - United States, 1950-2011

Source: National Notifiable Disease Surveillance System, CDC

Measles - United States, 1980-2011

Measles - United States, 1980-2011

Source: National Notifiable Disease Surveillance System, CDC

Measles Resurgence—United States, 1989-1991

- Cases
  - 55,622
- Age group affected
  - children younger than five years
- Deaths
  - 123

Temporal Pattern

In temperate areas, measles disease occurs primarily in late winter and spring.

Communicability

Measles is highly communicable, with greater than 90% secondary attack rates among susceptible persons. Measles may be transmitted from 4 days before to 4 days after rash onset. Maximum communicability occurs from onset of prodrome through the first 3–4 days of rash.

Secular Trends in the United States

Before 1963, approximately 500,000 cases and 500 deaths were reported annually, with epidemic cycles every 2–3 years. However, the actual number of cases was estimated at 3–4 million annually. More than 50% of persons had measles by age 6, and more than 90% had measles by age 15. The highest incidence was among 5–9-year-olds, who generally accounted for more than 50% of reported cases.

In the years following licensure of vaccine in 1963, the incidence of measles decreased by more than 95%, and 2–3-year epidemic cycles no longer occurred. Because of this success, a 1978 Measles Elimination Program set a goal to eliminate indigenous measles by October 1, 1982 (26,871 cases were reported in 1978). The 1982 elimination goal was not met, but in 1983, only 1,497 cases were reported (0.6 cases per 100,000 population), the lowest annual total ever reported up to that time.

During 1980–1988, a median of 57% of reported cases were among school-aged persons (5–19 years of age), and a median of 29% were among children younger than 5 years of age. A median of 8% of cases were among infants younger than 1 year of age.

From 1985 through 1988, 42% of cases occurred in persons who were vaccinated on or after their first birthday. During these years, 68% of cases in school-aged children (5–19 years) occurred among those who had been appropriately vaccinated. The occurrence of measles among previously vaccinated children (i.e., vaccine failure) led to a recommendation for a second dose in this age group.

Measles Resurgence in 1989–1991

From 1989 through 1991, a dramatic increase in reported measles cases occurred. During these 3 years a total of 55,622 cases were reported (18,193 in 1989; 27,786 in 1990; 9,643 in 1991). In addition to the increased number of cases, a change occurred in their age distribution. Prior to the resurgence, school-aged children had accounted for the largest proportion of reported cases. During the resurgence, 45% of all reported cases were in children younger than 5 years of age. In 1990, 48% of patients were in this age group, the first time that the proportion of cases in children younger than 5 years of age exceeded the proportion of cases in 5–19-year-olds (35%).

Overall incidence rates were highest for Hispanics and blacks and lowest for non-Hispanic whites. Among children younger than 5 years of age, the incidence of measles among blacks and Hispanics was four to seven times higher than among non-Hispanic whites.

A total of 123 measles-associated deaths were reported during this period (death-to-case ratio of 2.2 per 1,000 cases). Forty-nine percent of deaths were among children younger than 5 years of age. Ninety percent of fatal cases occurred among persons with no history of vaccination. Sixty-four deaths were reported in 1990, the largest annual number of deaths from measles since 1971.

The most important cause of the measles resurgence of 1989–1991 was low vaccination coverage. Measles vaccine coverage was low in many cities, including some that experienced large outbreaks among preschool-aged children throughout the early to mid-1980s. Surveys in areas experiencing outbreaks among preschool-aged children indicated that as few as 50% of children had been vaccinated against measles by their second birthday, and that black and Hispanic children were less likely to be age-appropriately vaccinated than were white children.

In addition, measles susceptibility of infants younger than 1 year of age may have increased. During the 1989–1991 measles resurgence, incidence rates for infants were more than twice as high as those in any other age group. The mothers of many infants who developed measles were young, and their measles immunity was most often due to vaccination rather than infection with wild virus. As a result, a smaller amount of antibody was transferred across the placenta to the fetus, compared with antibody transfer from mothers who had higher antibody titers resulting from wild-virus infection. The lower quantity of antibody resulted in immunity that waned more rapidly, making infants susceptible at a younger age than in the past.

The increase in measles in 1989–1991 was not limited to the United States. Large outbreaks of measles were reported by many other countries of North and Central America, including Canada, El Salvador, Guatemala, Honduras, Jamaica, Mexico, and Nicaragua.

13

Measles

Measles 1993-2011

- Endemic transmission interrupted

- Record low annual total in 2004 (37 total cases)

- Many cases among adults

- Most cases imported or linked to importation

- Most persons with measles were unvaccinated or unknown vaccination status

- In 2011, CDC reported 16 outbreaks of measles and 220 measles cases, most of which were imported cases in unvaccinated persons

Measles Since 1993

Reported cases of measles declined rapidly after the 1989–1991 resurgence. This decline was due primarily to intensive efforts to vaccinate preschool-aged children. Measles vaccination levels among 2-year-old children increased from 70% in 1990 to 91% in 1997.

Since 1993, fewer than 500 cases have been reported annually, and fewer than 200 cases per year have been reported since 1997. A record low annual total of 37 cases was reported in 2004. Available epidemiologic and virologic data indicate that measles transmission in the United States has been interrupted. The majority of cases are now imported from other countries or linked to imported cases. Most imported cases originate in Asia and Europe and occur both among U.S. citizens traveling abroad and persons visiting the United States from other countries. An aggressive measles vaccination program by the Pan American Health Organization (PAHO) has resulted in record low measles incidence in Latin America and the Caribbean, and the interruption of indigenous measles transmission in the Americas. Measles elimination from the Americas was achieved in 2002 and has been sustained since then, with only imported and importation-related measles cases occuring in the region.

Since the mid-1990s, no age group has predominated among reported cases of measles. Relative to earlier decades, an increased proportion of cases now occur among adults. In 1973, persons 20 years of age and older accounted for only about 3% of cases. In 1994, adults accounted for 24% of cases, and in 2001, for 48% of all reported cases.

The size and makeup of measles outbreaks has changed since the 1980s. Prior to 1989, the majority of outbreaks occurred among middle, high school and college student populations. As many as 95% of persons infected during these outbreaks had received one prior dose of measles vaccine. A second dose of measles vaccine was recommended for school-aged children in 1989, and all states now require two doses of measles vaccine for school-aged children. As a result, measles outbreaks in school settings are now uncommon.

In 2008 a total of 140 measles cases was reported, the largest annual total since 1996. Eighty nine percent of these cases were imported from or associated with importations from other countries, particularly countries in Europe where several outbreaks are ongoing. Persons younger than 20 years of age accounted for 76% of the cases; 91% were in persons who were unvaccinated (most because of personal or religious beliefs) or of unknown vaccination status. The increase in the number of cases of measles in 2008 was not a result of a greater number of imported measles cases. It was the result of more measles transmission after the virus was imported. The importation-associated cases occurred largely among school-aged children who were eligible for vaccination but whose parents chose not to have them vaccinated. Many of these children were home-schooled and not subject to school entry vaccination requirements.

In 2011, CDC reported 16 outbreaks of measles and 220 measles cases, most of which were imported cases in unvaccinated persons. Among the U.S. measles cases in persons 16 months through 19 years reported in 2011, 62% were in persons not vaccinated for a nonmedical reason.

For information about the clinical case definition, clinical classification and epidemiologic classification of measles see www.cdc.gov/vaccines/pubs/surv-manual/default.htm.

Measles Vaccine

Measles virus was first isolated by John Enders in 1954. The first measles vaccines were licensed in 1963. In that year, both an inactivated ("killed") and a live attenuated vaccine (Edmonston B strain) were licensed for use in the United States. The inactivated vaccine was withdrawn in 1967 because it did not protect against measles virus infection. Furthermore, recipients of inactivated measles vaccine frequently developed a unique syndrome, atypical measles, if they were infected with wild-type measles virus (see Atypical Measles, in the Complications section). The original Edmonston B vaccine was withdrawn in 1975 because of a relatively high frequency of fever and rash in recipients. A live, further attenuated vaccine (Schwarz strain) was first introduced in 1965 but also is no longer used in the United States. Another live, further attenuated strain vaccine (Edmonston-Enders strain) was licensed in 1968. These further attenuated vaccines caused fewer reactions than the original Edmonston B vaccine.

Characteristics

The only measles virus vaccine now available in the United States is a live, more attenuated Edmonston-Enders strain (formerly called "Moraten"). The vaccine is available combined with mumps and rubella vaccines as MMR, or combined with mumps, rubella, and varicella vaccine as MMRV (ProQuad). The Advisory Committee on Immunization Practices (ACIP) recommends that MMR be used when any of the individual components is indicated. Single-antigen measles vaccine is not available in the United States.

Measles vaccine is prepared in chick embryo fibroblast tissue culture. MMR and MMRV are supplied as a lyophylized

---

Measles Vaccines
- **1963**—Live attenuated and inactivated "killed" vaccines
- **1965**—Live further attenuated vaccine
- **1967**—Killed vaccine withdrawn
- **1968**—Live further attenuated vaccine (Edmonston-Enders strain)
- **1971**—Licensure of measles-mumps-rubella vaccine
- **1989**—Two dose schedule
- **2005**—Licensure of measles-mumps-rubella-varicella vaccine

Measles Vaccine
- Composition
  - live virus
- Efficacy
  - 95% at 12 months of age
  - 98% at 15 months of age
- Duration of Immunity
  - lifelong
- Schedule
  - 2 doses
  - should be administered with mumps and rubella as MMR or with mumps, rubella and varicella as MMRV
  - single-antigen measles vaccine not available in the United States

13

Measles

Measles Mumps Rubella (MMR) Vaccine Failure

- Measles, mumps, or rubella disease (or lack of immunity) in a previously vaccinated person
- 2%-5% of recipients do not respond to the first dose
- Caused by antibody, damaged vaccine, incorrect records
- Most persons with vaccine failure will respond to second dose

Measles (MMR) Vaccine Indications

- All children 12 months of age and older
- Susceptible adolescents and adults without documented evidence of immunity

(freeze-dried) powder and are reconstituted with sterile, preservative-free water. The vaccines contain small amounts of human albumin, neomycin, sorbitol, and gelatin.

Immunogenicity and Vaccine Efficacy

Measles vaccine produces an inapparent or mild, noncommunicable infection. Measles antibodies develop in approximately 95% of children vaccinated at 12 months of age and 98% of children vaccinated at 15 months of age. Seroconversion rates are similar for single-antigen measles vaccine, MMR, and MMRV. Approximately 2%–5% of children who receive only one dose of MMR vaccine fail to respond to it (i.e., primary vaccine failure). MMR vaccine failure may occur because of passive antibody in the vaccine recipient, damaged vaccine, incorrect records, or possibly other reasons. Most persons who fail to respond to the first dose will respond to a second dose. Studies indicate that more than 99% of persons who receive two doses of measles vaccine (with the first dose administered no earlier than the first birthday) develop serologic evidence of measles immunity.

Although the titer of vaccine-induced antibodies is lower than that following natural disease, both serologic and epidemiologic evidence indicate that vaccine-induced immunity appears to be long-term and probably lifelong in most persons. Most vaccinated persons who appear to lose antibody show an anamnestic immune response upon revaccination, indicating that they are probably still immune. Although revaccination can increase antibody titer in some persons, available data indicate that the increased titer may not be sustained. Some studies indicate that secondary vaccine failure (waning immunity) may occur after successful vaccination, but this appears to occur rarely and to play only a minor role in measles transmission and outbreaks.

Vaccination Schedule and Use

Two doses of measles-containing vaccine, as combination MMR, separated by at least 4 weeks, are routinely recommended for all children 12 months of age or older. All persons born during or after 1957 should have documentation of at least one dose of MMR or other evidence of measles immunity. Certain adolescents and adults should receive two doses of MMR.

The first dose of MMR should be given on or after the first birthday. Any dose of measles-containing vaccine given before 12 months of age should not be counted as part of the series. Children vaccinated with measles-containing vaccine before 12 months of age should be revaccinated with two doses of MMR vaccine, the first of which should be administered when the child is at least 12 months of age.

A second dose of MMR is recommended to produce immunity in those who failed to respond to the first dose. The second dose of MMR vaccine should routinely be given at age 4–6 years, before a child enters kindergarten or first grade. The recommended visit at age 11 or 12 years can serve as a catch-up opportunity to verify vaccination status and administer MMR vaccine to those children who have not yet received two doses of MMR.

The second dose of MMR may be administered as soon as 4 weeks (28 days) after the first dose. Children who have already received two doses of MMR vaccine at least 4 weeks apart, with the first dose administered no earlier than the first birthday, do not need an additional dose when they enter school. Children without documentation of adequate vaccination against measles, mumps, and rubella or other acceptable evidence of immunity to these diseases when they enter school should be admitted after receipt of the first dose of MMR. A second dose should be administered as soon as possible, but no less than 4 weeks after the first dose.

Only doses of vaccine with written documentation of the date of receipt should be accepted as valid. Self-reported doses or a parental report of vaccination is not considered adequate documentation. A healthcare provider should not provide an immunization record for a patient unless that healthcare provider has administered the vaccine or has seen a record that documents vaccination. Persons who lack adequate documentation of vaccination or other acceptable evidence of immunity should be vaccinated. Vaccination status and receipt of all vaccinations should be documented in the patient's permanent medical record and in a vaccination record held by the individual.

MMRV is approved by the Food and Drug Administration for children 12 months through 12 years of age (that is, until the 13th birthday). MMRV should not be administered to persons 13 years of age or older.

For the first dose of MMR and varicella vaccine at age 12 through 47 months, either MMR vaccine and varicella vaccine or MMRV vaccine may be used. Providers who are considering administering MMRV vaccine should discuss the benefits and risks of both vaccination options with the parents or caregivers. Unless the parent or caregiver expresses a preference for MMRV vaccine, CDC recommends that MMR vaccine and varicella vaccine should be administered at separate sites for the first dose in this age group. See "Adverse Reactions" for more information. For the second dose of MMR and varicella vaccine at any age (15 months through 12 years) and for the first dose at 48 months of age or older, use of MMRV vaccine generally

MMR Vaccine

- First dose of MMR at 12-15 months
- 12 months is the minimum age
- MMR given before 12 months should not be counted as a valid dose
- Revaccinate at 12 months of age or older

Second Dose of Measles Vaccine

- Second dose of MMR at 4-6 years
- Second dose may be given any time at least 4 weeks after the first dose
- Intended to produce measles immunity in persons who failed to respond to the first dose (primary vaccine failure)
- May boost antibody titers in some persons

MMR and MMRV Vaccine

- For the first dose of measles, mumps, rubella, and varicella vaccines either MMR and varicella vaccines or MMRV vaccine can be used
- Providers should discuss the benefits and risks of both vaccination options with the parents or caregivers
- Unless the parent or caregiver expresses preference for MMRV, CDC recommends using MMR and varicella vaccines for the first dose
- Providers who face barriers to clearly communicating benefits and risks for any reason, such as language barriers, should administer MMR and varicella vaccines separately
- For the second dose at any age, use of MMRV vaccine generally is preferred over separate injections of MMR and varicella vaccines

13

Measles

Adults at Increased Risk of Measles

- College students
- Persons working in medical facilities
- International travelers

Measles Immunity in Healthcare Personnel

- All persons who work within medical facilities should have evidence of immunity to measles

is preferred over separate injections of its equivalent component vaccines (i.e., MMR vaccine and varicella vaccine).

Vaccination of Adults

Adults born in 1957 or later who do not have a medical contraindication should receive at least one dose of MMR vaccine unless they have documentation of vaccination with at least one dose of measles-, mumps- and rubella-containing vaccine or other acceptable evidence of immunity to these three diseases. With the exception of women who might become pregnant (see Rubella chapter) and persons who work in medical facilities, birth before 1957 generally can be considered acceptable evidence of immunity to measles, mumps, and rubella.

Certain groups of adults may be at increased risk for exposure to measles and should receive special consideration for vaccination. These include persons attending colleges and other post-high school educational institutions, persons working in medical facilities, and international travelers.

Colleges and other post-high school educational institutions are potential high-risk areas for measles, mumps, and rubella transmission because of large concentrations of susceptible persons. Prematriculation vaccination requirements for measles immunity have been shown to significantly decrease the risk of measles outbreaks on college campuses where they are implemented and enforced. Colleges, universities, technical and vocational schools, and other institutions for post-high school education should require documentation of two doses of MMR vaccine or other acceptable evidence of measles, mumps, and rubella immunity before entry.

Students who have no documentation of live measles, mumps, or rubella vaccination or other acceptable evidence of measles, mumps, and rubella immunity at the time of enrollment should be admitted to classes only after receiving the first dose of MMR. A second dose of MMR should be administered no less than 4 weeks (28 days) later. Students with evidence of prior receipt of only one dose of MMR or other measles-containing vaccine on or after their first birthday should receive a second dose of MMR, provided at least 4 weeks have elapsed since their previous dose.

Persons who work in medical facilities are at higher risk for exposure to measles than the general population. All persons who work within medical facilities should have evidence of immunity to measles, mumps, and rubella. Because any healthcare personnel (i.e., medical or nonmedical, paid or volunteer, full time or part time, student or nonstudent, with or without patient-care responsibilities) who lack evidence of immunity to measles or rubella can contract and transmit these diseases, all medical facilities (i.e., inpatient and outpatient, private and public) should ensure measles and rubella immunity among those who work within their facilities.

Adequate vaccination for measles, mumps, and rubella for healthcare personnel born during or after 1957 consists of two doses of a live measles- and mumps-containing vaccine and at least one dose of a live rubella-containing vaccine. Healthcare personnel needing a second dose of measles-containing vaccine should be revaccinated at least 4 weeks after their first dose.

For unvaccinated personnel born before 1957 who lack laboratory evidence of measles, mumps and/or rubella immunity or laboratory confirmation of disease, healthcare facilities should consider vaccinating personnel with two doses of MMR vaccine at the appropriate interval (for measles and mumps) and one dose of MMR vaccine (for rubella), respectively. For unvaccinated personnel born before 1957 who lack laboratory evidence of measles, mumps and/or rubella immunity or laboratory confirmation of disease, healthcare facilities should recommend two doses of MMR vaccine during an outbreak of measles or mumps and one dose during an outbreak of rubella.

Serologic testing does not need to be done before vaccinating for measles and rubella unless the healthcare facility considers it cost-effective. Serologic testing is appropriate only if tracking systems are used to ensure that tested persons who are identified as susceptible are subsequently vaccinated in a timely manner. Serologic testing for immunity to measles and rubella is not necessary for persons documented to be appropriately vaccinated or who have other acceptable evidence of immunity. If the return and timely vaccination of those screened cannot be assured, serologic testing before vaccination should not be done.

Persons who travel outside the United States are at increased risk of exposure to measles. Measles is endemic or epidemic in many countries throughout the world. Although proof of immunization is not required for entry into the United States or any other country, persons traveling or living abroad should have evidence of measles immunity. Adequate vaccination of persons who travel outside the United States is two doses of MMR.

Revaccination

Revaccination is recommended for certain persons. The following groups should be considered unvaccinated and should receive at least one dose of measles vaccine: persons 1) vaccinated before the first birthday, 2) vaccinated with killed measles vaccine (KMV), 3) vaccinated from 1963 through 1967 with an unknown type of vaccine,

13

Measles Vaccine Indications for Revaccination

- Vaccinated before the first birthday
- Vaccinated with killed measles vaccine (KMV)
- Vaccinated from 1963 through 1967 with an unknown type of vaccine
- Vaccinated with IG in addition to a further attenuated strain or vaccine of unknown type

or 4) vaccinated with immune globulin (IG) in addition to a further attenuated strain or vaccine of unknown type. (Revaccination is not necessary if IG was given with Edmonston B vaccine).

Postexposure Prophylaxis

Live measles vaccine provides permanent protection and may prevent disease if given within 72 hours of exposure. IG may prevent or modify disease and provide temporary protection if given within 6 days of exposure. The dose is 0.5 mL/kg body weight, with a maximum of 15 mL intramuscularly and the recommended dose of IG given intravenously is 400mg/kg. IG may be especially indicated for susceptible household contacts of measles patients, particularly contacts younger than 1 year of age (for whom the risk of complications is highest). If the child is 12 months of age or older, live measles vaccine should be given about 5 months later when the passive measles antibodies have waned. IG should not be used to control measles outbreaks. Guidance for outbreak control for measles can be found in the Manual for the Surveillance of Vaccine-Preventable Diseases (http://www.cdc.gov/vaccines/pubs/surv-manual/index.html).

Contraindications and Precautions to Vaccination

Contraindications for MMR and MMRV vaccines include history of anaphylactic reactions to neomycin, history of severe allergic reaction to any component of the vaccine, pregnancy, and immunosuppression.

In the past, persons with a history of anaphylactic reactions following egg ingestion were considered to be at increased risk for serious reactions after receipt of measles- or mumps-containing vaccines, which are produced in chick embryo fibroblasts. However, data suggest that anaphylactic reactions to measles- and mumps-containing vaccines are not associated with hypersensitivity to egg antigens but to other components of the vaccines (such as gelatin). The risk for serious allergic reactions following receipt of these vaccines by egg-allergic persons is extremely low, and skin-testing with vaccine is not predictive of allergic reaction to vaccination. Therefore, MMR may be administered to egg-allergic children without prior routine skin testing or the use of special protocols.

MMR vaccine does not contain penicillin. A history of penicillin allergy is not a contraindication to vaccination with MMR or any other U.S. vaccine.

Women known to be pregnant should not receive measles vaccine. Pregnancy should be avoided for 4 weeks following MMR vaccine. Close contact with a pregnant

---

MMR Vaccine Contraindications and Precautions

- History of anaphylactic reactions to neomycin
- History of severe allergic reaction to any component of the vaccine
- Pregnancy
- Immunosuppression
- Moderate or severe acute illness
- Recent blood product
- Personal or family (i.e. sibling or parent) history of seizures of any etiology (MMRV only)

Measles and Mumps Vaccines and Egg Allergy

- Measles and mumps viruses grown in chick embryo fibroblast culture
- Studies have demonstrated safety of MMR in egg-allergic children
- Vaccinate without testing

13

woman is NOT a contraindication to MMR vaccination of the contact. Breastfeeding is NOT a contraindication to vaccination of either the woman or the breastfeeding child.

Replication of vaccine viruses can be prolonged in persons who are immunosuppressed or immunodeficient. Severe immunosuppression can be due to a variety of conditions, including congenital immunodeficiency, HIV infection, leukemia, lymphoma, generalized malignancy, or therapy with alkylating agents, antimetabolites, radiation, or large doses of corticosteroids. Evidence based on case reports has linked measles vaccine virus infection to subsequent death in at least six severely immunocompromised persons. For this reason, patients who are severely immunocompromised for any reason should not be given MMR vaccine. Healthy susceptible close contacts of severely immunocompromised persons should be vaccinated.

In general, persons receiving large daily doses of corticosteroids (2 mg/kg or more per day, or 20 mg or more per day of prednisone) for 14 days or more should not receive MMR vaccine because of concern about vaccine safety. MMR and its component vaccines should be avoided for at least 1 month after cessation of high-dose therapy. Persons receiving low-dose or short-course (less than 14 days) therapy, alternate-day treatment, maintenance physiologic doses, or topical, aerosol, intra-articular, bursal, or tendon injections may be vaccinated. Although persons receiving high doses of systemic corticosteroids daily or on alternate days for less than 14 days generally can receive MMR or its component vaccines immediately after cessation of treatment, some experts prefer waiting until 2 weeks after completion of therapy.

Patients with leukemia in remission who have not received chemotherapy for at least 3 months may receive MMR or its component vaccines.

Measles disease can be severe in persons with HIV infection. Available data indicate that vaccination with MMR has not been associated with severe or unusual adverse reactions in HIV-infected persons without evidence of severe immunosuppression, although antibody responses have been variable. MMR vaccine is recommended for all persons 12 months of age or older with HIV infection who do not have evidence of current severe immunosuppression [absence of severe immunosuppression is defined as CD4 percentages greater than or equal to 15% for 6 months or longer for persons five years of age or younger; and CD4 percentages greater than or equal to 15% and CD4 count greater than or equal to 200 cells/mm^3 for 6 months or longer for persons older than five years] or other current evidence of measles, rubella,

13

Measles Vaccine and HIV Infection
- MMR recommended for persons who do not have evidence of current severe immunosuppression
- Prevaccination HIV testing not recommended
- MMRV not for use in persons with HIV infection

Measles

and mumps immunity. Asymptomatic children do not need to be evaluated and tested for HIV infection before MMR or other measles-containing vaccines are administered. A theoretical risk of an increase (probably transient) in HIV viral load following MMR vaccination exists because such an effect has been observed with other vaccines. The clinical significance of such an increase is not known.

MMR and other measles-containing vaccines are not recommended for HIV-infected persons with evidence of severe immunosuppression. MMRV is not approved for and should not be administered to a person known to be infected with HIV.

Persons with moderate or severe acute illness should not be vaccinated until the patient has improved. This precaution is intended to prevent complicating the management of an ill patient with a potential vaccine adverse reaction, such as fever. Minor illness (e.g., otitis media, mild upper respiratory infections), concurrent antibiotic therapy, and exposure to or recovery from other illness are not contraindications to measles vaccination.

Receipt of antibody-containing blood products (e.g., immune globulin, whole blood or packed red blood cells, intravenous immune globulin) may interfere with seroconversion after measles vaccine. The length of time that such passively acquired antibody persists depends on the concentration and quantity of blood product received. For instance, it is recommended that vaccination be delayed for 3 months following receipt of immune globulin for prophylaxis of hepatitis A; a 7 to 11 month delay is recommended following administration of intravenous immune globulin, depending on the dose. For more information, see Chapter 2, General Recommendations on Immunization, and the table in Appendix A.

Persons who have a history of thrombocytopenic purpura or thrombocytopenia (low platelet count) may be at increased risk for developing clinically significant thrombocytopenia after MMR vaccination. No deaths have been reported as a direct consequence of vaccine-induced thrombocytopenia. The decision to vaccinate with MMR depends on the benefits of immunity to measles, mumps, and rubella and the risks for recurrence or exacerbation of thrombocytopenia after vaccination or during natural infection with measles or rubella. The benefits of immunization are usually greater than the potential risks, and administration of MMR vaccine is justified because of the even greater risk for thrombocytopenia after measles or rubella disease. However, deferring a subsequent dose of MMR vaccine may be prudent if the previous episode of thrombocytopenia occurred within

6 weeks after the previous dose of the vaccine. Serologic evidence of measles immunity in such persons may be sought in lieu of MMR vaccination.

A personal or family (i.e., sibling or parent) history of seizures of any etiology is a precaution for MMRV vaccination. Studies suggest that children who have a personal or family history of febrile seizures or family history of epilepsy are at increased risk for febrile seizures compared with children without such histories. Children with a personal or family history of seizures of any etiology generally should be vaccinated with MMR vaccine and varicella vaccine at separate sites because the risks for using MMRV vaccine in these children generally outweigh the benefits.

Tuberculin skin testing (TST) is not a prerequisite for vaccination with MMR or other measles-containing vaccine. TST has no effect on the response to MMR vaccination. However, measles vaccine (and possibly mumps, rubella, and varicella vaccines) may transiently suppress the response to TST in a person infected with *Mycobacterium tuberculosis*. If tuberculin skin testing is needed at the same time as administration of measles-containing vaccine, TST and vaccine can be administered at the same visit. Simultaneously administering TST and measles-containing vaccine does not interfere with reading the TST result at 48–72 hours and ensures that the person has received measles vaccine. If the measles-containing vaccine has been administered recently, TST screening should be delayed at least 4 weeks after vaccination. A delay in administering TST will remove the concern of any theoretical suppression of TST reactivity from the vaccine. TST screening can be performed and read before administering the measles-containing vaccine. This option is the least favored because it will delay receipt of the vaccine.

> **Tuberculin Skin Testing (TST)* and Measles Vaccine**
> - Apply TST at same visit as MMR
> - Delay TST at least 4 weeks if MMR given first
> - Apply TST first and administer MMR when skin test read (least favored option because receipt of MMR is delayed)
>
> *previously called PPD

Adverse Events Following Vaccination

Arthralgias and other joint symptoms are reported in up to 25% of susceptible adult women given MMR vaccine. This adverse event is associated with the rubella component (see Rubella chapter for more details).

Allergic reactions including rash, pruritus, and purpura have been temporally associated with mumps vaccination, but these are not common and usually mild and of brief duration.

To date there is no convincing evidence that any vaccine causes autism or autism spectrum disorder. Concern has been raised about a possible relation between MMR vaccine and autism by some parents of children with autism. Symptoms of autism are often noticed by parents during the second year of life, and may follow administration of MMR

> **MMR Adverse Events**
> - Arthralgias (susceptible women)
>   - 25%
> - Rash, pruritis, purpura
>   - not common
>
> **MMR Vaccine and Autism**
>
> To date there is no convincing evidence that any vaccine causes autism or autism spectrum disorder

13

Measles

by weeks or months. Two independent nongovernmental groups, the Institute of Medicine (IOM) and the American Academy of Pediatrics (AAP), have reviewed the evidence regarding a potential link between autism and MMR vaccine. Both groups independently concluded that available evidence does not support an association, and that the United States should continue its current MMR vaccination policy. Additional research on the causes of autism is needed.

Adverse Reactions Following Vaccination

Adverse reactions following measles vaccine (except allergic reactions) may be caused by replication of measles vaccine virus with subsequent mild illness. These events occur 5 to 12 days postvaccination and only in persons who are susceptible to infection. There is no evidence of increased risk of adverse reactions following MMR vaccination in persons who are already immune to the diseases.

Fever is the most common adverse reaction following MMR vaccination. Although measles, mumps, and rubella vaccines may cause fever after vaccination, the measles component of MMR vaccine is most often associated with fever. After MMR vaccination, 5% to 15% of susceptible persons develop a temperature of 103°F (39.4°C) or higher, usually occurring 7 to 12 days after vaccination and generally lasting 1 or 2 days. Most persons with fever are otherwise asymptomatic.

In MMRV vaccine prelicensure studies conducted among children 12–23 months of age, fever (reported as abnormal or elevated 102°F or higher oral equivalent) was observed 5-12 days after vaccination in 21.5% of MMRV vaccine recipients compared with 14.9% of MMR vaccine and varicella vaccine recipients. Two postlicensure studies indicated that among children 12–23 months of age, one additional febrile seizure occurred 5–12 days after vaccination per 2,300–2,600 children who had received the first dose of MMRV vaccine, compared with children who had received the first dose of MMR vaccine and varicella vaccine administered as separate injections at the same visit. Data from postlicensure studies do not suggest that children 4–6 years of age who received the second dose of MMRV vaccine had an increased risk for febrile seizures after vaccination compared with children the same age who received MMR vaccine and varicella vaccine administered as separate injections at the same visit.

Measles- and rubella-containing vaccines, including MMR, may cause a transient rash. Rashes, usually appearing 7 to 10 days after MMR or measles vaccination, have been reported in approximately 5% of vaccinees.

MMR Adverse Reactions

- Fever
  - 5%-15%
- Rash
  - 5%
- Thrombocytopenia
  - 1/30,000-40,000 doses
- Lymphadenopathy
  - rare
- Allergic reactions
  - rare

MMRV and Febrile Seizure

- Among children 12-23 months of age one additional febrile seizure occurred 5-12 days after vaccination per 2,300–2,600 children compared to children who received the first dose of MMR and varicella vaccine separately

- Data do not suggest that children 4-6 years of age who received the second dose had an increased risk

Rarely, MMR vaccine may cause thrombocytopenia within 2 months after vaccination. Estimates of the frequency of clinically apparent thrombocytopenia from Europe are one case per 30,000–40,000 vaccinated susceptible persons, with a temporal clustering of cases occurring 2 to 3 weeks after vaccination. The clinical course of these cases was usually transient and benign, although hemorrhage occurred rarely. The risk for thrombocytopenia during rubella or measles infection is much greater than the risk after vaccination. Based on case reports, the risk for MMR-associated thrombocytopenia may be higher for persons who have previously had immune thrombocytopenic purpura, particularly for those who had thrombocytopenic purpura after an earlier dose of MMR vaccine.

Transient lymphadenopathy sometimes occurs following receipt of MMR or other rubella-containing vaccine, and parotitis has been reported rarely following receipt of MMR or other mumps-containing vaccine.

Allergic reactions following the administration of MMR or any of its component vaccines are rare. Most of these reactions are minor and consist of a wheal and flare or urticaria at the injection site. Immediate, anaphylactic reactions to MMR or its component vaccines are extremely rare.

13

Vaccine Storage and Handling

MMR vaccine can be stored either in the freezer or the refrigerator and should be protected from light at all times. MMRV vaccine should be stored frozen between -58°F and +5°F (-50°C and -15°C). When MMR vaccine is stored in the freezer, the temperature should be the same as that required for MMRV, between -58°F and +5°F (-50°C and -15°C). Storing MMR in the freezer with MMRV may help prevent inadvertent storage of MMRV in the refrigerator.

Manufacturer package inserts contain additional information and can be found at http://www.fda.gov/ BiologicsBloodVaccines/Vaccines/ApprovedProducts/ ucm093830.htm. For complete information on best practices and recommendations please refer to CDC's Vaccine Storage and Handling Toolkit, http://www.cdc.gov/ vaccines/recs/storage/toolkit/storage-handling-toolkit.pdf.

Acknowledgment
The editors thank Drs. Gregory Wallace, and Zaney Leroy, CDC for their assistance in updating this chapter.

Selected References

American Academy of Pediatrics. Measles. In: Pickering L, Baker C, Kimberlin D, Long S, eds. *Red Book: 2009 Report of the Committee on Infectious Diseases*. 28th ed. Elk Grove Village, IL: American Academy of Pediatrics, 2009:444–55.

Atkinson WL, Orenstein WA, Krugman S. The resurgence of measles in the United States, 1989–1990. *Ann Rev Med* 1992;43:451–63.

Bellini WJ, Rota PA. Genetic diversity of wild-type measles viruses: implications for global measles elimination programs. *Emerg Infect Dis* 1998;4:29–35.

Bellini WJ, Rota JS, Lowe LE, et al. Subacute sclerosing panencephalitis: more cases of this fatal disease are prevented by measles immunization than was previously recognized. *J Infect Dis* 2005;192:1686–93.

CDC. Measles, mumps, and rubella—vaccine use and strategies for elimination of measles, rubella, and congenital rubella syndrome and control of mumps: recommendations of the Advisory Committee on Immunization Practices (ACIP). *MMWR* 1998;47(No. RR-8):1–57.

CDC. Prevention of measles, rubella, congenital rubella syndrome, and mumps, 2013: summary recommendations of the Advisory Committee on Immunization Practices (ACIP). *MMWR* 2013;62(No. 4):1-34.

CDC. Use of combination measles, mumps, rubella, and varicella vaccine: recommendations of the Advisory Committee on Immunization Practices (ACIP). *MMWR* 2010;59(No. RR-3):1–12.

CDC. Immunization of health-care personnel. Recommendations of the Advisory Committee on Immunization Practices (ACIP). *MMWR* 2011;60(RR-7):1-45.

CDC. Update: Measles — United States, January–July 2008. *MMWR* 2008;57:893–6.

CDC. Global measles mortality, 2000–2008. *MMWR* 2009;58:1321–6.

Gerber JS, Offit PA. Vaccines and autism: a tale of shifting hypotheses. *Clin Infect Dis* 2009;48:456–61.

Halsey NA, Hyman SL, Conference Writing Panel. Measles-mumps-rubella vaccine and autistic spectrum disorder: report from the New Challenges in Childhood Immunizations Conference convened in Oak Brook, IL, June 12–13, 2000. *Pediatrics* 2001;107(5).

13

Institute of Medicine. *Institute of Medicine immunization safety review: vaccines and autism.* Washington DC: National Academy Press, 2004.

Sugerman DE, Barskey AE, Delea MG et al. Measles outbreak in a highly vaccinated population, San Diego, 2008: role of the intentionally undervaccinated. *Pediatrics* 2010;125:747-52.

Vitek CR, Aduddel, M, Brinton MJ. Increased protection during a measles outbreak of children previously vaccinated with a second dose of measles-mumps-rubella vaccine. *Pediatr Infect Dis J* 1999;18:620–3.

13

Measles

Meningococcal disease is an acute, potentially severe illness caused by the bacterium *Neisseria meningitidis*. Illness believed to be meningococcal disease was first reported in the 16th century. The first definitive description of the disease was by Vieusseux in Switzerland in 1805. The bacterium was first identified in the spinal fluid of patients by Weichselbaum in 1887.

Neisseria meningitidis is a leading cause of bacterial meningitis and sepsis in the United States. It can also cause focal disease, such as pneumonia and arthritis. *N. meningitidis* is also a cause of epidemics of meningitis and bacteremia in sub-Saharan Africa. The World Health Organization has estimated that meningococcal disease was the cause of 171,000 deaths worldwide in 2000.

The first monovalent (serogroup C) polysaccharide vaccine was licensed in the United States in 1974. A quadrivalent polysaccharide vaccine was licensed in 1981. Monovalent serogroup C meningococcal conjugate vaccine has been licensed in United Kingdom since 1999 and has had a major impact on the incidence of serogroup C meningococcal disease. Quadrivalent conjugate vaccines were first licensed in the United States in 2005. A bivalent conjugate combination vaccine (with Hib) was licensed in the United States in 2012, and two serogroup B recombinant vaccines were licensed in early 2015.

Neisseria meningitidis

N. meningitidis, or meningococcus, is an aerobic, gram-negative diplococcus, closely related to *N. gonorrhoeae*, and to several nonpathogenic *Neisseria* species, such as *N. lactamica*. The organism has both an inner (cytoplasmic) and an outer membrane, separated by a cell wall. The outer membrane contains several protein structures that enable the bacteria to interact with the host cells as well as perform other functions.

The outer membrane is surrounded by a polysaccharide capsule that is necessary for pathogenicity because it helps the bacteria resist phagocytosis and complement-mediated lysis. The outer membrane proteins and the capsular polysaccharide make up the main surface antigens of the organism.

Meningococci are classified by using serologic methods based on the structure of the polysaccharide capsule. Thirteen antigenically and chemically distinct polysaccharide capsules have been described. Some strains, often those found to cause asymptomatic nasopharyngeal carriage, are not groupable and do not have a capsule. Almost all invasive disease is caused by one of five serogroups: A, B, C, W, and

Neisseria meningitidis

- Severe acute bacterial infection
- Cause of meningitis, sepsis, and focal disease (e.g. pneumonia and arthritis)
- Epidemic disease in sub-Saharan Africa
- Quadrivalent polysaccharide vaccine licensed in 1981
- Conjugate vaccine licensed in U.S. 2005
- Aerobic gram-negative bacteria
- 13 distinct polysaccharide capsules have been described
- Almost all invasive disease caused by serogroups A, B, C, Y, and W
- Relative importance of serogroups depends on geographic location and other factors (e.g. age)

14

Meningococcal Disease

Meningococcal Disease Pathogenesis

- Organism colonizes nasopharynx

- In some persons organism enters the bloodstream and causes infection at distant site

- Antecedent URI may be a contributing factor

Neisseria meningitidis Clinical Features

- Incubation period 3-4 days (range 2-10 days)

- Abrupt onset of fever, meningeal symptoms, hypotension, and rash

- Fatality rate 10%-15%, up to 40% in meningococcemia

Meningococcal Meningitis

- Most common presentation of invasive disease

- Results from hematogenous dissemination

- Clinical findings
  - fever
  - headache
  - stiff neck

Meningococcemia

- Bloodstream infection

- May occur with or without meningitis

- Clinical findings
  - fever
  - petechial or purpuric rash
  - hypotension
  - shock
  - acute adrenal hemorrhage
  - multiorgan failure

Y. The relative importance of each serogroup depends on geographic location, as well as other factors, such as age. For instance, serogroup A has historically been a major cause of disease in sub-Saharan Africa but is rarely isolated in the United States.

Meningococci are further classified on the basis of certain outer membrane proteins. Molecular subtyping using specialized laboratory techniques (e.g., pulsed-field gel electrophoresis) can provide useful epidemiologic information.

Pathogenesis

Meningococci are transmitted by droplet aerosol or secretions from the nasopharynx of colonized persons. The bacteria attach to and multiply on the mucosal cells of the nasopharynx. In a small proportion (less than 1%) of colonized persons, the organism penetrates the mucosal cells and enters the bloodstream. The bacteria spread by way of the blood to many organs. In about 50% of bacteremic persons, the organism crosses the blood–brain barrier into the cerebrospinal fluid and causes purulent meningitis. An antecedent upper respiratory infection (URI) may be a contributing factor.

Clinical Features

The incubation period of meningococcal disease is 3 to 4 days, with a range of 2 to 10 days.

Meningitis is the most common presentation of invasive meningococcal infection (meningococcal disease) and results from hematogenous dissemination of the organism. Meningeal infection is similar to other forms of acute purulent meningitis, with sudden onset of fever, headache, and stiff neck, often accompanied by other symptoms, such as nausea, vomiting, photophobia (eye sensitivity to light), and altered mental status. Meningococci can be isolated from the blood in up to 75% of persons with meningitis.

Meningococcal sepsis (bloodstream infection or meningococcemia) occurs without meningitis in 5% to 20% of invasive meningococcal infections. This condition is characterized by abrupt onset of fever and a petechial or purpuric rash, often associated with hypotension, shock, acute adrenal hemorrhage, and multiorgan failure.

Less common presentations of meningococcal disease include pneumonia (5% to 15% of cases), arthritis (2%), otitis media (1%), and epiglottitis (less than 1%).

The case-fatality ratio of meningococcal disease is 10% to 15%, even with appropriate antibiotic therapy. The case-fatality ratio of meningococcemia is up to 40%. As many as 20% of survivors have permanent sequelae, such as hearing loss, neurologic damage, or loss of a limb.

Risk factors for the development of meningococcal disease include deficiencies in the terminal common complement pathway, functional or anatomic asplenia, and underlying chronic disease. Persons with HIV infection are probably at increased risk for meningococcal disease. Certain genetic factors (such as polymorphisms in the genes for mannose-binding lectin and tumor necrosis factor) may also be risk factors.

Household crowding, and both active and passive smoking are associated with increased risk. Persons with antecedent viral infection are also at increased risk. Early studies in the United States demonstrated that blacks and persons of low socioeconomic status were at higher risk for meningococcal disease than other persons; however, race and low socio-economic status are likely markers for differences in factors such as smoking and household crowding rather than risk factors. As disease incidence has decreased, differences by race have also decreased, and no difference in disease incidence exists now between blacks and whites. During outbreaks, bar or nightclub patronage and alcohol use have also been associated with higher risk for disease.

Cases of meningococcal disease, including at least two fatal cases, have been reported among microbiologists. These persons have worked with *N. meningitidis* isolates rather than patient specimens.

Laboratory Diagnosis

Meningococcal disease is typically diagnosed by isolation of *N. meningitidis* from a normally sterile site. However, sensitivity of bacterial culture may be low, particularly when performed after initiation of antibiotic therapy. A Gram stain of cerebrospinal fluid (CSF) showing gram-negative diplococci strongly suggests meningococcal meningitis. Real-time polymerase chain reaction (rt-PCR) detects DNA of meningococci in blood, cerebrospinal fluid, or other clinical specimens. Although culture remains the criterion standard for diagnosis of meningococcal disease in the United States, PCR is useful for detection of *N. meningitidis* from clinical samples in which the organism could not be detected by culture methods, such as when a patient has been treated with antibiotics before obtaining a clinical specimen for culture.

Kits to detect polysaccharide antigen in cerebrospinal fluid are rapid and specific, but false-negative results are common, particularly in serogroup B disease. Antigen tests of urine or serum are unreliable.

Serologic testing (e.g., enzyme immunoassay) for antibodies to polysaccharide may be used as part of the evaluation if meningococcal disease is suspected, but should not be used to establish the diagnosis.

Neisseria meningitidis Risk Factors for Invasive Disease

- Host factors
  - deficiencies in the terminal common complement pathway
  - functional or anatomic asplenia
  - certain genetic factors
- Environmental factors
  - antecedent viral infection
  - household crowding
  - active and passive smoking
  - occupational (microbiologists)

Meningococcal Disease Laboratory Diagnosis

- Bacterial culture
- Gram stain
- Non-culture methods
  - PCR
  - antigen detection in CSF
  - serology

14

Meningococcal Disease

14

Medical Management

The clinical presentation of meningococcal meningitis is similar to other forms of bacterial meningitis. Consequently, empiric therapy with broad-spectrum antibiotics (e.g., third-generation cephalosporin, vancomycin) should be started promptly after appropriate cultures have been obtained.

Many antibiotics are effective for *N. meningitidis* infection, including penicillin. Few penicillin-resistant strains of meningococcus have been reported in the United States. Once *N. meningitidis* infection has been confirmed, penicillin alone is recommended.

Epidemiology
Occurrence

Meningococcal disease occurs worldwide in both endemic and epidemic form.

Reservoir

Humans are the only natural reservoir of meningococcus. As many as 10% of adolescents and adults are asymptomatic transient carriers of *N. meningitidis*, most strains of which are not pathogenic (i.e., strains that are not groupable).

Transmission

Primary mode is by respiratory droplet spread or by direct contact.

Temporal Pattern

Meningococcal disease occurs throughout the year, however, the incidence is highest in the late winter and early spring.

Communicability

The communicability of *N. meningitidis* is generally limited. In studies of households in which a case of meningococcal disease has occurred, only 3%–4% of households had secondary cases. Most households had only one secondary case. Estimates of the risk of secondary transmission are generally 2–4 cases per 1,000 household members at risk. However, this risk is 500–800 times that in the general population.

Secular Trends in the United States

During 2005-2011, an estimated 800-1,200 cases of meningococcal disease occurred annually in the United States, representing an incidence of 0.3 cases per 100,000 population. Incidence has declined annually since a peak of disease in the late 1990s. Since 2005, declines have occurred among all age groups and in all vaccine-

Meningococcal Disease - United States, 1972-2012*

*all serogroups

contained serogroups. In addition, incidence of disease attributable to serogroup B, a serogroup not included in the quadrivalent vaccine, declined for reasons that are not known. Serogroups B, C, and Y are the major causes of meningococcal disease in the United States, each being responsible for approximately one third of cases. The proportion of cases caused by each serogroup varies by age group. Approximately 60% of disease among children aged 0 through 59 months is caused by serogroup B, for which no conjugate vaccine is licensed or available in the United States. Serogroups C, W, or Y, which are included in vaccines available in the United States, cause 73% of all cases of meningococcal disease among persons 11 years of age or older.

The incidence of serogroups C and Y, which represent the majority of cases of meningococcal disease preventable by the conjugate vaccines, are at historic lows. However, a peak in disease incidence among adolescents and young adults 16 to 21 years of age has persisted, even after routine vaccination of adolescents was recommended in 2005. From 2000–2004 to 2005–2009, the estimated annual number of cases of serogroups C and Y meningococcal disease decreased 74% among persons aged 11 through 14 years but only 27% among persons aged 15 through 18 years.

During 2006-2010 (i.e., in the first 5 years after routine use of meningococcal vaccine was recommended) CDC received reports of approximately 30 cases of serogroups C and Y meningococcal disease among persons who had received the vaccine. The case-fatality ratio was similar among persons who had received vaccine compared with those who were unvaccinated. Of the 13 reports of breakthrough disease for which data on underlying conditions were available, four persons had underlying conditions or behaviors associated with increased risk for bacterial infections, including 1) Type 1 diabetes mellitus; 2) current smoking; 3) history of bacterial meningitis and recurrent infections; and 4) aplastic anemia, paroxysmal nocturnal hemoglobinuria, and receipt of eculizumab (which blocks complement protein C5).

In the United States, meningococcal outbreaks account for less than 2% of reported cases (98% of cases are sporadic). However, outbreaks of meningococcal disease continue to occur. During 2010, 2 serogroup C and 2 serogroup B outbreaks were reported to CDC. Cases associated with all reported outbreaks accounted for 108 (1.5%) of the 7,343 cases reported to CDC during 2005-2011. See www.cdc.gov/mmwr/pdf/rr/rr6202.pdf for additional information on the evaluation and management of meningococcal outbreaks.

14

Meningococcal Outbreaks in the United States

- Outbreaks account for less than 2% of reported cases

- Most recent outbreaks caused by serogroup C and B

Meningococcal Disease

14

Historically, large epidemics of serogroup A meningococcal disease occur in the African "meningitis belt," an area that extends from Ethiopia to Senegal. Rates of endemic meningococcal disease in this area are several times higher than in industrialized countries. In each epidemic, tens of thousands of cases and thousands of deaths may occur. Approximately 350 million people are at risk. The phased introduction in meningitis belt countries of MenAfriVac, a novel serogroup A meningococcal conjugate vaccine which is being implemented through preventive national campaigns of all individuals 1-29 years of age, holds great promise to end epidemic meningitis as a public health concern by 2016.

Meningococcal Vaccines
Characteristics

Meningococcal Polysaccharide Vaccine

The first meningococcal polysaccharide vaccine (MPSV4) was licensed in the United States in 1974. The current quadrivalent A, C, W, Y polysaccharide vaccine (Menomune, Sanofi Pasteur) was licensed in 1981. Each dose consists of 50 mcg of each of the four purified bacterial capsular polysaccharides. The vaccine contains lactose as a stabilizer.

MPSV4 is administered by subcutaneous injection. The vaccine is available in single-dose and 10-dose vials. Fifty-dose vials are no longer available. Diluent for the single-dose vial is sterile water without preservative. Diluent for the 10-dose vial is sterile water with thimerosal added as a preservative. After reconstitution the vaccine is a clear colorless liquid.

Meningococcal Conjugate Vaccines

Three meningococcal conjugate vaccines are licensed in the United States: two single-component vaccines (Menactra (MenACWY-D) and Menveo (MenACWY-CRM)) and one combination vaccine with Hib (MenHibrix (Hib-MenCY-TT)).

Menactra (MenACWY-D, sanofi pasteur) was licensed in 2005. Each 0.5-mL dose of vaccine is formulated in sodium phosphate buffered isotonic sodium chloride solution to contain 4 mcg each of meningococcal A, C, W, and Y polysaccharides conjugated to approximately 48 mcg of diphtheria toxoid protein carrier. MenACWY-D is approved for use in persons 9 months through 55 years of age. It is administered by intramuscular injection. MenACWY-D is supplied as a liquid in a single-dose vial and does not contain a preservative or an adjuvant.

Menveo (MenACWY-CRM, Novartis) was licensed in the United States in 2010. MenACWY-CRM consists of two portions: 10 μg of lyophilized meningococcal serogroup

A capsular polysaccharide conjugated to CRM$_{197}$ (MenA) and 5 μg each of capsular polysaccharide of serogroup C, W, and Y conjugated to CRM$_{197}$ in 0.5 mL of phosphate buffered saline, which is used to reconstitute the lyophilized MenA component before injection. MenACWY-CRM is approved for use in persons 2 through 55 years of age. It is administered by intramuscular injection. It does not contain a preservative or an adjuvant.

MenHibrix (Hib-MenCY-TT, GlaxoSmithKline) was licensed in the United States in 2012. Hib-MenCY-TT contains 5 micrograms of *N. meningitidis* serogroups C capsular polysaccharide conjugated to tetanus-toxoid, 5 micrograms of *N. meningitidis* serogroup Y capsular polysaccharide conjugated to tetanus-toxoid, and 2.5 micrograms of *Haemophilus influenzae* serogroup B capsular polysaccharide conjugated to tetanus-toxoid. The vaccine is lyophilized and should be reconstituted with a 0.9% saline diluent Hib-MenCY-TT is approved as a four dose series for children at 2, 4, 6, and 12 through 18 months.

Immunogenicity and Vaccine Efficacy

Meningococcal Polysaccharide Vaccine

The characteristics of MPSV4 are similar to other polysaccharide vaccines (e.g., pneumococcal polysaccharide). The vaccine is generally not effective in children younger than 18 months of age. The response to the vaccine is typical of a T-cell independent antigen, with an age-dependent response, and poor immunogenicity in children younger than 2 years of age. In addition, little boost in antibody titer occurs with repeated doses; the antibody which is produced is relatively low-affinity IgM, and "switching" from IgM to IgG production is poor.

The immunogenicity and clinical efficacy of serogroups A and C meningococcal polysaccharide vaccines are well-established. The serogroup A polysaccharide induces antibody response among children as young as 3 months, although a response comparable with that occurring in adults is not achieved until age 4 to 5 years; the serogroup C component is poorly immunogenic among recipients younger than 18 through 24 months. Serogroups A and C have demonstrated estimated clinical efficacies of 85% or more among school-aged children and adults during outbreaks. Although clinical protection has not been documented, vaccination with W and Y polysaccharides induces production of bactericidal antibodies. The antibody responses to each of the four polysaccharides in the quadrivalent vaccine are serogroup specific and independent (i.e., there is no cross-protection).

High-risk Groups: Functional or Anatomic Asplenia*

- Younger than 19 months
  - infant series at 2, 4, 6, and 12-15 months with HibMenCY-TT or MenACWY-CRM
- 19-23 months who have not received a complete series
  - 2-dose primary series of MenACWY-CRM at least 3 months apart**
- 24 months and older who have not received a complete series
  - 2-dose primary series of either MenACWY at least 3 months apart**

*Including sickle-cell disease
**Doses valid if 8 weeks apart

High-risk Groups: Persistent Complement Component Deficiency

- Children 2-18 months
- infant series at 2, 4, 6, and 12-15 months with HibMenCY-TT or MenACWY-CRM OR 2-dose primary series of MenACWY-D starting at 9 months at least 3 months apart *
- 19-23 months without complete series of HibMenCY-TT or MenACWY
  - 2-dose primary series of MenACWY at least 3 months apart*
- 24 months and older who have not received a complete series of HibMenCY-TT or MenACWY
  - 2-dose primary series of either MenACWY at least 3 months apart*

*Doses valid if 8 weeks apart

14

Meningococcal Disease

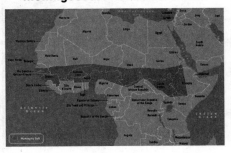
Meningococcal Conjugate Vaccines

Effectiveness of the three meningococcal conjugate vaccines, which were licensed after MPSV4, was inferred by comparing serum bactericidal antibody assay (SBA) measurements of the new vaccine with corresponding antibody responses of the U.S.-licensed meningococcal vaccine representing the standard of care at the time (among persons aged 2 through 55 years) or by achieving a seroresponse at or above a predefined bactericidal antibody titer (among children aged 2 through 23 months).

An advantage of conjugate vaccines is their ability to elicit immunologic memory. Meningococcal conjugate vaccines prime the immune system, and immunologic memory persists even in the absence of detectable bactericidal antibodies. However, while vaccine-induced immunologic memory might be protective against infection with other disease-causing encapsulated bacteria, the presence of detectable circulating antibody appears to be important for protection against *N. meningitidis*. In most cases, meningococcal infection progresses rapidly, with fulminant disease occurring within 1-4 days after invasion of normally sterile body sites.

When MenACWY-D vaccine was licensed in 2005 some experts predicted that the vaccine would be effective for up to 10 years, providing protection through the period of highest risk in late adolescence and early adulthood. Since the 2005 ACIP recommendations, additional data have led to improved understanding of meningococcal conjugate vaccines, including new data on duration of vaccine-induced immunity. Antibody persistence studies indicate that circulating antibody declines 3 to 5 years after a single dose of Menactra or Menveo (MenACWY). In addition, results from a vaccine effectiveness study demonstrate waning effectiveness, and many adolescents are not protected 5 years after vaccination. ACIP concluded that a single dose of meningococcal conjugate vaccine administered at age 11 or 12 years is unlikely to protect most adolescents through the period of increased risk at ages 16 through 21 years. On the basis of this information, in 2010, ACIP recommended adding a booster dose at age 16 years.

In 2010, ACIP revised the recommendations for dosing regimens (e.g., primary series and booster doses) for persons who have functional or anatomic asplenia, who have persistent complement component deficiencies, or who have HIV infection and are otherwise recommended to be vaccinated. For these immunosuppressed persons, a 2-dose primary series was recommended instead of a single dose. Booster doses after primary vaccination are important for persons with prolonged increased risk (persons with asplenia, persons with complement component deficiencies, and microbiologists) to ensure high levels of SBA are maintained over time.

Vaccination Schedule And Use

Meningococcal Polysaccharide Vaccine

Routine vaccination of civilians with MPSV4 is not recommended. Use of MPSV4 should be limited to persons older than 55 years of age, or when neither MenACWY is available.

Meningococcal Conjugate Vaccines

ACIP recommends routine vaccination with either MenACWY vaccine at 11 or 12 years of age, with a booster dose at 16 years of age. For adolescents who receive the first dose at 13 through 15 years of age, a one-time booster dose should be administered, preferably at age 16 through 18 years. Healthy persons who receive their first routine dose of meningococcal conjugate vaccine at or after age 16 years do not need a booster dose unless they become at increased risk for meningococcal disease. Routine vaccination of healthy persons who are not at increased risk for exposure to *N. meningitidis* is not recommended after age 21 years. A booster dose is not recommended for healthy persons 22 years of age or older even if the first dose was administered at 11 through 15 years of age. Although doses of MenACWY separated by 8 weeks can both be counted as valid it is preferable to use a longer interval between doses, 3 to 5 years if possible.

For children younger than 19 months of age with anatomic or functional asplenia (including sickle-cell disease), administer an infant series of Hib-MenCY-TT or MenACWY-CRM at 2, 4, 6, and 12-15 months.

For children 19 through 23 months of age with anatomic or functional asplenia (including sickle-cell disease), administer two primary doses of MenACWY-CRM at least 3 months apart (doses valid If 8 weeks apart).

For children 2 through 18 months of age with persistent complement component deficiencies, administer either an infant series of Hib-MenCY-TT or MenACWY-CRM at 2, 4, 6, and 12 through 15 months or a 2-dose primary series of MenACWY-D starting at 9 months, with at least 8 weeks between doses.

For children 19 through 23 months of age with persistent complement component deficiencies who have not received a complete series of Hib-MenCY-TT or MenACWY, administer 2 primary doses of MenACWY at least 3 months apart (doses valid if 8 weeks apart).

For children 24 months of age and older with persistent complement component deficiencies or anatomic or functional asplenia (including sickle cell disease), who have not received a complete series of Hib-MenCY-TT or

High-risk Boosters

- Children who receive primary immunization and remain at increased risk should receive booster doses

  - if primary immunization complete by 7 years of age
    - first booster should be 3 years after primary immunization and every 5 years thereafter if at continued risk

  - if primary immunization complete on or after 7 years of age
    - first booster should be 5 years after primary immunization and every 5 years thereafter if at continued risk

MenACWY and HIV Infection

- HIV infection is not currently an indication for MenACWY vaccination

- Some persons with HIV infection should receive MenACWY for other indications, such as adolescents or international travel

- Persons with HIV infection who are vaccinated with MenACWY should receive 2 primary series doses at least 8 weeks apart

14

Meningococcal Disease

Meningococcal Vaccine Use in Outbreaks

- Both MenACWY, and MPSV4 recommended for use in control of outbreaks caused by A, C, W, and Y

- HibMenCY-TT may be used for age-appropriate persons in outbreaks specifically caused by C and Y

- Outbreak definition:
  - at least 3 confirmed or probable primary cases of the same serogroup
  - period of 3 months or less
  - primary attack rate of more than 10 cases per 100,000 population

---

MenACWY, administer 2 primary doses of either MenACWY at least 3 months apart (doses valid if 8 weeks apart). Do not administer MenACWY-D to a child with asplenia (including sickle cell disease) until after the second birthday, and at least 4 weeks after completion of all PCV13 doses.

Meningococcal vaccination is recommended for persons at increased risk for meningococcal disease, including microbiologists who are routinely exposed to isolates of *N. meningitidis*, military recruits, and persons who travel to, and U.S. citizens who reside in, countries in which *N. meningitidis* is hyperendemic or epidemic, particularly countries in the sub-Saharan Africa "meningitis belt." Vaccination in the 3 years before the date of travel is required by the government of Saudi Arabia for all travelers to Mecca during the annual Hajj. Information concerning geographic areas for which vaccination is recommended can be obtained from the CDC Travelers Health website at http://www.cdc.gov/travel. These high-risk persons should be revaccinated every 5 years as long as their increased risk continues.

Infants and children who received Hib-MenCY-TT and are travelling to areas with high endemic rates of meningococcal disease are not protected against serogroups A and W and should receive a quadrivalent meningococcal vaccination.

Children who received primary immunization with Hib-MenCY-TT, MenACWY or MPSV4 before 7 years of age and remain at increased risk for meningococcal disease should receive a booster 3 years after primary immunization. Boosters should be repeated every five years thereafter. Persons who received primary immunization with MenACWY or MPSV4 at 7 years of age or older and remain at increased risk for meningococcal disease should receive a booster 5 years after their previous dose. Boosters should be repeated every five years thereafter.

Persons with persistent complement component deficiency, and persons with functional or anatomic asplenia should receive a 2-dose primary series administered 2 months apart and a booster dose every 5 years.

HIV infection is not currently considered to be an indication for MenACWY vaccination by itself. However, some persons with HIV infection should receive MenACWY for other indications, such as adolescents or international travel. Persons with HIV infection who are vaccinated with MenACWY should receive 2 primary doses at least 8 weeks apart.

Persons with complement component deficiency, functional or anatomic asplenia or HIV infection who have already received 1 dose of MenACWY should receive a second dose at the earliest opportunity, but at least 8 weeks after the previous dose.

MenACWY can be administered at the same visit as other indicated vaccines. All vaccines should be given at separate sites with separate syringes.

Both MenACWY and MPSV4 are recommended for use in control of meningococcal outbreaks caused by vaccine-preventable serogroups (A, C, W, Y). Hib-MenCY-TT may be used for age-appropriate persons in outbreaks specifically caused by vaccine-preventable serogroups C and Y. An outbreak is defined by the occurrence of at least three confirmed or probable primary cases of the same serogroup meningococcal disease during a period of 3 months or less, with a resulting primary attack rate of 10 or more cases per 100,000 population.

Contraindications and Precautions to Vaccination

Vaccination with MenACWY, MPSV4, or Hib-MenCY-TT is contraindicated for persons known to have had a severe allergic (anaphylactic) reaction to a vaccine component, including diphtheria toxoid. Recommended vaccinations can be administered to persons with minor acute illness (e.g. diarrhea or mild upper respiratory tract infection with or without low grade fever). Vaccination should be deferred for persons with moderate or severe acute illness until the condition has improved. After reviewing safety studies, ACIP voted in 2010 to remove a history Guillain-Barré syndrome (GBS) as a precaution for vaccination, because the benefits of meningococcal vaccination outweigh the risk for recurrent GBS in these persons. However, a history of GBS continues to be listed as a precaution in the package inserts for MenACWY. Breastfeeding and immunosuppression are not contraindications to vaccination. Pregnancy should not preclude vaccination with MenACWY or MPSV4, if indicated.

Adverse Events Following Vaccination
Meningococcal Conjugate Vaccine

The most frequently reported adverse events for MenACWY-D include fever (16.8%), headache (16.0%) injection site erythema (14.6%), and dizziness (13.4%). Syncope was reported in 10.0% of reports involving MenACWY-D. Of all reported MenACWY-D events, 6.6% were coded as serious (i.e., resulted in death, life-threatening illness, hospitalization, prolongation of hopitalization, or permanent disability). Serious events included headache, fever, vomiting, and nausea. A total of 24 deaths (0.3%) were reported.

Meningococcal Vaccines Contraindications and Precautions

- Severe allergic reaction to vaccine component or following a prior dose of vaccine
- Moderate or severe acute illness

14

MenACWY-D Adverse Events

- Fever
  - most frequently reported (16.8%)
- Headache (16.0%); injection-site erythema (14.6%); dizziness (13.4%)
- Syncope
  - reported in 10%
- Serious adverse events rare
  - death reported in 0.3%

MenACWY-CRM Adverse Events

- Injection site swelling (13.7%)
- Injection site reactions
  - most frequently reported (19.7%)
- Syncope
  - reported in 8.8%
  - Serious adverse events rare
    - death reported in 0.4%

Meningococcal Disease

HibMenCY-TT Adverse Events

- Rates comparable to adverse event rates after Hib-TT

- HibMenCY-TT safe and immunogenic for both Hib and serogroups C and Y

MPSV4 Adverse Reactions

- Local reactions
  - most common (48%)
  - Last for one to two days

Indications for Chemoprophylaxis

- Household members

- Child care center contacts

- Anyone directly exposed to the patient's oral secretions in 7 days before symptom onset

- Travelers with direct contact with respiratory secretions from an index patient or for anyone seated directly next to an index patient on a prolonged flight (more than 8 hours)

The most frequently reported adverse events for MenACWY-CRM were injection site erythema (19.7%) and injection-site swelling (13.7%). Syncope was reported in 8.8% of reports involving MenACWY-CRM. One death (0.4%) was reported.

Rates of local and systemic adverse events observed after administration of Hib-MenCY-TT were comparable to rates observed after administration of Hib-TT. Thus, Hib-MenCY-TT was found to be safe and immunogenic for both Hib and meningococcal serogroups C and Y.

Meningococcal Polysaccharide Vaccine

Fever (100°F - 103°F) within 7 days of vaccination is reported for up to 3% of recipients. Systemic reactions, such as headache and malaise, within 7 days of vaccination are reported for up to 60% of recipients. Fewer than 3% of recipients reported these systemic reactions as severe.

Adverse Reactions Following Vaccination
Meningococcal Polysaccharide Vaccine

Adverse reactions to MPSV4 are generally mild. The most frequent are local reactions, such as pain and redness at the injection site. These reactions last for 1 or 2 days, and occur in up to 48% of recipients.

Vaccine Storage and Handling

MPSV4, MenACWY, and Hib-MenCY-TT should be maintained at refrigerator temperature between 35°F and 46°F (2°C and 8°C). Manufacturer's package inserts contain additional information and can be found at http://www.fda.gov/BiologicsBloodVaccines/Vaccines/ApprovedProducts/ucm093830.htm. For complete information on best practices and recommendations please refer to CDC's Vaccine Storage and Handling Toolkit, http://www.cdc.gov/vaccines/recs/storage/toolkit/storage-handling-toolkit.pdf.

The MenA (lyophilized) component of MenACWY-CRM should only be reconstituted using the liquid C-W-Y component of MenACWY-CRM. No other vaccine or diluents can be used for this purpose. The reconstituted vaccine should be used immediately, but may be held at or below 77°F (25°C) for up to 8 hours. If the liquid C-W-Y component of MenACWY-CRM is administered alone (without using it to reconstitute the lyophilized A component) revaccination may not be needed. Serogroup A disease is rare in the U.S. so revaccination is not necessary if the person does not plan to travel outside the U.S. However, the person should be revaccinated with either a properly reconstituted dose of MenACWY-CRM or with MenACWY-D if international travel anticipated, especially travel to Africa. There is no minimum interval between the incomplete dose given in error and the repeat dose.

Surveillance and Reporting of Meningococcal Disease

Meningococcal disease is a reportable condition in most states. Healthcare personnel should report any case of invasive meningococcal infection (meningococcal disease) to local and state health departments.

Antimicrobial Chemoprophylaxis

In the United States, the primary means for prevention of sporadic meningococcal disease is antimicrobial chemoprophylaxis of close contacts of infected persons. Close contacts include household members, child care center contacts, and anyone directly exposed to the patient's oral secretions (e.g., through kissing, mouth-to-mouth resuscitation, endotracheal intubation, or endotracheal tube management) during the 7 days before symptom onset. Healthcare personnel should receive chemoprophylaxis if they were managing an airway or were exposed to respiratory secretions of a patient with meningococcal disease.

For travelers, antimicrobial chemoprophylaxis should be considered for any passenger who had direct contact with respiratory secretions from an index patient or for anyone seated directly next to an index patient on a prolonged flight (i.e., one lasting more than 8 hours). The attack rate for household contacts exposed to patients who have sporadic meningococcal disease was estimated to be four cases per 1,000 persons exposed, which is 500–800 times greater than the rate for the total population. In the United Kingdom, the attack rate among healthcare personnel exposed to patients with meningococcal disease was determined to be 25 times higher than among the general population.

Chemoprophylaxis is not recommended for close contacts of patients with evidence of *Neisseria meningitidis* only in nonsterile sites (e.g., oropharyngeal, endotracheal, or conjunctival). Reports of secondary cases after close contact to persons with noninvasive pneumonia or conjunctivitis are rare; there is no evidence of substantive excess risk. Furthermore, there is no indication to treat persons who are asymptomatic nasopharyngeal carriers.

Because the rate of secondary disease for close contacts is highest immediately after onset of disease in the index patient, antimicrobial chemoprophylaxis should be administered as soon as possible, ideally less than 24 hours after identification

Timing of Chemoprophylaxis

- Should be administered as soon as possible, ideally less than 24 hours after identification of the index patient
- Chemoprophylaxis administered more than 14 days after onset of illness in the index patient probably of limited or no value

14

Meningococcal Disease

Antimicrobials

- Rifampin, Ciprofloxacin, and Ceftriaxone 90%-95% effective in reducing nasopharyngeal carriage of N. meningitidis and are all acceptable for chemoprophylaxis

---

of the index patient. Conversely, chemoprophylaxis administered more than 14 days after onset of illness in the index patient is probably of limited or no value. Oropharyngeal or nasopharyngeal cultures are not helpful in determining the need for chemoprophylaxis and might unnecessarily delay institution of this preventive measure.

Rifampin, ciprofloxacin, and ceftriaxone are 90%–95% effective in reducing nasopharyngeal carriage of *N. meningitidis* and are all acceptable antimicrobial agents for chemoprophylaxis. Although sporadic resistance to rifampin and ciprofloxacin has been reported worldwide, meningococcal resistance to chemoprophylaxis antibiotics remains rare in the United States. Clinicians should report suspected chemoprophylaxis failures to their public health departments. Systemic antimicrobial therapy for meningococcal disease with agents other than ceftriaxone or other third-generation cephalosporins might not reliably eradicate nasopharyngeal carriage of *N. meningitidis*. If other agents have been used for treatment, the index patient should receive chemoprophylactic antibiotics for eradication of nasopharyngeal carriage before being discharged from the hospital.

Acknowledgement

The editors thank Drs. Amanda Cohn and Gina Mootrey, CDC for their assistance in updating this chapter.

Selected References

CDC. Active Bacterial Core surveillance (ABCs). Available at http://www.cdc.gov/ncidod/dbmd/abcs/survreports/htm.

CDC. Manual for the Prevention of Vaccine-Preventable Diseases. 5th edition, 2011. Available at www.cdc.gov/vaccines/pubs/surv-manual/chpt08-mening.html

CDC. Prevention and Control of Meningococcal Disease: Recommendations of the Advisory Committee on Immunization Practices (ACIP). *MMWR* 2013;62(No. RR-2):[1-30].

CDC. Updated recommendation from the Advisory Committee on Immunization Practices (ACIP) for revaccination of persons at prolonged increased risk for meningococcal disease. *MMWR* 2009;58(No.37):1042-3.

CDC. Updated recommendations for use of meningococcal conjugate vaccines -Advisory Committee on Immunization Practices (ACIP). *MMWR* 2011;60(No.3):72-6.

14

CDC. Recommendations of the Advisory Committee on Immunization Practices (ACIP) for use of quadrivalent meningococcal conjugate vaccine (MenACWY-D) among children aged 9 through 23 months at increased risk for invasive meningococcal disease. *MMWR* 2011;60(No.40):1391-2.

Granoff DM, Harrison L, Borrow R. Meningococcal vaccine. In: Plotkin SA, Orenstein WA, Offit PA, eds. *Vaccines*. 5th ed. China: Saunders; 2008:399–434.

Harrison LH, Pass MA, Mendelsohn AB, et al. Invasive meningococcal disease in adolescents and young adults. *JAMA* 2001;286:694–9.

Jodar L, Feavers IM, Salisbury D, Granoff DM. Development of vaccines against meningococcal disease. *Lancet* 2002;359(9316):1499–1508.

Rosenstein NE, Perkins BA, Stephens DS, et al. Meningococcal disease. *N Engl J Med* 2001;344:1378–88.

Shepard CW, Ortega-Sanchez IR, Scott RD, Rosenstein NE; ABCs Team. Cost-effectiveness of conjugate meningococcal vaccination strategies in the United States. *Pediatrics* 2005;115:1220–32.

Sejvar JJ, Johnson D, Popovic T, et al. Assessing the risk of laboratory-acquired meningococcal disease. *J Clin Microbiolol* 2005;43:4811–4.

14

Meningococcal Disease

Mumps is an acute viral illness. Parotitis and orchitis were described by Hippocrates in the 5th century BCE. In 1934, Johnson and Goodpasture showed that mumps could be transmitted from infected patients to rhesus monkeys and demonstrated that mumps was caused by a filterable agent present in saliva. This agent was later shown to be a virus. Mumps was a frequent cause of outbreaks among military personnel in the prevaccine era, and was one of the most common causes of aseptic meningitis and sensorineural deafness in childhood. During World War I, only influenza and gonorrhea were more common causes of hospitalization among soldiers. In 2006, a multistate mumps outbreak in the Midwest resulted in more than 6,000 reported cases. During 2009-2010, two large outbreaks occurred: one among Orthodox Jewish communities in the Northeast with 3,502 reported cases and the other on the U.S. Territory of Guam with 505 mumps cases reported.

Mumps Virus

Mumps virus is a paramyxovirus in the same group as parainfluenza and Newcastle disease virus. Parainfluenza and Newcastle disease viruses produce antibodies that cross-react with mumps virus. The virus has a single-stranded RNA genome.

The virus can be isolated or propagated in cultures of various human and monkey tissues and in embryonated eggs. It has been recovered from the saliva, cerebrospinal fluid, urine, blood, breastmilk, and infected tissues of patients with mumps.

Mumps virus is rapidly inactivated by formalin, ether, chloroform, heat, and ultraviolet light.

Pathogenesis

The virus is acquired by respiratory droplets. It replicates in the nasopharynx and regional lymph nodes. After 12 to 25 days a viremia occurs, which lasts from 3 to 5 days. During the viremia, the virus spreads to multiple tissues, including the meninges, and glands such as the salivary, pancreas, testes, and ovaries. Inflammation in infected tissues leads to characteristic symptoms of parotitis and aseptic meningitis.

Clinical Features

The incubation period of mumps is 12 to 25 days, but parotitis typically develops 16 to 18 days after exposure to mumps virus. The prodromal symptoms are nonspecific, and include myalgia, anorexia, malaise, headache, and low-grade fever.

Mumps
- Acute viral illness
- Parotitis and orchitis described by Hippocrates in 5th century BCE
- Viral etiology described by Johnson and Goodpasture in 1934
- Frequent cause of outbreaks among military personnel in prevaccine era

Mumps Virus
- Paramyxovirus
- RNA virus
- Rapidly inactivated by chemical agents, heat, and ultraviolet light

Mumps Pathogenesis
- Respiratory transmission of virus
- Replication in nasopharynx and regional lymph nodes
- Viremia 12 to 25 days after exposure with spread to tissues
- Multiple tissues infected during viremia

Mumps Clinical Features
- Incubation period 12 to 25 days
- Nonspecific prodrome of myalgia, malaise, headache, low-grade fever
- Parotitis in 9%-94%
- 15%-27% of infections asymptomatic in prevaccine era

15

Mumps

Parotitis is the most common manifestation. Rates of classical parotitis among all age groups typically range from 31% to 65%, but in specific age groups can be as low as 9% or as high as 94% depending on the age and immunity of the group. Parotitis may be unilateral or bilateral, and any combination of single or multiple salivary glands may be affected. Parotitis tends to occur within the first 2 days and may first be noted as earache and tenderness on palpation of the angle of the jaw. Symptoms tend to decrease after one week and usually resolve after 10 days.

Before the introduction of the mumps vaccine in the United States in 1967, 15% to 27% of infections were asymptomatic. In the postvaccine era, it is difficult to estimate the number of asymptomatic infections, because it is unclear how vaccine modifies clinical presentation. Serious complications can occur in the absence of parotitis. Several articles discuss mumps symptoms as nonspecific or primarily respiratory, however, findings in these articles were based on serologies taken every six months or a year, so it is difficult to prove that the respiratory symptoms were because of mumps or that the symptoms occurred at the same time as the mumps infection.

Mumps Complications

- Orchitis
  - 12%-66% in postpubertal males (prevaccine)
  - 3%-10% (postvaccine)
- Pancreatitis
  - 3.5% (prevaccine)
- Unilateral Deafness
  - 1/20,000 (prevaccine)
- Death
  - 2/10,000 from 1966-1971
  - No deaths in recent U.S. outbreaks

Complications

Orchitis (testicular inflammation) is the most common complication in postpubertal males. In the prevaccine era, orchitis was reported in 12% to 66% of postpubertal males infected with mumps. In 60% to 83% of males with mumps orchitis, only one testis was affected. With mumps-associated orchitis, there is usually abrupt onset of testicular swelling, tenderness, nausea, vomiting, and fever. Pain and swelling may subside in 1 week, but tenderness may last for weeks. Sterility from mumps orchitis, even bilateral orchitis, occurred infrequently. In U.S. outbreaks in 2006 and 2009–2010 (the postvaccine era), rates of orchitis among postpubertal males have ranged from 3.3% to 10%. Orchitis usually occurs after parotitis, but it may precede it, begin simultaneously, or occur alone.

In the 2006 and 2009–2010 U.S. mumps outbreaks, oophoritis (ovarian inflammation) rates were 1% or lower among postpubertal females. It may mimic appendicitis. There is no relationship to impaired fertility.

In the prevaccine era, mumps accounted for approximately 10% of cases of symptomatic aseptic meningitis (inflammatory cells in cerebrospinal fluid resulting in headache or stiff neck). Men were afflicted three times as often as women. Aseptic meningitis resolves without sequelae in 3 to 10 days. Mumps encephalitis accounted for 36% of all reported encephalitis cases in the United States in 1967.

The incidence of mumps encephalitis is reported to range from 1 in 6,000 mumps cases (0.02%) to 1 in 300 mumps cases (0.3%).

Prior to the vaccine, pancreatitis was reported in 3.5% of persons infected with mumps in one community during a two year period and was described in case reports. Pancreatitis is infrequent, but occasionally occurs without parotitis; the hyperglycemia is transient and is reversible. Although single instances of diabetes mellitus have been reported, a causal relationship with mumps virus infection has yet to be conclusively demonstrated; many cases of temporal association have been described both in siblings and individuals, and outbreaks of diabetes have been reported a few months or years after outbreaks of mumps.

In the prevaccine era, mumps caused transient deafness in 4.1% of infected adult males in a military population. Permanent unilateral deafness caused by mumps occurred in 1 of 20,000 infected persons; bilateral, severe hearing loss was very rare.

In the postvaccine era, among all persons infected with mumps, reported rates of meningitis, encephalitis, pancreatitis, and deafness have all been less than 1%. Permanent sequelae such as paralysis, seizures, cranial nerve palsies, and hydrocephalus occurred very rarely, even in the prevaccine era. Although, in the United States during 1966–1971 there were two deaths per 10,000 reported mumps cases, there were no mumps-related deaths in recent U.S. outbreaks.

Laboratory Diagnosis

The diagnosis of mumps is usually suspected based on clinical manifestations, in particular the presence of parotitis. However, if mumps is suspected, laboratory testing should be performed. Acute mumps infection can be detected by the presence of serum mumps IgM, a significant rise in IgG antibody titer in acute and convalescent-phase serum specimens, IgG seroconversion, positive mumps virus culture, or detection of virus by real-time reverse transcriptase polymerase chain reaction (rRT-PCR). However, in both unvaccinated and vaccinated persons, false positive results can occur because assays may be affected by other diagnostic entities that cause parotitis. In addition, laboratory confirming the diagnosis of mumps in highly vaccinated populations may be challenging, and serologic tests should be interpreted with caution because false negative results in vaccinated persons (i.e., a negative serologic test in a person with true mumps) are common. With previous contact with mumps virus either through vaccination (particularly with two doses) or natural

15

Mumps Laboratory Diagnosis
- rRT-PCR
- Culture
- Serology

infection, serum mumps IgM test results may be negative; IgG test results may be positive at the initial blood draw; and viral detection in rRT-PCR or culture may have low yield if the buccal swab is collected more than three days after parotitis onset. Therefore, mumps cases should not be ruled out by negative laboratory results.

Mumps virus can be isolated from the parotid duct, other affected salivary gland ducts, the throat, from urine, and from cerebrospinal fluid (CSF). The preferred sample for viral isolation is a swab from the parotid duct, or the duct of another affected salivary gland. Collection of viral samples from persons suspected of having mumps is strongly recommended. Clinical specimens should ideally be obtained within three days and not more than eight days after parotitis onset. Mumps virus can also be detected by real-time reverse transcriptase polymerase chain reaction (rRT-PCR). Molecular typing is recommended because it provides important epidemiologic information, including transmission pathways of mumps strains circulating in the United States and it is a tool for distinguishing wild-type mumps virus from vaccine virus.

Serology is the simplest method for confirming mumps virus infection and enzyme immunoassay (EIA), is the most commonly used test. EIA is widely available and is more sensitive than other serologic tests. It is available for both IgM and IgG. In unvaccinated persons, IgM antibodies usually become detectable during the first 5 days of illness, reach a peak about a week after onset, and remain elevated for several weeks or months. However, as with measles and rubella, mumps IgM may be transient or missing in persons who have had any doses of mumps-containing vaccine. Sera should be collected as soon as possible after symptom onset for IgM testing or as the acute-phase specimen for IgG seroconversion. Convalescent-phase sera should be collected 2 weeks later. A negative serologic test, especially in a vaccinated person, should not be used to rule out a mumps diagnosis because the tests are not sensitive enough to detect infection in all persons with clinical illness. In the absence of another diagnosis, a person meeting the clinical case definition should be reported as a suspect mumps case. Additional information about specimen collection and shipping for mumps specimens may be obtained from the CDC mumps website at http://www.cdc.gov/mumps/lab/specimen-collect.html.

Epidemiology

Occurrence

Mumps occurs worldwide.

Reservoir

Mumps is a human disease. Although persons with asymptomatic or nonclassical infection can transmit the virus, no carrier state is known to exist.

Transmission

Mumps is spread through airborne transmission or by direct contact with infected droplet nuclei or saliva.

Temporal Pattern

Mumps incidence peaks predominantly in late winter and spring, but the disease has been reported throughout the year.

Communicability

Contagiousness is similar to that of influenza and rubella, but is less than that for measles or varicella. Although mumps virus has been isolated from seven days before, through 11–14 days after parotitis onset, the highest percentage of positive isolations and the highest virus loads occur closest to parotitis onset and decrease rapidly thereafter. Mumps is therefore most infectious in the several days before and after parotitis onset. Most transmission likely occurs several days before and after parotitis onset. Transmission also likely occurs from persons with asymptomatic infections and from persons with prodromal symptoms.

Secular Trends in the United States

Mumps became a nationally reportable disease in the United States in 1968. However, an estimated 212,000 cases occurred in the United States in 1964. Following vaccine licensure, reported mumps decreased rapidly. Approximately 3,000 cases were reported annually in 1983–1985 (1.3–1.55 cases per 100,000 population).

In 1986 and 1987, there was a relative resurgence of mumps, which peaked in 1987, when 12,848 cases were reported. The highest incidence of mumps during the resurgence was among older school-age and college-age youth (10–19 years of age), who were born before routine mumps vaccination was recommended. Mumps incidence in this period correlated with the absence of comprehensive state requirements for mumps immunization. Several mumps outbreaks among highly vaccinated school populations were reported, indicating that high coverage with a single dose of mumps vaccine did not always prevent disease transmission, probably because of vaccine failure.

Mumps Epidemiology

- Reservoir
  - human
  - asymptomatic infections may transmit
- Transmission
  - airborne
  - direct contact with droplet nuclei or saliva
- Temporal pattern
  - peak in late winter and spring
- Communicability
  - several days before and after onset of parotitis

15

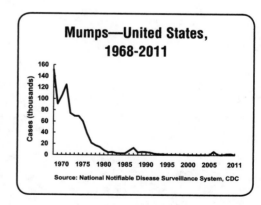

Mumps—United States, 1968-2011

Source: National Notifiable Disease Surveillance System, CDC

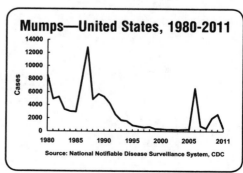

Mumps—United States, 1980-2011

Source: National Notifiable Disease Surveillance System, CDC

Mumps

Since 1989 when two doses of MMR vaccine were recommended for school-aged children for improved measles control, the number of reported mumps cases steadily declined, from 5,712 cases in 1989 to 258 cases in 2004. In 2006, the United States experienced a multi-state outbreak involving 6,584 reported cases of mumps. This resurgence predominantly affected Midwestern college students with the highest attack rates occurring among those living in dormitories. In the following two years, the number of reported cases returned to usual levels, and outbreaks involved fewer than 20 cases.

Beginning in June 2009, the largest U.S. mumps outbreak since 2006 has occurred. The index case was an 11 year old male infected in the United Kingdom, where approximately 7,400 reports of laboratory-confirmed mumps were received by the Health Protection Agency in 2009. A total of 3,502 outbreak-related cases were reported, primarily from New York. The outbreak was confined primarily to Orthodox Jewish communities, with less than 3% of cases occurring among persons outside these communities. The largest percentage of cases (53%) occurred among persons aged 5–17 years, and 71% of the patients were male. Among the patients for whom vaccination status was reported, 90% had received at least 1 dose of mumps-containing vaccine, and 76% had received 2 doses.

From December 2009, through December 2010, the U.S. Territory of Guam also experienced an outbreak, with 505 mumps cases reported; the median age was 12 years. Of the 287 school-aged children aged 6–18 years with reported mumps, 270 (94%) had received at least two doses of MMR vaccine, 8 (3%) had received one dose, 2 (1%) were unvaccinated, and 7 (2%) had unknown vaccination status. Two-dose MMR vaccine coverage in the most highly affected schools ranged from 99.3%–100%.

Like the mumps outbreaks that occurred in 2006, much of the 2009-2010 outbreaks occurred in congregate settings, where prolonged, close contact among persons facilitated transmission. Although school settings and large household sizes likely promoted transmission, the high vaccination coverage in the affected communities likely limited the size of the outbreaks. In addition, high vaccination coverage and less intense exposures in surrounding communities are the most plausible reasons that the few cases outside of the affected communities did not cause other outbreaks.

In 2011, there were 404 cases of mumps reported, and in 2012 there were 229 cases reported.

For information about the clinical case definition, clinical classification and epidemiologic classification of mumps see http://www.cdc.gov/vaccines/pubs/surv-manual/chpt09-mumps.html.

15

Mumps Vaccine

Characteristics

Mumps virus was isolated in 1945, and an inactivated vaccine was developed in 1948. This vaccine produced only short-lasting immunity, and its use was discontinued in the mid-1970s. The currently used Jeryl Lynn strain of live attenuated mumps virus vaccine was licensed in December 1967. The vaccine was recommended for routine use in the United States in 1977.

Mumps vaccine is available combined with measles and rubella vaccines (as MMR), or combined with measles, rubella, and varicella vaccine as MMRV (ProQuad). Single-antigen mumps vaccine is not available in the United States.

Mumps vaccine is prepared in chick embryo fibroblast tissue culture. MMR and MMRV are supplied as a lyophilized (freeze-dried) powder and are reconstituted with sterile, preservative-free water. The vaccine contains small amounts of human albumin, neomycin, sorbitol, and gelatin.

Immunogenicity and Vaccine Efficacy

Mumps vaccine produces an inapparent, or mild, noncommunicable infection. Approximately 94% (89% to 97%) of recipients of a single dose develop measurable mumps antibody. Seroconversion rates are similar for single antigen mumps vaccine, MMR, and MMRV. Postlicensure studies determined that one dose of mumps or MMR vaccine was 78% (49% to 92%) effective. Two dose mumps vaccine effectiveness is 88% (66% to 95%).

Vaccination Schedule and Use

In 1977, one dose of mumps-containing vaccine was routinely recommended for all children 12 months of age and older. In 1989, children began receiving two doses of mumps vaccine because of the implementation of a two-dose measles vaccination policy using the combined measles, mumps, and rubella (MMR) vaccine. In 2006, a two-dose mumps vaccine policy was recommended for school-aged children, students at post high school educational institutions, healthcare personnel, and international travelers.

The first dose of mumps-containing vaccine should be given on or after the first birthday. Mumps-containing vaccine given before 12 months of age should not be counted as part of the series. Children vaccinated with mumps-containing vaccine before 12 months of age should be revaccinated with two doses of MMR vaccine, the first of which should be administered when the child is at least 12 months of age.

Mumps Vaccine

- Composition
  - live virus (Jeryl Lynn strain)
- Effectiveness
  - 88% (Range, 66%-95%) – 2 doses
- Duration of Immunity
  - lifelong
- Schedule
  - at least 1 Dose
  - should be administered with measles and rubella (MMR) or with measles, rubella and varicella (MMRV)
- Single-antigen vaccine not available in the United States

15

Mumps (MMR) Vaccine Indications

- One dose (as MMR) for preschool-age children 12 months of age and older and persons born during or after 1957 not at high risk of mumps exposure
- Second dose (as MMR) for school-age children and adults at high risk of mumps exposure (i.e., healthcare personnel, international travelers and students at post-high school educational institutions)

Mumps

The second dose should be given routinely at age 4 through 6 years, before a child enters kindergarten or first grade. The recommended health visit at age 11 or 12 years can serve as a catch-up opportunity to verify vaccination status and administer MMR vaccine to those children who have not yet received two doses of MMR. The second dose of MMR may be administered as soon as 4 weeks (i.e., 28 days) after the first dose. The combined MMR vaccine is recommended for both doses to ensure immunity to all three viruses.

Only doses of vaccine with written documentation of the date of receipt should be accepted as valid. Self-reported doses or a parental report of vaccination is not considered adequate documentation. A clinician should not provide an immunization record for a patient unless that clinician has administered the vaccine or has seen a record that documents vaccination. Persons who lack adequate documentation of vaccination or other acceptable evidence of immunity should be vaccinated. Vaccination status and receipt of all vaccinations should be documented in the patient's permanent medical record and in a vaccination record held by the individual.

MMRV is approved by the Food and Drug Administration for children 12 months through 12 years of age (that is, until the 13th birthday). MMRV should not be administered to persons 13 years of age or older.

For the first dose of measles, mumps, rubella, and varicella vaccines at age 12 through 47 months, either separate MMR and varicella vaccines or MMRV vaccine may be used. Providers who are considering administering MMRV vaccine should discuss the benefits and risks of both vaccination options with the parents or caregivers. Unless the parent or caregiver expresses a preference for MMRV vaccine, ACIP recommends that MMR vaccine and varicella vaccine should be administered for the first dose in this age group (see Measles chapter for more information). For the second dose of measles, mumps, rubella, and varicella vaccines at any age (15 months through 12 years) and for the first dose at 48 months of age or older, use of MMRV vaccine generally is preferred over separate injections of its equivalent component vaccines (i.e., MMR vaccine and varicella vaccine).

Mumps Immunity

Generally, persons can be considered immune to mumps if they were born before 1957, have serologic evidence of mumps immunity or laboratory confirmation of disease, or have written documentation of adequate vaccination for mumps at age 12 months or older. Demonstration of mumps IgG antibody by any commonly used serologic

---

Mumps Immunity

- Birth before 1957
- Serologic evidence of mumps immunity
- Laboratory confirmation of disease
- Documentation of adequate vaccination

assay is acceptable evidence of mumps immunity. Persons who have an "equivocal" serologic test result should be considered susceptible to mumps.

For unvaccinated health-care personnel born before 1957 who lack laboratory evidence of measles, mumps and/or rubella immunity or laboratory confirmation of disease, healthcare facilities should consider vaccination with two doses of MMR vaccine at the appropriate interval (for measles and mumps) and one dose of MMR vaccine (for rubella), respectively. For unvaccinated personnel born before 1957 who lack laboratory evidence of measles, mumps and/or rubella immunity or laboratory confirmation of disease, healthcare facilities should recommend two doses of MMR vaccine during an outbreak of measles or mumps and one dose during an outbreak of rubella.

Postexposure Prophylaxis

Immune globulin (IG) is not effective postexposure prophylaxis. Vaccination after exposure is not harmful and may possibly avert later disease.

Contraindications and Precautions to Vaccination

Contraindications for MMR and MMRV vaccines include history of anaphylactic reactions to neomycin, history of severe allergic reaction to any component of the vaccine, pregnancy, and immunosuppression.

In the past, persons with a history of anaphylactic reactions following egg ingestion were considered to be at increased risk of serious reactions after receipt of measles- or mumps-containing vaccines, which are produced in chick embryo fibroblasts. However, data suggest that most anaphylactic reactions to measles- and mumps-containing vaccines are not associated with hypersensitivity to egg antigens but to other components of the vaccines (such as gelatin). The risk for serious allergic reactions such as anaphylaxis following receipt of these vaccines by egg-allergic persons is extremely low, and skin-testing with vaccine is not predictive of allergic reaction to vaccination. As a result, MMR may be administered to egg-allergic children without prior routine skin-testing or the use of special protocols.

MMR vaccine does not contain penicillin. A history of penicillin allergy is not a contraindication to MMR vaccination.

Pregnant women should not receive mumps vaccine, although the risk is theoretical. There is no evidence that mumps vaccine virus causes fetal damage. Pregnancy should be avoided for 4 weeks after vaccination with MMR vaccine.

15

MMR Vaccine Contraindications and Precautions

- History of anaphylactic reactions to neomycin
- History of severe allergic reaction to any component of the vaccine
- Pregnancy
- Immunosuppression
- Moderate or severe acute illness
- Recent blood product
- Personal or family (i.e., sibling or parent) history of seizures of any etiology (MMRV only)

Measles and Mumps Vaccines and Egg Allergy

- Measles and mumps viruses grown in chick embryo fibroblast culture
- Studies have demonstrated safety of MMR in egg allergic children
- Vaccinate without testing

Mumps

Persons with immunodeficiency or immunosuppression resulting from leukemia, lymphoma, generalized malignancy, immune deficiency disease, or immunosuppressive therapy should not be vaccinated. However, treatment with low-dose (less than 2 mg/kg/day), alternate-day, topical, or aerosolized steroid preparations is not a contraindication to mumps vaccination. Persons whose immunosuppressive therapy with steroids has been discontinued for 1 month (3 months for chemotherapy) may be vaccinated. See Measles chapter for additional details on vaccination of immunosuppressed persons, including those with HIV infection.

Persons with moderate or severe acute illness should not be vaccinated until the illness has improved. Minor illness (e.g., otitis media, mild upper respiratory infections), concurrent antibiotic therapy, and exposure or recovery from other illnesses are not contraindications to mumps vaccination.

Receipt of antibody-containing blood products (e.g., immune globulin, whole blood or packed red blood cells, intravenous immune globulin) may interfere with seroconversion following mumps vaccination. Vaccine should be given 2 weeks before, or deferred for at least 3 months following, administration of an antibody-containing blood product. See Chapter 2, General Recommendations on Immunization, for details.

A personal or family (i.e., sibling or parent) history of seizures of any etiology is a precaution for MMRV vaccination. Studies suggest that children who have a personal or family history of febrile seizures or family history of epilepsy are at increased risk for febrile seizures compared with children without such histories. Children with a personal or family history of seizures of any etiology generally should be vaccinated with MMR vaccine and varicella vaccine because the risks for using MMRV vaccine in this group of children generally outweigh the benefits. A family history of diabetes is not a contraindication to vaccination with MMR vaccine.

Adverse Events Following Vaccination

Most adverse events reported following MMR vaccine (such as fever, rash, and joint symptoms) are attributable to the measles or rubella components. No adverse reactions were reported in large-scale field trials. Subsequently, parotitis and fever have been reported rarely. A few cases of orchitis (all suspect) also have been reported.

Rare cases of central nervous system (CNS) dysfunction, including cases of deafness, within 2 months of mumps vaccination have been reported. The Institute of Medicine (1994) concluded that evidence is inadequate to accept or

---

MMR Adverse Events

- Fever
  - not common
- Rash
  - not common
- Joint symptoms
  - 25%
- Orchitis
  - not common
- Parotitis
  - rare
- CNS reactions
  - 1/800,000 doses

reject a causal relationship between the Jeryl Lynn strain of mumps vaccine and aseptic meningitis, encephalitis, sensori-neural deafness, or orchitis.

Adverse Reactions Following Vaccination

Allergic reactions, including rash, pruritus, and purpura, have been temporally associated with vaccination, but these are transient and generally mild. The calculated incidence of CNS reactions is approximately one per 800,000 doses of Jeryl Lynn strain of mumps vaccine virus.

See the Measles and Varicella chapters for information about adverse reactions following MMRV vaccine.

> **MMR Adverse Reactions**
> - Allergic reactions (rash, pruritis, purpura)
>   - not common
> - CNS reactions
>   - 1/800,000 doses

Vaccine Storage and Handling

MMR vaccine can be stored either in the freezer or the refrigerator and should be protected from light at all times. MMRV vaccine should be stored frozen between -58°F and +5°F (-50°C and -15°C). When MMR vaccine is stored in the freezer, the temperature should be the same as that required for MMRV, between -58°F and +5°F (-50°C and -15°C). Storing MMR in the freezer with MMRV may help prevent inadvertent storage of MMRV in the refrigerator.

Manufacturer package inserts contain additional information and can be found at http://www.fda.gov/BiologicsBloodVaccines/Vaccines/ApprovedProducts/ucm093830.htm. For complete information on best practices and recommendations please refer to CDC's Vaccine Storage and Handling Toolkit, http://www.cdc.gov/vaccines/recs/storage/toolkit/storage-handling-toolkit.pdf.

15

Acknowledgments

The editors thank Amy Parker Fiebelkorn, CDC for her assistance in updating this chapter.

Selected References

Barskey AE, Schulte C, Rosen JB, Handschur EF, Rausch-Phung E, Doll MK, et al. Mumps Outbreak in Orthodox Jewish Communities in the United States. *New Engl J Med.* 2012 Nov 1;367(18):1704-13.

CDC. Prevention of measles, rubella, congenital rubella syndrome, and mumps, 2013: summary recommendations of the Advisory Committee on Immunization Practices (ACIP), *MMWR* 2013:62(No. 4): 1-34.

CDC. General recommendations on immunization. recommendations of the Advisory Committee on Immunization Practices (ACIP). *MMWR.* 2011; 60(RR-2); 1-61.

CDC. Notice to readers: Updated recommendations of the Advisory Committee on Immunization Practices (ACIP) for the control and elimination of mumps. *MMWR* 2006;55:629–30.

CDC. Measles, mumps, and rubella—vaccine use and strategies for elimination of measles, rubella, and congenital rubella syndrome and control of mumps. Recommendations of the Advisory Committee on Immunization Practices (ACIP). *MMWR* 1998;47(No. RR-8):1–57.

CDC. Mumps surveillance: January 1972–June 1974. Atlanta, GA: U.S. Department of Health, Education, and Welfare, Public Health Service, 1974.

CDC. Mumps vaccine. 1977. *MMWR* 26(48):393–94.

CDC. Update: Mumps outbreak—New York and New Jersey, June 2009–January 2010. *MMWR* 2010;59:125–9.

CDC. Updated recommendations for isolation of persons with mumps. *MMWR* 2008. 57(40):1103–5.

CDC. Use of combination measles, mumps, rubella, and varicella vaccine: recommendations of the Advisory Committee on Immunization Practices (ACIP). *MMWR* 2010;59(No. RR-3):1–12.

Dayan GH, Quinlisk MP, Parker AA, Barskey AE, Harris ML, Schwartz JM, et al. Recent resurgence of mumps in the United States. *N Engl J Med*. 2008 Apr 10;358(15):1580-9.

Dayan GH and Rubin S. Mumps outbreaks in unvaccinated populations: are available mumps vaccines effective enough to prevent outbreaks? *Clin Infect Dis* 2008;47:1458-67.

Everberg G. Deafness following mumps. *Acta Otolaryngol* 1957;48(5–6):397–403.

Falk WA, et al. The epidemiology of mumps in southern Alberta 1980–1982. *Am J Epidemiol* 1989;130(4):736–49.

Hirsh BS, Fine PEM, Kent WK, et al. Mumps outbreak in a highly vaccinated population. *J Pediatr* 1991;119:187–93.

Kutty PK, et al. Guidance for isolation precautions for mumps in the United States: a review of the scientific basis for policy change. *Clin Infect Dis* 2010;50(12):1619–28.

Lee CM. Primary virus mastitis from mumps. *Va Med Mon* (1918) 1946;73:327.

15

Litman N and Baum SG. Mumps virus. In: Mandell GL, Bennett JE, and Dolin R, editors. *Mandell, Douglas, and Bennett's principles and practice of infectious diseases*. 7th ed. Philadelphia, PA: Churchill Livingstone Elsiever; 2010. p. 2201–06.

Morrison JC, et al. Mumps oophoritis: a cause of premature menopause. *Fertil Steril* 1975;26(7)655–9.

Miller HG, Stanton JB, Gibbons JL. Parainfectious encephalomyelitis and related syndromes; a critical review of neurological complications of certain specific fevers. *Q J Med* 1956;25:427–505.

Nelson GE, Aguon A, Valencia E, Oliva R, Guerrero ML, Reyes R, et al. Epidemiology of a Mumps Outbreak in a Highly Vaccinated Island Population and Use of a Third Dose of Measles-Mumps-Rubella Vaccine for Outbreak Control- Guam 2009-2010. *Pediatr Infect Dis J*. 2012 Oct 24.

Ogbuanu IU, Kutty PK, Hudson JM, Blog D, Abedi GR, Goodell S, et al. Impact of a third dose of measles-mumps-rubella vaccine on a mumps outbreak. *Pediatrics*. 2012 Dec;130(6):e1567-74

Orenstein WA, Hadler S, Wharton M. Trends in vaccine-preventable diseases. *Semin Pediatr Infect Dis* 1997;8:23–33.

Philip RN, Reinhard KR, Lackman DB. Observations on a mumps epidemic in a virgin population. *Am J Hyg* 1959;69(2):91–111.

Plotkin SA, Rubin SA. Mumps vaccine. In: Plotkin SA, Orenstein, WA, Offit PA, eds. *Vaccines*. 5th ed. China: Saunders;2008:435–65.

Rambar AC. Mumps; use of convalescent serum in the treatment and prophylaxis of orchitis. *Am J Dis Child* 1946;71:1–13.

Reed D, et al. A mumps epidemic on St. George Island, Alaska. *JAMA* 1967; 199(13):113–7.

Russell RR and Donald JC. The neurological complications of mumps. *Br Med J* 1958;2(5087):27–30.

Taparelli F, et al. Isolation of mumps virus from vaginal secretions in association with oophoritis. *J Infect* 1988;17(3)255–8.

15

Mumps

Van Loon FPL, Holmes SJ, Sirotkin BI, et al. Mumps surveillance—United States, 1988–1993. In: CDC Surveillance Summaries, August 11, 1995. *MMWR* 1995;44(No. SS-3): 1-14.

Veghelyi PV. Secondary pancreatitis. *Am J Dis Child* 1947;74(1):45–51.

Weaver RJ and Petry TN. Mumps mastitis in the nursing female, with a case report. *J Indiana State Med Assoc* 1958;51(5)644–5.

Werner CA. Mumps orchitis and testicular atrophy; occurrence. *Ann Intern Med* 1950;32(6):1066–74.

Witte CL and Schanzer B. Pancreatitis due to mumps. *JAMA* 1968;203(12):1068–9.

15

Pertussis, or whooping cough, is an acute infectious disease caused by the bacterium *Bordetella pertussis*. Outbreaks of pertussis were first described in the 16th century, and the organism was first isolated in 1906.

In the 20th century, pertussis was one of the most common childhood diseases and a major cause of childhood mortality in the United States. Before the availability of pertussis vaccine in the 1940s, more than 200,000 cases of pertussis were reported annually. Since widespread use of the vaccine began, incidence has decreased more than 80% compared with the prevaccine era.

Pertussis remains a major health problem among children in developing countries, with 195,000 deaths resulting from the disease in 2008 (World Health Organization estimate).

Bordetella pertussis

B. pertussis is a small, aerobic gram-negative rod. It is fastidious and requires special media for isolation (see Laboratory Diagnosis).

B. pertussis produces multiple antigenic and biologically active products, including pertussis toxin (PT), filamentous hemagglutinin (FHA), agglutinogens, adenylate cyclase, pertactin, and tracheal cytotoxin. These products are responsible for the clinical features of pertussis disease, and an immune response to one or more produces immunity following infection. Immunity following *B. pertussis* infection does not appear to be permanent.

Pathogenesis

Pertussis is primarily a toxin-mediated disease. The bacteria attach to the cilia of the respiratory epithelial cells, produce toxins that paralyze the cilia, and cause inflammation of the respiratory tract, which interferes with the clearing of pulmonary secretions. Pertussis antigens appear to allow the organism to evade host defenses, in that lymphocytosis is promoted but chemotaxis is impaired. Until recently it was thought that *B. pertussis* did not invade the tissues. However, recent studies have shown the bacteria to be present in alveolar macrophages.

Clinical Features

The incubation period of pertussis is commonly 7–10 days, with a range of 4–21 days, and rarely may be as long as 42 days. The clinical course of the illness is divided into three stages.

Pertussis
- Acute infectious disease caused by *Bordetella pertussis*
- Outbreaks first described in 16th century
- *Bordetella pertussis* isolated in 1906
- Estimated 195,000 deaths worldwide in 2008

Bordetella pertussis
- Fastidious gram-negative bacteria
- Antigenic and biologically active components:
  - pertussis toxin (PT)
  - filamentous hemagglutinin (FHA)
  - agglutinogens
  - adenylate cyclase
  - pertactin
  - tracheal cytotoxin

Pertussis Pathogenesis
- Primarily a toxin-mediated disease
- Bacteria attach to cilia of respiratory epithelial cells
- Inflammation occurs which interferes with clearance of pulmonary secretions
- Pertussis antigens allow evasion of host defenses (lymphocytosis promoted but impaired chemotaxis)

16

Pertussis

Pertussis Clinical Features

- Incubation period 7-10 days (range 4-21 days)
- Insidious onset, similar to the common cold with nonspecific cough
- Fever usually minimal throughout course of illness
- Catarrhal stage
  - 1-2 weeks
- Paroxysmal cough stage
  - 1-6 weeks
- Convalescence
  - weeks to months

Pertussis Among Children, Adolescents and Adults

- Disease often milder than in infants and young children
- Infection may be asymptomatic, or may present as classic pertussis
- Persons with mild disease may transmit the infection
- Older persons often source of infection for children

The first stage, the catarrhal stage, is characterized by the insidious onset of coryza (runny nose), sneezing, low-grade fever, and a mild, occasional cough, similar to the common cold. The cough gradually becomes more severe, and after 1–2 weeks, the second, or paroxysmal stage, begins. Fever is generally minimal throughout the course of the illness.

It is during the paroxysmal stage that the diagnosis of pertussis is usually suspected. Characteristically, the patient has bursts, or paroxysms, of numerous, rapid coughs, apparently due to difficulty expelling thick mucus from the tracheobronchial tree. At the end of the paroxysm, a long inspiratory effort is usually accompanied by a characteristic high-pitched whoop. During such an attack, the patient may become cyanotic (turn blue). Children and young infants, especially, appear very ill and distressed. Vomiting and exhaustion commonly follow the episode. The person does not appear to be ill between attacks.

Paroxysmal attacks occur more frequently at night, with an average of 15 attacks per 24 hours. During the first 1 or 2 weeks of this stage, the attacks increase in frequency, remain at the same level for 2 to 3 weeks, and then gradually decrease. The paroxysmal stage usually lasts 1 to 6 weeks but may persist for up to 10 weeks. Infants younger than 6 months of age may not have the strength to have a whoop, but they do have paroxysms of coughing.

In the convalescent stage, recovery is gradual. The cough becomes less paroxysmal and disappears in 2 to 3 weeks. However, paroxysms often recur with subsequent respiratory infections for many months after the onset of pertussis.

Adolescents, adults and children partially protected by the vaccine may become infected with B. pertussis but may have milder disease than infants and young children. Pertussis infection in these persons may be asymptomatic, or present as illness ranging from a mild cough illness to classic pertussis with persistent cough (i.e., lasting more than 7 days). Inspiratory whoop is not common.

Even though the disease may be milder in older persons, those who are infected may transmit the disease to other susceptible persons, including unimmunized or incompletely immunized infants. Older persons are often found to have the first case in a household with multiple pertussis cases, and are often the source of infection for children.

Complications

The most common complication, and the cause of most pertussis-related deaths, is secondary bacterial pneumonia. Young infants are at highest risk for acquiring pertussis-associated complications. Data from 1997–2000 indicate that pneumonia occurred in 5.2% of all reported pertussis cases, and among 11.8% of infants younger than 6 months of age.

Neurologic complications such as seizures and encephalopathy (a diffuse disorder of the brain) may occur as a result of hypoxia (reduction of oxygen supply) from coughing, or possibly from toxin. Neurologic complications of pertussis are more common among infants. Other less serious complications of pertussis include otitis media, anorexia, and dehydration. Complications resulting from pressure effects of severe paroxysms include pneumothorax, epistaxis, subdural hematomas, hernias, and rectal prolapse.

In 2008 through 2011 a total of 72 deaths from pertussis were reported to CDC. Children 3 months of age or younger accounted for 60 (83%) of these deaths. During 2008-2011, the annual mean of pertussis cases in infants was 3,132 (range 2,230 - 4,298), the mean of hospitalizations was 1,158 (range 687-1,459) and the mean of deaths was 16 (range 11-25).

Adolescents and adults may also develop complications of pertussis, such as difficulty sleeping, urinary incontinence, pneumonia, and rib fracture.

Laboratory Diagnosis

The diagnosis of pertussis is based on a characteristic clinical history (cough for more than 2 weeks with whoop, paroxysms, or posttussive vomiting) as well as a variety of laboratory tests (culture, polymerase chain reaction [PCR], and serology).

Culture is considered the gold standard laboratory test and is the most specific of the laboratory tests for pertussis. However, fastidious growth requirements make *B. pertussis* difficult to culture. The yield of culture can be affected by specimen collection, transportation, and isolation techniques. Specimens from the posterior nasopharynx, not the throat, should be obtained using Dacron® or calcium alginate (not cotton) swabs. Isolation rates are highest during the first 2 weeks of illness (catarrhal and early paroxysmal stages). Cultures are variably positive (30%–50%) and may take as long as 2 weeks, so results may be too late for clinical usefulness. Cultures are less likely to be positive if performed later in the course of illness (more than 2 weeks after cough onset) or on specimens from persons who have received antibiotics or have been vaccinated. Since adolescents and adults have often been coughing for several weeks before they seek medical attention, it is often too late for culture to be useful.

Pertussis Complications in Children

- Secondary bacterial pneumonia – most common
- Neurologic complications – seizures, encephalopathy more common among infants
- Otitis media
- Anorexia
- Dehydration
- Pneumothorax
- Epistaxis
- Subdural hematomas
- Hernias
- Rectal prolapse

Pertussis Complications in Adolescents and Adults

- Difficulty sleeping
- Urinary incontinence
- Pneumonia
- Rib fracture

Pertussis Laboratory Diagnosis

- Culture – gold standard
- Polymerase Chain Reaction (PCR)
  - can confirm pertussis in an outbreak
  - highly sensitive
  - high false-positive rate
- Serology
  - can confirm illness late in the course of infection
  - many tests have unproven or unknown clinical accuracy
- Direct fluorescent antibody test
  - low sensitivity
  - variable specificity
  - should not be used for laboratory confirmation

16

Pertussis

Polymerase chain reaction (PCR) is a rapid test and has excellent sensitivity. PCR tests vary in specificity, so obtaining culture confirmation of pertussis for at least one suspicious case is recommended any time there is suspicion of a pertussis outbreak. Results should be interpreted along with the clinical symptoms and epidemiological information. PCR should be tested from nasopharyngeal specimens taken at 0-3 weeks following cough onset, but may provide accurate results for up to 4 weeks of cough in infants or unvaccinated persons. After the fourth week of cough, the amount of bacterial DNA rapidly diminishes, which increases the risk of obtaining falsely-negative results. PCR assay protocols that include multiple targets allow for speciation among *Bordetella* species. The high sensitivity of PCR increases the risk of false-positivity, but following some simple best practices can reduce the risk of obtaining inaccurate results (http://www.cdc.gov/pertussis/clinical/diagnostic-testing/diagnosis-pcr-bestpractices.html).

Serologic testing could be useful for adults and adolescents who present late in the course of their illness, when both culture and PCR are likely to be negative. CDC and FDA have developed a serologic assay that has been extremely useful for confirming diagnosis, especially during suspected outbreaks. Many state public health labs have included this assay as part of their testing regimen for pertussis. Commercially, there are many different serologic tests used in United States with unproven or unknown clinical accuracy. CDC is actively engaged in better understanding the usefulness of these commercially available assays. Generally, serologic tests are more useful for diagnosis in later phases of the disease. For the CDC single point serology, the optimal timing for specimen collection is 2 to 8 weeks following cough onset, when the antibody titers are at their highest; however, serology may be performed on specimens collected up to 12 weeks following cough onset.

Because direct fluorescent antibody testing of nasopharyngeal secretions has been demonstrated in some studies to have low sensitivity and variable specificity, such testing should not be relied on as a criterion for laboratory confirmation.

An elevated white blood cell count with a lymphocytosis is usually present in classical disease of infants. The absolute lymphocyte count often reaches 20,000 or greater. However, there may be no lymphocytosis in some infants and children or in persons with mild or modified cases of pertussis. More information on the laboratory diagnosis of pertussis is available at http://www.cdc.gov/vaccines/pubs/surv-manual/default.pdf

Medical Management

The medical management of pertussis cases is primarily supportive, although antibiotics are of some value. This therapy eradicates the organism from secretions, thereby decreasing communicability and, if initiated early, may modify the course of the illness. Recommended antibiotics are azithromycin, clarithromycin, and erythromycin. Trimethoprim-sulfamethoxasole can also be used.

An antibiotic effective against pertussis should be administered to all close contacts of persons with pertussis, regardless of age and vaccination status. Revised treatment and postexposure prophylaxis recommendations were published in December 2005 (see reference list). All close contacts younger than 7 years of age who have not completed the four-dose primary series should complete the series with the minimal intervals. (see table in Appendix A). Close contacts who are 4–6 years of age and who have not yet received the second booster dose (usually the fifth dose of DTaP) should be vaccinated. The administration of Tdap to persons who have been exposed to a person with pertussis is not contraindicated, but the efficacy of postexposure use of Tdap is unknown.

Epidemiology

Occurrence

Pertussis occurs worldwide.

Reservoir

Pertussis is a human disease. No animal or insect source or vector is known to exist. Adolescents and adults are an important reservoir for *B. pertussis* and are often the source of infection for infants.

Transmission

Transmission most commonly occurs by the respiratory route through contact with respiratory droplets, or by contact with airborne droplets of respiratory secretions. Transmission occurs less frequently by contact with freshly contaminated articles of an infected person.

Temporal Pattern

Pertussis has no distinct seasonal pattern, but it may increase in the summer and fall.

Communicability

Pertussis is highly communicable, as evidenced by secondary attack rates of 80% among susceptible household contacts. Persons with pertussis are most infectious during the catarrhal period and the first 2 weeks after cough onset (i.e., approximately 21 days).

Pertussis Epidemiology

- Reservoir
  - Human Adolescents and adults
- Transmission
  - Respiratory droplets
- Communicability
  - Maximum in catarrhal stage
  - Secondary attack rate up to 80%

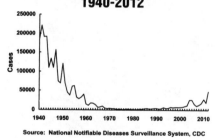

Pertussis—United States, 1940-2012

Source: National Notifiable Diseases Surveillance System, CDC

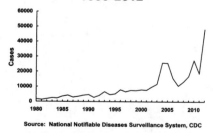

Pertussis—United States, 1980-2012

Source: National Notifiable Diseases Surveillance System, CDC

16

Pertussis

Secular Trends in the United States

Before the availability of vaccine, pertussis was a common cause of morbidity and mortality among children. During the 6-year period from 1940 through 1945, more than 1 million cases of pertussis were reported, an average of 175,000 cases per year (incidence of approximately 150 cases per 100,000 population).

Following introduction of whole-cell pertussis vaccine in the 1940s, pertussis incidence gradually declined, reaching 15,000 reported cases in 1960 (approximately 8 per 100,000 population). By 1970, annual incidence was fewer than 5,000 cases per year, and during 1980–1990, an average of 2,900 cases per year were reported (approximately 1 per 100,000 population).

Pertussis incidence has been gradually increasing since the early 1980s. A total of 25,827 cases was reported in 2004, the largest number since 1959. The reasons for the increase are not clear. A total of 27,550 pertussis cases and 27 pertussis-related deaths were reported in 2010. Case counts for 2012 have surpassed 2010, with 48,277 pertussis cases, with 13 deaths in infants (provisional).

During 2001–2003, the highest average annual pertussis incidence was among infants younger than 1 year of age (55.2 cases per 100,000 population), and particularly among children younger than 6 months of age (98.2 per 100,000 population). In 2002, 24% of all reported cases were in this age group. However, in recent years, adolescents (11–18 years of age) and adults (19 years and older) have accounted for an increasing proportion of cases. During 2001–2003, the annual incidence of pertussis among persons aged 10–19 years increased from 5.5 per 100,000 in 2001, to 6.7 in 2002, and 10.9 in 2003. In 2004 and 2005, approximately 60% of reported cases were among persons 11 years of age and older. Increased recognition and diagnosis of pertussis in older age groups probably contributed to this increase of reported cases among adolescents and adults. In 2010, the United States experienced another peak in cases with approximately 27,000 cases and the emergence of disease in children 7-10 years of age. In 2012, case counts continued to be elevated among children 7-10 years; however, reports of disease were also elevated among adolescents aged 13 and 14, which has not been observed since the introduction of Tdap. The epidemiology of pertussis has changed in recent years, with an increasing burden of disease among fully-vaccinated children and adolescents, which is likely being driven by the transition to acellular vaccines in the 1990s.

Pertussis Surveillance

For information about pertussis surveillance and information about the case definition, and case classification see www.cdc.gov/vaccines/pubs/surv-manual/default.htm.

Pertussis Vaccines

Whole-Cell Pertussis Vaccine

Whole-cell pertussis vaccine is composed of a suspension of formalin-inactivated *B. pertussis* cells. Whole-cell pertussis vaccines were first licensed in the United States in 1914 and became available combined with diphtheria and tetanus toxoids (as DTP) in 1948.

Based on controlled efficacy trials conducted in the 1940s and on subsequent observational efficacy studies, a primary series of four doses of whole-cell DTP vaccine was 70%–90% effective in preventing serious pertussis disease. Protection decreased with time, resulting in little or no protection 5 to 10 years following the last dose. Local reactions such as redness, swelling, and pain at the injection site occurred following up to half of doses of whole-cell DTP vaccines. Fever and other mild systemic events were also common. Concerns about safety led to the development of more purified (acellular) pertussis vaccines that are associated with a lower frequency of adverse reactions. Whole-cell pertussis vaccines are no longer available in the United States but are still used in many other countries.

Acellular Pertussis Vaccine

Characteristics

Acellular pertussis vaccines are subunit vaccines that contain purified, inactivated components of *B. pertussis* cells. Several acellular pertussis vaccines have been developed for different age groups; these contain different pertussis components in varying concentrations. Acellular pertussis vaccines are available only as combinations with tetanus and diphtheria toxoids.

Pediatric Formulation (DTaP)

Two pediatric acellular pertussis vaccines are currently available for use in the United States. Both vaccines are combined with diphtheria and tetanus toxoids as DTaP and are approved for children 6 weeks through 6 years of age (to age 7 years). Infanrix (GlaxoSmithKline) contains three antigens, mostly pertussis toxin (PT) and FHA. Daptacel (sanofi pasteur) contains five components, PT, FHA, pertactin, and fimbriae types 2 and 3. Neither of the available DTaP vaccines contains thimerosal as a preservative. Infanrix is supplied in single-dose vials or syringes, and Daptacel is supplied in single-dose vials only.

Whole-Cell Pertussis Vaccine

- Developed in 1930s and used widely in clinical practice through mid-1940s
- DTP - 70%-90% effective after 4 doses
- Little to no protection after 5-10 years
- Local adverse reactions common

16

Pertussis-containing Vaccines

- DTaP (pediatric)
- approved for children 6 weeks through 6 years (to age 7 years)
- Tdap (adolescent and adult)
- approved for persons 10 years and older (Boostrix) and 10 through 64 years (Adacel)

Composition* of Acellular Pertussis Vaccines

Product	PT	FHA	PERT	FIM
Infanrix	25	25	8	--
Daptacel	10	5	3	5
Boostrix	8	8	2.5	--
Adacel	2.5	5	3	5

*mcg per dose

16

Adolescent and Adult Formulation (Tdap)

Acellular pertussis–containing vaccines were first licensed for adolescents and adults in 2005. Two vaccines are currently available. Both vaccines are combined with tetanus toxoid and a reduced amount of diphtheria toxoid compared with pediatric DTaP (that is, similar quantities of tetanus and diphtheria toxoid to adult formulation Td). Boostrix (GlaxoSmithKline) is approved for persons 10 years of age and older, and contains three pertussis antigens (PT, FHA, and pertactin) in a reduced quantity compared with the GlaxoSmithKline pediatric formulation. The vaccine contains aluminum hydroxide as an adjuvant and does not contain a preservative. Adacel (sanofi pasteur) is approved for persons 10 through 64 years of age. It contains the same five pertussis components as Daptacel but with a reduced quantity of PT. Adacel contains aluminum phosphate as an adjuvant and does not contain a preservative. Both vaccines are supplied in single-dose vials or syringes.

Immunogenicity and Vaccine Efficacy

DTaP

Since 1991, several studies conducted in Europe and Africa have evaluated the efficacy of DTaP vaccines administered to infants. These studies varied in type and number of vaccines, design, case definition, and laboratory method used to confirm the diagnosis of pertussis, so comparison among studies must be made with caution. Point estimates of vaccine efficacy ranged from 80% to 85% for vaccines currently licensed in the United States. Confidence intervals for vaccine efficacy overlap, suggesting that none of the vaccines is significantly more effective than the others. When studied, the acellular pertussis vaccine was significantly more effective than whole-cell DTP. Mild local and systemic adverse reactions and more serious adverse reactions (such as high fever, persistent crying, hypotonic-hyporesponsive episodes, and seizures) occurred less frequently among infants vaccinated with acellular pertussis vaccines than among those vaccinated with whole-cell DTP.

Tdap

Adolescent and adult formulation Tdap vaccines were licensed on the basis of noninferiority of the serologic response to the various components compared with each company's pediatric DTaP formulation (Infanrix and Daptacel) among persons who had received pediatric DTaP or DTP in childhood. For both vaccines, the antibody response to a single dose of Tdap was similar to that following three doses of DTaP in infants. This type of study is known as "bridging." The new vaccines are assumed to have similar clinical efficacy as DTaP vaccine since a similar level of antibody to the components was achieved.

Routine DTaP Primary Vaccination Schedule

Dose	Age	Minimum Interval
Primary 1	6 weeks - 2 months	---
Primary 2	4 months	4 wks
Primary 3	6 months	4 wks
Primary 4	15-18 months	6 mos

Vaccination Schedule and Use
DTaP

The primary series of DTaP vaccine consists of four doses, the first three doses given at 4- to 8-week intervals (minimum of 4 weeks), beginning at 6 weeks to 2 months of age. The fourth dose is given 6–12 months after the third to maintain adequate immunity for the ensuing preschool years. DTaP should be administered simultaneously with all other indicated vaccines.

The fourth dose of all brands of DTaP is licensed, and recommended by ACIP, to be administered at 15–18 months of age (15–20 months for Daptacel). However, ACIP recommends that in certain circumstances the fourth dose be given earlier than 15 months of age. The fourth dose of DTaP may be given if the child is at least 12 months of age, and at least 6 months have elapsed since the third dose of pertussis vaccine was given, and, in the opinion of the immunization provider, the child is unlikely to return for an additional visit at 15–18 months of age. All three of these criteria should be met in order to administer the fourth dose of DTaP at 12–14 months of age.

Children who received all four primary doses before the fourth birthday should receive a fifth (booster) dose of DTaP before entering school. This booster dose is not necessary (but may be given) if the fourth dose in the primary series was given on or after the fourth birthday. The booster dose increases antibody levels and may decrease the risk of school-age children transmitting the disease to younger siblings who are not fully vaccinated.

ACIP recommends that the series be completed with the same brand of DTaP vaccine if possible. However, limited data suggest that "mix and match" DTaP schedules do not adversely affect safety and immunogenicity. If the vaccine provider does not know or have available the type of DTaP vaccine previously administered to a child, any available DTaP vaccine should be used to continue or complete the vaccination series. Unavailability of the vaccine used for earlier doses is not a reason for missing the opportunity to administer a dose of acellular pertussis vaccine for which the child is eligible.

Interruption of the recommended schedule or delayed doses does not lead to a reduction in the level of immunity reached on completion of the primary series. There is no need to restart a series regardless of the time that has elapsed between doses.

DTaP Fourth Dose

- Recommended at 15-18 months*

- May be given at 12 months of age if:

  - 6 months since DTaP3, and

  - unlikely to return at 15-18 months

*15-20 months for Daptacel

School Entry (Fifth) Dose

- Fifth dose recommended when 4th dose given before age 4 years

- All DTaP vaccines are licensed for 5th dose after DTaP series

Interchangeability of Different Brands of DTaP Vaccine

- Series should be completed with same brand of vaccine if possible

- Limited data suggest that "mix and match" DTaP schedules do not adversely affect safety and immunogenicity

- Use different brand of DTaP if necessary

Tdap Vaccines

- Boostrix (GlaxoSmithKline)

  - approved for persons 10 years of age and older

- Adacel (sanofi pasteur)

  - approved for persons 10 through 64 years of age

16

Pertussis

Tdap Recommendations

- A single dose of Tdap is recommended for

  - adolescents 11 through 18 years of age

  - adults 19 ~~through 64 years of age~~ *and older (See 9/2015 Errata)*

  - children 7-10 years of age who are not fully vaccinated against pertussis*

  - ~~adults 65 years of age and older who have or anticipate having close contact with an infant less than 12 months of age~~ *See 9/2015 Errata*

* "Not fully vaccinated" against pertussis is defined as having received fewer than 4 doses of DTaP, or having received 4 doses of DTaP but the last dose was prior to age 4 years. See *MMWR* 2011;60(No.1):13-5.

Tdap Recommendations for Pregnant Women

- Providers of prenatal care should implement a Tdap vaccination program for pregnant women who previously have not received Tdap

- Administer Tdap in each pregnancy, preferably at 27 through 36 weeks gestation

- If not administered during pregnancy, Tdap should be administered immediately postpartum, for women not previously vaccinated with Tdap

MMWR 2013;62(No. 7):131-5

Tdap

Both Tdap vaccines are approved by the Food and Drug Administration for a single (booster) dose for persons who have completed the recommended childhood DTP/DTaP vaccination series. Boostrix is approved for persons 10 years of age and older; Adacel is approved for persons ~~11~~ *10, See 9/2015 Errata* through 64 years of age.

ACIP recommends a single Tdap dose for persons aged 11 through 18 years who have completed the recommended childhood diphtheria and tetanus toxoids and pertussis/diphtheria and tetanus toxoids and acellular pertussis (DTP/DTaP) vaccination series and for adults aged 19 through 64 years.

Children 7 through 10 years of age who are not fully vaccinated against pertussis (defined as having received fewer than 4 doses of DTaP, or having received 4 doses of DTaP but the last dose was prior to age 4 years) and who do not have a contraindication to pertussis vaccine should receive a single dose of Tdap to provide protection against pertussis. If additional doses of tetanus and diphtheria toxoid- containing vaccines are needed, then children 7 through 10 years of age should be vaccinated according to the catch-up schedule, with Tdap preferred as the first dose. Either brand of Tdap may be used. Currently, Tdap is recommended only for a single dose across all age groups.

Adults 19 years of age and older who previously have not received Tdap should receive a single dose of Tdap to protect against pertussis and reduce the likelihood of transmission. For adults 19-64 years of age either brand of Tdap may be used. Adults 65 years or older should be vaccinated with Boostrix if feasible. However, either vaccine administered to a person 65 years or older is immunogenic and would provide protection. A dose of either vaccine would be considered valid.

Tdap can be administered regardless of interval since the last tetanus- or diphtheria-toxoid containing vaccine. After receipt of Tdap, persons should continue to receive Td for routine booster immunization against tetanus and diphtheria, generally every 10 years.

ACIP recommends that providers of prenatal care implement a Tdap immunization program for all pregnant women. Healthcare personnel should administer a dose of Tdap during each pregnancy, irrespective of the patient's prior history of receiving Tdap. To maximize the maternal antibody response and passive antibody transfer to the infant, optimal timing for Tdap administration is between 27 and 36 weeks gestation although Tdap may be given at any time during pregnancy. For women not previously vaccinated with Tdap, if Tdap is not administered during pregnancy, Tdap should be administered immediately postpartum. No study has assessed the safety of repeated doses of Tdap in pregnant women. CDC will monitor and assess the safety of Tdap use during pregnancy.

Studies on the persistence of antipertussis antibodies following a dose of Tdap show antibody levels in healthy, nonpregnant adults peak during the first month after vaccination, with antibody levels declining after 1 year. The decline in antibody levels in pregnant women likely would be similar. Because antibody levels wane substantially during the first year after vaccination, ACIP concluded a single dose of Tdap at one pregnancy would be insufficient to provide protection for subsequent pregnancies.

ACIP also recommends that adolescents and adults (e.g., parents, siblings, grandparents, childcare providers, and healthcare personnel) who have or anticipate having close contact with an infant younger than 12 months of age should receive a single dose of Tdap to protect against pertussis if they have not previously received Tdap. Ideally, these persons should receive Tdap at least 2 weeks before beginning close contact with the infant.

Healthcare personnel should receive a single dose of Tdap as soon as feasible if they have not previously received Tdap and regardless of the time since their most recent Td vaccination.. Priority should be given to vaccination of healthcare personnel who have direct contact with infants 12 months of age and younger.

Tdap vaccine may be given at the same visit, or any time before or after any other vaccine.

Immunity following pertussis is not permanent. Persons with a history of pertussis should receive a single dose of Tdap if it is otherwise indicated.

All adolescents and adults should have documentation of having received a primary series of at least three doses of tetanus and diphtheria toxoids during their lifetime. A person without such documentation should receive a series of three doses of tetanus- and diphtheria-containing vaccine. One of these doses, preferably the first, should be Tdap. The remaining two doses should be adult formulation Td.

Tdap Vaccine and Healthcare Personnel

- Healthcare personnel should receive a single dose of Tdap as soon as feasible*

- Priority should be given to vaccination of healthcare personnel who have direct contact with infants 12 months of age and younger

*if they have not previously received Tdap. *MMWR* 2006;55(RR-17):1-37

Tdap For Persons Without A History of DTP or DTaP

- All adolescents and adults should have documentation of having received a series of DTaP, DTP, DT, or Td

- Persons without documentation should receive a series of 3 vaccinations

- One dose should be Tdap, preferably the first

16

Pertussis

Combination Vaccines Containing DTaP

Pediarix

In 2002, the FDA approved Pediarix (GlaxoSmithKline), the first pentavalent (5 component) combination vaccine licensed in the United States. Pediarix contains DTaP (Infanrix), hepatitis B (Engerix-B), and inactivated polio vaccines.

The minimum age for the first dose of Pediarix is 6 weeks, so it cannot be used for the birth dose of the hepatitis B series. Pediarix is approved for the first three doses of the DTaP and inactivated polio vaccine (IPV) series, which are usually given at about 2, 4, and 6 months of age; it is not approved for fourth or fifth (booster) doses of the DTaP or IPV series. However, Pediarix is approved for use through 6 years of age. A child who is behind schedule can receive Pediarix as long as it is given for doses 1, 2, or 3 of the series, and the child is younger than 7 years of age.

A dose of Pediarix inadvertently administered as the fourth or fifth dose of the DTaP or IPV series does not need to be repeated.

Pediarix may be used interchangeably with other pertussis-containing vaccines if necessary (although ACIP prefers the use of the same brand of DTaP for all doses of the series, if possible). It can be given at 2, 4, and 6 months to infants who received a birth dose of hepatitis B vaccine (total of four doses of hepatitis B vaccine). Although not labeled for this indication by FDA, Pediarix may be used in infants whose mothers are HBsAg positive or whose HBsAg status is not known.

Pentacel

Pentacel is a combination vaccine that contains lyophilized Hib (ActHIB) vaccine that is reconstituted with a liquid DTaP-IPV solution. The vaccine was licensed by FDA in June 2008. Pentacel is licensed by FDA for doses 1 through 4 of the DTaP series among children 6 weeks through 4 years of age. The minimum intervals for Pentacel are determined by the DTaP component. The first three doses must be separated by at least 4 weeks. The fourth dose must be separated from the third by at least 6 calendar months, and not administered before 12 months of age. Pentacel should not be used for the fifth dose of the DTaP series, or for children 5 years or older regardless of the number of prior doses of the component vaccines.

The DTaP-IPV solution is licensed only for use as the diluent for the lyophilized Hib component and should not be used separately.

Kinrix

Kinrix is a combination vaccine that contains DTaP and inactivated poliovirus vaccine (IPV) that is produced by GlaxoSmithKline. It was approved by the FDA in 2008. Kinrix is licensed only for the fifth dose of DTaP and fourth dose of IPV in children 4 through 6 years of age whose previous DTaP vaccine doses have been with Infanrix and/or Pediarix for the first three doses and Infanrix for the fourth dose. However, if Kinrix is administered to children who received another brand of DTaP for prior DTaP doses the Kinrix dose does not need to be repeated.

Other DTaP Issues

In certain circumstances, vaccination with DTaP vaccine should be delayed until a child with a known or suspected neurologic condition has been evaluated, treatment initiated, and the condition stabilized. These conditions include the presence of an evolving neurologic disorder (e.g., uncontrolled epilepsy, infantile spasms, and progressive encephalopathy), a history of seizures that has not been evaluated, or a neurologic event that occurs between doses of pertussis vaccine.

A family history of seizures or other neurologic diseases, or stable or resolved neurologic conditions (e.g., controlled idiopathic epilepsy, cerebral palsy, developmental delay) are not contraindications to pertussis vaccination.

Reducing the dose of DTaP vaccine or giving the full dose in multiple smaller doses may result in an altered immune response and inadequate protection. Furthermore, there is no evidence that the chance of a significant vaccine reaction is likely to be reduced by this practice. The use of multiple reduced doses that together equal a full immunizing dose, or the use of smaller, divided doses is not endorsed or recommended. Any vaccination using less than the standard dose should not be counted, and the person should be revaccinated according to age.

Because immunity from pertussis disease wanes, children who have recovered from documented pertussis should be vaccinated with pertussis vaccines according to the routine schedules.

Pertussis Vaccine Use in Children with Underlying Neurologic Disorders

Underlying Condition	Recommendation
Prior seizure	Delay and assess*
Suspected neurologic disorder	Delay and assess*
Neurologic event between doses	Delay and assess*
Stable/resolved neurologic condition	Vaccinate

*vaccinate after treatment initiated and condition stabilized

16

Pertussis

DTaP Contraindications

- Severe allergic reaction to vaccine component or following a prior dose

- Encephalopathy not due to another identifiable cause occurring within 7 days after vaccination

DTaP Precautions*

- Moderate or severe acute illness

- Temperature 105°F (40.5°C) or higher within 48 hours with no other identifiable cause

- Collapse or shock-like state (hypotonic-hyporesponsive episode) within 48 hours

- Persistent, inconsolable crying lasting 3 hours or longer, occurring within 48 hours

- Convulsions with or without fever occurring within 3 days

*may consider use in outbreaks

Tdap Contraindications

- Severe allergic reaction to vaccine component or following a prior dose

- Encephalopathy not due to another identifiable cause occurring within 7 days after vaccination with a pertussis-containing vaccine

Contraindications and Precautions to Vaccination

DTaP

Contraindications to further vaccination with DTaP are a severe allergic reaction (anaphylaxis) to a vaccine component or following prior dose of vaccine, and encephalopathy not due to another identifiable cause occurring within 7 days after vaccination.

Moderate or severe acute illness is a precaution to vaccination. Children with mild illness, such as otitis media or upper respiratory infection, should be vaccinated. Children for whom vaccination is deferred because of moderate or severe acute illness should be vaccinated when their condition improves.

Certain infrequent adverse reactions following DTaP vaccination are considered to be precautions for subsequent doses of pediatric pertussis vaccine. These adverse reactions are a temperature of 105°F (40.5°C) or higher within 48 hours that is not due to another identifiable cause; collapse or shock-like state (hypotonic-hyporesponsive episode) within 48 hours; persistent, inconsolable crying lasting 3 hours or longer, occurring within 48 hours; and convulsions with or without fever occurring within 3 days.

There are circumstances (e.g., during a communitywide outbreak of pertussis) in which the benefit of vaccination outweighs the risk, even if one of the four precautionary adverse reactions occurred following a prior dose. In these circumstances, one or more additional doses of pertussis vaccine should be considered. DTaP should be used in these circumstances.

Tdap

Tdap is contraindicated for persons with a history of a severe allergic reaction to a vaccine component or following a prior dose of vaccine. Tdap is also contraindicated for persons with a history of encephalopathy not due to another identifiable cause occurring within 7 days after administration of a pertussis-containing vaccine.

Precautions to Tdap include a history of Guillain-Barré syndrome within 6 weeks after a previous dose of tetanus toxoid-containing vaccine and a progressive neurologic disorder (such as uncontrolled epilepsy or progressive encephalopathy) until the condition has stabilized. Persons with a history of a severe local reaction (Arthus reaction) following a prior dose of a tetanus and/or diphtheria toxoid-containing vaccine should generally not receive Tdap or Td vaccination until at least 10 years have elapsed after the last Td-containing vaccine. Moderate or severe acute illness is a precaution to vaccination. Persons for whom vaccination is deferred because of moderate or severe acute illness should be vaccinated when their condition improves.

As noted above, certain conditions following DTaP vaccine, such as temperature of 105°F or higher, collapse or shock-like state, persistent crying, or convulsions with or without fever are a precaution to subsequent doses of DTaP. However, occurrence of one of these adverse reactions following DTaP vaccine in childhood is not a contraindication or precaution to administration of Tdap to an adolescent or adult. A history of extensive limb swelling following DTaP is not a contraindication to Tdap vaccination. A stable neurologic disorder (such as controlled seizures or cerebral palsy), breastfeeding, and immunosuppression are not contraindications or precautions to administration of Tdap.

Adverse Reactions Following Vaccination
DTaP

As with all injected vaccines, administration of DTaP may cause local reactions, such as pain, redness, or swelling. Local reactions have been reported in 20%–40% of children after the first three doses. Local reactions appear to be more frequent after the fourth and/or fifth doses. Mild systemic reactions such as drowsiness, fretfulness, and low-grade fever may also occur. Temperature of 101°F or higher is reported in 3%–5% of DTaP recipients. These reactions are self-limited and can be managed with symptomatic treatment with acetaminophen or ibuprofen. Moderate or severe systemic reactions (such as fever [105°F or higher], febrile seizures, persistent crying lasting 3 hours or longer, and hypotonic-hyporesponsive episodes) have been reported after administration of DTaP but occur less frequently than among children who received whole-cell DTP. Rates of these less common reactions vary by symptom and vaccine but generally occur in fewer than 1 in 10,000 doses. See the Pertussis chapter in the textbook *Vaccines* (Plotkin, Orenstein, and Offit eds., 2013) for a comprehensive review of DTaP adverse event data.

Information on adverse reactions following a full series of DTaP is also limited. Available data suggest a substantial increase in the frequency and magnitude of local reactions after the fourth and fifth doses. For example, swelling at the site of injection occurred in 2% of patients after the first dose of Tripedia, and in 29% following the fourth dose. Increases in the frequency of fever after the fourth dose have also been reported, although the increased frequencies of other systemic reactions (e.g., fretfulness, drowsiness, or decreased appetite) have not been observed. Further details

Tdap Precautions

- History of Guillain-Barré syndrome within 6 weeks after a prior dose of tetanus toxoid-containing vaccine

- Progressive neurologic disorder until the condition has stabilized

- History of a severe local reaction (Arthus reaction) following a prior dose of a tetanus and/or diphtheria toxoid-containing vaccine

- Moderate or severe acute illness

DTaP Adverse Reactions

- Local reactions (pain, redness, swelling)
  - 20%-40%
- Temp of 101°F
  - 3%-5% or higher
- More severe adverse reactions
  - not common
- Local reactions more common following 4th and 5th doses

Adverse Reactions Following the 4th and 5th DTaP Dose

- Local adverse reactions and fever increased with 4th and 5th doses of DTaP

- Reports of swelling of entire limb

- Extensive swelling after 4th dose NOT a contraindication to 5th dose

16

on this issue can be found in a supplemental ACIP statement published in 2000 (*MMWR* 2000;49(No RR-13):1–8).

Swelling involving the entire thigh or upper arm has been reported after booster doses of certain acellular pertussis vaccines. The limb swelling may be accompanied by erythema, pain and fever. Although the swelling may interfere with walking, most children have no limitation of activity. The pathogenesis and frequency of substantial local reactions and limb swelling are not known, but these conditions appear to be self-limited and resolve without sequelae.

ACIP recommends that a fifth dose of DTaP be administered before a child enters school. It is not known whether children who experience entire limb swelling after a fourth dose of DTaP are at increased risk for this reaction after the fifth dose. Because of the importance of this dose in protecting a child during school years, ACIP recommends that a history of extensive swelling after the fourth dose should not be considered a contraindication to receipt of a fifth dose at school entry. Parents should be informed of the increase in reactogenicity that has been reported following the fourth and fifth doses of DTaP.

Tdap

The safety of Tdap vaccines was evaluated as part of prelicensure studies. The most common adverse reaction following both brands of Tdap vaccine is a local reaction, such as pain (66%), redness (25%) or swelling (21%) at the site of injection. Temperature of 100.4°F or higher was reported by 1.4% of Tdap recipients and 1.1% of Td recipients. Tdap recipients also reported a variety of nonspecific systemic events, such as headache, fatigue and gastrointestinal symptoms. Local reactions, fever, and nonspecific systemic symptoms occurred at approximately the same rate in recipients of Tdap and the comparison group that received Td without acellular pertussis vaccine. No serious adverse events have been attributed to Tdap.

Vaccine Storage and Handling

DTaP, Td and Tdap vaccines should be stored at 35°–46°F (2°–8°C) at all times. The vaccines must never be frozen. Vaccine exposed to freezing temperature must not be administered and should be discarded. DTaP, Td and Tdap should not be used after the expiration date printed on the box or label.

Acknowledgment

The editors thank Drs. Jennifer Liang, Cindy Weinbaum, and Pedro Moro; and Stacey Martin, CDC for their assistance in updating this chapter.

16

Tdap Adverse Reactions

- Local reactions (pain, redness, swelling)
  - 21%-66%
- Temp of 100.4° F or higher
  - 1.4%
- Adverse reactions occur at approximately the same rate as Td alone (without acellular pertussis vaccine)

Selected References

American Academy of Pediatrics. Pertussis. In: Pickering L, Baker CJ, Kimberlin D, Long SS, eds Red Book: *2009 Report of the Committee on Infectious Diseases*. 28th ed. Elk Grove Village, IL: American Academy of Pediatrics, 2009:504–19.

CDC. Pertussis vaccination: use of acellular pertussis vaccines among infants and young children. Recommendations of the Advisory Committee on Immunization Practices (ACIP). *MMWR* 1997;46(No. RR-7):1–25.

CDC. Recommended antimicrobial agents for the treatment and postexposure prophylaxis of pertussis. 2005 CDC Guidelines. *MMWR* 2005;54(No. RR-14):1–16.

CDC. Preventing tetanus, diphtheria, and pertussis among adolescents: use of tetanus toxoid, reduced diphtheria toxoid and acellular pertussis vaccine: recommendations of the Advisory Committee on Immunization Practices (ACIP). *MMWR* 2006;55(No. RR-3):1–43.

CDC. Preventing tetanus, diphtheria, and pertussis among adults: use of tetanus toxoid, reduced diphtheria toxoid and acellular pertussis vaccine: recommendations of the Advisory Committee on Immunization Practices (ACIP). *MMWR* 2006;55(No. RR-17):1–33.

CDC. Updated recommendations for use of tetanus toxoid, reduced diphtheria toxoid and acellular pertussis (Tdap) Vaccine from the Advisory Committee on Immunization Practices (ACIP), 2011. *MMWR* 2011;60(No.1):13-15.

CDC. Updated Recommendations for Use of Tetanus Toxoid, Reduced Diphtheria Toxoid, and Acellular Pertussis Vaccine (Tdap) in Pregnant Women — Advisory Committee on Immunization Practices (ACIP), 2012. *MMWR* 2012; 62(07);131-135.

CDC. Updated recommendations for use of tetanus toxoid, reduced diphtheria toxoid and acellular pertussis vaccine (Tdap) in pregnant women and persons who have or anticipate having close contact with an infant <12 months of age – Advisory Committee on Immunization Practices (ACIP), 2011.

Cherry JD, The epidemiology of pertussis: a comparison of the epidemiology of the disease pertussis with the epidemiology of *Bordetella pertussis* infection. *Pediatrics* 2005;115:1422–7.

Edwards KM, Decker MD. Pertussis Vaccines. In: Plotkin SA, Orenstein, WA, and Offit PA, eds. *Vaccines*. 6th ed. China: Saunders; 2013.

16

Pertussis

Greenberg DP. Pertussis in adolescents: increasing incidence brings attention to the need for booster immunization of adolescents. *Pediatr Infect Dis J* 2005;24:721–8.

Ward JI, Cherry JD, Chang SJ, et al. Efficacy of an acellular pertussis vaccine among adolescents and adults. *N Engl J Med* 2005;353:1555–63.

Woo EJ, Burwen DR, Gatumu SNM, et al. Extensive limb swelling after immunization: Reports to the Vaccine Adverse Event Reporting System. *Clin Infect Dis* 2003;37:351–8.

16

Streptococcus pneumoniae causes an acute bacterial infection. The bacterium, also called pneumococcus, was first isolated by Pasteur in 1881 from the saliva of a patient with rabies. The association between the pneumococcus and lobar pneumonia was first described by Friedlander and Talamon in 1883, but pneumococcal pneumonia was confused with other types of pneumonia until the development of the Gram stain in 1884. From 1915 to 1945, the chemical structure and antigenicity of the pneumococcal capsular polysaccharide, its association with virulence, and the role of bacterial polysaccharides in human disease were explained. More than 80 serotypes of pneumococci had been described by 1940.

Efforts to develop effective pneumococcal vaccines began as early as 1911. However, with the advent of penicillin in the 1940s, interest in pneumococcal vaccination declined, until it was observed that many patients still died despite antibiotic treatment. By the late 1960s, efforts were again being made to develop a polyvalent pneumococcal vaccine. The first pneumococcal vaccine was licensed in the United States in 1977. The first conjugate pneumococcal vaccine was licensed in 2000.

Streptococcus pneumoniae

Streptococcus pneumoniae bacteria are lancet-shaped, gram-positive, facultative anaerobic organisms. They are typically observed in pairs (diplococci) but may also occur singularly or in short chains. Most pneumococci are encapsulated, their surfaces composed of complex polysaccharides. Capsular polysaccharides are one determinant of the pathogenicity of the organism. They are antigenic and form the basis for classifying pneumococci by serotypes. Ninety-two serotypes have been documented as of 2011, based on their reaction with type-specific antisera. Type-specific antibody to capsular polysaccharide is protective. These antibodies and complement interact to opsonize pneumococci, which facilitates phagocytosis and clearance of the organism. Antibodies to some pneumococcal capsular polysaccharides may cross-react with related types as well as with other bacteria, providing protection against additional serotypes.

Most *S. pneumoniae* serotypes have been shown to cause serious disease, but only a few serotypes produce the majority of pneumococcal infections. The 10 most common serotypes are estimated to account for about 62% of invasive disease worldwide. The ranking and serotype prevalence differ by patient age group and geographic area. In the United States, prior to widespread use of 7-valent pneumococcal conjugate vaccine (PCV7), the seven most common serotypes isolated from blood or cerebrospinal fluid (CSF)

Pneumococcal Disease

- *S. pneumoniae* first isolated by Pasteur in 1881
- Confused with other causes of pneumonia until discovery of Gram stain in 1884
- More than 80 serotypes described by 1940
- First U.S. vaccine in 1977

17

Streptococcus pneumonia

- Gram-positive organisms
- Polysaccharide capsule important pathogenicity factor
- 92 serotypes documented as of 2011
- Type-specific antibody is protective

Pneumococcal Disease

of children younger than 5 years of age accounted for 80% of infections. These seven serotypes accounted for only about 50% of isolates from older children and adults.

Pneumococci are common inhabitants of the respiratory tract and may be isolated from the nasopharynx of 5% to 90% of healthy persons. Rates of asymptomatic carriage vary with age, environment, and the presence of upper respiratory infections. Among school-aged children, 20%–60% may be colonized. Only 5%–10% of adults without children are colonized although, on military installations, as many as 50%–60% of service personnel may be colonized. The duration of carriage varies and is generally longer in children than adults. In addition, the relationship of carriage to the development of natural immunity is poorly understood.

Clinical Features

The major clinical syndromes of pneumococcal disease are pneumonia, bacteremia, and meningitis.

Pneumococcal pneumonia is the most common clinical presentation of pneumococcal disease among adults. The incubation period of pneumococcal pneumonia is short, about 1 to 3 days. Symptoms generally include an abrupt onset of fever and chills or rigors. Classically there is a single rigor, and repeated shaking chills are uncommon. Other common symptoms include pleuritic chest pain, cough productive of mucopurulent, rusty sputum, dyspnea (shortness of breath), tachypnea (rapid breathing), hypoxia (poor oxygenation), tachycardia (rapid heart rate), malaise, and weakness. Nausea, vomiting, and headaches occur less frequently.

Approximately 400,000 hospitalizations from pneumococcal pneumonia are estimated to occur annually in the United States. Pneumococci account for up to 36% of adult community-acquired pneumonia. Pneumococcal pneumonia has been demonstrated to complicate influenza infection. About 25-30% of patients with pneumococcal pneumonia also experience pneumococcal bacteremia. The case-fatality rate is 5%–7% and may be much higher among elderly persons. Other complications of pneumococcal pneumonia include empyema (i.e., infection of the pleural space), pericarditis (inflammation of the sac surrounding the heart), and endobronchial obstruction, with atelectasis and lung abscess formation.

More than 12,000 cases of pneumococcal bacteremia without pneumonia occur each year. The overall case-fatality rate for bacteremia is about 20% but may be as high as 60% among elderly patients. Patients with asplenia who develop bacteremia may experience a fulminant clinical course.

Pneumococcal Pneumonia Clinical Features

- Abrupt onset of fever
- Chills or rigors
- Pleuritic chest pain
- Productive cough
- Dyspnea, tachypnea, hypoxia
- Tachycardia, malaise, weakness

Pneumococcal Pneumonia

- Estimated 400,000 hospitalizations per year in the United States
- Up to 36% of adult community-acquired pneumonias
- Common bacterial complication of influenza
- Case-fatality rate 5%–7%, higher in elderly

Pneumococcal Bacteremia

- More than 12,000 cases per year in the United States
- Case-fatality rate ~20%; up to 60% among the elderly

17

Pneumococci cause over 50% of all cases of bacterial meningitis in the United States. An estimated 3,000 to 6,000 cases of pneumococcal meningitis occur each year. Some patients with pneumococcal meningitis also have pneumonia. The clinical symptoms, cerebrospinal fluid (CSF) profile and neurologic complications are similar to other forms of purulent bacterial meningitis. Symptoms may include headache, lethargy, vomiting, irritability, fever, nuchal rigidity, cranial nerve signs, seizures and coma. The case-fatality rate of pneumococcal meningitis is about 8% among children and 22% among adults. Neurologic sequelae are common among survivors.

Adults with certain medical conditions are at highest risk for invasive pneumococcal disease. For adults aged 18-64 years with hematologic cancer, the rate of invasive pneumococcal disease in 2010 was 186 per 100,000, and for persons with human immunodeficiency virus (HIV) the rate was 173 per 100,000. Other conditions that place adults at highest risk for invasive pneumococcal disease include other immunocompromising conditions, either from disease or drugs, functional or anatomic asplenia, and renal disease. Other conditions that increase the risk of invasive pneumococcal disease include chronic heart disease, pulmonary disease (including asthma in adults), liver disease, smoking cigarettes (in adults) CSF leak, and having a cochlear implant.

Pneumococcal Disease in Children

Bacteremia without a known site of infection is the most common invasive clinical presentation of pneumococcal infection among children 2 years of age and younger, accounting for approximately 70% of invasive disease in this age group. Bacteremic pneumonia accounts for 12%–16% of invasive pneumococcal disease among children 2 years of age and younger. With the decline of invasive Hib disease, S. pneumoniae has become the leading cause of bacterial meningitis among children younger than 5 years of age in the United States. Before routine use of pneumococcal conjugate vaccine, children younger than 1 year had the highest rates of pneumococcal meningitis, approximately 10 cases per 100,000 population.

Pneumococci are a common cause of acute otitis media and are detected in 28%–55% of middle ear aspirates. By age 12 months, more than 60% of children have had at least one episode of acute otitis media. Middle ear infections are the most frequent reasons for pediatric office visits in the United States, resulting in more than 20 million visits annually. Complications of pneumococcal otitis media may include mastoiditis and meningitis.

Pneumococcal Meningitis

- Estimated 3,000–6,000 cases per year in the United States
- Case-fatality rate 8% among children
- Case-fatality rate 22% among adults
- Neurologic sequelae common among survivors

Conditions That Increase Risk for Invasive Pneumococcal Disease

- Decreased immune function — including hematologic cancer and HIV infection
- Asplenia (functional or anatomic)
- Chronic heart, pulmonary (including asthma in adults), liver or renal disease
- Cigarette smoking (in adults)
- Cerebrospinal fluid (CSF) leak
- Cochlear implant

Pneumococcal Disease in Children

- Bacteremia without known site of infection most common clinical presentation
- S. pneumoniae leading cause of bacterial meningitis among children younger than 5 years of age
- Common cause of acute otitis media

17

Pneumococcal Disease

Before routine use of pneumococcal conjugate vaccine, the burden of pneumococcal disease among children younger than 5 years of age was significant. An estimated 17,000 cases of invasive disease occurred each year, of which 13,000 were bacteremia without a known site of infection and about 700 were meningitis. An estimated 200 children died every year as a result of invasive pneumococcal disease. Although not considered invasive disease, an estimated 5 million cases of acute otitis media occured each year among children younger than 5 years of age.

Children with functional or anatomic asplenia, particularly those with sickle cell disease, and children with immune compromise including human immunodeficiency virus (HIV) infection are at very high risk for invasive disease, with rates in some studies more than 50 times higher than those among children of the same age without these conditions (i.e., incidence rates of 5,000–9,000 per 100,000 population). Rates are also increased among children of certain racial and ethnic groups, including Alaska Natives, African Americans, and certain American Indian groups (Navajo and White Mountain Apache). The reason for this increased risk by race and ethnicity is not known with certainty but was also noted for invasive *Haemophilus influenzae* infection (also an encapsulated bacterium). Attendance at a child care center has also been shown to increase the risk of invasive pneumococcal disease and acute otitis media 2–3-fold among children younger than 59 months of age. Children with cochlear implants are at increased risk for pneumococcal meningitis.

Burden of Pneumococcal Disease in Children*

Syndrome	Cases
Bacteriemia	13,000
Meningitis	700
Death	200
Otitis media	5,000,000

*Prior to routine use of pneumococcal conjugate vaccine

Children at Increased Risk of Invasive Pneumococcal Disease

- Functional or anatomic asplenia, particularly sickle cell disease
- Immune compromise, including HIV infection
- Alaska Native, African American, American Indian (Navajo and White Mountain Apache)
- Child care attendance
- Cochlear implant

Laboratory Diagnosis

A definitive diagnosis of infection with *S. pneumoniae* generally relies on isolation of the organism from blood or other normally sterile body sites. Tests are also available to detect capsular polysaccharide antigen in body fluids.

The appearance of lancet-shaped diplococci on Gram stain is suggestive of pneumococcal infection, but interpretation of stained sputum specimens may be difficult because of the presence of normal nasopharyngeal bacteria. The suggested criteria for obtaining a diagnosis of pneumococcal pneumonia using gram-stained sputum includes more than 25 white blood cells and fewer than 10 epithelial cells per high-power field, and a predominance of gram-positive diplococci.

A urinary antigen test based on an immunochromatographic membrane technique to detect the C-polysaccharide antigen of *Streptococcus pneumoniae* as a cause of community-acquired pneumonia among adults is commercially available and has

17

been cleared by FDA. The test is rapid and simple to use, has a reasonable specificity in adults, and has the ability to detect pneumococcal pneumonia after antibiotic therapy has been started.

Medical Management

Resistance to penicillin and other antibiotics was previously very common. However, following introduction of PCV7, antibiotic resistance declined and then began to increase again. Then, in 2008, the definition of penicillin resistance was changed such that a much larger proportion of pneumococci are now considered susceptible to penicillin. The revised susceptibility breakpoints for *S. pneumoniae*, published by the Clinical and Laboratory Standards Institute (CLSI) in January 2008, were the result of a reevaluation that showed clinical response to penicillin was being preserved in clinical studies of pneumococcal infection, despite reduced susceptibility response in vitro. Guidelines for treatment of meningitis and pneumonia are available from professional societies.

Epidemiology

Occurrence

Pneumococcal disease occurs throughout the world.

Reservoir

S. pneumoniae is a human pathogen. The reservoir for pneumococci is the nasopharynx of asymptomatic humans. There is no animal or insect vector.

Transmission

Transmission of *S. pneumoniae* occurs as the result of direct person-to-person contact via respiratory droplets and by autoinoculation in persons carrying the bacteria in their upper respiratory tract. Different pneumococcal serotypes have different propensities for causing asymptomatic colonization, otitis media, meningitis, and pneumonia. The spread of the organism within a family or household is influenced by such factors as household crowding and viral respiratory infections.

Temporal Pattern

Pneumococcal infections are more common during the winter and in early spring when respiratory diseases are more prevalent.

Communicability

The period of communicability for pneumococcal disease is unknown, but presumably transmission can occur as long as the organism appears in respiratory secretions.

Pneumococcal Disease Epidemiology

Reservoir	Human Carriers
Transmission	Respiratory and Autoinoculation
Temporal pattern	Winter and early spring
Communicability	Unknown (Probably as long as organism appears in respiratory secretions)

17

Pneumococcal Disease

Secular Trends in the United States

Estimates of the incidence of pneumococcal disease have been made from a variety of population-based studies. More than 35,000 cases and more than 4,200 deaths from invasive pneumococcal disease (bacteremia and meningitis) are estimated to have occurred in the United States in 2011. More than half of these cases occurred in adults who had an indication for pneumococcal polysaccharide vaccine.

Data from the Active Bacterial Core surveillance (ABCs) system suggest that the use of pneumococcal conjugate vaccine has had a major impact on the incidence of invasive disease among young children. The reductions in incidence resulted from a 99% decrease in disease caused by the seven serotypes in PCV7 and serotype 6A, a serotype against which PCV7 provides some cross-protection. The decreases have been offset partially by increases in invasive disease caused by serotypes not included in PCV7, in particular 19A.

Pneumococcal Vaccines
Characteristics
Pneumococcal Polysaccharide Vaccine

Pneumococcal polysaccharide vaccine is composed of purified preparations of pneumococcal capsular polysaccharide. The first polysaccharide pneumococcal vaccine was licensed in the United States in 1977. It contained purified capsular polysaccharide antigen from 14 different types of pneumococcal bacteria. In 1983, a 23-valent polysaccharide vaccine (PPSV23) was licensed and replaced the 14-valent vaccine, which is no longer produced. PPSV23 contains polysaccharide antigen from 23 types of pneumococcal bacteria that cause 60-76% of invasive disease.

The polysaccharide vaccine currently available in the United States (Pneumovax 23, Merck) contains 25 mcg of each antigen per dose and contains 0.25% phenol as a preservative. The vaccine is available in a single-dose vial or syringe, and in a 5-dose vial. Pneumococcal vaccine is given by injection and may be administered either intramuscularly or subcutaneously.

Pneumococcal Conjugate Vaccine

The first pneumococcal conjugate vaccine (PCV7) was licensed in the United States in 2000. It includes purified capsular polysaccharide of seven serotypes of *S. pneumoniae* (4, 9V, 14, 19F, 23F, 18C, and 6B) conjugated to a nontoxic variant of diphtheria toxin known as CRM197. In 2010 a 13-valent pneumococcal conjugate vaccine (PCV13) was licensed in the United States. It contains the 7 serotypes of *S pneumoniae* as PCV7 plus serotypes 1, 3, 5, 6A, 7F and 19A

Pneumococcal Vaccines

Year	Vaccine
1977	14-valent polysaccharide vaccine licensed
1983	23-valent polysaccharide vaccine licensed (PPSV23)
2000	7-valent polysaccharide conjugate vaccine licensed (PCV7)
2010	13-valent PCV licensed

Pneumococcal Polysaccharide Vaccine

- Purified capsular polysaccharide antigen from 23 types of pneumococcus

- Account for 60% –76% of bacteremic pneumococcal disease

Pneumococcal Conjugate Vaccine

- Purified capsular polysaccharide from 13 types of pneumococcus conjugated to nontoxic diphtheria toxin (CRM197)

- In 2008 vaccine serotypes contained in PCV13 accounted for 61% of invasive pneumococcal disease cases among children younger than 5 years

17

which are also conjugated to CRM197. A 0.5-mL PCV13 dose contains approximately 2.2 µg of polysaccharide from each of 12 serotypes and approximately 4.4 µg of polysaccharide from serotype 6B; the total concentration of CRM197 is approximately 34 µg. The vaccine contains 0.02% polysorbate 80 (P80), 0.125 mg of aluminum as aluminum phosphate (AlPO4) adjuvant, 5mL of succinate buffer, and no thimerosal preservative. Except for the addition of six serotypes, P80, and succinate buffer, the formulation of PCV13 is the same as that of PCV7.

ABCs data indicate that in 2008, before PCV13 replaced PCV7 for routine use among children, approximately 61% of invasive pneumococcal disease cases among children younger than 5 years were attributable to the serotypes included in PCV13, with serotype 19A accounting for 43% of cases; PCV7 serotypes caused less than 2% of cases.

Indirect effects from PCV13 use among children, if similar to those observed after PCV7 introduction, might further reduce the remaining burden of adult pneumococcal disease caused by PCV13-types. A preliminary analysis using a probabilistic model following a single cohort of persons 65 years old or older demonstrated that adding a dose of PCV13 to the current PPSV23 recommendations, would lead to additional health benefits. This strategy would prevent an estimated 230 cases of IPD and approximately 12,000 cases of community-acquired pneumonia over the lifetime of a single cohort of persons 65 years old, assuming current indirect effects from the child immunization program and PPSV23 vaccination coverage among adults 65 years old or older (approximately 60%). In a setting of fully realized indirect effects assuming the same vaccination coverage, the expected benefits of PCV13 use among this cohort will likely decline to an estimated 160 cases of IPV and 4,500 cases of community-acquired pneumonia averted among persons 65 years old or older.

In December 2011 the Food and Drug Administration approved PCV13 as a single dose for the prevention of pneumonia and invasive disease caused by vaccine serotypes of *S. pneumoniae* in persons 50 years of age and older. Licensure was based on serological studies comparing immune response of PCV13 recipients to a response following a dose of PPSV23. In two randomized, multicenter immunogenicity studies conducted in the United States and Europe, immunocompetent adults aged 50 years and older received a single dose of PCV13 or PPSV23. In adults age 60 through 64 years and age 70 years and older, PCV13 elicited opsonophagocytic activity (OPA) geometric mean antibody titers (GMTs) that were comperable with, or higher than, responses elicited by PPSV23. Persons who received PPSV23 as the initial study dose had lower opsonophago-

17

Pneumococcal Disease

cytic antibody responses after subsequent administration of a PCV13 dose 1 year later than those who had received PCV13 as the initial dose. Approximately, 20%–25% of IPD cases and 10% of community-acquired pneumonia cases in adults aged ≥65 years are caused by PCV13 serotypes and are potentially preventable with the use of PCV13 in this population.

Immunogenicity and Vaccine Efficacy

Pneumococcal Polysaccharide Vaccine

More than 80% of healthy adults who receive PPSV23 develop antibodies against the serotypes contained in the vaccine, usually within 2 to 3 weeks after vaccination. Older adults, and persons with some chronic illnesses or immunodeficiency may not respond as well, if at all. In children younger than 2 years of age, antibody response to PPSV23 is generally poor. Elevated antibody levels persist for at least 5 years in healthy adults but decline more quickly in persons with certain underlying illnesses.

PPSV23 vaccine efficacy studies have resulted in various estimates of clinical effectiveness. Overall, the vaccine is 60%–70% effective in preventing invasive disease caused by serotypes included in the vaccine. Despite the vaccine's reduced effectiveness among immunocompromised persons, PPSV23 is still recommended for such persons because they are at high risk of developing severe disease. There is no consensus regarding the ability of PPSV23 to prevent non-bacteremic pneumococcal pneumonia. For this reason, providers should avoid referring to PPSV23 as "pneumonia vaccine".

Studies comparing patterns of pneumococcal carriage before and after PPSV23 vaccination have not shown clinically significant decreases in carrier rates among vaccinees. In addition, no population-level change in the distribution of vaccine-type and non–vaccine-type organisms causing invasive disease has been observed despite modest increases in PPSV23 coverage among adults.

Pneumococcal Conjugate Vaccine

In a large clinical trial, PCV7 was shown to reduce invasive disease caused by vaccine serotypes by 97%. Children who received PCV7 had 20% fewer episodes of chest X-ray confirmed pneumonia, 7% fewer episodes of acute otitis media and underwent 20% fewer tympanostomy tube placements than did unvaccinated children. There is evidence that PCV7 reduces nasopharyngeal carriage, among children, of pneumococcal serotypes included in the vaccine.

PCV13 was licensed in the United States based upon studies that compared the serologic response of children who

---

Pneumococcal Polysaccharide Vaccine

- Purified pneumococcal polysaccharide (23 types)
- Not effective in children younger than 2 years
- 60%–70% against invasive disease
- Less effective in preventing pneumococcal pneumonia

Pneumococcal Conjugate Vaccine

- More than 90% effective against invasive disease caused by vaccine serotypes in children
- 45% effective against vaccine-type non-bacteremic pneumococcal pneumonia in adults older than 65 years
- 75% effective against vaccine-type invasive disease in adults older than 65 years

received PCV13 to those who received PCV7. These studies showed that PCV13 induced levels of antibodies that were comparable to those induced by PCV7 and shown to be protective against invasive disease.

In another study of PCV13, children 7-11 months, 12-23 months, and 24-71 months of age who had not received pneumococcal conjugate vaccine doses previously were administered 1, 2, or 3 doses of PCV13 according to age-appropriate immunization schedules. These schedules resulted in antibody responses to each of the 13 serotypes that were comparable to those achieved after the 3-dose infant PCV13 series in the U.S. immunogenicity trial, except for serotype 1, for which IgG geometric mean concentration (GMC) was lower among children aged 24-71 months.

A randomized placebo-controlled trial (CAPiTA trial) was conducted in the Netherlands among approximately 85,000 adults 65 years old or older during 2008-2013 to evaluate the clinical benefit of PCV13 in the prevention of pneumococcal pneumonia. The results of the CAPiTA trial demonstrated 45.6% efficacy of PCV13 against vaccine-type pneumococcal pneumonia, 45.0% efficacy against vaccine-type nonbacteremic pneumococcal pneumonia and 75.0% efficacy of PCV13 against vaccine-type invasive pneumococcal disease (IPD).

Vaccination Schedule and Use
Pneumococcal Conjugate Vaccine

All children 2 through 59 months of age should be routinely vaccinated with PCV13. The primary series beginning in infancy consists of three doses routinely given at 2, 4, and 6 months of age. The first dose can be administered as early as 6 weeks of age. A fourth (booster) dose is recommended at 12–15 months of age. PCV13 should be administered at the same time as other routine childhood immunizations, using a separate syringe and injection site. For children vaccinated at younger than 12 months of age, the minimum interval between doses is 4 weeks. Doses given at 12 months of age and older should be separated by at least 8 weeks. A PCV schedule begun with PCV7 should be completed with PCV13.

A detailed PCV13 vaccination schedule by age and number of previous doses is available in the December 2010 PCV13 ACIP statement.

Unvaccinated children 7 months of age and older do not require a full series of four doses. The number of doses a child needs to complete the series depends on the child's current age and the age at which the first dose of PCV13

Pneumococcal Conjugate Vaccine Recommendations

- Routine vaccination of children 2 through 59 months of age

- Doses at 2, 4, 6, months of age, booster dose at 12–15 months of age

- First dose as early as 6 weeks

- Unvaccinated children 7 months of age or older require fewer doses

- Adults 65 years old and older

Pneumococcal Conjugate Vaccine Schedule for Unvaccinated Older Children-Primary Series

Age at first dose	# of Doses	Booster
7–11 months	2 doses	Yes
12–23 months	2 doses*	No
24–59 months, healthy	1 dose	No
24–71months, medical conditions**	2 doses*	No

*separated by at least 8 weeks *MMWR* 2010;59(RR-11):1–19

** chronic heart, lung disease, diabetes, CSF leak, cochlear implant, sickle-cell disease, other hemoglobinopathies, functional or anatomic asplenia, HIV infection, immunocompromising conditions

17

was received. Unvaccinated children aged 7 through 11 months should receive two doses of vaccine at least 4 weeks apart, followed by a booster dose at age 12 through 15 months. Unvaccinated children aged 12 through 23 months should receive two doses of vaccine, at least 8 weeks apart. Previously unvaccinated healthy children 24 through 59 months of age should receive a single dose of PCV13.

Unvaccinated children 24 through 71 months of age with certain chronic medical conditions should receive 2 doses of PCV13 separated by at least 8 weeks. These conditions include chronic heart and lung disease, diabetes, CSF leak, cochlear implant, sickle cell disease and other hemoglobin-opathies, functional or anatomic asplenia, HIV infection, or immunocompromising conditions resulting from disease or treatment of a disease.

A single supplemental dose of PCV13 is recommended for all children 14 through 59 months of age who have received 4 doses of PCV7 or another age-appropriate, complete PCV7 schedule. For children who have an underlying medical condition, a single supplemental PCV13 dose is recommended through 71 months. This includes children who have received PPSV23 previously. PCV13 should be administered at least 8 weeks after the most recent dose of PCV7 or PPSV23. This will constitute the final dose of PCV for these children.

A single dose of PCV13 should be administered for children 6 through 18 years of age who have not received PCV13 previously and are at increased risk for invasive pneumo-coccal disease because of anatomic or functional asplenia (including sickle cell disease), immunocompromising conditions such as HIV-infection, cochlear implant, or cerebrospinal fluid leaks, regardless of whether they have previously received PCV7 or PPSV23. Routine use of PCV13 is not recommended for healthy children 5 years of age or older.

Children who have received PPSV23 previously also should receive the recommended PCV13 doses. Children 24 through 71 months of age with an underlying medical condition who received fewer than 3 doses of PCV7 before age 24 months should receive a series of 2 doses of PCV13 followed by 1 dose of PPSV23 administered at least 8 weeks later. Children 24 through 71 months of age with an underlying medical condition who received any incomplete schedule of 3 doses of PCV7 before age 24 months should receive 1 dose of PCV13 followed by 1 dose of PPSV23 administered at least 8 weeks later. When elective splenectomy, immunocompromising therapy, or cochlear implant placement is being planned, PCV13 and/or PPSV23 vaccination should be completed at least 2 weeks before surgery or initiation of therapy.

Pneumococcal Conjugate Vaccine High-risk Schedule — Children 6 years through 18 years

- Single dose if no dose of PCV13 received previously
- Anatomic asplenia (including sickle-cell disease)
- Immunocompromising conditions (e.g. HIV infection)
- Cochlear implant
- Cerebrospinal fluid leak

Pneumococcal Conjugate Vaccine for Persons 65 Years Old and Older

- For those who have not received PCV13 previously, administer a dose of PCV13
- A dose of PPSV23 should be administered 6-12 months after the dose of PCV13
- Do not administer the two vaccines simultaneously
- Adults who previously received a dose of PPSV23 should receive PCV13 no earlier than 1 year after the dose of PPSV23

17

Adults 65 years old or older who have not previously received pneumococcal vaccine or whose previous vaccination history is unknown should received a dose of PCV13. A dose of PPSV23 should be given 6-12 months after the dose of PCV13. If PPSV23 cannot be given during this time window, the dose of PPSV23 should be given during the next visit after 12 months. The two vaccines should not be administered simultaneously (the same clinic day) and the minimum acceptable interval between PCV13 and PPSV23 is 8 weeks.

Adults 65 years old or older who have previously received one or more doses of PPSV23 should receive a dose of PCV13 if they have not received it. A dose of PCV13 should be given one or more years after receipt of the most recent PPSV23 dose. For those for whom an additional dose of PPSV23 is indicated, this subsequent PPSV23 dose should be given 6 -12 months after PCV13 and five or more years after the most recent dose of PPSV23. Only one dose of PPSV23 is recommended on or after the 65th birthday.

The recommendations for routine use of PCV13 among adults 65 years old or older will be reevaluated in 2018 and revised as needed.

In June 2012, ACIP recommended vaccination of adults with specific risk factors. All PCV13-naïve adults 19 years and older with functional or anatomic asplenia (e.g., from sickle cell disease or splenectomy), HIV infection, leukemia, lymphoma, Hodgkin disease, multiple myeloma, generalized malignancy, chronic renal failure, nephrotic syndrome, or other conditions associated with immunosuppression (e.g., organ or bone marrow transplantation) and those receiving immunosuppressive chemotherapy, including long-term corticosteroids, or those with CSF leak or cochlear implants, should receive a dose of PCV13 vaccine. PCV13 should be administered to eligible adults with one of these risk factors prior to PPSV23, the vaccine recommended for these groups of adults since 1997. Eligible adults with one of these risk factors who have not previously received PPSV23 should receive a dose of PCV13 first followed by a dose of PPSV23 at least 8 weeks later. Subsequent doses of PPSV23 should follow PPSV23 recommendations for these adults. Adults 19 years of age or older with the aforementioned conditions who have previously received one or more doses of PPSV23 should be given a dose of PCV13 one or more years after the last PPSV23 dose was received. For those who require additional doses of PPSV23, the first such dose should be given no sooner than 8 weeks after PCV13 and at least 5 years since the most recent dose of PPSV23.

Providers should not withhold vaccination in the absence of an immunization record or complete record. The patient's

Pneumococcal Conjugate Vaccine High-risk Schedule – Adults 19 through 64 years old

- Anatomic asplenia (including sickle-cell disease)
- Immunocompromising conditions (e.g. HIV infection)
- Cochlear implant
- Cerebrospinal fluid leak
- PPSV23 should also be recommended, if not received previously
- PCV13 administered first followed by a dose of PPSV23 8 weeks later

17

Pneumococcal Disease

Pneumococcal Polysaccharide Vaccine Recommendations

- Adults 65 years and older
- Persons 2 years ~~and older with~~ 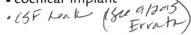 *through 64 see Errata 9/2015*
  - chronic illness
  - anatomic or functional asplenia
  - immunocompromised (disease, chemotherapy, steroids)
  - HIV infection
  - environments or settings with increased risk
  - cochlear implant
  - *CSF Leak (see 9/2015 Errata)*

Pneumococcal Polysaccharide Vaccine Revaccination — High-risk Immunocompetent Persons

- Routine revaccination of immunocompetent persons is not recommended
- Revaccination recommended for immunocompetent persons 2 years of age or older who are at high risk of serious pneumococcal infection
  - chronic heart disease
  - pulmonary disease (including asthma, 19 years and older)
  - liver disease
  - alcoholism
  - CSF leaks
  - cochlear implants
  - those who smoke cigarettes (19 years and older)
- Single revaccination dose at least 5 years after the first dose and after the 65th birthday

verbal history may be used to determine vaccination status. Persons with uncertain or unknown vaccination status should be vaccinated.

The target groups for pneumococcal vaccines (polysaccharide or conjugate) and influenza vaccine overlap. Both pneumococcal vaccines can be given at the same time as influenza vaccine but at different sites if indicated. Pneumococcal polysaccharide vaccine should never be given during the same visit as pneumococcal conjugate vaccine. Most adults need only a single lifetime dose of each PCV13 and PPSV23 (see Revaccination).

Pneumococcal Polysaccharide Vaccine

Pneumococcal polysaccharide vaccine should be administered routinely to all adults 65 years of age and older, regardless of previous PCV receipt. A single dose of the vaccine is also indicated for immunocompetent persons 2 years of age and older with a normal immune system who have a chronic illness, including cardiovascular disease, pulmonary disease, diabetes, alcoholism, chronic liver disease, cirrhosis, cerebrospinal fluid leak, or a cochlear implant.

Immunocompromised persons 2 years of age and older who are at highest risk of pneumococcal disease or its complications should also be vaccinated. This group includes persons with splenic dysfunction or absence (either from disease or surgical removal), Hodgkin disease, lymphoma, multiple myeloma, chronic renal failure, nephrotic syndrome (a type of kidney disease), asymptomatic or symptomatic HIV infection, or conditions such as organ transplantation associated with immunosuppression. Persons immunosuppressed from chemotherapy or high-dose corticosteroid therapy (14 days or longer) should be vaccinated. Pneumococcal vaccine should be considered for persons living in special environments or social settings with an identified increased risk of pneumococcal disease or its complications, such as certain Native American (i.e., Alaska Native, Navajo, and Apache) populations.

In 2010 ACIP added asthma and cigarette smoking to the list of indications for receipt of PPSV23 due to increased risk of invasive pneumococcal disease among these groups. Available data do not support asthma or cigarette smoking as indications for PPSV23 among persons younger than 19 years.

If elective splenectomy or cochlear implant is being considered, the vaccine should be given at least 2 weeks before the procedure. If vaccination prior to the procedure is not feasible, the vaccine should be given as soon as possible after surgery. Similarly, there should also be a 2-week interval between vaccination and initiation of cancer chemotherapy or other immunosuppressive therapy, if possible.

Revaccination with PPSV23

Following vaccination with PPSV23, antibody levels decline after 5–10 years and decrease more rapidly in some groups than others. However, the relationship between antibody titer and protection from invasive disease is not certain for adults, so the ability to define the need for revaccination based only on serology is limited. In addition, currently available pneumococcal polysaccharide vaccines elicit a T-cell-independent response, and do not produce a sustained increase ("boost") in antibody titers. Available data do not indicate a substantial increase in antibody level in the majority of revaccinated persons.

For immunocompetent adults 19 through 64 years of age with chronic heart disease, pulmonary disease (including asthma), liver disease, alcoholism, CSF leaks, cochlear implants, or those who smoke cigarettes only one dose of PPSV23 is recommended before the 65th birthday. Additionally those who received a dose of PPSV23 before age 65 years for any indication should receive another dose of the vaccine at age 65 years of later if at least 5 years have elapsed since their previous PPSV23 dose.

A second PPSV23 dose is recommended 5 years after the first PPSV23 dose for persons aged 19-64 years with functional or anatomic asplenia (e.g. from sickle cell disease or splenectomy) and for persons with immunocompromising conditions such as HIV infection, leukemia, lymphoma, Hodgkin disease, multiple myeloma, generalized malignancy, chronic renal failure, nephrotic syndrome, or other conditions associated with immunosuppression (e.g., organ or bone marrow transplantation) and those receiving immuno-suppressive chemotherapy, including long-term cortico-steroids. The above group includes the same conditions as those that are adult indications for PCV13, with the exception of CSF leak and cochlear implants. Persons with CSF leaks or cochlear implants should receive no additional doses of PPSV23 until age 65 years. Additionally, those who received 1 or 2 doses of PPSV23 before age 65 years for any indication should receive another dose of the vaccine at age 65 years or later if at least 5 years have elapsed since their previous PPSV23 dose.

Contraindications and Precautions to Vaccination

For both pneumococcal polysaccharide and conjugate vaccines, a severe allergic reaction (anaphylaxis) to a vaccine component or following a prior dose is a contraindication

---

Pneumococcal Polysaccharide Vaccine Revaccination — Highest-risk Persons

- Persons 2 years of age or older with:
  - functional or anatomic asplenia
  - immunosuppression
  - transplant
  - chronic renal failure
  - nephrotic syndrome
  - A revaccination dose 5 years after the first dose
  - For those who receive 2nd dose prior to the 65th birthday, a third dose is recommended after the 65th birthday (and at least 5 years from the second dose)

17

Pneumococcal Vaccines Contraindications and Precautions

- Severe allergic reaction to vaccine component or following prior dose of vaccine
- Moderate or severe acute illness

Pneumococcal Disease

> ## Pneumococcal Conjugate Vaccine Adverse Events
>
> - Events reported after PCV7 include
> - apnea
> - hypersensitivity reactions
> - dyspnea
> - bronchospasm
> - anaphylactic/anaphylactoid reactions
> - angioneurotic edema
> - erythema multiforme
> - injection site reactions
>
> ## Pneumococcal Vaccines Adverse Reactions
>
> - Local reactions
>   - polysaccharide
>   - 30%–50%
>   - conjugate
>   - 5%–49%
> - Fever, myalgia
>   - polysaccharide
>   - <1%
>   - conjugate
>   - 24%–35%
> - Febrile seizures
>   - conjugate
>   - 1.2–13.7/100,000
>   - conjugate (with TIV)
>   - 4–44.9/100,000
> - Severe adverse reactions
>   - polysaccharide
>   - rare
>   - conjugate
>   - 8%

to further doses of vaccine. Such allergic reactions are rare. Persons with moderate or severe acute illness should not be vaccinated until their condition improves. However, minor illnesses, such as upper respiratory infections, are not a contraindication to vaccination.

The safety of PPSV23 vaccine for pregnant women has not been studied, although no adverse consequences have been reported among newborns whose mothers were inadvertently vaccinated during pregnancy. Women who are at high risk of pneumococcal disease and who are candidates for pneumococcal vaccine should be vaccinated before pregnancy, if possible.

Adverse Events Following Vaccination
Pneumococcal Conjugate Vaccine

Certain rare adverse events observed during PCV7 postmarketing surveillance included, apnea, hypersensitivity reaction including facial edema, dyspnea, bronchospasm, anaphylactic/anaphylactoid reaction including shock, angioneurotic edema, erythema multiforme, injection-site dermatitis, injection-site pruritus, injection-site urticaria, and lymphadenopathy localized to the region of the injection site. The causal relation of these events to vaccination is unknown.

Adverse Reactions Following Vaccination
Pneumococcal Polysaccharide Vaccine

The most common adverse events following either pneumococcal polysaccharide or conjugate vaccine are local reactions. For PPSV23, 30%–50% of vaccinees report pain, swelling, or erythema at the site of injection. These reactions usually persist for less than 48 hours.

Local reactions are reported more frequently following a second dose of PPSV23 vaccine than following the first dose. Moderate systemic reactions (such as fever and myalgia) are not common (fewer than 1% of vaccinees), and more severe systemic adverse reactions are rare.

A transient increase in HIV replication has been reported following PPSV23 vaccine. No clinical or immunologic deterioration has been reported in these persons.

Pneumococcal Conjugate Vaccine

Local reactions (such as pain, swelling or redness) following PCV13 occur in up to half of recipients. Approximately 8% of local reactions are considered to be severe (e.g., tenderness that interferes with limb movement). Local reactions are generally more common with the fourth dose than with the first three doses. In clinical trials of pneumococcal conjugate vaccine, fever (higher than 100.4°F [38°C]) within 7 days of any dose of the primary series was reported for 24%-35% of children. High fever was reported in less than 1% of vaccine recipients. Nonspecific symptoms such as decreased appetite or irritability were reported in up to 80% of recipients.

A study of 200,000 children 6 months through 4 years of age, conducted through the Vaccine Safety Datalink in 2010-2011, found that febrile seizures occurred in some children following receipt of inactivated influenza and PCV13 vaccines. Among children 6-59 months of age, the incidence rate ratio (IRR) for trivalent influenza vaccine (TIV) adjusted for concomitant PCV13 was 2.4 (95% CI, 1.2, 4.7) while the IRR for PCV13 adjusted for concomitant TIV was 2.5 (95% CI 1.3, 4.7); the IRR for concomitant TIV and PCV13 was 5.9 (95% CI 3.1, 11.3). Risk difference estimates varied by age due to the varying baseline risk for seizures in young children, with the highest estimates occurring at 16 months (12.5 per 100,000 doses for TIV without concomitant PCV13, 13.7 per 100,000 doses for PCV13 without concomitant TIV, and 44.9 per 100,000 doses for concomitant TIV and PCV13) and the lowest estimates occurring at 59 months (1.1 per 100,000 doses for TIV without concomitant PCV13, 1.2 per 100,000 doses for PCV13 without concomitant TIV, and 4.0 per 100,000 doses for concomitant TIV and PCV13). After evaluating the data on febrile seizures and taking into consideration benefits and risks of vaccination, ACIP made no change in its recommendations for use of TIV or PCV13.

Vaccine Storage and Handling

PCV13 and PPSV23 should be maintained at refrigerator temperature between 35°F and 46°F (2°C and 8°C). Manufacturer package inserts contain additional information and can be found at http://www.fda.gov/BiologicsBloodVaccines/Vaccines/ApprovedProducts/ucm093830.htm. For complete information on best practices and recommendations please refer to CDC's Vaccine Storage and Handling Toolkit, http://www.cdc.gov/vaccines/recs/storage/toolkit/storage-handling-toolkit.pdf.

Goals and Coverage Levels

The *Healthy People 2020* goal is to achieve at least 90% coverage for pneumococcal polysaccharide vaccine among persons 65 years of age and older. Data from the 2005 Behavioral Risk Factor Surveillance System (BRFSS, a population-based, random-digit-dialed telephone survey of the noninstitutionalized U.S. population 18 years of age and older) estimate that 64% of persons 65 years of age or older

17

Pneumococcal Polysaccharide Vaccine Coverage

- Healthy People 2020 goal: 90% coverage for persons 65 years of age or older

- 2005 BRFSS: 64% of persons 65 years of age or older ever vaccinated

- Vaccination coverage levels were lower among persons 18-64 years of age with a chronic illness

Pneumococcal Polysaccharide Vaccine Missed Opportunities

- >65% of patients with severe pneumococcal disease had been hospitalized within preceding 3–5 years yet few had received vaccine had ever received pneumococcal polysaccharide. Vaccination coverage levels were lower among persons 18–64 years of age with a chronic illness.

Opportunities to vaccinate high-risk persons are missed both at the time of hospital discharge and during visits to clinicians' offices. Effective programs for vaccine delivery are needed, including offering the vaccine in hospitals at discharge and in clinicians' offices, nursing homes, and other long-term care facilities.

More than 65% of the persons who have been hospitalized with severe pneumococcal disease had been admitted to a hospital in the preceding 3–5 years, yet few had received pneumococcal vaccine. In addition, persons who frequently visit physicians and who have chronic conditions are more likely to be at high risk of pneumococcal infection than those who require infrequent visits. Screening and subsequent immunization of hospitalized persons found to be at high risk could have a significant impact on reducing complications and death associated with pneumococcal disease.

Acknowledgment

The editors thank Dr. Matthew Moore and Tamara Pilishvilli, CDC for their assistance in updating this chapter.

Selected References

Black S, Shinefield HR, Fireman B, et al. Efficacy, safety and immunogenicity of heptavalent pneumococcal conjugate vaccine in children. *Pediatr Infect Dis J* 2000;19:187–95.

CDC. Active Bacterial Core surveillance. Available at http://www.cdc.gov/ncidod/dbmd/abcs/.

CDC. Prevention of pneumococcal disease among infants and children - use of 13-valent pneumococcal conjugate vaccine and 23-valent pneumococcal polysaccharide vaccine. Recommendations of the Advisory Committee on Immunization Practices (ACIP). *MMWR* 2010;59(No. RR-11):1–1.

CDC. Updated recommendations for prevention of invasive pneumococcal disease among adults using the 23-valent pneumococcal polysaccharide vaccine (PPSV23). *MMWR* 2010;59(No.34):1102–6.

CDC. Invasive pneumococcal disease in young children before licensure of 13-valent pneumococcal conjugate vaccine — United States, 2007. *MMWR* 2010;59(No. 9):253–7.

17

Jackson LA, Benson P, Sneller VP, et al. Safety of revaccination with pneumococcal polysaccharide vaccine. *JAMA* 1999;281:243–8.

Pilishvili T, Lexau C, Farley MM, et al. Sustained reductions in invasive pneumococcal disease in the era of conjugate vaccine. *J Infect Dis* 2010;201:32–41.

Robinson KA, Baughman W, Rothrock G. Epidemiology of invasive Streptococcus pneumoniae infections in the United States, 1995–1998. Opportunities for prevention in the conjugate vaccine era. *JAMA* 2001;285:1729–35.

Tomczyk S, Bennett N, Stoecker C, et. Al. Use of 13-valent pneumococcal conjugate vaccine and 23-valent pneumococcal polysaccharide vaccine among adults aged ≥ 65 years: Recommendations of the Advisory Committee on Immunization Practices (ACIP). *MMWR* 2014; 63:822–825.

Tsai CJ, Griffin MR, Nuorti JP et al. Changing epidemiology of pneumococcal meningitis after the introduction of pneumococcal conjugate vaccine in the United States. *Clin Infect Dis* 2008;46:1664–72.

Whitney CG. The potential of pneumococcal conjugate vaccines for children. *Pediatr Infect Dis J* 2002;21:961–70.

Whitney CG, Shaffner W, Butler JC. Rethinking recommendations for use of pneumococcal vaccines in adults. *Clin Infect Dis* 2001;33:662–75.

Whitney CG. Impact of conjugate pneumococcal vaccines. *Pediatr Infect Dis J* 2005;24:729–30.

Alison Tse , Hung Fu Tseng , et al. Signal identification and evaluation for risk of febrile seizures in children following trivalent inactivated influenza vaccine in the Vaccine Safety Datalink Project, 2010–2011. *Vaccine*. 2012 Mar 2;30(11):2024–31.

17

Pneumococcal Disease

The words polio (grey) and myelon (marrow, indicating the spinal cord) are derived from the Greek. It is the effect of poliomyelitis virus on the spinal cord that leads to the classic manifestation of paralysis.

Records from antiquity mention crippling diseases compatible with poliomyelitis. Michael Underwood first described a debility of the lower extremities in children that was recognizable as poliomyelitis in England in 1789. The first outbreaks in Europe were reported in the early 19th century, and outbreaks were first reported in the United States in 1843. For the next hundred years, epidemics of polio were reported from developed countries in the Northern Hemisphere each summer and fall. These epidemics became increasingly severe, and the average age of persons affected rose. The increasingly older age of persons with primary infection increased both the disease severity and number of deaths from polio. Polio reached a peak in the United States in 1952, with more than 21,000 paralytic cases. However, following introduction of effective vaccines, polio incidence declined rapidly. The last case of wild-virus polio acquired in the United States was in 1979, and global polio eradication may be achieved within this decade.

> **Poliomyelitis**
> - First described by Michael Underwood in 1789
> - First outbreak described in U.S. in 1843
> - More than 21,000 paralytic cases reported in the U. S. in 1952
> - Global eradication within this decade

Poliovirus

Poliovirus is a member of the enterovirus subgroup, family Picornaviridae. Enteroviruses are transient inhabitants of the gastrointestinal tract, and are stable at acid pH. Picornaviruses are small, ether-insensitive viruses with an RNA genome.

There are three poliovirus serotypes (P1, P2, and P3). There is minimal heterotypic immunity between the three serotypes. That is, immunity to one serotype does not produce significant immunity to the other serotypes.

The poliovirus is rapidly inactivated by heat, formaldehyde, chlorine, and ultraviolet light.

> **Poliovirus**
> - Enterovirus (RNA)
> - Three serotypes: 1, 2, 3
> - Minimal heterotypic immunity between serotypes
> - Rapidly inactivated by heat, formaldehyde, chlorine, ultraviolet light

18

Pathogenesis

The virus enters through the mouth, and primary multiplication of the virus occurs at the site of implantation in the pharynx and gastrointestinal tract. The virus is usually present in the throat and in the stool before the onset of illness. One week after onset there is less virus in the throat, but virus continues to be excreted in the stool for several weeks. The virus invades local lymphoid tissue, enters the bloodstream, and then may infect cells of the central nervous system. Replication of poliovirus in motor neurons of the anterior horn and brain stem results in cell destruction and causes the typical manifestations of poliomyelitis.

> **Poliomyelitis Pathogenesis**
> - Entry into mouth
> - Replication in pharynx, GI tract
> - Hematologic spread to lymphatics and central nervous system
> - Viral spread along nerve fibers
> - Destruction of motor neurons

Poliomyelitis

Clinical Features

The incubation period for nonparalytic poliomyelitis is 3-6 days. For the onset of paralysis in paralytic poliomyelitis, the incubation period usually is 7 to 21 days.

The response to poliovirus infection is highly variable and has been categorized on the basis of the severity of clinical presentation.

Up to 72% of all polio infections in children are asymptomatic. Infected persons without symptoms shed virus in the stool and are able to transmit the virus to others.

Approximately 24% of polio infections in children consist of a minor, nonspecific illness without clinical or laboratory evidence of central nervous system invasion. This clinical presentation is known as abortive poliomyelitis, and is characterized by complete recovery in less than a week. This is characterized by a low grade fever and sore throat.

Nonparalytic aseptic meningitis (symptoms of stiffness of the neck, back, and/or legs), usually following several days after a prodrome similar to that of minor illness, occurs in 1%–5% of polio infections in children. Increased or abnormal sensations can also occur. Typically these symptoms will last from 2 to 10 days, followed by complete recovery.

Fewer than 1% of all polio infections in children result in flaccid paralysis. Paralytic symptoms generally begin 1 to 18 days after prodromal symptoms and progress for 2 to 3 days. Generally, no further paralysis occurs after the temperature returns to normal. The prodrome may be biphasic, especially in children, with initial minor symptoms separated by a 1- to 7-day period from more major symptoms. Additional prodromal signs and symptoms can include a loss of superficial reflexes, initially increased deep tendon reflexes and severe muscle aches and spasms in the limbs or back. The illness progresses to flaccid paralysis with diminished deep tendon reflexes, reaches a plateau without change for days to weeks, and is usually asymmetrical. Strength then begins to return. Patients do not experience sensory losses or changes in cognition.

Many persons with paralytic poliomyelitis recover completely and, in most, muscle function returns to some degree. Weakness or paralysis still present 12 months after onset is usually permanent.

Paralytic polio is classified into three types, depending on the level of involvement. Spinal polio is most common, and during 1969–1979, accounted for 79% of paralytic cases. It is characterized by asymmetric paralysis that most often involves the legs. Bulbar polio leads to weakness of muscles

Outcomes of Poliovirus Infection

Legend: Asymptomatic, Minor non-CNS illness, Aseptic menigitis, Paralytic

Percent (0, 20, 40, 60, 80, 100)

18

innervated by cranial nerves and accounted for 2% of cases during this period. Bulbospinal polio, a combination of bulbar and spinal paralysis, accounted for 19% of cases.

The death-to-case ratio for paralytic polio is generally 2%–5% among children and up to 15%–30% for adults (depending on age). It increases to 25%–75% with bulbar involvement.

Laboratory Testing
Viral Isolation

Poliovirus may be recovered from the stool, is less likely recovered from the pharynx, and only rarely recovered from cerebrospinal fluid (CSF) or blood. If poliovirus is isolated from a person with acute flaccid paralysis, it must be tested further, using reverse transcriptase - polymerase chain reaction (RT-PCR) or genomic sequencing, to determine if the virus is "wild type" (that is, the virus that causes polio disease) or vaccine type (virus that could derive from a vaccine strain).

Serology

Serology may be helpful in establishing a diagnosis of disease if obtained early in the course of disease. Two specimens are needed, one early in the course of the illness and another three weeks later. A four-fold rise in the titer suggests poliovirus infection. Two specimens in which no antibody is detected may rule out poliovirus infection. There are limitations to antibody titers. Patients who are immunocompromised may have two titers with no antibody detected and still be infected with poliovirus. For any patient, neutralizing antibodies appear early and may be at high levels by the time the patient is hospitalized; therefore, a four-fold rise in antibody titer may not be demonstrated. Someone who has been vaccinated and does not have poliovirus infection may have a specimen with detectable antibody from the vaccine.

Cerebrospinal Fluid (CSF)

In poliovirus infection, the CSF usually contains an increased number of white blood cells (10–200 cells/mm^3, primarily lymphocytes) and a mildly elevated protein (40–50 mg/100 mL).

Epidemiology
Occurrence

At one time poliovirus infection occurred throughout the world. Transmission of wild poliovirus was interrupted in the United States in 1979 or possibly earlier. A polio eradication program conducted by the Pan American Health

18

Poliovirus Epidemiology
- Reservoir
  - human
- Transmission
  - fecal-oral
  - oral-oral possible
- Communicability
  - most infectious 7-10 days before and after onset of symptoms
  - virus present in stool 3-6 weeks

Poliomyelitis

Organization led to elimination of polio in the Western Hemisphere in 1991. The Global Polio Eradication Program has dramatically reduced poliovirus transmission throughout the world. In 2012, only 223 confirmed cases of polio were reported globally and polio was endemic only in three countries.

Reservoir

Humans are the only known reservoir of poliovirus, which is transmitted most frequently by persons with inapparent infections. There is no asymptomatic carrier state except in immune deficient persons.

Transmission

Person-to-person spread of poliovirus via the fecal-oral route is the most important route of transmission, although the oral-oral route is possible.

Temporal Pattern

Poliovirus infection typically peaks in the summer months in temperate climates. There is no seasonal pattern in tropical climates.

Communicability

Poliovirus is highly infectious, with seroconversion rates among susceptible household contacts of children nearly 100%, and greater than 90% among susceptible household contacts of adults. Persons infected with poliovirus are most infectious from 7 to 10 days before and after the onset of symptoms, but poliovirus may be present in the stool from 3 to 6 weeks.

Secular Trends in the United States

Before the 18th century, polioviruses probably circulated widely. Initial infections with at least one type probably occurred in early infancy, when transplacentally acquired maternal antibodies were high. Exposure throughout life probably provided continual boosting of immunity, and paralytic infections were probably rare. (This view has been challenged based on data from lameness studies in developing countries).

In the immediate prevaccine era, improved sanitation allowed less frequent exposure and increased the age of primary infection. Boosting of immunity from natural exposure became more infrequent and the number of susceptible persons accumulated, ultimately resulting in the occurrence of epidemics, with 13,000 to 20,000 paralytic cases reported annually.

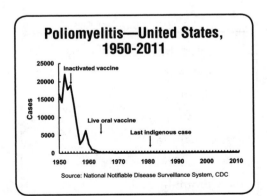

Poliomyelitis—United States, 1950-2011

Source: National Notifiable Disease Surveillance System, CDC

In the early vaccine era, the incidence dramatically decreased after the introduction of inactivated polio vaccine (IPV) in 1955. The decline continued following oral polio vaccine (OPV) introduction in 1961. In 1960, a total of 2,525 paralytic cases were reported, compared with 61 in 1965.

The last cases of paralytic poliomyelitis caused by endemic transmission of wild virus in the United States were in 1979, when an outbreak occurred among the Amish in several Midwest states. The virus was imported from the Netherlands.

From 1980 through 1999, a total of 162 confirmed cases of paralytic poliomyelitis were reported, an average of 8 cases per year. Six cases were acquired outside the United States and imported. The last imported case was reported in 1993. Two cases were classified as indeterminant (no poliovirus isolated from samples obtained from the patients, and patients had no history of recent vaccination or direct contact with a vaccine recipient). The remaining 154 (95%) cases were vaccine-associated paralytic polio (VAPP) caused by live oral polio vaccine.

In order to eliminate VAPP from the United States, ACIP recommended in 2000 that IPV be used exclusively in the United States. The last case of VAPP acquired in the United States was reported in 1999. In 2005, an unvaccinated U.S. resident was infected with polio vaccine virus in Costa Rica and subsequently developed VAPP. A second case of VAPP from vaccine-derived poliovirus in a person with long-standing combined immunodeficiency was reported in 2009. The patient was probably infected approximately 12 years prior to the onset of paralysis. Also in 2005, several asymptomatic infections with a vaccine-derived poliovirus were detected in unvaccinated children in Minnesota. The source of the vaccine virus has not been determined, but it appeared to have been circulating among humans for at least 2 years based on genetic changes in the virus. No VAPP has been reported from this virus.

Poliovirus Vaccines

Inactivated poliovirus vaccine (IPV) was licensed in 1955 and was used extensively from that time until the early 1960s. In 1961, type 1 and 2 monovalent oral poliovirus vaccine (MOPV) was licensed, and in 1962, type 3 MOPV was licensed. In 1963, trivalent OPV was licensed and largely replaced IPV use. Trivalent OPV was the vaccine of choice in the United States and most other countries of the world after its introduction in 1963. An enhanced-potency IPV was licensed in November 1987 and first became available in 1988. Use of OPV was discontinued in the United States in 2000.

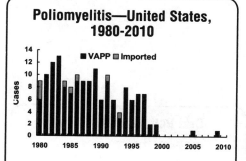

Poliomyelitis—United States, 1980-2010

Poliovirus Vaccine

- **1955**—Inactivated vaccine
- **1961**—Types 1 and 2 monovalent OPV
- **1962**—Type 3 monovalent OPV
- **1963**—Trivalent OPV
- **1987**—Enhanced-potency IPV (IPV)

Inactivated Polio Vaccine (IPV)

- Contains 3 serotypes of vaccine virus
- Grown in monkey kidney (Vero) cells
- Inactivated with formaldehyde
- Contains 2-phenoxyethanol, neomycin, streptomycin, polymyxin B

18

Poliomyelitis

Oral Polio Vaccine (OPV)

- Contains 3 serotypes of vaccine virus
- Grown in monkey kidney (Vero) cells
- Contains neomycin and streptomycin
- Shed in stool for up to 6 weeks following vaccination

IPV Efficacy

- Highly effective in producing immunity to poliovirus
- 90% or more immune after 2 doses
- At least 99% immune after 3 doses
- Duration of immunity not known with certainty

Characteristics

Inactivated poliovirus vaccine

Two enhanced forms of inactivated poliovirus vaccine are currently licensed in the U.S., but only one vaccine (IPOL, sanofi pasteur) is actually distributed. This vaccine contains all three serotypes of polio vaccine virus. For sanofi's single component vaccine the viruses are grown in a type of monkey kidney tissue culture (Vero cell line) and inactivated with formaldehyde. The vaccine contains 2-phenoxyethanol as a preservative, and trace amounts of neomycin, streptomycin, and polymyxin B. It is supplied in a single-dose prefilled syringe and should be administered by either subcutaneous or intramuscular injection. For sanofi's combination DTaP-IPV/Hib vaccine (Pentacel) the IPV component is grown in a human diploid cell line and does not contain 2-phenoxyethanol at preservative level concentrations. GlaxoSmithKline's combination vaccine DTaP-IPV (Kinrix) uses IPV grown in the Vero cell line. Kinrix does not contain any preservative.

Oral poliovirus vaccine (not available in the United States)

Trivalent OPV contains live attenuated strains of all three serotypes of poliovirus in a 10:1:3 ratio. The vaccine viruses are grown in monkey kidney tissue culture (Vero cell line). The vaccine is supplied as a single 0.5-mL dose in a plastic dispenser. The vaccine contains trace amounts of neomycin and streptomycin. OPV does not contain a preservative.

Live attenuated polioviruses replicate in the intestinal mucosa and lymphoid cells and in lymph nodes that drain the intestine. Vaccine viruses are excreted in the stool of the vaccinated person for up to 6 weeks after a dose. Maximum viral shedding occurs in the first 1–2 weeks after vaccination, particularly after the first dose.

Vaccine viruses may spread from the recipient to contacts. Persons coming in contact with fecal material of a vaccinated person may be exposed and infected with vaccine virus.

Immunogenicity and Vaccine Efficacy

Inactivated poliovirus vaccine

IPV is highly effective in producing immunity to poliovirus and protection from paralytic poliomyelitis. Ninety percent or more of vaccine recipients develop protective antibody to all three poliovirus types after two doses, and at least 99% are immune following three doses. Protection against paralytic disease correlates with the presence of antibody.

IPV appears to produce less local gastrointestinal immunity than does OPV, so persons who receive IPV are more readily infected with wild poliovirus than OPV recipients.

The duration of immunity with IPV is not known with certainty, although it probably provides lifelong immunity after a complete series.

Oral poliovirus vaccine

OPV is highly effective in producing immunity to poliovirus. A single dose of OPV produces immunity to all three vaccine viruses in approximately 50% of recipients. Three doses produce immunity to all three poliovirus types in more than 95% of recipients. As with other live-virus vaccines, immunity from oral poliovirus vaccine is probably lifelong. OPV produces excellent intestinal immunity, which helps prevent infection with wild virus.

Serologic studies have shown that seroconversion following three doses of either IPV or OPV is nearly 100% to all three vaccine viruses. However, seroconversion rates after three doses of a combination of IPV and OPV are lower, particularly to type 3 vaccine virus (as low as 85% in one study). A fourth dose (most studies used OPV as the fourth dose) usually produces seroconversion rates similar to three doses of either IPV or OPV.

Vaccination Schedule and Use

Trivalent OPV was the vaccine of choice in the United States (and most other countries of the world) since it was licensed in 1963. The nearly exclusive use of OPV led to elimination of wild-type poliovirus from the United States in less than 20 years. However, one case of VAPP occurred for every 2 to 3 million doses of OPV administered, which resulted in 8 to 10 cases of VAPP each year in the United States (see Adverse Events section for more details on VAPP). From 1980 through 1999, VAPP accounted for 95% of all cases of paralytic poliomyelitis reported in the United States.

In 1996, ACIP recommended an increase in use of IPV through a sequential schedule of IPV followed by OPV. This recommendation was intended to reduce the occurrence of vaccine-associated paralytic polio. The sequential schedule was expected to eliminate VAPP among vaccine recipients by producing humoral immunity to polio vaccine viruses with inactivated polio vaccine prior to exposure to live vaccine virus. Since OPV was still used for the third and fourth doses of the polio vaccination schedule, a risk of VAPP would continue to exist among contacts of vaccinees, who were exposed to live vaccine virus in the stool of vaccine recipients.

OPV Efficacy

- Highly effective in producing immunity to poliovirus
- Approximately 50% immune after 1 dose
- More than 95% immune after 3 doses
- Immunity probably lifelong

Polio Vaccination Recommendations, 1996-1999

- Increased use of IPV (sequential IPV- OPV schedule) recommended in 1996
- Intended to reduce the risk of vaccine-associated paralytic polio (VAPP)
- Continued risk of VAPP for contacts of OPV recipients

Polio Vaccination Recommendations

- Exclusive use of IPV recommended in 2000
- OPV no longer routinely available in the United States
- Indigenous VAPP eliminated

18

Poliomyelitis

Polio Vaccination Schedule

Age	Vaccine	Minimum Interval
2 months	IPV	---
4 months	IPV	4 weeks
6-18 months	IPV	4 weeks
4-6 years	IPV	6 months

Schedules that Include Both IPV and OPV

- Only IPV is available in the United States

- Schedule begun with OPV should be completed with IPV

- Any combination of 4 doses of IPV and OPV by 4-6 years of age constitutes a complete series

The sequential IPV–OPV polio vaccination schedule was widely accepted by both providers and parents. Fewer cases of VAPP were reported in 1998 and 1999, suggesting an impact of the increased use of IPV. However, only the complete discontinuation of use of OPV would lead to complete elimination of VAPP. To further the goal of complete elimination of paralytic polio in the United States, ACIP recommended in July 1999 that inactivated polio vaccine be used exclusively in the United States beginning in 2000. OPV is no longer routinely available in the United States. Exclusive use of IPV eliminated the shedding of live vaccine virus, and eliminated any indigenous VAPP.

A primary series of IPV consists of three doses. In infancy, these primary doses are integrated with the administration of other routinely administered vaccines. The first dose may be given as early as 6 weeks of age but is usually given at 2 months of age, with a second dose at 4 months of age. The third dose should be given at 6–18 months of age. The recommended interval between the primary series doses is 2 months. However, if accelerated protection is needed, the minimum interval between each of the first 3 doses of IPV is 4 weeks.

The final dose in the IPV series should be administered at 4 years of age or older. A dose of IPV on or after age 4 years is recommended regardless of the number of previous doses. The minimum interval from the next-to-last to final dose is 6 months.

When DTaP-IPV/Hib (Pentacel) is used to provide 4 doses at ages 2, 4, 6, and 15-18 months, an additional booster dose of age-appropriate IPV-containing vaccine (IPV or DTaP-IPV [Kinrix]) should be administered at age 4-6 years. This will result in a 5-dose IPV vaccine series, which is considered acceptable by ACIP. DTaP-IPV/Hib is not indicated for the booster dose at 4-6 years of age. ACIP recommends that the minimum interval from dose 4 to dose 5 should be at least 6 months to provide an optimum booster response.

Shorter intervals between doses and beginning the series at a younger age may lead to lower seroconversion rates. Consequently, ACIP recommends the use of the minimum age (6 weeks) and minimum intervals between doses in the first 6 months of life only if the vaccine recipient is at risk for imminent exposure to circulating poliovirus (e.g., during an outbreak or because of travel to a polio-endemic region).

Only IPV is available for routine polio vaccination of children in the United States. A polio vaccination schedule begun with OPV should be completed with IPV. If a child receives both types of vaccine, four doses of any combination of IPV or OPV by 4-6 years of age is considered a complete poliovirus vaccination series. A minimum interval of 4 weeks should separate all doses of the series.

There are three combination vaccines that contain inactivated polio vaccine. Pediarix is produced by GlaxoSmithKline and contains DTaP, hepatitis B and IPV vaccines. Pediarix is licensed for the first 3 doses of the DTaP series among children 6 weeks through 6 years of age. Kinrix is also produced by GSK and contains DTaP and IPV. Kinrix is licensed only for the fifth dose of DTaP and fourth dose of IPV among children 4 through 6 years of age. Pentacel is produced by sanofi pasteur and contains DTaP, Hib and IPV. It is licensed for the first four doses of the component vaccines among children 6 weeks through 4 years of age. Pentacel is not licensed for children 5 years or older. Additional information about these combination vaccines is in the Pertussis chapter of this book.

Polio Vaccination of Adults

Routine vaccination of adults (18 years of age and older) who reside in the United States is not necessary or recommended because most adults are already immune and have a very small risk of exposure to wild poliovirus in the United States.

Some adults, however, are at increased risk of infection with poliovirus. These include travelers to areas where poliomyelitis is endemic or epidemic (see CDC Health Information for International Travel 2014 (the Yellow Book) at http://wwwnc.cdc.gov/travel/page/yellowbook-home-2014/?s_cid=cdc_homepage_topmenu_003 for specific regions), and laboratory workers handling specimens that may contain polioviruses.

Recommendations for poliovirus vaccination of adults in the above categories depend upon the previous vaccination history and the time available before protection is required.

For unvaccinated adults (including adults without a written record of prior polio vaccination) at increased risk of exposure to poliomyelitis, primary immunization with IPV is recommended. The recommended schedule is two doses separated by 1 to 2 months, and a third dose given 6 to 12 months after the second dose. The minimum interval between the second and the third doses is 6 months.

In some circumstances time will not allow completion of this schedule. If 8 weeks or more are available before protection is needed, three doses of IPV should be given at least 4 weeks apart. If 4 to 8 weeks are available before protection is needed, two doses of IPV should be given at least 4 weeks apart. If less than 4 weeks are available before protection is needed, a single dose of IPV is recommended. In all instances, the remaining doses of vaccine should be given later, at the recommended intervals, if the person remains at increased risk.

Combination Vaccines That Contain IPV

- Pediarix
  - DTaP, Hepatitis B and IPV
- Kinrix
  - DTaP and IPV
- Pentacel
  - DTaP, Hib and IPV

Polio Vaccination of Adults

- Routine vaccination of U.S. residents 18 years of age and older not necessary or recommended
- May consider vaccination of travelers to polio-endemic countries and selected laboratory workers

Polio Vaccination of Unvaccinated Adults

- Use standard IPV schedule if possible (0, 1-2 months, 6-12 months)
- May separate first and second doses by 4 weeks if accelerated schedule needed
- The minimum interval between the second and third doses is 6 months

Polio Vaccination of Previously Vaccinated Adults

- Previously complete primary series of three or more doses
  - administer one dose of IPV
- Incomplete series
  - administer remaining doses in series
  - no need to restart series

18

Poliomyelitis

Adults who have previously completed a primary series of 3 or more doses and who are at increased risk of exposure to poliomyelitis should receive one dose of IPV. The need for further supplementary doses has not been established. Only one supplemental dose of polio vaccine is recommended for adults who have received a complete series (i.e., it is not necessary to administer additional doses for subsequent travel to a polio endemic country).

Adults who have previously received less than a full primary course of OPV or IPV and who are at increased risk of exposure to poliomyelitis should be given the remaining doses of IPV, regardless of the interval since the last dose and type of vaccine previously received. It is not necessary to restart the series of either vaccine if the schedule has been interrupted.

Contraindications And Precautions To Vaccination

Severe allergic reaction (e.g. anaphylaxis) to a vaccine component, or following a prior dose of vaccine, is a contraindication to further doses of that vaccine. Since IPV contains trace amounts of streptomycin, neomycin, and polymyxin B, there is a possibility of allergic reactions in persons sensitive to these antibiotics. Persons with allergies that are not anaphylactic, such as skin contact sensitivity, may be vaccinated.

Persons with a moderate or severe acute illness normally should not be vaccinated until their symptoms have decreased.

Breastfeeding does not interfere with successful immunization against poliomyelitis with IPV. IPV may be administered to a child with diarrhea. Minor upper respiratory illnesses with or without fever, mild to moderate local reactions to a prior dose of vaccine, current antimicrobial therapy, and the convalescent phase of an acute illness are not contraindications for vaccination with IPV.

Contraindications to combination vaccines that contain IPV are the same as the contraindications to the individual components (e.g., DTaP, hepatitis B).

Adverse Reactions Following Vaccination

Minor local reactions (pain, redness) most commonly occur following IPV. Because IPV contains trace amounts of streptomycin, polymyxin B, and neomycin, allergic reactions may occur in persons allergic to these antibiotics.

Polio Vaccine Contraindications and Precautions
- Severe allergic reaction to a vaccine component or following a prior dose of vaccine
- Moderate or severe acute illness

Polio Vaccine Adverse Reactions
- Local reactions (IPV)
- Paralytic poliomyelitis (OPV)

18

Vaccine-Associated Paralytic Poliomyelitis

Vaccine-associated paralytic polio is a rare adverse event following live oral poliovirus vaccine. Inactivated poliovirus vaccine does not contain live virus, so it cannot cause VAPP. The mechanism of VAPP is believed to be a mutation, or reversion, of the vaccine virus to a more neurotropic form. These mutated viruses are called revertants. Reversion is believed to occur in almost all vaccine recipients, but it only rarely results in paralytic disease. The paralysis that results is identical to that caused by wild virus, and may be permanent.

The risk of VAPP is not equal for all OPV doses in the vaccination series. The risk of VAPP is 7 to 21 times higher for the first dose than for any other dose in the OPV series. VAPP is more likely to occur in persons 18 years of age and older than in children, and is much more likely to occur in immunodeficient children than in those who are immunocompetent. Compared with immunocompetent children, the risk of VAPP is almost 7,000 times higher for persons with certain types of immunodeficiencies, particularly B-lymphocyte disorders (e.g., agammaglobulinemia and hypogammaglobulinemia), which reduce the synthesis of immune globulins. There is no procedure available for identifying persons at risk of paralytic disease, except excluding older persons and screening for immunodeficiency.

From 1980 through 1999, 162 cases of paralytic polio were reported in the United States; 2 cases were indeterminate as to source, and 154 (95%) of these cases were VAPP, and the remaining six were in persons who acquired documented or presumed wild-virus polio outside the United States. Some cases occurred in vaccine recipients and some cases occurred in contacts of vaccine recipients. None of the vaccine recipients were known to be immunologically abnormal prior to vaccination. Since 1999, only 2 cases of VAPP have been reported in the United States: one acquired outside the United States and one who likely was infected prior to the cessation of OPV in the United States.

Vaccine Storage and Handling

Polio vaccine should be maintained at refrigerator temperature between 35°F and 46°F (2°C and 8°C). Manufacturer package inserts contain additional information and can be found at http://www.fda.gov/BiologicsBloodVaccines/Vaccines/ApprovedProducts/ucm093830.htm. For complete information on best practices and recommendations please refer to CDC's Vaccine Storage and Handling Toolkit, http://www.cdc.gov/vaccines/recs/storage/toolkit/storage-handling-toolkit.pdf.

Vaccine-Associated Paralytic Poliomyelitis

- More likely in persons 18 years of age and older
- Much more likely in persons with immunodeficiency
- No procedure available for identifying persons at risk of paralytic disease

18

Poliomyelitis

Outbreak Investigation and Control

Collect preliminary clinical and epidemiologic information (including vaccine history and contact with OPV vaccines) on any suspected case of paralytic polio. Notify CDC, (Emergency Operations Center (EOC), 770-488-7100). Follow-up should occur in close collaboration with local and state health authorities. Paralytic polio is designated "immediately notifiable, extremely urgent", requiring state and local health authorities to notify CDC within 4 hours of their notification. Non-paralytic polio is designated "immediately notifiable and urgent" requiring state and local health authorities to notify CDC within 24 hours of their notification. CDC's EOC will provide consultation regarding the collection of appropriate clinical specimens for virus isolation and serology, the initiation of appropriate consultations and procedures to rule out or confirm poliomyelitis, the compilation of medical records, and most importantly, the evaluation of the likelihood that the disease may be caused by wild poliovirus.

Polio Eradication

Following the widespread use of poliovirus vaccine in the mid-1950s, the incidence of poliomyelitis declined rapidly in many industrialized countries. In the United States, the number of cases of paralytic poliomyelitis reported annually declined from more than 20,000 cases in 1952 to fewer than 100 cases in the mid-1960s. The last documented indigenous transmission of wild poliovirus in the United States was in 1979.

In 1985, the member countries of the Pan American Health Organization adopted the goal of eliminating poliomyelitis from the Western Hemisphere by 1990. The strategy to achieve this goal included increasing vaccination coverage; enhancing surveillance for suspected cases (i.e., surveillance for acute flaccid paralysis); and using supplemental immunization strategies such as national immunization days, house-to-house vaccination, and containment activities. Since 1991, when the last wild-virus–associated indigenous case was reported from Peru, no additional cases of poliomyelitis have been confirmed despite intensive surveillance. In September 1994, an international commission certified the Western Hemisphere to be free of indigenous wild poliovirus. The commission based its judgment on detailed reports from national certification commissions that had been convened in every country in the region.

In 1988, the World Health Assembly (the governing body of the World Health Organization) adopted the goal of global eradication of poliovirus by the year 2000. Although this goal was not achieved, substantial progress has been made.

Polio Eradication

- Last case in United States in 1979
- Western Hemisphere certified polio free in 1994
- Last isolate of type 2 poliovirus in India in October 1999
- Global eradication goal

18

In 1988, an estimated 350,000 cases of paralytic polio occurred, and the disease was endemic in more than 125 countries. By 2012, only 223 cases were reported globally—a reduction of more than 99% from 1988—and polio remained endemic in only three countries. In addition, one type of poliovirus appears to have already been eradicated. The last isolation of type 2 virus was in India in October 1999.

The polio eradication initiative is led by a coalition of international organizations that includes WHO, the United Nations Children's Fund (UNICEF), CDC, and Rotary International. Other bilateral and multilateral organizations also support the initiative. Rotary International has contributed more than $600 million to support the eradication initiative. Current information on the status of the global polio eradication initiative is available on the World Health Organization website at www.polioeradication.org/.

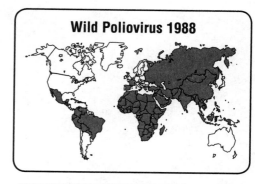

Wild Poliovirus 1988

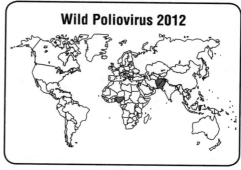

Wild Poliovirus 2012

Post-polio Syndrome

After an interval of 15–40 years, 25%–40% of persons who contracted paralytic poliomyelitis in childhood experience new muscle pain and exacerbation of existing weakness, or develop new weakness or paralysis. This disease entity is referred to as post-polio syndrome. Factors that increase the risk of post-polio syndrome include increasing length of time since acute poliovirus infection, presence of permanent residual impairment after recovery from the acute illness, and female sex. The pathogenesis of post-polio syndrome is thought to involve the failure of oversized motor units created during the recovery process of paralytic poliomyelitis. Post-polio syndrome is not an infectious process, and persons experiencing the syndrome do not shed poliovirus.

For more information, or for support for persons with post-polio syndrome and their families, contact:

Post-Polio Health International
4207 Lindell Boulevard #110
St. Louis, MO 63108-2930
314-534-0475

info@post-polio.org
www.post-polio.org

Acknowledgment

The editors thank Drs. Greg Wallace, and Jim Alexander, CDC for their assistance in updating this chapter.

18

Poliomyelitis

Selected References

CDC. Imported vaccine-associated paralytic poliomyelitis—United States, 2005. *MMWR* 2006;55:97–9.

CDC. Tracking Progress Toward Global Polio Eradication — Worldwide, 2009–2010. *MMWR* 2011;60(No. 14):441-5.

CDC. Poliomyelitis prevention in the United States: updated recommendations of the Advisory Committee on Immunization Practices. (ACIP). *MMWR* 2000;49 (No. RR-5):1–22.

CDC. Apparent global interruption of wild poliovirus type 2 transmission. *MMWR* 2001;50:222–4.

CDC. Updated recommendations of the Advisory Committee on Immunization Practices (ACIP) regarding routine poliovirus vaccination. *MMWR* 2009;58 (No. 30):829–30.

18

Diarrheal disease has been recognized in humans since antiquity. Until the early 1970s, a bacterial, viral, or parasitic etiology of diarrheal disease in children could be detected in fewer than 30% of cases. In 1973, Bishop and colleagues observed a virus particle in the intestinal tissue of children with diarrhea by using electron micrography. This virus was subsequently called "rotavirus" because of its similarity in appearance to a wheel (*rota* is Latin for wheel). By 1980, rotavirus was recognized as the most common cause of severe gastroenteritis in infants and young children in the United States. It is now known that infection with rotavirus is nearly universal, with almost all children infected by 5 years of age. Prior to vaccine implemenation, rotavirus was responsible for 20–60 deaths per year in the United States and up to 500,000 deaths from diarrhea worldwide. A vaccine to prevent rotavirus gastroenteritis was first licensed in August 1998 but was withdrawn in 1999 because of its association with intussusception. Second-generation vaccines were licensed in 2006 and 2008.

Rotavirus

Rotavirus is a double-stranded RNA virus of the family *Reoviridae*. The virus is composed of three concentric shells that enclose 11 gene segments. The outermost shell contains two important proteins—VP7, or G-protein, and VP4, or P-protein. VP7 and VP4 define the serotype of the virus and induce neutralizing antibody that is probably involved in immune protection. From 1996 through 2005, five strains of rotavirus (G1–4, G9) accounted for 90% of isolates from children younger than 5 years in the United States. Of these, the G1 strain accounted for more than 75% of isolates.

Rotavirus is very stable and may remain viable in the environment for weeks or months if not disinfected.

Rotaviruses cause infection in many species of mammals, including cows and monkeys. These animal strains are antigenically distinct from those causing human infection, and they rarely cause infection in humans.

Pathogenesis

The virus enters the body through the mouth. Viral replication occurs in the villous epithelium of the small intestine. Recent evidence indicates that up to two-thirds of children with severe rotavirus gastroenteritis show the presence of rotavirus antigen in serum (antigenemia). Infection may result in decreased intestinal absorption of sodium, glucose, and water, and decreased levels of intestinal lactase, alkaline phosphatase, and sucrase activity, and may lead to isotonic diarrhea.

Rotavirus

- First identified as cause of diarrhea in 1973
- Most common cause of severe gastroenteritis in infants and children
- Nearly universal infection by age 5 years
- Responsible for up to 500,000 diarrheal deaths each year worldwide

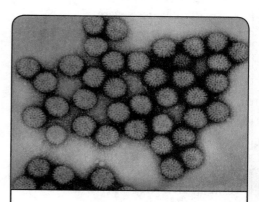

Rotavirus

- Reovirus (RNA)
- VP7 and VP4 proteins define virus serotype and induce neutralizing antibody
- From 1996-2005, five predominant strains in U.S. (G1-G4, G9) accounted for 90% of isolates
- G1 strain accounts for 75% of infections
- Very stable and may remain viable for weeks or months if not disinfected

19

Rotavirus

Rotavirus Pathogenesis

- Entry through mouth
- Replication in epithelium of small intestine
- In severe infections – rotavirus antigen detectable in serum
- Infection leads to isotonic diarrhea

Rotavirus Immunity

- Antibody against VP7 and VP4 probably important for protection
- First infection usually does not lead to permanent immunity
- Reinfection can occur at any age
- Subsequent infections generally less severe

Rotavirus Clinical Features

- Short incubation period (usually less than 48 hours)
- First infection after age 3 months generally most severe
- May be asymptomatic or result in severe dehydrating diarrhea with fever and vomiting
- Gastrointestinal symptoms generally resolve in 3 to 7 days

Rotavirus Complications

- Severe diarrhea
- Dehydration
- Electrolyte imbalance
- Metabolic acidosis
- Immunodeficient children may have more severe or persistent disease

The immune correlates of protection from rotavirus are poorly understood. Serum and mucosal antibodies against VP7 and VP4 are probably important for protection from disease. Cell-mediated immunity probably plays a role in recovery from infection and in protection.

Recovery from a first rotavirus infection usually does not lead to permanent immunity. After a single natural infection, 38% of children are protected against any subsequent rotavirus infection, 77% are protected against rotavirus diarrhea, and 87% are protected against severe diarrhea. Reinfection can occur at any age. Subsequent infections confer progressively greater protection and are generally less severe than the first.

Clinical Features

The incubation period for rotavirus diarrhea is short, usually less than 48 hours. The clinical manifestations of infection vary and depend on whether it is the first infection or reinfection. The first infection after 3 months of age is generally the most severe. Infection may be asymptomatic, may cause self-limited watery diarrhea, or may result in severe dehydrating diarrhea with fever and vomiting. Up to one-third of infected children may have a temperature greater than 102°F (39°C). The gastrointestinal symptoms generally resolve in 3 to 7 days.

The clinical features and stool characteristics of rotavirus diarrhea are nonspecific, and similar illness may be caused by other pathogens. As a result, confirmation of a diarrheal illness as rotavirus requires laboratory testing.

Complications

Rotavirus infection in infants and young children can lead to severe diarrhea, dehydration, electrolyte imbalance, and metabolic acidosis. Children who are immunocompromised because of congenital immunodeficiency or because of bone marrow or solid organ transplantation may experience severe or prolonged rotavirus gastroenteritis and may have evidence of abnormalities in multiple organ systems, particularly the kidney and liver.

Laboratory Diagnosis

The most widely available method for confirmation of rotavirus infection is detection of rotavirus antigen in stool by enzyme-linked immunoassay (EIA). Several commercial test kits are available that detect an antigen common to human rotaviruses. These kits are simple to use, inexpensive, and very sensitive. Other techniques (such as electron microscopy, reverse transcription polymerase chain reaction, nucleic acid hybridization, sequence analysis, and culture) are used primarily in research settings. Rotavirus antigen has also been identified in the serum of patients 3–7 days after disease onset, but at present, routine diagnostic testing is based primarily on testing of fecal specimens.

Epidemiology

Occurrence

Rotavirus occurs throughout the world. The incidence of rotavirus is similar in developed and developing countries, suggesting that improved sanitation alone is not sufficient to prevent the infection. The prevalence of specific rotavirus strains varies by geographic area.

Reservoir

The reservoir of rotavirus is the gastrointestinal tract and stool of infected humans. Although rotavirus infection occurs in many nonhuman mammals, transmission of animal rotaviruses to humans is believed to be rare and probably does not lead to clinical illness. Although immunodeficient persons may shed rotavirus for a prolonged period, a true carrier state has not been described.

Transmission

Rotaviruses are shed in high concentration in the stool of infected persons. Transmission is by fecal-oral route, both through close person-to-person contact and by fomites (such as toys and other environmental surfaces contaminated by stool). Transmission of rotavirus through contaminated water or food appears to be uncommon.

Temporal Pattern

In temperate climates, disease is more prevalent during fall and winter. In the United States in the prevaccine period, annual epidemic peaks usually progressed from the Southwest during November and December to the Northeast by April and May. Following vaccine introduction, the seasons have become shorter with overall less notable differences in timing by geographic region. In tropical climates, the disease is less seasonal than in temperate areas.

Communicability

Rotavirus is highly communicable, as evidenced by the nearly universal infection of children by age 5 years in the prevaccine era. Infected persons shed large quantities of virus in their stool beginning 2 days before the onset of diarrhea and for up to 10 days after onset of symptoms. Rotavirus may be detected in the stool of immunodeficient persons for more than 30 days after infection. Spread within families, institutions, hospitals, and child care settings is common.

Rotavirus Epidemiology

- Reservoir
  - Human –GI tract and stool
- Transmission
  - Fecal-oral, fomites
- Temporal pattern
  - Fall and winter (temperate areas)
- Communicability
  - 2 days before to 10 days after onset of symptoms

19

Rotavirus

> ## Rotavirus Disease in the United States
>
> - Estimated 3 million cases per year*
> - 95% of children infected by 5 years of age
> - Annually* responsible for:
>   - more than 400,000 physician visits
>   - more than 200,000 emergency dept visits
>   - 55,000 to 70,000 hospitalizations
>   - 20 to 60 deaths
> - Annual direct and indirect costs are estimated at approximately $1 billion
> - Highest incidence among children 3 to 35 months of age
>
> *Prevaccine era

Rotavirus Disease in the United States Pre and Post Vaccine Introduction

Rotavirus infection is not nationally notifiable in the United States. Estimates of incidence and disease burden are based on special surveys, cohort studies, and hospital discharge data.

In the prevaccine era an estimated 3 million rotavirus infections occurred every year in the United States and 95% of children experienced at least one rotavirus infection by age 5 years. Rotavirus infection was responsible for more than 400,000 physician visits, more than 200,000 emergency department (ED) visits, 55,000 to 70,000 hospitalizations, and 20 to 60 deaths each year in children younger than 5 years. Annual direct and indirect costs were estimated at approximately $1 billion, primarily due to the cost of time lost from work to care for an ill child.

In the prevaccine era, rotavirus accounted for 30% to 50% of all hospitalizations for gastroenteritis among U.S. children younger than 5 years of age; the incidence of clinical illness was highest among children 3 to 35 months of age. Infants younger than 3 months of age have relatively low rates of rotavirus infection, probably because of passive maternal antibody, and possibly breastfeeding. Rotavirus infection of adults is usually asymptomatic but may cause diarrheal illness.

Rotavirus activity has been monitored through data on routine testing for rotavirus performed at a set of clinical laboratories across the country. Rotavirus activity in the United States decreased significantly after introduction of rotavirus vaccine in 2006. The 2010-2011 rotavirus season was 8 weeks shorter in duration than the prevaccine baseline. The threshold for the start of the rotavirus season was never achieved nationally during the 2011-2012 season. During these seasons, nationally, the number of positive rotavirus tests declined 74-90% compared with the prevaccine baseline and the total number of tests performed annually declined 28%-36%. The annual proportion positive at the 25 consistently reporting laboratories remained below 10% in both seasons compared with a prevaccine baseline median of 26%. A pattern of biennial increases in rotavirus activity emerged during the 5 postvaccine seasons from 2007-2012, but activity remained substantially below prevaccine levels.

The reduction in rotavirus disease burden in the United States following vaccine introduction has been documented in many different evaluations, including those using data on hospitalizations and emergency room care for diarrhea among young children. Following RV5 introduction in 2006, an estimated 40,000 to 60,000 fewer diarrhea-associated hospitalizations occurred in 2008 in the United States among young children, compared with the prevaccine period. In this season, there was evidence that disease reduction also occurred among children too old to have received vaccine, suggesting indirect protection to unvaccinated and previously uninfected children. Diarrhea hospitalizations during the 2009 rotavirus season were also lower than in the prevaccine period, but greater than the number in 2008, suggesting no indirect benefit in 2009.

Rotavirus Vaccines

The first rotavirus vaccines were derived from either bovine (cow) or rhesus (monkey) origin. Studies demonstrated that these live oral vaccines could prevent rotavirus diarrhea in young children, but efficacy varied widely. Because immunity to G (VP7) or P (VP4) proteins was associated with disease protection and recovery, new live virus vaccines were developed that incorporated G proteins or both G and P proteins for each of the predominant serotypes.

In 1998, a rhesus-based tetravalent rotavirus vaccine (RRV-TV, Rotashield) was licensed and recommended for routine immunization of U.S. infants. However, RRV-TV was withdrawn from the U.S. market within 1 year of its introduction because of its association with intussusception. The risk of intussusception was most elevated (more than a 20-fold increase) within 3 to 14 days after receipt of the first dose of RRV-TV, with a smaller (approximately 5-fold) increase in risk within 3 to 14 days after the second dose. Overall, the risk associated with the first dose of RRV-TV was estimated to be about one case per 10,000 vaccine recipients. Some researchers have suggested that the relative risk of intussusception associated with the first dose of RRV-TV increased with increasing age at vaccination.

Characteristics

There are currently two rotavirus vaccines licensed for use in the United States. RV5 (RotaTeq) is a live oral vaccine manufactured by Merck and licensed by the Food and Drug Administration in February 2006. RV5 contains five reassortant rotaviruses developed from human and bovine parent rotavirus strains. Each 2-mL vial of vaccine contains approximately 2 x 106 infectious units of each of the five reassortant strains. The vaccine viruses are suspended in a buffer solution that contains sucrose, sodium citrate, sodium phosphate monobasic monohydrate, sodium hydroxide, polysorbate 80, and tissue culture media. Trace amounts of fetal bovine serum might be present. The vaccine contains no preservatives or thimerosal.

Rotavirus Vaccines

- RV5 (RotaTeq)
  - contains five reassortant rotaviruses developed from human and bovine parent rotavirus strains
  - vaccine viruses suspended in a buffer solution
  - contains no preservatives or thimerosal
- RV1 (Rotarix)
  - contains one strain of live attenuated human rotavirus (type G1PA[8])
  - provided as a lyophilized powder that is reconstituted before administration
  - contains no preservatives or thimerosal

19

Rotavirus

Fecal shedding of vaccine virus was evaluated in a subset of persons enrolled in the phase III trials. Vaccine virus was shed by 9% of 360 infants after dose 1, but none of 249 and 385 infants after doses 2 and 3, respectively. Shedding was observed as early as 1 day and as late as 15 days after a dose. The potential for transmission of vaccine virus was not assessed in trials. In a post-licensure evaluation in the United States, stool samples were collected from infants for 9 days following the first dose. Rotavirus antigen was detected in stool of 21% of 103 infants, as early as day 3 post vaccination and as late as day 9.

RV1 (Rotarix), a live oral vaccine manufactured by GlaxoSmithKline, was licensed by the FDA in April 2008. RV1 contains one strain of live attenuated human strain 89-12 (type G1P1A[8]) rotavirus. RV1 is provided as a lyophilized powder that is reconstituted before administration. Each 1-mL dose of reconstituted vaccine contains at least 106 median cell culture infective units of virus. The vaccine contains amino acids, dextran, Dulbecco's modified Eagle medium, sorbitol and sucrose. The diluent contains calcium carbonate, sterile water and xanthan. The vaccine contains no preservatives or thimerosal.

Fecal shedding of rotavirus antigen was evaluated in all or a subset of infants from seven studies in various countries. After dose 1, rotavirus antigen shedding was detected by EIA in 50% to 80% (depending on the study) of infants at approximately day 7 and 0 to 24% at approximately day 30. After dose 2, rotavirus antigen shedding was detected in 4% to 18% of infants at approximately day 7, and 0 to 1.2% at approximately day 30. The potential for transmission of vaccine virus was assessed in a clinical trial among twin pairs (with one twin receiving the vaccine and the other not receiving vaccine) in the Dominican Republic. This study showed evidence of vaccine strain transmission in 19% of the unvaccinated twins, and seroconversion in 21% of the unvaccinated twins. .

Porcine circovirus type 1 has been detected in RV1 and porcine circovirus type 1 and type 2 DNA fragments have been detected in RV5. There is no evidence that the virus is a safety risk or causes illness in humans.

Vaccine Efficacy

In the main Phase III RV5 clinical efficacy evaluation, conducted in Finland and United States, the efficacy of the three-dose series against G1-G4 rotavirus gastroenteritis of any severity was 74%, and against severe G1-G4 rotavirus gastroenteritis (defined by severity of fever, vomiting, diarrhea and changes in behavior) was 98% during the first full rotavirus season after vaccination. In a large healthcare

---

Rotavirus Vaccine Efficacy

~~Condition~~ *See 9/2015 Errata*

- ~~Efficacy~~
- Any rotavirus gastroenteritis
  - 74%-87%
- Severe gastroenteritis
  - 85%-98%
- Both vaccines significantly reduced physician visits for diarrhea, and reduced rotavirus-related hospitalization

19

utilization study evaluating children during the first 2 years of life, RV5 vaccine reduced the incidence of office visits for G1-G4 rotavirus gastroenteritis by 86%, ED visits for that outcome by 94%, and hospitalizations for that outcome by 96%.

The main Phase III clinical efficacy trials of RV1 were conducted in Latin America and Europe. In the Latin American study, the efficacy of the 2-dose series against severe (a clinical definition) rotavirus gastroenteritis to age 1 year was 85%. In the European study, the efficacy against severe rotavirus gastroenteritis (based on a clinical scoring system that evaluated fever, vomiting, diarrhea, dehydration and treatment) was 96% through the first rotavirus season, and against any rotavirus gastroenteritis was 87%. In the European study, RV1 reduced hospitalization for rotavirus gastroenteritis by 96% through the second season.

RV5 was introduced in the United States in 2006 and RV1 was introduced in 2008; hence most post-introduction data from the United States are based on RV5. Several RV5 case-control vaccine effectiveness evaluations have been performed in the United States and have demonstrated the 3-dose series is highly effective (~85% or greater) against rotavirus disease resulting in emergency department care/hospitalization in young children. US vaccine effectiveness evaluations for RV1 are being completed.

Duration of Immunity

The duration of immunity from rotavirus vaccine is not precisely known. In the main clinical trials described above, good efficacy was demonstrated through 2 rotavirus seasons or to age 2 years (depending on the study design) for both vaccines. In case-control vaccine effectiveness evaluations conducted in the United States after vaccine introduction, high effectiveness for RV5 has been demonstrated during the first 3 years of life against rotavirus disease resulting in emergency department care/hospitalization. US vaccine effectiveness evaluations for RV1 are being completed. In low-income countries, rotavirus vaccine efficacy or effectiveness has generally been lower in the second year of life compared with the first year.

Vaccination Schedule and Use

Revised ACIP recommendations for the use of rotavirus vaccine were published in *MMWR* in February 2009. Because of similar estimates of efficacy and safety, neither The Advisory Committee on Immunization Practices (ACIP) nor the Academies of Pediatrics or Family Physicians state a preference for one vaccine over the other.

19

> **Rotavirus Vaccine Recommendations**
>
> - Similar estimates of efficacy and safety between RV1 and RV5
>
> - No preference for one vaccine over the other

Rotavirus

19

ACIP recommends routine rotavirus vaccination of all infants without a contraindication. The vaccine should be administered as a series of either two (at ages 2 and 4 months) or three (at ages 2, 4, and 6 months) oral doses, for RV1 and RV5, respectively. The vaccination series for both vaccines may be started as early as 6 weeks of age. The minimum interval between doses is 4 weeks. Rotavirus vaccine should be given at the same visit as other vaccines given at these ages.

The ACIP developed age recommendations that vary from those of the manufacturers. ACIP recommendations state that the maximum age for the first dose of both vaccines is 14 weeks 6 days. This is an off-label recommendation for RV5 since the product information states a maximum age of 12 weeks. The minimum interval between doses of both rotavirus vaccines is 4 weeks. The maximum age for any dose of either rotavirus vaccine is 8 months 0 days. No rotavirus vaccine should be administered to infants older than 8 months 0 days of age. This is an off-label recommendation for both vaccines, because the labeled maximum age for RV1 is 24 weeks, and the labeled maximum age for RV5 is 32 weeks.

ACIP did not define a maximum interval between doses. It is preferable to adhere to the recommended interval of 8 weeks. But if the interval is prolonged, the infant can still receive the vaccine as long as it can be given on or before the 8-month birthday. It is not necessary to restart the series or add doses because of a prolonged interval between doses.

There are few data on the safety or efficacy of giving more than one dose, even partial doses close together. ACIP recommends that providers do not repeat the dose if the infant spits out or regurgitates the vaccine. Any remaining doses should be administered on schedule. Doses of rotavirus vaccine should be separated by at least 4 weeks.

ACIP recommends that the rotavirus vaccine series should be completed with the same product whenever possible. However, vaccination should not be deferred if the product used for a prior dose or doses is not available or is not known. In this situation, the provider should continue or complete the series with the product that is available. If any dose in the series was RV5 (RotaTeq) or the vaccine brand used for any prior dose in the series is not known, a total of three doses of rotavirus vaccine should be administered.

Breastfeeding does not appear to diminish immune response to rotavirus vaccine. Infants who are being breastfed should be vaccinated on schedule.

Infants documented to have had rotavirus gastroenteritis before receiving the full course of rotavirus vaccinations should still begin or complete the 2- or 3-dose schedule following the age recommendations, because the initial infection may provide only partial protections against subsequent rotavirus disease.

Contraindications and Precautions to Vaccination

Rotavirus vaccine is contraindicated for infants who are known to have had a severe (anaphylactic) allergic reaction to a vaccine component or following a prior dose of rotavirus vaccine. Latex rubber is contained in the RV1 oral applicator, so infants with a severe allergy to latex should not receive RV1. The RV5 dosing tube is latex free.

Some postmarketing studies of the currently licensed vaccines have detected an increased risk for intussusception following rotavirus vaccine administration, particularly during the first week following the first dose of vaccine. As a result, in October 2011, ACIP added a history of intussusception as a contraindication to rotavirus vaccination.

In response to reported cases of vaccine-acquired rotavirus infection in infants with severe combined immunodeficiency (SCID) following rotavirus vaccine administration, ACIP added SCID as a contraindication to rotavirus vaccination in June 2010.

For children with known or suspected altered immunocompetence, ACIP advises consultation with an immunologist or infectious diseases specialist before administration of rotavirus vaccine. Children who are immunocompromised because of congenital immunodeficiency, or hematopoietic stem cell or solid organ transplantation sometimes experience severe, prolonged, and even fatal wild-type rotavirus gastroenteritis.

Limited data are available from clinical trials on the safety of rotavirus vaccines in infants known to be HIV-infected; these infants were clinically asymptomatic or mildly symptomatic (clinical stages I and II according to WHO classification) when vaccinated. The limited data available do not indicate that rotavirus vaccines have a substantially different safety profile in HIV-infected infants that are clinically asymptomatic or mildly symptomatic compared with infants that are not HIV infected. Two other considerations support vaccination of HIV-exposed or infected infants in the United States. First, the HIV diagnosis might not be established in infants born to HIV-infected mothers by the time they reach the age of the first rotavirus vaccine dose. Only 3% percent or less of HIV-exposed infants in the United States will be determined to be HIV infected. Second, vaccine strains of rotavirus are considerably attenuated.

Rotavirus Vaccine Recommendations

- ACIP recommends that providers do not repeat the dose if the infant spits out or regurgitates the vaccine

- Any remaining doses should be administered on schedule

  - Doses of rotavirus vaccine should be separated by at least 4 weeks.

- Complete the series with the same product whenever possible

- If product used for a prior dose or doses is not available or not known, continue or complete the series with the product that is available

- If any dose in the series was RV5 (RotaTeq) or the vaccine brand used for any prior dose is not known, a total of 3 doses of rotavirus vaccine should be administered

- Infants documented to have had rotavirus gastroenteritis before receiving the full course of rotavirus vaccinations should still begin or complete the 2- or 3-dose schedule

Rotavirus Vaccine Contraindications

- Severe allergic reaction to a vaccine component (including latex) or following a prior dose of vaccine

  - latex rubber is contained in the RV1 oral applicator

- History of intussusception

- Severe combined immunodeficiency (SCID)

19

Rotavirus

Rotavirus Vaccine Precautions*

- Altered immunocompetence, (except severe combined immunodeficiency, which is a contraindication)
  - Limited data do not indicate a different safety profile in HIV-infected versus HIV-uninfected infants
  - HIV diagnosis not established in infants due for rotavirus vaccine
  - Vaccine strains of rotavirus are attenuated
  - These considerations support rotavirus vaccination of HIV-exposed or infected infants
- Acute, moderate or severe gastroenteritis or other acute illness

*The decision to vaccinate if a precaution is present should be made on a case-by-case risk and benefit basis.

Rotavirus Vaccine - Conditions Not Considered to be Precautions

- Pre-existing chronic gastrointestinal conditions
  - no data available
  - ACIP considers the benefits of vaccination to outweigh the theoretic risks

Rotavirus Vaccine and Preterm Infants

- ACIP supports vaccination of a preterm infant if:
  - chronological age is at least 6 weeks
  - clinically stable; and
  - vaccine is administered at time of discharge or after discharge from neonatal intensive care unit or nursery

Rotavirus vaccine should generally not be administered to infants with acute, moderate or severe gastroenteritis, or other acute illness until the condition improves. However, infants with mild acute gastroenteritis or other mild acute illness can be vaccinated, particularly if a delay in vaccination will postpone the first dose of vaccine beyond 15 weeks 0 days of age.

Available data suggest that preterm infants (i.e., infants born at less than 37 weeks' gestation) are at increased risk for hospitalization from rotavirus during the first 1 to 2 years of life. In clinical trials, rotavirus vaccine appeared to be generally well tolerated in preterm infants, although relatively small numbers of preterm infants were evaluated. ACIP considers the benefits of rotavirus vaccination of preterm infants to outweigh the risks of adverse events. ACIP supports vaccination of a preterm infant according to the same schedule and precautions as a full-term infant, provided the following conditions are met: the infant's chronological age is at least 6 weeks, the infant is clinically stable, and the vaccine is administered at the time of discharge or after discharge from the neonatal intensive care unit or nursery. Infants living in households with persons who have or are suspected of having an immunodeficiency disorder or impaired immune status can be vaccinated. ACIP believes that the indirect protection of the immunocompromised household member provided by vaccinating the infant in the household, and thereby preventing wild-type rotavirus disease, outweighs the small risk for transmitting vaccine virus to the immunocompromised household member.

Infants living in households with pregnant women should be vaccinated according to the same schedule as infants in households without pregnant women. Because the majority of women of childbearing age have pre-existing immunity to rotavirus, the risk for infection by the attenuated vaccine virus is considered to be very low. It is prudent for all members of the household to employ measures such as good hand washing after changing a diaper or otherwise coming in contact with the feces of the vaccinated infant.

Adverse Events following Vaccination
Intussusception

The phase III clinical trials of both vaccines were very large (>60,000 infants each) to be able to study the occurrence of intussusception in vaccine compared with placebo recipients, and no increased risk for intussusception was observed for either vaccine. However, post-licensure monitoring is necessary to evaluate for a possible risk of intussusception at a lower level than that able to be evaluated in the clinical trials. Post-licensure evaluations of RV1 in Mexico identified a low-level increased risk of intussusception in week 1 after dose 1 (approximately 1 to 3 excess intussusception cases per 100,000 first doses). In Australia, a possible risk was identified with both RV5 and RV1, although based on small numbers of cases. US data on RV5 available through February 2010 from the Vaccine Safety Datalink (VSD) did not identify an increased risk of intussusception, but were not able to exclude a risk of the magnitude observed in these other settings. The VSD was unable to assess RV1 at that time because too few doses had been administered. Monitoring in the United States is ongoing. Parents and health care providers should be aware of a possible low-level increased risk of intussusception following rotavirus vaccine.

Adverse Reactions following Vaccination

In the subset of infants in RV5 clinical trials that were studied in detail for potential adverse events, for the first week after any dose, RV5 recipients had a small but statistically significant increased rate of diarrhea (18.1% in RV5 group, 15.3% in placebo group) and vomiting (11.6% in RV5, 9.9% in placebo). During the 42-day period following any dose, statistically significantly greater rates of diarrhea, vomiting, otitis media, nasopharyngitis and bronchospasm occurred in RV5 recipients compared with placebo recipients.

In the subset of infants in RV1 clincial studies with details on adverse events, for the first week after vaccination, Grade 3 (i.e., those that prevented normal everyday activities) cough or runny nose occurred at a slightly but statsitically higher rate in the RV1 group (3.6 %) compared with placebo group (3.2%). During the 31 day period after vaccination, the following unsolicited adverse events occurred at a statstically higher incidence among vaccine recipients: irritability (11.4% in RV1 group, 8.7% in placebo group) and flatulence (2.2% in RV1 group, 1.3% in placebo group)

Post-marketing strain surveillance in the United States and other countries has occasionally detected RV5 vaccine reassortant strains in stool samples of children with diarrhea. In some of these reports, the reassortant virus seemed to be the likely cause of the diarrheal illness.

Vaccine Storage and Handling

Rotavirus vaccine should be maintained at refrigerator temperature: 35°F–46°F (2°C–8°C). For complete information on best practices and recommendations please refer to CDC's Vaccine Storage and Handling Toolkit, http://www.cdc.gov/vaccines/recs/storage/toolkit/storage-handling-toolkit.pdf

Immunosuppressed Household Contacts of Rotavirus Vaccine Recipients

- Infants living in households with persons who have or are suspected of having an immunodeficiency disorder or impaired immune status can be vaccinated

- Protection provided by vaccinating the infant outweighs the small risk of transmitting vaccine virus

Pregnant Household Contacts of Rotavirus Vaccine Recipients

- Infants living in households with pregnant women should be vaccinated

  - majority of women of childbearing age have preexisting immunity to rotavirus

  - risk for infection by vaccine virus is considered to be very low

Rotavirus Vaccine Adverse Events

- Intussusception

  - Postlicensure-evaluation RV1 – 1-3 excess cases per 100,000 first doses, possible risk for RV5 cases too small to confirm

  - VAERS – reports show events cluster in 3-6 days following RV5

  - Vaccine Safety Datalink – no increased risk of intussusception – unable to assess RV1

19

Rotavirus

Rotavirus Vaccine Adverse Reactions

- RV5
  - Diarrhea 18.1%
  - Vomiting 11.6%
  - Also greater rates of otitis media, nasopharyngitis and bronchospasm
- RV1
  - Irritability 11.4%
  - Cough or runny nose 3.6%
  - Flatulence 2.2%

Rotavirus Surveillance

Rotavirus gastroenteritis is not a reportable disease in the United States. Methods of surveillance for rotavirus disease at the national level include review of national hospital discharge databases for rotavirus-specific or rotavirus-compatible diagnoses, surveillance for rotavirus disease at sites that participate in the New Vaccine Surveillance Network, and reports of rotavirus detection from a sentinel system of laboratories. Special evaluations (e.g.,. case control and retrospective cohort methods) have been used to measure the effectiveness of rotavirus vaccine under routine use in the United States. CDC has established a national strain surveillance system of sentinel laboratories that monitors circulating rotavirus strains.

Acknowledgment

The editors thank Dr. Margaret Cortese, CDC for her assistance in updating this chapter.

Selected References

American Academy of Pediatrics. Rotavirus infections. In:Pickering LK, Baker CJ, Long SS, eds. *RedBook: 2009 Report of the Committee on Infectious Diseases*. 28th ed. Elk Grove Village, IL: American Academy of Pediatrics, 2009:576–9.

CDC. Prevention of rotavirus gastroenteritis among infants and children. Recommendations of the Advisory Committee on Immunization Practices (ACIP). *MMWR* 2009;58 (No. RR-2):1–24.

CDC. Addition of severe combined immunodeficiency as a contraindication for administration of rotavirus vaccine. *MMWR* 2010;59(No. 22):687–8.

CDC. Addition of history of intussusception as a contraindication for rotavirus vaccination. *MMWR* 2010;59 (No. 22);687-8.

Cortes JE, Curns AT, Tate JE, Cortese MM, Patel MM, Zhou F, Parashar UD. Rotavirus vaccine and health care utilization for diarrhea in U.S. children. *N Engl J Med*. 2011 Sep 22;365(12):1108-17

Cortese MM, Leblanc J, White KE, Jerris RC, Stinchfield P, Preston KL, Meek J, Odofin L, Khizer S, Miller CA, Buttery V, Mijatovic-Rustempasic S, Lewis J, Parashar UD, Immergluck LC. Leveraging state immunization information systems to measure the effectiveness of rotavirus vaccine. *Pediatrics*. 2011 Dec;128(6):e1474-81

Curns AT, Steiner CA, Barrett M, Hunter K, Wilson E, Parashar UD. Reduction in acute gastroenteritis hospitalizations among US children after introduction of rotavirus vaccine: analysis of hospital discharge data from 18 US states. *J Infect Dis*. 2010 Jun 1;201(11):1617-24.

19

Fischer TK, Viboud C, Parashar U, et al. Hospitalizations and deaths from diarrhea and rotavirus among children <5 years of age in the United States, 1993-2003. *J Infect Dis* 2007;195:1117–25.

Haber P, Patel M, Pan Y, et. Al. Intusussception after rotavirus vaccines reported to U.S. VAERS, 2006-2012. *Pediatrics*, 2013 May; 131:1042-1049.

Parashar UD, Hummelman EG, Bresee JS, et al. Global illness and deaths caused by rotavirus disease in children. *Emerg Infect Dis* 2003;9:565–72.

Patel MM, López-Collada VR, Bulhões MM, et al. Intussusception risk and health benefits of rotavirus vaccination in Mexico and Brazil. *N Engl J Med*. 2011 Jun 16;364(24):2283-92.

Patel MM, Glass R, Desai R, Tate JE, Parashar UD. Fulfilling the promise of rotavirus vaccines: how far have we come since licensure? *Lancet Infect Dis*. 2012 Jul;12(7):561-70

Payne DC, Staat MA, Edwards KM, Szilagyi PG, Weinberg GA, Hall CB, Chappell J, Curns AT, Wikswo M, Tate JE, Lopman BA, Parashar UD; New Vaccine Surveillance Network (NVSN). Direct and indirect effects of rotavirus vaccination upon childhood hospitalizations in 3 US Counties, 2006-2009. *Clin Infect Dis*. 2011 Aug 1;53(3): 245-53.

Shui IM, Baggs J, Patel M, Parashar UD, Rett M, Belongia EA, Hambidge SJ, Glanz JM, Klein NP, Weintraub E. Risk of intussusception following administration of a pentavalent rotavirus vaccine in US infants. *JAMA*. 2012 Feb 8;307(6):598-604. doi: 10.1001/jama.2012.97

Staat MA, Payne DC, Donauer S, Weinberg GA, Edwards KM, Szilagyi PG, Griffin MR, Hall CB, Curns AT, Gentsch JR, Salisbury S, Fairbrother G, Parashar UD; New Vaccine Surveillance Network (NVSN). Effectiveness of pentavalent rotavirus vaccine against severe disease. *Pediatrics*. 2011 Aug;128(2):e267-75. doi: 10.1542/peds.2010-3722.

Tate J, Mutue J, Panozzo C, et al. Sustained decline in rotavirus detections in the United States following the intro-duction of rotavirus vaccine in 2006. *Pediatric Inf Dis* 2011, 30:530–4.

Vesikari T, Matson DO, Dennehy P, et al. Safety and efficacy of a pentavalent human–bovine (WC3) reassortant rotavirus vaccine. *N Engl J Med* 2006;354:23–33.

Vesikari T, Karvonen A, Prymula R, et al. Efficacy of human rotavirus vaccine against rotavirus gastroenteritis during the first 2 years of life in European infants: randomized, double-blind controlled study. *Lancet* 2007;370:1757-63.

19

Rotavirus

The name rubella is derived from Latin, meaning "little red." Rubella was initially considered to be a variant of measles or scarlet fever and was called "third disease". It was not until 1814 that it was first described as a separate disease in the German medical literature, hence the common name "German measles". In 1914, Hess postulated a viral etiology based on his work with monkeys. Hiro and Tosaka in 1938 confirmed the viral etiology by passing the disease to children using filtered nasal washings from persons with acute cases.

Following a widespread epidemic of rubella infection in 1940, Norman Gregg, an Australian ophthalmologist, reported in 1941 the occurrence of congenital cataracts among 78 infants born following maternal rubella infection in early pregnancy. This was the first published recognition of congenital rubella syndrome (CRS). Rubella virus was first isolated in 1962 by Parkman and Weller. The first rubella vaccines were licensed in 1969.

Rubella Virus

Rubella virus is classified as a togavirus, genus Rubivirus. It is most closely related to group A arboviruses, such as eastern and western equine encephalitis viruses. It is an enveloped RNA virus, with a single antigenic type that does not cross-react with other members of the togavirus group. Rubella virus is relatively unstable and is inactivated by lipid solvents, trypsin, formalin, ultraviolet light, low pH, heat, and amantadine.

Pathogenesis

Following respiratory transmission of rubella virus, replication of the virus is thought to occur in the nasopharynx and regional lymph nodes. A viremia occurs 5 to 7 days after exposure with spread of the virus throughout the body. Transplacental infection of the fetus occurs during viremia. Fetal damage occurs through destruction of cells as well as mitotic arrest.

Clinical Features
Acquired Rubella

The incubation period of rubella is 14 days, with a range of 12 to 23 days. Symptoms are often mild, and up to 50% of infections may be subclinical or inapparent. In children, rash is usually the first manifestation and a prodrome is rare. In older children and adults, there is often a 1 to 5 day prodrome with low-grade fever, malaise, lymphadenopathy, and upper respiratory symptoms preceding the rash. The rash of rubella is maculopapular and occurs 14 to 17 days

---

Rubella

- From Latin meaning "little red"

- Discovered in 18th century –thought to be variant of measles

- First described as distinct clinical entity in German literature

- Congenital rubella syndrome (CRS) described by Gregg in 1941

- Rubella virus first isolated in 1962 by Parkman and Weller

Rubella Virus

- Togavirus

- RNA virus

- One antigenic type

- Inactivated by lipid solvents, trypsin, formalin, ultraviolet light, low pH, heat, and amantadine

Rubella Pathogenesis

- Respiratory transmission of virus

- Replication in nasopharynx and regional lymph nodes

- Viremia 5 to 7 days after exposure with spread throughout body

- Transplacental infection of fetus during viremia

20

Rubella

after exposure. The rash usually occurs initially on the face and then progresses from head to foot. It lasts about 3 days and is occasionally pruritic. The rash is fainter than measles rash and does not coalesce. The rash is often more prominent after a hot shower or bath. Lymphadenopathy may begin a week before the rash and last several weeks. Postauricular, posterior cervical, and suboccipital nodes are commonly involved.

Arthralgia and arthritis occur so frequently in adults that they are considered by many to be an integral part of the illness rather than a complication. Other symptoms of rubella include conjunctivitis, testalgia, or orchitis. Forschheimer spots may be noted on the soft palate but are not diagnostic for rubella.

Complications

Complications of rubella are not common, but they generally occur more often in adults than in children.

Arthralgia or arthritis may occur in up to 70% of adult women who contract rubella, but it is rare in children and adult males. Fingers, wrists, and knees are often affected. Joint symptoms tend to occur about the same time or shortly after appearance of the rash and may last for up to 1 month; chronic arthritis is rare.

Encephalitis occurs in one in 6,000 cases, more frequently in adults (especially in females) than in children. Mortality estimates vary from 0 to 50%.

Hemorrhagic manifestations occur in approximately one per 3,000 cases, occurring more often in children than in adults. These manifestations may be secondary to low platelets and vascular damage, with thrombocytopenic purpura being the most common manifestation. Gastrointestinal, cerebral, or intrarenal hemorrhage may occur. Effects may last from days to months, and most patients recover.

Additional complications include orchitis, neuritis, and a rare late syndrome of progressive panencephalitis.

Congenital Rubella Syndrome

Prevention of CRS is the main objective of rubella vaccination programs in the United States.

A rubella epidemic in the United States in 1964–1965 resulted in 12.5 million cases of rubella infection and about 20,000 newborns with CRS. The estimated cost of the epidemic was $840 million. This does not include the emotional toll on the families involved.

Infection with rubella virus is most severe in early gestation. The virus may affect all organs and cause a variety of congenital defects. Infection may lead to fetal death, spontaneous abortion, or preterm delivery. The severity of the effects of rubella virus on the fetus depends largely on the time of gestation at which infection occurs. As many as 85% of infants infected in the first trimester of pregnancy will be found to be affected if followed after birth. While fetal infection may occur throughout pregnancy, defects are rare when infection occurs after the 20th week of gestation. The overall risk of defects during the third trimester is probably no greater than that associated with uncomplicated pregnancies.

Congenital infection with rubella virus can affect virtually all organ systems. Deafness is the most common and often the sole manifestation of congenital rubella infection, especially after the fourth month of gestation. Eye defects, including cataracts, glaucoma, retinopathy, and microphthalmia may occur. Cardiac defects such as patent ductus arteriosus, ventricular septal defect, pulmonic stenosis, and coarctation of the aorta are possible. Neurologic abnormalities, including microcephaly and mental retardation, and other abnormalities, including bone lesions, splenomegaly, hepatitis, and thrombocytopenia with purpura may occur.

Manifestations of CRS may be delayed from 2 to 4 years. Diabetes mellitus appearing in later childhood occurs frequently in children with CRS. In addition, progressive encephalopathy resembling subacute sclerosing panencephalitis has been observed in some older children with CRS. Children with CRS have a higher than expected incidence of autism.

Infants with CRS may have low titers by hemagglutination inhibition (HI) but may have high titers of neutralizing antibody that may persist for years. Reinfection may occur. Impaired cell-mediated immunity has been demonstrated in some children with CRS.

Laboratory Diagnosis

Many rash illnesses can mimic rubella infection, and as many as 50% of rubella infections may be subclinical. The only reliable evidence of acute rubella infection is a positive viral culture for rubella or detection of rubella virus by polymerase chain reaction (PCR), the presence of rubella-specific IgM antibody, or demonstration of a significant rise in IgG antibody from paired acute- and convalescent-phase sera.

Rubella virus can be isolated from nasal, blood, throat, urine and cerebrospinal fluid specimens from rubella and CRS patients. Virus may be isolated from the pharynx 1 week

Congenital Rubella Syndrome

- Infection may affect all organs
- May lead to fetal death or premature delivery
- Severity of damage to fetus depends on gestational age
- Up to 85% of infants affected if infected during first trimester
- Deafness
- Eye defects
- Cardiac defects
- Microcephaly
- Mental retardation
- Bone alterations
- Liver and spleen damage

Rubella Laboratory Diagnosis

- Isolation of rubella virus from clinical specimen (e.g., nasopharynx, urine)
- Serologic tests available vary among laboratories
- Positive serologic test for rubella IgM antibody
- Significant rise in rubella IgG by any standard serologic assay (e.g., enzyme immunoassay)

20

Rubella

before and until 2 weeks after rash onset. Although isolation of the virus is diagnostic of rubella infection, viral cultures are labor intensive, and therefore not done in many laboratories; they are generally not used for routine diagnosis of rubella. Viral isolation is an extremely valuable epidemiologic tool and should be attempted for all suspected cases of rubella or CRS. Information about rubella virus isolation can be found on the CDC website at www.cdc.gov/rubella/lab/lab-protocols.htm.

Serology is the most common method of confirming the diagnosis of rubella. Acute rubella infection can be serologically confirmed by a significant rise in rubella antibody titer in acute- and convalescent-phase serum specimens or by the presence of serum rubella IgM. Serum should be collected as early as possible (within 7–10 days) after onset of illness, and again 14–21 days (minimum of 7) days later.

False-positive serum rubella IgM tests have occurred in persons with parvovirus infections, with a positive heterophile test for infectious mononucleosis, or with a positive rheumatoid factor.

The serologic tests available for laboratory confirmation of rubella infections vary among laboratories. The state health department can provide guidance on available laboratory services and preferred tests.

Enzyme-linked immunosorbent assay (ELISA) is sensitive, widely available, and relatively easy to perform. It can also be modified to measure IgM antibodies. Most of the diagnostic testing done for rubella antibodies uses some variation of ELISA.

Epidemiology

Occurrence

Rubella occurs worldwide. For information about the clinical case definition, clinical classification and epidemiologic classification of rubella and congenital rubella syndrome see www.cdc.gov/vaccines/pubs/surv-manual/default.htm.

Reservoir

Rubella is a human disease. There is no known animal reservoir. Although infants with CRS may shed rubella virus for an extended period, a true carrier state has not been described.

Transmission

Rubella is spread from person to person via droplets shed from the respiratory secretions of infected persons. There is no evidence of insect transmission.

20

Rubella Epidemiology

- Reservoir
  - human
- Transmission
  - respiratory (Subclinical cases may transmit)
- Temporal pattern
  - peak in late winter and spring
- Communicability
  - 7 days before 5 to 7 days after rash onset
- Infants with CRS may shed virus for up to a year

Rubella may be transmitted by persons with subclinical or asymptomatic cases (up to 50% of all rubella virus infections).

Temporal Pattern

In temperate areas, incidence is usually highest in late winter and early spring.

Communicability

Rubella is only moderately contagious. The disease is most contagious when the rash first appears, but virus may be shed from 7 days before to 5–7 days or more after rash onset.

Infants with CRS shed large quantities of virus from body secretions for up to 1 year and can therefore transmit rubella to persons caring for them who are susceptible to the disease.

Secular Trends in the United States

Rubella and congenital rubella syndrome became nationally notifiable diseases in 1966. The largest annual total of cases of rubella in the United States was in 1969, when 57,686 cases were reported (58 cases per 100,000 population). Following vaccine licensure in 1969, rubella incidence declined rapidly. By 1983, fewer than 1,000 cases per year were reported (less than 0.5 cases per 100,000 population). A moderate resurgence of rubella occurred in 1990–1991, primarily due to outbreaks in California (1990) and among the Amish in Pennsylvania (1991). In 2003, a record low annual total of seven cases was reported. In October 2004, CDC convened an independent expert panel to review available rubella and CRS data. After a careful review, the panel unanimously agreed that rubella was no longer endemic in the United States. The number of reported cases of rubella in the United States remains low with a median of 11 cases annually in 2005-2011.

Until recently, there was no predominant age group for rubella cases. During 1982 through 1992, approximately 30% of cases occurred in children younger than 5 years, 30% occurred in children 5 through 14 years, and 30% occurred in persons 15 through 39 years. Adults 40 years of age and older typically accounted for less than 10% of cases. Since 2004 when endemic rubella was declared eliminated in the U.S., persons 20-49 years of age have accounted for 60 percent of the cases (median age 32 years).

Most reported rubella in the United States in the mid-1990s has occurred among Hispanic young adults who were born in areas where rubella vaccine is routinely not given. In 1998,

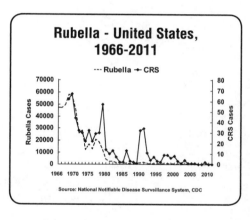

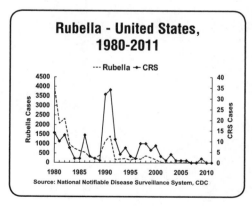

20

Rubella

<table>
<tr><td>

Rubella and CRS in the United States

- Most reported rubella in the U.S. in the mid-1990s has occurred among foreign-born Hispanic young adults

- Indigenous transmission of rubella determined to have ended in 2004

- In 2010 PAHO announced region of the Americas achieved rubella and CRS elimination goal

</td></tr>
</table>

Latin America nations and Mexico began major rubella control efforts, which resulted in a marked decrease in the number of rubella cases.

CRS surveillance is maintained through the National Congenital Rubella Registry, which is managed by the National Center for Immunization and Respiratory Diseases. The largest annual total of reported CRS cases to the registry was in 1970 (67 cases). An average of 2-3 CRS cases were reported annually during 1998-2012. Although reported rubella activity has consistently and significantly decreased since vaccine has been used in the United States, the incidence of CRS has paralleled the decrease in rubella cases only since the mid-1970s. The decline in CRS since the mid-1970s was due to an increased effort to vaccinate susceptible adolescents and young adults, especially women. Rubella outbreaks are almost always followed by an increase in CRS.

Rubella outbreaks in California and Pennsylvania in 1990–1991 resulted in 25 cases of CRS in 1990 and 33 cases in 1991. From 2004-2012, a total of 6 CRS cases were reported in the U.S., 5 of which where the mother was likely infected while in Asia or Africa. In 2010, the Pan American Health Organization (PAHO) announced that the Region of the Americas had achieved the rubella and CRS elimination goals set in 2003 based on surveillance data. Although regional documentation of elimination is ongoing, an expert panel unanimously agreed in December 2011 that rubella elimination has been maintained in the United States.

Rubella Vaccine

Three rubella vaccines were licensed in the United States in 1969: HPV-77:DE-5 Meruvax (duck embryo), HPV-77:DK-12 Rubelogen (dog kidney), and GMK-3:RK53 Cendevax (rabbit kidney) strains. HPV-77:DK-12 was later removed from the market because there was a higher rate of joint complaints following vaccination with this strain. In 1979, the RA 27/3 (human diploid fibroblast) strain (Meruvax-II, Merck) was licensed and all other strains were discontinued.

Rubella Vaccine

Vaccine	Trade Name	Licensure	Discontinued
HPV-77:DE5	Meruvax	1969	1979
HPV-77:DK12	Rubelogen	1969	1979
GMK-3:RK53	Cendevax	1969	1979
RA 27/3*	Meruvax II	1979	Still in use

*Only vaccine currently licensed in U.S.

Characteristics

The RA 27/3 rubella vaccine is a live attenuated virus. It was first isolated in 1965 at the Wistar Institute from a rubella-infected aborted fetus. The virus was attenuated by 25–30 passages in tissue culture, using human diploid fibroblasts. It does not contain duck, chicken or egg protein.

Vaccine virus is not communicable except in the setting of breastfeeding (see Contraindications Section), even though virus may be cultured from the nasopharynx of vaccinees.

Rubella vaccine is available combined with measles and mumps vaccines as MMR, or combined with mumps, measles, and varicella vaccine as MMRV (ProQuad). The Advisory Committee on Immunization Practices (ACIP) recommends that combined measles-mumps-rubella vaccine (MMR) be used when any of the individual components is indicated. Single-antigen rubella vaccine is not available in the U.S.

MMR and MMRV are supplied as a lyophylized (freeze-dried) powder and are reconstituted with sterile, preservative-free water. The vaccines contains a small amount of human albumin, neomycin, sorbitol, and gelatin.

Immunogenicity and Vaccine Efficacy

RA 27/3 rubella vaccine is safe and more immunogenic than rubella vaccines used previously. In clinical trials, 95% or more of vaccinees aged 12 months and older developed serologic evidence of rubella immunity after a single dose. More than 90% of vaccinated persons have protection against both clinical rubella and viremia for at least 15 years. Follow-up studies indicate that one dose of vaccine confers long-term, probably lifelong, protection. Seroconversion rates are similar for single-antigen rubella vaccine, MMR, and MMRV.

Several reports indicate that viremic reinfection following exposure may occur in vaccinated persons who have low levels of detectable antibody. The frequency and consequences of this phenomenon are unknown, but it is believed to be uncommon. Rarely, clinical reinfection and fetal infection have been reported among women with vaccine-induced immunity. Rare cases of CRS have occurred among infants born to women who had documented serologic evidence of rubella immunity before they became pregnant.

Vaccination Schedule and Use

At least one dose of rubella-containing vaccine, as combination MMR (or MMRV) vaccine, is routinely recommended for all children 12 months of age or older. MMRV is approved for ages 12 months through 12

Rubella Vaccine

- Composition
  - live virus (RA 27/3 strain)
- Efficacy
  - 95% or more
- Duration of Immunity
  - lifelong
- Schedule
  - at least 1 dose
- Should be administered with measles and mumps as MMR or with measles, mumps and varicella as MMRV

20

Rubella

Rubella Vaccine (MMR)
Indications

- All infants 12 months of age and older
- Susceptible adolescents and adults without documented evidence of rubella immunity
- Emphasis on nonpregnant women of childbearing age, particularly those born outside the U.S.
- Emphasis on males and females in college, places of employment, and health care settings

years (that is, until the 13th birthday) and should not be adminstered to persons 13 years or older. All persons born during or after 1957 should have documentation of at least one dose of MMR. The first dose of MMR should be given on or after the first birthday. Any dose of rubella-containing vaccine given before 12 months of age should not be counted as part of the series. Children vaccinated with rubella-containing vaccine before 12 months of age should be revaccinated when the child is at least 12 months of age.

A second dose of MMR is recommended to produce immunity to measles and mumps in those who failed to respond to the first dose. Data indicate that almost all persons who do not respond to the measles component of the first dose will respond to a second dose of MMR. Few data on the immune response to the rubella and mumps components of a second dose of MMR are available. However, most persons who do not respond to the rubella or mumps component of the first MMR dose would be expected to respond to the second dose. The second dose is not generally considered a booster dose because a primary immune response to the first dose provides long-term protection. Although a second dose of vaccine may increase antibody titers in some persons who responded to the first dose, available data indicate that these increased antibody titers are not sustained. The combined MMR vaccine is recommended for both doses to ensure immunity to all three viruses.

The second dose of MMR vaccine should routinely be given at age 4 through 6 years, before a child enters kindergarten or first grade. The recommended health visit at age 11 or 12 years can serve as a catch-up opportunity to verify vaccination status and administer MMR vaccine to those children who have not yet received two doses of MMR (with the first dose administered no earlier than the first birthday). The second dose of MMR may be administered as soon as 1 month (i.e., minimum of 28 days) after the first dose. The minimum interval between doses of MMRV is 3 months.

All older children not previously immunized should receive at least one dose of rubella vaccine as MMR or MMRV if 12 years of age or younger.

Adults born in 1957 or later who do not have a medical contraindication should receive at least one dose of MMR vaccine unless they have documentation of vaccination with at least one dose of measles-, mumps-, and rubella-containing vaccine or other acceptable evidence of immunity to these three diseases. Some adults at high risk of measles and mumps exposure may require a second dose. This second dose should be administered as combined MMR vaccine (see Measles chapter for details). Efforts should be made to identify and vaccinate susceptible adolescents and adults, particularly women of childbearing age who are not pregnant. Particular emphasis should be placed on vaccinating both males and females in colleges, places of employment, and healthcare settings.

Only doses of vaccine with written documentation of the date of receipt should be accepted as valid. Self-reported doses or a parental report of vaccination is not considered adequate documentation. A healthcare provider should not provide an immunization record for a patient unless that healthcare provider has administered the vaccine or has seen a record that documents vaccination. Persons who lack adequate documentation of vaccination or other acceptable evidence of immunity should be vaccinated. Vaccination status and receipt of all vaccinations should be documented in the patient's permanent medical record and in a vaccination record held by the individual.

For the first dose of measles, mumps, rubella, and varicella vaccines at age 12 through 47 months, either MMR vaccine and varicella vaccine or MMRV vaccine may be used. Providers who are considering administering MMRV vaccine should discuss the benefits and risks of both vaccination options with the parents or caregivers. Unless the parent or caregiver expresses a preference for MMRV vaccine, CDC recommends that MMR vaccine and varicella vaccine should be administered for the first dose in this age group. For the second dose of measles, mumps, rubella, and varicella vaccines at any age (15 months through 12 years) and for the first dose at 48 months of age or older, use of MMRV vaccine generally is preferred over separate injections of its equivalent component vaccines (i.e., MMR vaccine and varicella vaccine).

Rubella Immunity

Persons generally can be considered immune to rubella if they have documentation of vaccination with at least one dose of MMR (or MMRV) or other live rubella-containing vaccine administered on or after their first birthday, have serologic evidence of rubella immunity, or were born before 1957. Persons who have an "equivocal" serologic test result should be considered rubella-susceptible. Although only one dose of rubella-containing vaccine is required as acceptable evidence of immunity to rubella, children should receive two doses of MMR vaccine according to the routine childhood vaccination schedule.

Birth before 1957 provides only presumptive evidence of rubella immunity; it does not guarantee that a person is immune to rubella. Because rubella can occur in some

20

Rubella Immunity

- Documentation of one dose of rubella-containing vaccine on or after the first birthday

- Serologic evidence of immunity

- Birth before 1957 (except women of childbearing age)

- Birth before 1957 is not acceptable evidence of rubella immunity for women who might become pregnant

- Only serology or documented vaccination should be accepted

Rubella

unvaccinated persons born before 1957 and because congenital rubella and congenital rubella syndrome can occur in the offspring of women infected with rubella during pregnancy, birth before 1957 is not acceptable evidence of rubella immunity for women who might become pregnant. Only a positive serologic test for rubella antibody or documentation of appropriate vaccination should be accepted for women who may become pregnant.

Healthcare personnel born before 1957 also should not be presumed to be immune. Medical facilities should consider recommending at least one dose of MMR vaccine to unvaccinated healthcare personnel born before 1957 who do not have laboratory evidence of rubella immunity. Rubella vaccination or laboratory evidence of rubella immunity is particularly important for healthcare personnel who could become pregnant, including those born before 1957. This recommendation is based on serologic studies which indicate that among hospital personnel born before 1957, 5% to 9% had no detectable measles antibody.

Clinical diagnosis of rubella is unreliable and should not be considered in assessing immune status. Because many rash illnesses may mimic rubella infection and many rubella infections are unrecognized, the only reliable evidence of previous rubella infection is the presence of serum rubella IgG antibody. Laboratories that regularly perform antibody testing are generally the most reliable because their reagents and procedures are strictly standardized.

Serologic screening need not be done before vaccinating for measles and rubella unless the medical facility considers it cost-effective. Serologic testing is appropriate only if tracking systems are used to ensure that tested persons who are identified as susceptible are subsequently vaccinated in a timely manner. If the return and timely vaccination of those screened cannot be assured, vaccination should be done without prior testing. Serologic testing for immunity to measles and rubella is not necessary for persons documented to be appropriately vaccinated or who have other acceptable evidence of immunity.

Neither rubella vaccine nor immune globulin is effective for postexposure prophylaxis of rubella. Vaccination after exposure is not harmful and may possibly avert later disease.

Contraindications and Precautions to Vaccination

Contraindications for MMR and MMRV vaccines include history of anaphylactic reactions to neomycin, history of severe allergic reaction to any component of the vaccine, and immunosuppression. Women known to be pregnant or attempting to become pregnant should not receive rubella

---

MMR Vaccine Contraindications and Precautions

- History of anaphylactic reactions to neomycin
- History of severe allergic reaction to any component of the vaccine
- Pregnancy
- Immunosuppression
- Moderate or severe acute illness
- Recent blood product
- Personal or family (i.e., sibling or parent) history of seizures of any etiology (MMRV only)

vaccine. Although there is no evidence that rubella vaccine virus causes fetal damage, pregnancy should be avoided for 4 weeks (28 days) after rubella or MMR vaccination.

Persons with immunodeficiency or immunosuppression, resulting from leukemia, lymphoma, generalized malignancy, immune deficiency disease, or immunosuppressive therapy should not be vaccinated. However, treatment with low-dose (less than 2 mg/kg/day), alternate-day, topical, or aerosolized steroid preparations is not a contraindication to rubella vaccination. Persons whose immunosuppressive therapy with steroids has been discontinued for 1 month (3 months for chemotherapy) may be vaccinated. Rubella vaccine should be considered for persons with asymptomatic or mildly symptomatic HIV infection. See Measles chapter for additional details on vaccination of immunosuppressed persons, including those with human immunodeficiency virus infection.

Persons with moderate or severe acute illness should not be vaccinated until the illness has improved. Minor illness (e.g., otitis media, mild upper respiratory infections), concurrent antibiotic therapy, and exposure or recovery from other illnesses are not contraindications to rubella vaccination.

Receipt of antibody-containing blood products (e.g., immune globulin, whole blood or packed red blood cells, intravenous immune globulin) may interfere with seroconversion to rubella vaccine. Vaccine should be given 2 weeks before, or deferred for at least 3 months following administration of an antibody-containing blood product. If rubella vaccine is given as combined MMR, a longer delay may be necessary before vaccination. For more information, see Chapter 2, General Recommendations on Immunization.

Previous administration of human anti-Rho(D) immune globulin (RhoGam) does not generally interfere with an immune response to rubella vaccine and is not a contra-indication to postpartum vaccination. However, women who have received anti-Rho immune globulin should be serologically tested 6–8 weeks after vaccination to ensure that seroconversion has occurred.

A personal or family (i.e., sibling or parent) history of seizures of any etiology is a precaution for MMRV vaccination. Studies suggest that children who have a personal or family history of febrile seizures or family history of epilepsy are at increased risk for febrile seizures compared with children without such histories. Children with a personal or family history of seizures of any etiology generally should be vaccinated with MMR vaccine and varicella vaccine (for the first dose) because the risks for using MMRV vaccine in this group of children generally outweigh the benefits.

20

Rubella

Although vaccine virus may be isolated from the pharynx, vaccinees do not transmit rubella to others, except occasionally in the case of the vaccinated breastfeeding woman. In this situation, the infant may be infected, presumably through breast milk, and may develop a mild rash illness, but serious effects have not been reported. Infants infected through breastfeeding have been shown to respond normally to rubella vaccination at 12–15 months of age. Breastfeeding is not a contraindication to rubella vaccination and does not alter rubella vaccination recommendations.

Adverse Events Following Vaccination

Rubella vaccine is very safe. Most adverse events reported following MMR vaccination (such as fever and rash) are attributable to the measles component. Data from studies in the United States and experience from other countries using the RA 27/3 strain rubella vaccine have not supported an association between the vaccine and chronic arthritis. The Institute of Medicine found that evidence was inadequate to accept or reject a causal relationship between MMR vaccine and chronic arthralgia or arthritis in women. Rarely, transient peripheral neuritic complaints, such as paresthesias and pain in the arms and legs, have been reported. One study among 958 seronegative immunized and 932 seronegative unimmunized women aged 15–39 years found no association between rubella vaccination and development of recurrent joint symptoms, neuropathy, or collagen disease.

Adverse Reactions Following Vaccination

The most common complaints following rubella vaccination are fever, lymphadenopathy, and arthralgia. These reactions only occur in susceptible persons and are more common in adults, especially in women.

Joint symptoms, such as arthralgia (joint pain) and arthritis (joint redness and/or swelling), are associated with the rubella component of MMR. Arthralgia and transient arthritis occur more frequently in susceptible adults than in children and more frequently in susceptible women than in men. Acute arthralgia or arthritis is rare following vaccination of children with RA 27/3 vaccine. By contrast, approximately 25% of susceptible postpubertal females develop acute arthralgia following RA 27/3 vaccination, and approximately 10% have been reported to have acute arthritis-like signs and symptoms.

When acute joint symptoms occur, or when pain or paresthesias not associated with joints occur, the symptoms

---

MMR Adverse Events
- Fever
- Rash
- Chronic arthralgias
- Chronic arthritis
- Transient peripheral neuritic complaints
- Recurrent joint symptoms
- Collagen disease

MMR Adverse Reactions
- Fever
- Lymphadenopathy
- Arthralgia – associated with rubella component
- Arthritis- associated with rubella component
- Pain, paresthesia – begins 1-3 weeks after vaccination, persist for 1 day to three weeks, and rarely recurs

Rubella Vaccine Arthropathy
- Acute arthralgia in about 25% of vaccinated, susceptible adult women
- Acute arthritis-like signs and symptoms occurs in about 10% of recipients
- Rare reports of chronic or persistent symptoms

generally begin 1–3 weeks after vaccination, persist for 1 day to 3 weeks, and rarely recur. Adults with acute joint symptoms following rubella vaccination rarely have had to disrupt work activities.

The ACIP continues to recommend the vaccination of all adult women who do not have evidence of rubella immunity.

See the Measles and Varicella chapters for information about adverse reactions following MMRV vaccine.

Rubella Vaccination of Women of Childbearing Age

Women who are pregnant or who intend to become pregnant within 4 weeks should not receive rubella vaccine. ACIP recommends that vaccine providers ask a woman if she is pregnant or likely to become pregnant in the next 4 weeks. Those who are pregnant or intend to become pregnant should not be vaccinated. All other women should be vaccinated after being informed of the theoretical risks of vaccination during pregnancy and the importance of not becoming pregnant during the 4 weeks following vaccination. ACIP does not recommend routine pregnancy screening of women before rubella vaccination.

If a pregnant woman is inadvertently vaccinated or if she becomes pregnant within 4 weeks after vaccination, she should be counseled about the concern for the fetus (see below), but MMR vaccination during pregnancy should not ordinarily be a reason to consider termination of the pregnancy.

When rubella vaccine was licensed, concern existed about women being inadvertently vaccinated while they were pregnant or shortly before conception. This concern came from the known teratogenicity of the wild-virus strain. To determine whether CRS would occur in infants of such mothers, CDC maintained a registry from 1971 to 1989 of women vaccinated during pregnancy. This was called the Vaccine in Pregnancy (VIP) Registry.

Although subclinical fetal infection has been detected serologically in approximately 1%–2% of infants born to susceptible vaccinees, regardless of the vaccine strain, the data collected by CDC in the VIP Registry showed no evidence of CRS occurring in offspring of the 321 susceptible women who received rubella vaccine and who continued pregnancy to term. The observed risk of vaccine-induced malformation was 0%, with a maximum theoretical risk of 1.6%, based on 95% confidence limits (1.2% for all types of rubella vaccine). Since the risk of the vaccine to the fetus appears to be extremely low, if it exists at all, routine

---

Vaccination of Women of Childbearing Age

- Ask if pregnant or likely to become so in next 4 weeks
- Exclude those who say "yes"
- For others
  - explain theoretical risks
  - vaccinate

Vaccination in Pregnancy Study 1971-1989

- 321 women vaccinated
- 324 live births
- No observed CRS
- Maximum theoretical risk of 1.6%, based on confidence limits (1.2% for all types of rubella vaccine)

20

termination of pregnancy is not recommended. Individual counseling for these women is recommended. As of April 30, 1989, CDC discontinued the VIP registry.

The ACIP continues to state that because of the small theoretical risk to the fetus of a vaccinated woman, pregnant women should not be vaccinated.

Vaccine Storage and Handling

MMR vaccine can be stored either in the freezer or the refrigerator and should be protected from light at all times. MMRV vaccine should be stored frozen between -58°F and +5°F (-50°C to -15°C). When MMR vaccine is stored in the freezer, the temperature should be the same as that required for MMRV, between -58°F and +5°F (-50°C to -15°C). Storing MMR in the freezer with MMRV may help prevent inadvertent storage of MMRV in the refrigerator.

Manufacturer package inserts contain additional information and can be found at http://www.fda.gov/BiologicsBloodVaccines/Vaccines/ApprovedProducts/ucm093830.htm. For complete information on best practices and recommendations please refer to CDC's Vaccine Storage and Handling Toolkit, http://www.cdc.gov/vaccines/recs/storage/toolkit/storage-handling-toolkit.pdf.

Strategies to Decrease Rubella and CRS
Vaccination of Susceptible Postpubertal Females

Elimination of indigenous rubella and CRS can be maintained by continuing efforts to vaccinate susceptible adolescents and young adults of childbearing age, particularly those born outside the United States. These efforts should include vaccinating in family planning clinics, sexually transmitted disease (STD) clinics, and as part of routine gynecologic care; maximizing use of premarital serology results; emphasizing immunization for college students; vaccinating women postpartum and postabortion; immunizing prison staff and, when possible, prison inmates, especially women inmates; offering vaccination to at-risk women through the special supplemental program for Women, Infants and Children (WIC); and implementing vaccination programs in the workplace, particularly those employing persons born outside the United States.

Hospital Rubella Programs

Emphasis should be placed on vaccinating susceptible hospital personnel, both male and female (e.g., volunteers, trainees, nurses, physicians.) Ideally, all hospital employees should be immune. It is important to note that screening programs alone are not adequate. Vaccination of susceptible staff must follow.

Acknowledgement

The editors thank Drs. Greg Wallace, and Zaney Leroy, CDC for their assistance in updating this chapter.

Selected References

American Academy of Pediatrics. Rubella. In: Pickering L, Baker C, Kimberlin D, Long S, eds. *Red Book: 2009 Report of the Committee on Infectious Diseases*. 28th ed. Elk Grove Village, IL: American Academy of Pediatrics, 2009:579–84.

CDC. Measles, mumps, and rubella—vaccine use and strategies for elimination of measles, rubella, and congenital rubella syndrome and control of mumps. Recommendations of the Advisory Committee on Immunization Practices (ACIP). *MMWR* 1998;47(No. RR-8):1–57.

CDC. Immunization of health-care personnel. Recommendations of the Advisory Committee on Immunization Practices (ACIP). *MMWR* 2011;60(RR-7):1–45.

CDC. Control and prevention of rubella: evaluation and management of suspected outbreaks, rubella in pregnant women, and surveillance for congenital rubella syndrome. *MMWR* 2001;50(No. RR-12):1–30.

CDC. Rubella vaccination during pregnancy—United States, 1971–1988. *MMWR* 1989;38:289–93.

CDC. Notice to readers. Revised ACIP recommendations for avoiding pregnancy after receiving rubella-containing vaccine. *MMWR* 2001;50:1117.

CDC. Use of combination measles, mumps, rubella, and varicella vaccine: recommendations of the Advisory Committee on Immunization Practices (ACIP). *MMWR* 2010;59(No. RR-3):1–12.

Frenkel LM, Nielsen K, Garakian A, et al. A search for persistent rubella virus infection in persons with chronic symptoms after rubella and rubella immunization and in patients with juvenile rheumatoid arthritis. *Clin Infect Dis* 1996;22:287–94.

Mellinger AK, Cragan JD, Atkinson WL, et al. High incidence of congenital rubella syndrome after a rubella outbreak. *Pediatr Infect Dis J* 1995;14:573–78.

Orenstein WA, Hadler S, Wharton M. Trends in vaccine-preventable diseases. *Semin Pediatr Infect Dis* 1997;8:23–33.

Reef SE, Frey TK, Theall K, et al. The changing epidemiology of rubella in the 1990s. *JAMA* 2002;287:464–72.

20

Rubella

Institute of Medicine. 2012. Adverse Events of Vaccines: Evidence and Causality. Washington D.C. : The National Academies Press.

Tetanus is an acute, often fatal, disease caused by an exotoxin produced by the bacterium *Clostridium tetani*. It is characterized by generalized rigidity and convulsive spasms of skeletal muscles. The muscle stiffness usually involves the jaw (lockjaw) and neck and then becomes generalized.

Although records from antiquity (5th century BCE) contain clinical descriptions of tetanus, it was Carle and Rattone in 1884 who first produced tetanus in animals by injecting them with pus from a fatal human tetanus case. During the same year, Nicolaier produced tetanus in animals by injecting them with samples of soil. In 1889, Kitasato isolated the organism from a human victim, showed that it produced disease when injected into animals, and reported that the toxin could be neutralized by specific antibodies. In 1897, Nocard demonstrated the protective effect of passively transferred antitoxin, and passive immunization in humans was used for treatment and prophylaxis during World War I. A method for inactivating tetanus toxin with formaldehyde was developed by Ramon in the early 1920's which led to the development of tetanus toxoid by Descombey in 1924. It was first widely used during World War II.

> **Tetanus**
> - Etiology discovered in 1884 by Carle and Rattone
> - Passive immunization used for treatment and prophylaxis during World War I
> - Tetanus toxoid first widely used during World War II

Clostridium tetani

C. tetani is a slender, gram-positive, anaerobic rod that may develop a terminal spore, giving it a drumstick appearance. The organism is sensitive to heat and cannot survive in the presence of oxygen. The spores, in contrast, are very resistant to heat and the usual antiseptics. They can survive autoclaving at 249.8°F (121°C) for 10–15 minutes. The spores are also relatively resistant to phenol and other chemical agents.

The spores are widely distributed in soil and in the intestines and feces of horses, sheep, cattle, dogs, cats, rats, guinea pigs, and chickens. Manure-treated soil may contain large numbers of spores. In agricultural areas, a significant number of human adults may harbor the organism. The spores can also be found on skin surfaces and in contaminated heroin.

C. tetani produces two exotoxins, tetanolysin and tetanospasmin. The function of tetanolysin is not known with certainty. Tetanospasmin is a neurotoxin and causes the clinical manifestations of tetanus. On the basis of weight, tetanospasmin is one of the most potent toxins known. The estimated minimum human lethal dose is 2.5 nanograms per kilogram of body weight (a nanogram is one billionth of a gram), or 175 nanograms for a 70-kg (154lb) human.

> **Clostridium tetani**
> - Anaerobic gram-positive, spore-forming bacteria
> - Spores found in soil, animal feces
> - Two exotoxins produced with growth of bacteria
> - Tetanospasmin estimated human lethal dose = 2.5 ng/kg

21

Tetanus

Tetanus Pathogenesis

- Anaerobic conditions allow germination of spores and production of toxins
- Toxin binds in central nervous system
- Interferes with neurotransmitter release to block inhibitor impulses
- Leads to unopposed muscle contraction and spasm

Tetanus Clinical Features

- Incubation period; 8 days (range, 3-21 days)
- Three clinical forms: local (uncommon), cephalic (rare), generalized (most common)
- Generalized tetanus: descending pattern of trismus (lockjaw), stiffness of the neck, difficulty swallowing, rigidity of abdominal muscles
  - spasms continue for 3-4 weeks
  - complete recovery may take months

Neonatal Tetanus

- Generalized tetanus in newborn infant
- Infant born without protective passive immunity
- 58,000 neonates died in 2010 worldwide

21

Pathogenesis

C. tetani usually enters the body through a wound. In the presence of anaerobic (low oxygen) conditions, the spores germinate. Toxins are produced and disseminated via blood and lymphatics. Toxins act at several sites within the central nervous system, including peripheral motor end plates, spinal cord, and brain, and in the sympathetic nervous system. The typical clinical manifestations of tetanus are caused when tetanus toxin interferes with release of neurotransmitters, blocking inhibitor impulses. This leads to unopposed muscle contraction and spasm. Seizures may occur, and the autonomic nervous system may also be affected.

Clinical Features

The incubation period ranges from 3 to 21 days, usually about 8 days. In general the further the injury site is from the central nervous system, the longer is the incubation period. Shorter incubation periods are associated with a higher chance of death. In neonatal tetanus, symptoms usually appear from 4 to 14 days after birth, averaging about 7 days.

On the basis of clinical findings, three different forms of tetanus have been described.

Local tetanus is an uncommon form of the disease, in which patients have persistent contraction of muscles in the same anatomic area as the injury. These contractions may persist for many weeks before gradually subsiding. Local tetanus may precede the onset of generalized tetanus but is generally milder. Only about 1% of cases are fatal.

Cephalic tetanus is a rare form of the disease, occasionally occurring with otitis media (ear infections) in which *C. tetani* is present in the flora of the middle ear, or following injuries to the head. There is involvement of the cranial nerves, especially in the facial area.

The most common type (about 80%) of reported tetanus is generalized tetanus. The disease usually presents with a descending pattern. The first sign is trismus or lockjaw, followed by stiffness of the neck, difficulty in swallowing, and rigidity of abdominal muscles. Other symptoms include elevated temperature, sweating, elevated blood pressure, and episodic rapid heart rate. Spasms may occur frequently and last for several minutes. Spasms continue for 3–4 weeks. Complete recovery may take months.

Neonatal tetanus (NT) is a form of generalized tetanus that occurs in newborn infants. Neonatal tetanus occurs in infants born without protective passive immunity, because the mother is not immune. It usually occurs through infection of the unhealed umbilical stump, particularly when the stump is cut with an unsterile instrument. Neonatal tetanus is common in some developing countries but very rare in the United States. World Health Organization (WHO) estimates that in 2010, 58,000 newborns died from NT, a 93% reduction from the situation in the late 1980s.

Complications

Laryngospasm (spasm of the vocal cords) and/or spasm of the muscles of respiration leads to interference with breathing. Fractures of the spine or long bones may result from sustained contractions and convulsions. Hyperactivity of the autonomic nervous system may lead to hypertension and/or an abnormal heart rhythm.

Nosocomial infections are common because of prolonged hospitalization. Secondary infections may include sepsis from indwelling catheters, hospital-acquired pneumonias, and decubitus ulcers. Pulmonary embolism is particularly a problem in drug users and elderly patients. Aspiration pneumonia is a common late complication of tetanus, found in 50%–70% of autopsied cases. In recent years, tetanus has been fatal in approximately 11% of reported cases. Cases most likely to be fatal are those occurring in persons 60 years of age and older (18%) and unvaccinated persons (22%). In about 20% of tetanus deaths, no obvious pathology is identified and death is attributed to the direct effects of tetanus toxin.

Laboratory Diagnosis

No laboratory findings are characteristic of tetanus. The diagnosis is entirely clinical and does not depend upon bacteriologic confirmation. *C. tetani* is recovered from the wound in only 30% of cases and can be isolated from patients who do not have tetanus. Laboratory identification of the organism depends most importantly on the demonstration of toxin production in mice.

Medical Management

All wounds should be cleaned. Necrotic tissue and foreign material should be removed. If tetanic spasms are occurring, supportive therapy and maintenance of an adequate airway are critical.

Tetanus immune globulin (TIG) is recommended for persons with tetanus. TIG can only help remove unbound tetanus toxin. It cannot affect toxin bound to nerve endings. A single intramuscular dose of 500 units is generally recommended for children and adults, with part of the dose infiltrated

> ### Tetanus Complications
> - Laryngospasm
> - Fractures
> - Hypertension and/or abnormal heart rhythm
> - Nosocomial infections
> - Pulmonary embolism
> - Aspiration pneumonia
> - Death

21

Tetanus

around the wound if it can be identified. Intravenous immune globulin (IVIG) contains tetanus antitoxin and may be used if TIG is not available.

Because of the extreme potency of the toxin, tetanus disease does not result in tetanus immunity. Active immunization with tetanus toxoid should begin or continue as soon as the person's condition has stabilized.

Wound Management

Antibiotic prophylaxis against tetanus is neither practical nor useful in managing wounds; proper immunization plays the more important role. The need for active immunization, with or without passive immunization, depends on the condition of the wound and the patient's immunization history (see *MMWR* 2006;55[RR-17] for details). Rarely have cases of tetanus occurred in persons with a documented primary series of tetanus toxoid.

Persons with wounds that are neither clean nor minor, and who have had fewer than 3 prior doses of tetanus toxoid or have an unknown history of prior doses should receive TIG as well as Td or Tdap. This is because early doses of toxoid may not induce immunity, but only prime the immune system. The TIG provides temporary immunity by directly providing antitoxin. This ensures that protective levels of antitoxin are achieved even if an immune response has not yet occurred.

Epidemiology
Occurrence

Tetanus occurs worldwide but is most frequently encountered in densely populated regions in hot, damp climates with soil rich in organic matter.

Reservoir

Organisms are found primarily in the soil and intestinal tracts of animals and humans.

Mode of Transmission

Transmission is primarily by contaminated wounds (apparent and inapparent). The wound may be major or minor. In recent years, however, a higher proportion of patients had minor wounds, probably because severe wounds are more likely to be properly managed. Tetanus may follow elective surgery, burns, deep puncture wounds, crush wounds, otitis media (ear infections), dental infection, animal bites, abortion, and pregnancy.

Tetanus Wound Management

Vaccination History	Clean, minor wounds		All other wounds*	
	Tdap or Td[†]	TIG	Tdap or Td[†]	TIG
Unknown or fewer than 3 doses	Yes	No	Yes	Yes
3 or more doses	No[§]	No	No[¶]	No

*Such as, but not limited to, wounds contaminated with dirt, feces, soil, and saliva; puncture wounds; avulsions; and wounds resulting from missiles, crushing, burns, and frostbite.

[†]Tdap is preferred to Td for adults who have never received Tdap. Single antigen tetanus toxoid (TT) is no longer available in the United States.

[§]Yes, if more than ten years since the last tetanus toxoid-containing vaccine dose.

[¶]Yes, if more than five years since the last tetanus toxoid-containing vaccine dose.

Tetanus Epidemiology

- Reservoir
  - soil and intestine of animals and humans
- Transmission
  - contaminated wounds
  - tissue injury
- Temporal pattern
  - peak in summer or wet season
- Communicability
  - not contagious

21

Communicability

Tetanus is not contagious from person to person. It is the only vaccine-preventable disease that is infectious but not contagious.

Secular Trends in the United States

A marked decrease in mortality from tetanus occurred from the early 1900s to the late 1940s. In the late 1940s, tetanus toxoid was introduced into routine childhood immunization and tetanus became nationally notifiable. At that time, 500–600 cases (approximately 0.4 cases per 100,000 population) were reported per year.

After the 1940s, reported tetanus incidence rates declined steadily. Since the mid-1970s, 50–100 cases (~0.05 cases per 100,000) have been reported annually. From 2000 through 2007 an average of 31 cases were reported per year. The death-to-case ratio has declined from 30% to approximately 10% in recent years. An all-time low of 18 cases (0.01 cases per 100,000) was reported in 2009.

During 2001 through 2008, the last years for which data have been compiled, a total of 233 tetanus cases were reported, an average of 29 cases per year. Among the 197 cases with known outcomes the case-fatality rate was 13%. Age of onset was reported for all 233 cases, of which, 49% were among persons 50 years of age or older. The median age was 49 years (range 5-94 years). A total of 138 (59%) were male. Incidence was similar among races. The incidence among Hispanics was almost twice that among non-Hispanics. However, when intravenous drug users (IDUs) were excluded the incidence was almost the same among Hispanics and non-Hispanics. Between 18 and 37 cases of tetanus were reported annually in the United States between 2009 and 2012 (average 29 cases per year).

Almost all reported cases of tetanus are in persons who have either never been vaccinated, or who completed a primary series but have not had a booster in the preceding 10 years.

Heroin users, particularly persons who inject themselves subcutaneously, appear to be at high risk for tetanus. Quinine is used to dilute heroin and may support the growth of *C. tetani*.

Neonatal tetanus is rare in the United States, with only two cases reported since 1989. Neither of the infants' mothers had ever received tetanus toxoid.

Tetanus toxoid vaccination status was reported for 92 (40%) of the 233 patients. Thirty-seven patients (41%) had never received a tetanus toxoid-containing product, 26 (28%)

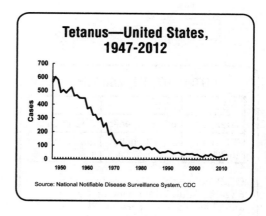

Tetanus—United States, 1947-2012

Source: National Notifiable Disease Surveillance System, CDC

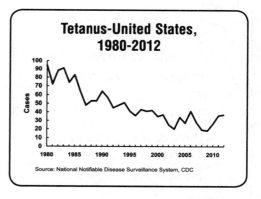

Tetanus-United States, 1980-2012

Source: National Notifiable Disease Surveillance System, CDC

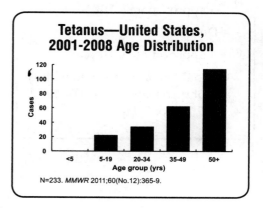

Tetanus—United States, 2001-2008 Age Distribution

N=233. *MMWR* 2011;60(No.12):365-9.

21

Tetanus

had received 1 dose, five (5%) had received 3 doses, and 24 (26%) had received 4 or more doses. Seven (24%) of 29 patients with 3 or more doses had received their last dose within the previous 10 years, 18 (62%) between 10 and 54 years previously, and four (14%) reported an unknown interval since their last dose.

Among 195 patients whose medical history was known, 30 (15%) were reported to have diabetes. Twenty-seven (15%) of 176 patients whose status was known were IDUs, of whom 16 (59%) were Hispanic. An acute wound preceded disease onset in 167 (72%) patients. Of those patients' wounds, 132 (79%) were either punctures or contaminated, infected, or devitalized wounds considered tetanus-prone and eligible to receive TIG. Case reports for 51 (84%) of those who sought care were sufficiently complete to evaluate prophylaxis received; 49 (96%) did not receive appropriate tetanus toxoid prophylaxis or tetanus toxoid plus TIG, as is currently recommended. Among all 233 patients, 31 (13%) reported a chronic wound or infection (e.g., diabetic ulcer or dental abscess) before disease onset. Twenty-two (9%) reported no wounds or infections. Of these, 14 were IDUs.

Tetanus Toxoid
Characteristics

Tetanus toxoid was first produced in 1924, and tetanus toxoid immunizations were used extensively in the armed services during World War II. Tetanus cases among this population declined from 70 in World War I (13.4/100,000 wounds and injuries) to 12 in World War II (0.44/100,000). Of the 12 case-patients, half had received no prior toxoid.

Tetanus toxoid consists of a formaldehyde-treated toxin. The toxoid is standardized for potency in animal tests according to Food and Drug Administration (FDA) regulations. Occasionally, potency is mistakenly equated with Lf units, which are a measure of the quantity of toxoid, not its potency in inducing protection.

There are two types of toxoid available—adsorbed (aluminum salt precipitated) toxoid and fluid toxoid. Although the rates of seroconversion are about equal, the adsorbed toxoid is preferred because the antitoxin response reaches higher titers and is longer lasting than that following the fluid toxoid.

Tetanus toxoid is available combined with diphtheria toxoid as pediatric diphtheria-tetanus toxoid (DT) or adult tetanus-diphtheria (Td), and with both diphtheria toxoid and acellular pertussis vaccine as DTaP or Tdap. Tetanus toxoid is also available as combined DTaP-HepB-IPV (Pediarix) and DTaP-IPV/Hib (Pentacel) —see Pertussis

---

DTaP, DT, Td, and Tdap

Type	Diphtheria	Tetanus
DTaP, DT	6.7-25 Lf units	5-10 Lf units
Td, Tdap (adults)	2-2.5 Lf units	2-5 Lf units

DTaP and pediatric DT used through age 6 years. Adult Td for persons 7 years and older. Tdap for persons 10 years and older (Boostrix) or 10 through 64 years (Adacel)

Tetanus Toxoid

- Formalin-inactivated tetanus toxin
- Schedule
  - three or four doses plus booster
  - booster every 10 years
- Efficacy
  - approximately 100%
- Duration
  - approximately 10 years
- Should be administered with diphtheria toxoid as DTaP, DT, Td, or Tdap

chapter for more information. Pediatric formulations (DT and DTaP) contain a similar amount of tetanus toxoid as adult Td, but contain 3 to 4 times as much diphtheria toxoid. Children younger than 7 years of age should receive either DTaP or pediatric DT. Persons 7 years of age or older should receive the adult formulation (adult Td), even if they have not completed a series of DTaP or pediatric DT. Tetanus toxoid is given in combination with diphtheria toxoid, since periodic boosting is needed for both antigens. Two brands of Tdap are available: Boostrix (approved for persons 10 and older) and Adacel (approved for persons 10 through 64 years of age). DTaP and Tdap vaccines do not contain thimerosal as a preservative.

Immunogenicity and Vaccine Efficacy

After a primary series (three properly spaced doses of tetanus toxoid in persons 7 years of age and older, or four doses in children younger than 7 years of age) essentially all recipients achieve antitoxin levels considerably greater than the protective level of 0.1 IU/mL.

Efficacy of the toxoid has never been studied in a vaccine trial. It can be inferred from protective antitoxin levels that a complete tetanus toxoid series has a clinical efficacy of virtually 100%; cases of tetanus occurring in fully immunized persons whose last dose was within the last 10 years are extremely rare.

Antitoxin levels decrease with time. While some persons may be protected for life, by 10 years after the last dose, most persons have antitoxin levels that only approach the minimal protective level. As a result, routine boosters are recommended every 10 years.

In a small percentage of individuals, antitoxin levels fall below the minimal protective level before 10 years have elapsed. To ensure adequate protective antitoxin levels, persons who sustain a wound that is other than clean and minor should receive a tetanus booster if more than 5 years have elapsed since their last dose. (See Wound Management for details on persons who previously received less than three doses).

Vaccination Schedule and Use

DTaP (diphtheria and tetanus toxoids and acellular pertussis vaccine) is the vaccine of choice for children 6 weeks through 6 years of age. The usual schedule is a primary series of four doses at 2, 4, 6, and 15–18 months of age. The first, second, and third doses of DTaP should be separated by a minimum of 4 weeks. The fourth dose should follow the third dose by no less than 6 months and should not be administered before 12 months of age.

21

Routine DTaP Primary Vaccination Schedule

Dose	Age	Interval
Primary 1	2 months	---
Primary 2	4 months	4 weeks
Primary 3	6 months	4 weeks
Primary 4	15-18 months	6 months

Children Who Receive DT

- The number of doses of DT needed to complete the series depends on the child's age at the first dose:
  - if first dose given at younger than 12 months of age, 4 doses are recommended
  - if first dose given at 12 months or older, 3 doses complete the primary series

Tetanus

If a child has a valid contraindication to pertussis vaccine, pediatric DT should be used to complete the vaccination series. If the child was younger than 12 months old when the first dose of DT was administered (as DTaP or DT), the child should receive a total of four primary DT doses. If the child was 12 months of age or older at the time that the first dose of DT was administered, three doses (third dose 6–12 months after the second) completes the primary DT series.

If the fourth dose of DTaP, DTP, or DT is administered before the fourth birthday, a booster dose is recommended at 4–6 years of age. The fifth dose is not required if the fourth dose was given on or after the fourth birthday.

Because of waning antitoxin titers, most persons have antitoxin levels below the optimal level 10 years after the last dose of DTaP, DTP, DT, or Td. Additional booster doses of tetanus and diphtheria toxoids are required every 10 years to maintain protective antitoxin titers. The first booster dose of Td may be given at 11 or 12 years of age if at least 5 years have elapsed since the last dose of DTaP, DTP, or DT. The Advisory Committee on Immunization Practices (ACIP) recommends that this dose be administered as Tdap. If a dose is given sooner as part of wound management, the next booster is not needed for 10 years thereafter. More frequent boosters are not indicated and have been reported to result in an increased incidence and severity of local adverse reactions.

Tetanus, Diphtheria and Pertussis Booster Doses

- 4 through 6 years of age, before entering school (DTaP)
- 11 or 12 years of age (Tdap)
- Every 10 years thereafter (Td)

Routine Td Schedule Unvaccinated Persons 7 Years of Age or Older

Dose*	Interval
Primary 1	---
Primary 2	4 weeks
Primary 3	6 to 12 months
Booster dose every 10 years	

*ACIP recommends that one of these doses (preferably the first) be administered as Tdap

Td is the vaccine of choice for children 7 years and older and for adults. A primary series is three or four doses, depending on whether the person has received prior doses of diphtheria-containing vaccine and the age these doses were administered. The number of doses recommended for children who received one or more doses of DTP, DTaP, or DT before age 7 years is discussed above. For unvaccinated persons 7 years and older (including persons who cannot document prior vaccination), the primary series is three doses. The first two doses should be separated by at least 4 weeks, and the third dose given 6 to 12 months after the second. ACIP recommends that *one* of these doses (preferably the first) be administered as Tdap. A booster dose of Td should be given every 10 years. Tdap is approved for a single dose at this time (i.e., it should not be used for all the doses of Td in a previously unvaccinated person 7 years or older). Refer to the Pertussis chapter for more information about Tdap.

Interruption of the recommended schedule or delay of subsequent doses does not reduce the response to the vaccine when the series is finally completed. There is no need to restart a series regardless of the time elapsed between doses.

21

Tetanus disease does not confer immunity because of the very small amount of toxin required to produce illness. Persons recovering from tetanus should begin or complete active immunization with a tetanus toxoid-containing vaccine during convalescence.

Contraindications and Precautions to Vaccination

A severe allergic reaction (anaphylaxis) to a vaccine component or following a prior dose of tetanus toxoid is a contraindication to receipt of tetanus toxoid. If a generalized reaction is suspected to represent allergy, it may be useful to refer an individual for appropriate skin testing before discontinuing tetanus toxoid immunization. A moderate or severe acute illness is a precaution to routine vaccination, but a minor illness is not. *See Errata 9/2015.*

If a contraindication to using tetanus toxoid-containing preparations exists, passive immunization with tetanus immune globulin (TIG) should be considered whenever an injury other than a clean minor wound is sustained.

See the Pertussis chapter for additional information on contraindications and precautions to Tdap.

Adverse Events Following Vaccination

Severe systemic reactions such as generalized urticaria (hives), anaphylaxis, or neurologic complications have been reported after receipt of tetanus toxoid. A few cases of peripheral neuropathy and Guillain-Barré syndrome (GBS) have been reported following tetanus toxoid vaccine administration. A 2011 Institute of Medicine review found evidence to be inadequate to accept or reject a causal relationship between tetanus toxoid vaccine and peripheral neuropathy and GBS, and favored rejection of a causal relationship between tetanus toxoid and type 1 diabetes, and supported a causal relationship between tetanus toxoid and anaphylaxis.

Adverse Reactions Following Vaccination

Local reactions (e.g., erythema, induration, pain at the injection site) are common but are usually self-limited and require no therapy. A nodule may be palpable at the injection site of adsorbed products for several weeks. Abscess at the site of injection has been reported. Fever and other systemic symptoms are not common.

Exaggerated local (Arthus-like) reactions are not common following receipt of a diphtheria- or tetanus- containing vaccine. These reactions present as extensive painful swelling,

---

Diphtheria and Tetanus Toxoids Contraindications and Precautions

- Severe allergic reaction to vaccine component or following a prior dose
- Moderate or severe acute illness

Tetanus Toxoid Adverse Events

- Institute of Medicine favors a causal relationship
  - anaphylaxis
- Institute of Medicine rejects a causal relationship
  - type 1 diabetes
- Institute of Medicine finds evidence inadequate to support or reject a causal relationship
  - peripheral neuropathy
  - Guillain-Barré syndrome (GBS)

Diphtheria and Tetanus Toxoids Adverse Reactions

- Local reactions (erythema, induration) are common
- Fever and systemic symptoms not common
- Exaggerated local reactions (Arthus-type) occasionally reported
- Brachial neuritis

21

often from shoulder to elbow. They generally begin from 2 to 8 hours after injections and are reported most often in adults, particularly those who have received frequent doses of diphtheria or tetanus toxoid. Persons experiencing these severe reactions usually have very high serum antitoxin levels; they should not be given further routine or emergency booster doses of Td more frequently than every 10 years. Less severe local reactions may occur in persons who have multiple prior boosters.

In 1994 the Institute of Medicine concluded that the available evidence favors a causal relationship between tetanus toxoid and brachial neuritis in the 1 month after immunization at a rate of 0.5 to 1 case per 100,000 toxoid recipients.

Vaccine Storage and Handling

All tetanus-toxoid containing vaccines should be maintained at refrigerator temperature between 35°F and 46°F (2°C and 8°C). Manufacturer package inserts contain additional information and can be found at http://www.fda.gov/BiologicsBloodVaccines/Vaccines/ApprovedProducts/ucm093830.htm. For complete information on best practices and recommendations please refer to CDC's Vaccine Storage and Handling Toolkit, http://www.cdc.gov/vaccines/recs/storage/toolkit/storage-handling-toolkit.pdf.

Acknowledgment

The editors thank Drs. Gina Mootrey, Tejpratap Tiwari, and Cindy Weinbaum, CDC for their assistance in updating this chapter.

Selected References

CDC. Diphtheria, tetanus, and pertussis: Recommendations for vaccine use and other preventive measures. Recommendations of the Immunization Practices Advisory Committee (ACIP). *MMWR* 1991;40(No. RR-10):1–28.

CDC. Pertussis vaccination: use of acellular pertussis vaccines among infants and young children. Recommendations of the Advisory Committee on Immunization Practices (ACIP). *MMWR* 1997;46 (No. RR-7):1–25.

CDC. Preventing tetanus, diphtheria, and pertussis among adolescents: use of tetanus toxoid, reduced diphtheria toxoid and acellular pertussis vaccines. Recommendations of the Advisory Committee on Immunization Practices (ACIP). *MMWR* 2006;55(No. RR-3):1–34.

21

CDC. Preventing tetanus, diphtheria, and pertussis among adults: use of tetanus toxoid, reduced diphtheria toxoid and acellular pertussis vaccines. Recommendations of the Advisory Committee on Immunization Practices (ACIP) and Recommendation of ACIP, supported by the Healthcare Infection Control Practices Advisory Committee (HICPAC), for Use of Tdap Among Health-Care Personnel. *MMWR* 2006;55(No. RR-17):1–33.

CDC. Tetanus surveillance—United States, 1998–2000. *MMWR* 2003;52(No. SS-3):1–12.

CDC. Updated Recommendations for Use of Tetanus Toxoid, Reduced Diphtheria Toxoid and Acellular Pertussis (Tdap) Vaccine from the Advisory Committee on Immunization Practices, 2011. *MMWR* 2011;60(No.1): 13-15.

IOM (Institute of Medicine) 2011. Adverse Effects of Vaccines: Evidence and Causality. Washington DC: The National Academies Press

Wassilak SGF, Roper MH, Kretsinger K, Orenstein WA. Tetanus toxoid. In: Plotkin SA, Orenstein WA, Offit PA, eds. *Vaccines*. 5th ed. China: Saunders, 2008:805–39.

World Health Organization. The "high-risk" approach: the WHO-recommended strategy to accelerate elimination of neonatal tetanus. Wlky *Epidemiol Rec* 1996;71:33–36.

21

Tetanus

Varicella is an acute infectious disease caused by varicella zoster virus (VZV). The recurrent infection (herpes zoster, also known as shingles) has been recognized since ancient times. Primary varicella infection (chickenpox) was not reliably distinguished from smallpox until the end of the 19th century. In 1875, Steiner demonstrated that chickenpox was caused by an infectious agent by inoculating volunteers with the vesicular fluid from a patient with acute varicella. Clinical observations of the relationship between varicella and herpes zoster were made in 1888 by von Bokay, when children without evidence of varicella immunity acquired varicella after contact with herpes zoster. VZV was isolated from vesicular fluid of both chickenpox and zoster lesions in cell culture by Thomas Weller in 1954. Subsequent laboratory studies of the virus led to the development of a live attenuated varicella vaccine in Japan in the 1970s. The vaccine was licensed for use in the United States in March 1995. The first vaccine to reduce the risk of herpes zoster was licensed in May 2006.

Varicella Zoster Virus

VZV is a DNA virus and is a member of the herpesvirus group. Like other herpesviruses, VZV has the capacity to persist in the body after the primary (first) infection as a latent infection. VZV persists in sensory nerve ganglia. Primary infection with VZV results in chickenpox. Herpes zoster (shingles) is the result of reactivation of latent VZV infection. The virus is believed to have a short survival time in the environment.

Pathogenesis

VZV enters through the respiratory tract and conjunctiva. The virus is believed to replicate at the site of entry in the nasopharynx and in regional lymph nodes. A primary viremia occurs 4 to 6 days after infection and disseminates the virus to other organs, such as the liver, spleen, and sensory ganglia. Further replication occurs in the viscera, followed by a secondary viremia, with viral infection of the skin. Virus can be cultured from mononuclear cells of an infected person from 5 days before to 1 or 2 days after the appearance of the rash.

Clinical Features

The incubation period is 14 to 16 days after exposure, with a range of 10 to 21 days. The incubation period may be prolonged in immunocompromised patients and those who have received postexposure treatment with a varicella antibody–containing product.

Varicella Zoster Virus (VZV)

- Herpesvirus (DNA)
- Primary infection results in varicella (chickenpox)
- Reactivation of latent infection results in herpes zoster (shingles)
- Short survival in environment

Varicella Pathogenesis

- Respiratory transmission of virus
- Replication in nasopharynx and regional lymph nodes
- Primary viremia 4 to 6 days after infection
- Multiple tissues, including sensory ganglia, infected during viremia

22

Varicella

Varicella Clinical Features

- Incubation period 14 to 16 days (range 10 to 21 days)
- Mild prodrome for 1 to 2 days (adults)
- Rash generally appears first on head; most concentrated on trunk
- Successive crops over several days with lesions present in several stages of development

---

Primary Infection (Chickenpox)

A mild prodrome may precede the onset of a rash. Adults may have 1 to 2 days of fever and malaise prior to rash onset, but in children the rash is often the first sign of disease.

In individuals who have not been vaccinated with varicella vaccine, the rash is generalized and pruritic and progresses rapidly from macules to papules to vesicular lesions before crusting. The rash usually appears first on the head, then on the trunk, and then the extremities; the highest concentration of lesions is on the trunk. Lesions also can occur on mucous membranes of the oropharynx, respiratory tract, vagina, conjunctiva, and the cornea. Lesions are usually 1 to 4 mm in diameter. The vesicles are superficial and delicate and contain clear fluid on an erythematous base. Vesicles may rupture or become purulent before they dry and crust. Successive crops appear over several days, with lesions present in several stages of development. For example, macular lesions may be observed in the same area of skin as mature vesicles. Healthy children usually have 200 to 500 lesions in 2 to 4 successive crops.

Breakthrough varicella is defined as a case of varicella due to infection with wild-type VZV occurring more than 42 days after varicella vaccination. With decreasing incidence of varicella overall and increasing varicella vaccination coverage, more than half of varicella cases reported in the varicella active surveillance sites in 2010 were breakthrough varicella. In clinical trials, breakthrough varicella was substantially less severe with the median number of skin lesions commonly less than 50; vesicular lesions are less common and the lesions are commonly papules that do not progress to vesicles. Varicella in vaccinated persons is typically shorter in duration and has a lower incidence of fever than in unvaccinated persons. Breakthrough varicella has been reported in both one- and two-dose vaccine recipients.

The clinical course in healthy children is generally mild, with malaise, pruritus (itching), and temperature up to 102°F for 2 to 3 days. Adults may have more severe disease and have a higher incidence of complications. Respiratory and gastrointestinal symptoms are absent. Children with lymphoma and leukemia may develop a severe progressive form of varicella characterized by high fever, extensive vesicular eruption, and high complication rates. Children infected with human immunodeficiency virus (HIV) also may have severe, prolonged illness.

Recovery from primary varicella infection usually results in lifetime immunity. In otherwise healthy persons, a second occurrence of chickenpox is not common, but it can happen, particularly in immunocompromised persons. As with other viral diseases, reexposure to natural (wild) varicella may lead to reinfection that boosts antibody titers without causing clinical illness or detectable viremia.

Recurrent Disease (Herpes Zoster)

Herpes zoster, or shingles, occurs when latent VZV reactivates and causes recurrent disease. The immunologic mechanism that controls latency of VZV is not well understood. However, factors associated with recurrent disease include aging, immunosuppression, intrauterine exposure to VZV, and having had varicella at a young age (younger than 18 months). In immunocompromised persons, zoster may disseminate, causing generalized skin lesions and central nervous system, pulmonary, and hepatic involvement.

The vesicular eruption of zoster generally occurs unilaterally in the distribution of a sensory nerve. Most often, this involves the trunk or the fifth cranial nerve. Two to four days prior to the eruption, there may be pain and paresthesia in the involved area. There are few systemic symptoms.

Complications
Varicella

Acute varicella is generally mild and self-limited, but it may be associated with complications. Secondary bacterial infections of skin lesions with *Staphylococcus* or *Streptococcus* are the most common cause of hospitalization and outpatient medical visits. Secondary infection with invasive group A streptococci may cause serious illness and lead to hospitalization or death. Pneumonia following varicella is usually viral but may be bacterial. Secondary bacterial pneumonia is more common in children younger than 1 year of age. Central nervous system manifestations of varicella range from aseptic meningitis to encephalitis. Involvement of the cerebellum, with resulting cerebellar ataxia, is the most common central nervous system manifestation and generally has a good outcome. Encephalitis is an infrequent complication of varicella (estimated 1.8 per 10,000 cases) and may lead to seizures and coma. Diffuse cerebral involvement is more common in adults than in children. Reye syndrome is an unusual complication of varicella and influenza and occurs almost exclusively in children who take aspirin during the acute illness. The etiology of Reye syndrome is unknown. There has been a dramatic decrease in the incidence of Reye syndrome, presumably related to decreased use of aspirin by children.

Rare complications of varicella include aseptic meningitis, transverse myelitis, Guillain-Barré syndrome, thrombocyto-

---

Herpes Zoster (Shingles)
- Reactivation of varicella zoster virus (VZV)
- Associated with:
  - aging
  - immunosuppression
  - intrauterine exposure
  - varicella at younger than 18 months of age

Varicella Complications
- Bacterial infection of skin lesions
- Pneumonia (viral or bacterial)
- Central nervous system manifestations
- Reye syndrome
- Hospitalization: 2-3 per 1,000 cases (children)
- Death: 1 per 60,000 cases

22

Varicella

penia, hemorrhagic varicella, purpura fulminans, glomerulo-nephritis, myocarditis, arthritis, orchitis, uveitis, iritis, and hepatitis.

In the prevaccine era, approximately 11,000 persons with varicella required hospitalization each year. Hospitalization rates were approximately 2 to 3 per 1,000 cases among healthy children and 8 per 1,000 cases among adults. Death occurred in approximately 1 in 60,000 cases. From 1990 through 1996, an average of 103 deaths from varicella were reported each year. Most deaths occur in immunocompetent children and adults. Since 1996, hospitalizations and deaths from varicella have declined more than 70% and 88% respectively.

The risk of complications from varicella varies with age. Complications are infrequent among healthy children. They occur much more frequently in persons older than 15 years of age and infants younger than 1 year of age. Prior to the introduction of varicella vaccination, the fatality rates for varicella were approximately 1 per 100,000 cases among children 1-14 years of age, 2.7 per 100,000 cases among persons 15-19 years of age, and 25.2 per 100,000 cases among adults 30-49 years of age. Adults accounted for only 5% of reported cases of varicella but approximately 35% of mortality.

> **Groups at Increased Risk of Complications of Varicella**
> - Persons older than 15 years
> - Infants younger than 1 year
> - Immunocompromised persons
> - Newborns of women with rash onset within 5 days before to 2 days after delivery

Immunocompromised persons have a high risk of disseminated disease (up to 36% in one report). These persons may have multiple organ system involvement, and the disease may become fulminant and hemorrhagic. The most frequent complications in immunocompromised persons are pneumonia and encephalitis. Children with HIV infection are at increased risk for morbidity from varicella and herpes zoster.

The onset of maternal varicella from 5 days before to 2 days after delivery may result in overwhelming infection of the neonate and a fatality rate as high as 30%. This severe disease is believed to result from fetal exposure to varicella virus without the benefit of passive maternal antibody. Infants born to mothers with onset of maternal varicella 5 days or more prior to delivery usually have a benign course, presumably due to passive transfer of maternal antibody across the placenta.

Herpes Zoster

Postherpetic neuralgia (PHN), or pain in the area of the ocurrence that persists after the lesions have resolved, is a distressing complication of zoster. There is currently no adequate therapy available. PHN may last a year or longer after the episode of zoster. Ocular nerve and other organ involvement with zoster can occur, often with severe sequelae.

22

Congenital VZV Infection

Primary maternal varicella infection in the first 20 weeks of gestation is occasionally associated with abnormalities in the newborn, including low birth weight, hypoplasia of an extremity, skin scarring, localized muscular atrophy, encephalitis, cortical atrophy, chorioretinitis, and microcephaly. This constellation of abnormalities, collectively known as congenital varicella syndrome, was first recognized in 1947. The risk of congenital abnormalities from primary maternal varicella infection appears to be very low (less than 2%). Rare reports of congenital birth defects following maternal zoster exist, but virologic confirmation of maternal lesions is lacking.

Laboratory Diagnosis

Laboratory testing, whenever possible, or epidemiological linkage to a typical case or laboratory-confirmed case should be sought to confirm – or rule out – varicella.

Varicella zoster virus polymerase chain reaction (PCR) is the method of choice for diagnosis of varicella. VZV may also be isolated in tissue culture, although this is less sensitive and requires several days to obtain a result. The most frequent source of VZV isolation is vesicular fluid. Laboratory techniques allow differentiation of wild-type and vaccine strains of VZV.

Rapid varicella virus identification techniques are indicated for a case with severe or unusual disease to initiate specific antiviral therapy. VZV PCR is the method of choice for rapid clinical diagnosis. Real-time PCR methods are widely available and are the most sensitive and specific method of the available tests. Results are available within several hours. If real-time PCR is unavailable, the direct fluorescent antibody (DFA) method can be used, although it is less sensitive than PCR and requires more meticulous specimen collection and handling.

Specimens are best collected by unroofing a vesicle, preferably a fresh fluid-filled vesicle, and then rubbing the base of a skin lesion with a polyester swab. Crusts from lesions are also excellent specimens for PCR. Because viral proteins persist after cessation of viral replication, PCR and DFA may be positive when viral cultures are negative. Additional information concerning virus isolation and strain differentiation can be found at http://www.cdc.gov/chickenpox/lab-testing/index.html. A variety of serologic tests for varicella antibody are available commercially including a latex agglutination assay (LA) and a number of enzyme-linked immunosorbent assays (ELISA) that can be used to assess disease-induced immunity. Currently available ELISA methods are not sufficiently sensitive to

> ### Congenital Varicella Syndrome
> - Results from maternal infection during pregnancy
> - Period of risk may extend through first 20 weeks of pregnancy
> - Low birth weight, hypoplasia of extremity, skin scarring, eye and neurologic abnormalities
> - Risk appears to be very low (less than 2%)

> ### Varicella Laboratory Diagnosis
> - Isolation of varicella virus from clinical specimen
> - Rapid varicella virus identification using real-time PCR (preferred, if available) or DFA
> - Significant rise in varicella IgG by any standard serologic assay

22

Varicella

reliably detect seroconversion to vaccine, but are robust enough to screen persons for VZV susceptibility. ELISA is sensitive and specific, simple to perform, and widely available commercially. A commercially available LA is sensitive, simple, and rapid to perform. LA is somewhat more sensitive than commercial ELISAs, although it can result in false-positive results, leading to failure to identify persons without evidence of varicella immunity. This latter concern can be minimized by performing LA as a dilution series. Either of these tests would be useful for screening for varicella immunity.

Antibody resulting from vaccination is generally of lower titer than antibody resulting from varicella disease. Commercial antibody assays, particularly the LA test, may not be sensitive enough to detect vaccine-induced antibody in some recipients. Because of the potential for false-negative serologic tests, routine postvaccination serologic testing is not recommended. For diagnosis of acute varicella infection, serologic confirmation would include a significant rise in varicella IgG by any standard serologic assay. Testing using commercial kits for IgM antibody is not recommended since available methods lack sensitivity and specificity; false-positive IgM results are common in the presence of high IgG levels. The National VZV Laboratory at CDC has developed a reliable IgM capture assay. Contact the laboratory by e-mail at vzvlab@cdc.gov for details about collecting and submitting specimens for testing.

Epidemiology

Occurrence

Varicella and herpes zoster occur worldwide. Some data suggest that in tropical areas varicella infection occurs more commonly among adults than children. The reason(s) for this difference in age distribution are not known with certainty.

Reservoir

Varicella is a human disease. No animal or insect source or vector is known to exist.

Transmission

Infection with VZV occurs through the respiratory tract. The most common mode of transmission of VZV is believed to be person to person from infected respiratory tract secretions. Transmission may also occur by respiratory contact with airborne droplets or by direct contact or inhalation of aerosols from vesicular fluid of skin lesions of acute varicella or zoster.

Varicella Epidemiology

- Reservoir
  - human
- Transmission
  - person to person – respiratory tract secretions
  - direct contact with lesions
- Temporal pattern
  - peak in winter and early spring (U.S.)
- Communicability
  - 1 to 2 days before until lesions have formed crusts
  - may be longer in immunocompromised

Temporal Pattern

In temperate areas, varicella has a distinct seasonal fluctuation, with the highest incidence occurring in winter and early spring. In the United States, incidence is highest between March and May and lowest between September and November. Less seasonality is reported in tropical areas. Herpes zoster has no seasonal variation and occurs throughout the year.

Communicability

The period of communicability extends from 1 to 2 days before the onset of rash until lesions have formed crusts. Vaccinated persons with varicella may develop lesions that do not crust (macules and papules only). Isolation guidance for these persons is to exclude until no new lesions appear within a 24-hour period. Immunocompromised patients with varicella are probably contagious during the entire period new lesions are appearing. The virus has not been isolated from crusted lesions.

Varicella is highly contagious. It is less contagious than measles, but more so than mumps and rubella. Secondary attack rates among susceptible household contacts of persons with varicella are as high as 90% (that is, 9 of 10 susceptible household contacts of persons with varicella will become infected).

Secular Trends in the United States

Varicella

In the prevaccine era, varicella was endemic in the United States, and virtually all persons acquired varicella by adulthood. As a result, the number of cases occurring annually was estimated to approximate the birth cohort, or approximately 4 million per year. Varicella was removed from the list of nationally notifiable conditions in 1981, but some states continued to report cases to CDC. The majority of cases (approximately 90%) occurred among children younger than 15 years of age. The highest age-specific incidence of varicella was among children 1–4 years of age, who accounted for 39% of all cases. This age distribution was probably a result of earlier exposure to VZV in preschool and child care settings. Children 5–9 years of age accounted for 38% of cases. Adults 20 years of age and older accounted for only 7% of cases (National Health Interview Survey data, 1990–1994).

The incidence of varicella, as well as varicella-related hospitalizations, has decreased significantly since licensure of vaccine in 1995. Despite high one-dose vaccination coverage and success of the vaccination program in reducing varicella morbidity and mortality, varicella surveillance indicated

22

Varicella

that the number of reported varicella cases appeared to have plateaued in the early 2000s. An increasing proportion of cases represent breakthrough infection (chickenpox occurring in a previously vaccinated person). In 2001–2005, outbreaks were reported in schools with high varicella vaccination coverage (96%–100%). These outbreaks had many similarities: all occurred in elementary schools; vaccine effectiveness was within the expected range (72%–85%); the highest attack rates occurred among the younger students; each outbreak lasted about 2 months; and persons with breakthrough infection transmitted the virus although the breakthrough disease was mild. Overall attack rates among vaccinated children were 11%–17%, with attack rates in some classrooms as high as 40%. These data indicate that even in settings where almost everyone was vaccinated and vaccine performed as expected, varicella outbreaks could not be prevented with the one-dose vaccination policy. These observations led to the recommendation in 2006 for a second routine dose of varicella vaccine.

In 2010, varicella vaccination coverage among children 19–35 months in two of the active surveillance areas was estimated to be 95%. Varicella cases declined 97% between 1995 and 2010. Cases declined most among children 5–9 years of age, but a decline occurred in all age groups including infants and adults, indicating reduced transmission of the virus in these groups since implementation of the routine two-dose varicella vaccination program. One-dose varicella vaccine coverage among 19–35-month-old children was estimated by the National Immunization Survey to be 90.8% in 2011.

Herpes Zoster

Herpes zoster is not a notifiable condition. An estimated 500,000 to 1 million episodes of zoster occur annually in the United States. The lifetime risk of zoster is estimated to be at least 32%. Increasing age and cellular immunosuppression are the most important risk factors; 50% of persons living until age 85 years will develop zoster.

Vaccines Containing Varicella Virus

Three VZV-containing vaccines are now licensed in the United States: varicella vaccine (Varivax), combination measles-mumps-rubella-varicella (MMRV) vaccine (ProQuad), and herpes zoster vaccine (Zostavax).

Characteristics

Varicella Vaccine

Varicella vaccine (Varivax, Merck) is a live-attenuated viral vaccine, derived from the Oka strain of VZV. The vaccine virus was isolated by Takahashi in the early 1970s

---

Herpes Zoster

- 500,000 to 1 million episodes occur annually in the United States

- Lifetime risk of zoster estimated to be 32%

- 50% of persons living until age 85 years will develop zoster

from vesicular fluid from an otherwise healthy child with varicella disease. Varicella vaccine was licensed for general use in Japan and Korea in 1988. It was licensed in the United States in 1995 for persons 12 months of age and older. The virus was attenuated by sequential passage in human embryonic lung cell culture, embryonic guinea pig fibroblasts, and in WI-38 human diploid cells. The Oka/Merck vaccine has undergone further passage through MRC-5 human diploid cell cultures for a total of 31 passages. The reconstituted vaccine contains small amounts of sucrose, processed porcine gelatin, sodium chloride, monosodium L-glutamate, sodium diphosphate, potassium phosphate, and potassium chloride, and trace quantities of residual components of MRC-5 cells (DNA and protein), EDTA, neomycin, and fetal bovine serum. The vaccine is reconstituted with sterile water and contains no preservative.

Varicella-Containing Vaccines
- Varicella vaccine (Varivax)
  - approved for persons 12 months and older
- Measles-mumps-rubella-varicella vaccine (ProQuad)
  - approved for children 12 months through 12 years
- Herpes zoster vaccine (Zostavax)
  - approved for persons 50 years and older

Measles-Mumps-Rubella-Varicella Vaccine

In September 2005, the Food and Drug Administration (FDA) licensed a combined live-attenuated measles-mumps-rubella and varicella vaccine (ProQuad, Merck) for use in persons 12 months through 12 years of age. The attenuated measles, mumps, and rubella vaccine viruses in MMRV are identical and of equal titer to those in the measles-mumps-rubella (MMR) vaccine. The titer of Oka/Merck varicella zoster virus is higher in MMRV vaccine than in single-antigen varicella vaccine, a minimum of 9,772 (3.99 log10) plaque-forming units (PFU) versus 1,350 PFU (~3.13 log10), respectively. Each 0.5-mL dose contains small quantities of sucrose, hydrolyzed gelatin, sodium chloride, sorbitol, monosodium L-glutamate, sodium phosphate dibasic, human albumin, sodium bicarbonate, potassium phosphate monobasic, potassium chloride; potassium phosphate dibasic; residual components of MRC-5 cells (DNA and protein) neomycin, bovine calf serum, and other buffer and media ingredients. The vaccine is reconstituted with sterile water and contains no preservative.

Herpes Zoster Vaccine

In May 2006, the FDA approved herpes zoster vaccine (Zostavax, Merck) for use in persons 60 years of age and older. In March 2011, the FDA approved a label change for zoster vaccine to include persons 50 through 59 years of age. The vaccine contains the same Oka/Merck varicella zoster virus used in varicella and MMRV vaccines but at a much higher titer (a minimum of 19,400 PFU versus 1,350 PFU in varicella vaccine). Each 0.65-mL dose contains small quantities of sucrose, hydrolyzed porcine gelatin, sodium chloride, monosodium L-glutamate, sodium phosphate dibasic, potassium phosphate monobasic, potassium chloride; residual components of MRC-5 cells including (DNA and protein); neomycin and bovine calf serum. The vaccine is reconstituted with sterile water and contains no preservative.

22

Varicella

22

Varicella Vaccine Immunogenicity and Efficacy

- Detectable antibody
  - 97% of children 12 months through 12 years following 1 dose
  - 99% of persons 13 years and older after 2 doses
- 70% to 90% effective against any varicella disease
- 90%-100% effective against severe varicella disease

Varicella Breakthrough Infection

- Breakthrough infection is significantly milder, with fewer lesions
- No consistent evidence that risk of breakthrough infection increases with time since vaccination
- Retrospective cohort study of 115,000 children vaccinated in 2 HMOs during January 1995 through December 1999
- Risk of breakthrough varicella 2.5 times higher if varicella vaccine administered less than 30 days following MMR
- No increased risk if varicella vaccine given simultaneously or more than 30 days after MMR

Immunogenicity and Vaccine Efficacy

Varicella Vaccine

After one dose of single-antigen varicella vaccine, 97% of children 12 months through 12 years of age develop detectable antibody titers. More than 90% of vaccine responders maintain antibody for at least 6 years. In Japanese studies, 97% of children had antibody 7 to 10 years after vaccination. Vaccine efficacy is estimated to be 70% to 90% against infection, and 90% to 100% against moderate or severe disease.

Among healthy adolescents and adults 13 years of age and older, an average of 78% develop antibody after one dose, and 99% develop antibody after a second dose given 4 to 8 weeks later. Antibody persisted for at least 1 year in 97% of vaccinees after the second dose given 4 to 8 weeks after the first dose.

Immunity appears to be long-lasting, and is probably permanent in the majority of vaccinees. Breakthrough infection is significantly milder than infection among unvaccinated persons, with fewer lesions (generally fewer than 50), many of which are maculopapular rather than vesicular. Most persons with breakthrough infection do not have fever.

Although findings of some studies have suggested otherwise, most investigations have not identified time since vaccination as a risk factor for breakthrough varicella. Some, but not all, recent investigations have identified the presence of asthma, use of steroids, and vaccination at younger than 15 months of age as risk factors for breakthrough varicella. Classification of varicella infection as breakthrough could be a result of several factors, including interference of vaccine virus replication by circulating antibody, impotent vaccine resulting from storage or handling errors, or inaccurate recordkeeping.

Interference from live viral vaccine administered before varicella vaccine could also reduce vaccine effectiveness. A study of 115,000 children in two health maintenance organizations during 1995–1999 found that children who received varicella vaccine less than 30 days after MMR vaccination had a 2.5-fold increased risk of breakthrough varicella compared with those who received varicella vaccine before, simultaneously with, or more than 30 days after MMR.

Studies have shown that a second dose of varicella vaccine boosts immunity and reduces the risk of breakthrough disease in children.

MMRV Vaccine

MMRV vaccine was licensed on the basis of equivalence of immunogenicity of the antigenic components rather than the clinical efficacy. Clinical studies involving healthy children age 12 through 23 months indicated that those who received a single dose of MMRV vaccine developed similar levels of antibody to measles, mumps, rubella and varicella as children who received MMR and varicella vaccines concomitantly at separate injection sites.

Herpes Zoster Vaccine

The primary clinical trial for zoster vaccine included more than 38,000 adults 60 to 80 years of age with no prior history of shingles. Participants were followed for a median of 3.1 years after a single dose of vaccine. Compared with the placebo group, the vaccine group had 51% fewer episodes of zoster. Efficacy was highest for persons 60–69 years of age (64%) and declined with increasing age. Efficacy was 18% for participants 80 years or older. Vaccine recipients who developed zoster generally had less severe disease. Vaccine recipients also had about 66% less postherpetic neuralgia, the pain that can persist long after the shingles rash has resolved. In a subsequent clinical trial that included more than 22,000 persons 50 through 59 years of age, zoster vaccine was shown to reduce the risk of zoster by 69.8% in this age group. The duration of reduction of risk of zoster is not known.

Vaccination Schedule and Use
Varicella Vaccine

Varicella vaccine is recommended for all children without contraindications at 12 through15 months of age. The vaccine may be given to all children at this age regardless of prior history of varicella.

A second dose of varicella vaccine should be administered at 4 through 6 years of age, at the same visit as the second dose of MMR vaccine. The second dose may be administered earlier than 4 through 6 years of age if at least 3 months have elapsed following the first dose (i.e., the minimum interval between doses of varicella vaccine is 3 months for children younger than 13 years). However, if the second dose is administered at least 28 days following the first dose, it does not need to be repeated. A second dose of varicella vaccine is also recommended for persons older than 6 years of age who have received only one dose. Varicella vaccine doses administered to persons 13 years or older should be separated by 4-8 weeks.

All varicella-containing vaccines should be administered by the subcutaneous route. Varicella vaccine has been shown to be safe and effective in healthy children when administered at the same time as MMR vaccine at separate sites and with separate syringes. If varicella and MMR vaccines are not administered at the same visit, they should be separated

---

Herpes Zoster Vaccine Efficacy

- Vaccine recipients 60 to 80 years of age had 51% fewer episodes of zoster

  - efficacy declines with increasing age

  - significantly reduces the risk of postherpetic neuralgia

- Reduces the risk of zoster 69.8% in persons 50 through 59 years of age

---

Varicella Vaccine Recommendations Children

- Routine vaccination at 12 through 15 months of age

- Routine second dose at 4 through 6 years of age

- Minimum interval between doses of varicella vaccine is 3 months for children younger than 13 years of age

Varicella Vaccine Recommendations Adolescents and Adults

- All persons 13 years of age and older without evidence of varicella immunity

- 2 doses separated by at least 4 weeks

- Do not repeat first dose because of extended interval between doses

22

Varicella

by at least 28 days. Varicella vaccine may also be administered simultaneously (but at separate sites with separate syringes) with all other childhood vaccines. ACIP strongly recommends that varicella vaccine be administered simultaneously with all other vaccines recommended at 12 through 15 months of age.

Children with a clinician-diagnosed or verified history of typical chickenpox can be assumed to be immune to varicella. Serologic testing of such children prior to vaccination is not warranted because the majority of children between 12 months and 12 years of age without a clinical history of chickenpox are not immune. Prior history of chickenpox is not a contraindication to varicella vaccination.

Varicella vaccine should be administered to all adolescents and adults 13 years of age and older who do not have evidence of varicella immunity (see Varicella Immunity section). Persons 13 years of age and older should receive two doses of varicella vaccine separated by 4-8 weeks. If there is a lapse of more than 4 weeks after the first dose, the second dose may be administered at any time without repeating the first dose.

Assessment of varicella immunity status of all adolescents and adults and vaccination of those who lack evidence of varicella immunity are important to protect these individuals from their higher risk of complications from varicella. Vaccination may be offered at the time of routine healthcare visits. However, specific assessment efforts should be focused on adolescents and adults who are at highest risk of exposure and those most likely to transmit varicella to others.

The ACIP recommends that all healthcare personnel be immune to varicella. In healthcare settings, serologic screening of personnel who are uncertain of their varicella history, or who claim not to have had the disease is likely to be cost-effective. Testing for varicella immunity following two doses of vaccine is not necessary because 99% of persons are seropositive after the second dose. Moreover, available commercial assays are not sensitive enough to detect antibody following vaccination in all instances.

Seroconversion does not always result in full protection against disease, although no data regarding correlates of protection are available for adults. Vaccinated healthcare personnel exposed to VZV should be monitored daily from day 10 to day 21 after exposure through the employee health or infection control program to screen for fever, skin lesions, and systemic symptoms. Persons with varicella may be infectious starting 2 days before rash onset. In addition,

---

Varicella Vaccination Recommendations Healthcare Personnel

- ACIP recommends all healthcare personnel be immune to varicella

- Prevaccination serologic screening likely cost-effective for persons with uncertain history

- Postvaccination testing not necessary or recommended

healthcare personnel should be instructed to immediately report fever, headache, or other constitutional symptoms and any skin lesions (which may be atypical). The person should be placed on sick leave immediately if symptoms occur.

The risk of transmission of vaccine virus from a vaccinated person to a susceptible contact appears to be very low (see Transmission of Varicella Vaccine Virus section), and the benefits of vaccinating susceptible healthcare personnel clearly outweigh this potential risk. Transmission of vaccine virus appears to occur primarily if and when the vaccinee develops a vaccine-associated rash. As a safeguard, medical facilities may wish to consider protocols for personnel who develop a rash following vaccination (e.g., avoidance of contact with persons at high risk of serious complications, such as immunosuppressed persons who do not have evidence of varicella immunity).

MMRV Vaccine

MMRV vaccine is approved for vaccination against measles, mumps, rubella and varicella in children 12 months through 12 years of age. Persons 13 years of age and older should not receive MMRV. When used, MMRV vaccine should be administered on or after the first birthday, preferably as soon as the child becomes eligible for vaccination. MMRV may be used for both the first and second doses of MMR and varicella in children younger than 13 years. The minimum interval between doses of MMRV is 3 months. However, if the second dose is administered at least 28 days following the first dose, it does not need to be repeated.

For the first dose of measles, mumps, rubella, and varicella vaccines at age 12 through 47 months, either MMR vaccine and varicella vaccine or MMRV vaccine may be used. Providers who are considering administering MMRV vaccine should discuss the benefits and risks of both vaccination options with the parents or caregivers. Unless the parent or caregiver expresses a preference for MMRV vaccine, CDC recommends that MMR vaccine and varicella vaccine should be administered for the first dose in this age group. See the Adverse Recations section of this chapter for more information. For the second dose of measles, mumps, rubella, and varicella vaccines at any age (15 months through 12 years) and for the first dose at 48 months of age or older, use of MMRV vaccine generally is preferred over separate injections of its equivalent component vaccines (i.e., MMR vaccine and varicella vaccine).

Herpes Zoster Vaccine

Zoster vaccine is approved by FDA for persons 50 years and older. However, ACIP does not currently recommend vaccination of persons younger than 60 years because of

> **MMRV Vaccine**
> - Approved for children 12 months through 12 years of age (to age 13 years)
> - Do not use for persons 13 years and older
> - May be used for both first and second doses of MMR and varicella vaccines
> - Minimum interval between doses is 3 months

22

Varicella

Herpes Zoster Vaccine

- Approved for persons 50 years and older

- ACIP does not recommend vaccination of persons younger than 60 years because of supply and lower risk of zoster in this age group

Varicella Vaccine Postexposure Prophylaxis

- Varicella vaccine is recommended for use in persons without evidence of varicella immunity after exposure to varicella

  - 70%-100% effective if given within 3 days of exposure (possibly up to 5 days)

  - not effective if administered more than 5 days after exposure but will produce immunity if recipient is not infected

concerns about vaccine supply and the lower risk of zoster in this age group. ACIP recommends a single dose of zoster vaccine for adults 60 years of age and older whether or not they report a prior episode of herpes zoster. Persons with a chronic medical condition may be vaccinated unless a contraindication or precaution exists for the condition (see Conraindications and Precautions to Vaccination).

In June 2011, the package insert for zoster vaccine was revised to advise that in a randomized clinical study, a reduced immune response to Zostavax as measured by glycoprotein-based ELISA (gpELISA) was observed in individuals who received Pneumovax 23 (PPSV23) and Zostavax concurrently compared with individuals who received these vaccines 4 weeks apart. A subsequent clinical study did not find a significant increase in the incidence of zoster among persons who received zoster vaccine and PPSV23 at the same visit compared with persons who received the vaccines 30 or more days apart. Consequently, to avoid introducing barriers to patients and providers who are interested in these two important vaccines, CDC has not changed its recommendation for either vaccine, and continues to recommend that zoster vaccine and PPSV be administered at the same visit if the person is eligible for both vaccines.

Postexposure Prophylaxis

Varicella Vaccine

Data from the United States and Japan in a variety of settings indicate that varicella vaccine is 70% to 100% effective in preventing illness or modifying the severity of illness if used within 3 days, and possibly up to 5 days, after exposure. ACIP recommends the vaccine for postexposure prophylaxis in persons who do not have evidence of varicella immunity. If exposure to varicella does not cause infection, postexposure vaccination should induce protection against subsequent exposure. If the exposure results in infection, there is no evidence that administration of varicella vaccine during the incubation period or prodromal stage of illness increases the risk for vaccine-associated adverse reactions. Although postexposure use of varicella vaccine has potential applications in hospital settings, preexposure vaccination of all healthcare personnel without evidence of varicella immunity is the recommended and preferred method for preventing varicella in healthcare settings.

Varicella outbreaks in some settings (e.g., child care facilities and schools) can persist up to 6 months. Varicella vaccine has been used successfully to control these outbreaks. The ACIP recommends a second dose of varicella vaccine for outbreak control. During a varicella outbreak, persons who have received one dose of varicella vaccine should receive a second dose, provided the appropriate vaccination interval has elapsed since the first dose (3 months for persons aged 12 months through 12 years and at least 4 weeks for persons aged 13 years of age and older).

MMRV Vaccine

MMRV vaccine may be used as described for varicella vaccine, and for measles as described in the Measles chapter.

Herpes Zoster Vaccine

Exposure to a person with either primary varicella (chickenpox) or herpes zoster does not cause zoster in the exposed person. Herpes zoster vaccine has no role in the postexposure management of either chickenpox or zoster and should not be used for this purpose.

Varicella Immunity

In 2007, the ACIP published a revised definition for evidence of immunity to varicella. Evidence of immunity to varicella includes any of the following:

- Documentation of age-appropriate vaccination:

  - Preschool-aged children 12 months of age or older: one dose

  - School-aged children, adolescents, and adults: two doses

- Laboratory evidence of immunity or laboratory confirmation of disease: commercial assays can be used to assess disease-induced immunity, but they lack adequate sensitivity to reliably detect vaccine-induced immunity (i.e., they may yield false-negative results).

- Birth in the United States before 1980: for healthcare personnel and pregnant women, birth before 1980 should not be considered evidence of immunity. Persons born outside the United States should meet one of the other criteria for varicella immunity.

- A healthcare provider diagnosis or verification of varicella disease: verification of history or diagnosis of typical disease can be done by any healthcare provider (e.g., school or occupational clinic nurse, nurse practitioner, physician assistant, physician). For persons reporting a history of or presenting with atypical and/or mild cases, assessment by a physician or designee is recommended, and one of the following should be sought: a) an epidemiologic link to a typical varicella case, or b) evidence of laboratory confirmation if laboratory testing was performed at the time of acute

---

Varicella Immunity

- Written documentation of age-appropriate vaccination

- Laboratory evidence of immunity or laboratory confirmation of disease

- Born in the United States before 1980

- Healthcare personnel diagnosis or verification of varicella disease

- History of herpes zoster based on healthcare provider diagnosis

22

Varicella

disease. When such documentation is lacking, a person should not be considered as having a valid history of disease, because other diseases may mimic mild or atypical varicella.

- History of herpes zoster based on healthcare provider diagnosis.

Contraindications and Precautions to Vaccination
Varicella and MMRV Vaccines

Contraindications and precautions are similar for all varicella-containing vaccines. Persons with a severe allergic reaction (e.g. anaphylaxis) to a vaccine component or following a prior dose of varicella containing vaccine should not receive varicella vaccine. Varicella, MMRV, and zoster vaccines all contain minute amounts of neomycin and hydrolyzed gelatin but do not contain egg protein or preservative.

Persons with immunosuppression due to leukemia, lymphoma, generalized malignancy, immune deficiency disease, or immunosuppressive therapy should not be vaccinated with a varicella-containing vaccine. However, treatment with low-dose (less than 2 mg/kg/day), alternate-day, topical, replacement, or aerosolized steroid preparations is not a contraindication to vaccination. Persons whose immunosuppressive therapy with steroids has been discontinued for 1 month (3 months for chemotherapy) may be vaccinated.

Single-antigen varicella vaccine may be administered to persons with impaired humoral immunity (e.g., hypogammaglobulinemia). However, the blood products used to treat humoral immunodeficiency may interfere with the response to vaccination. Recommended spacing between administration of the blood product and receipt of varicella vaccine should be observed (see Chapter 2, General Recommendations on Immunization, for details).

Persons with moderate or severe cellular immunodeficiency resulting from infection with human immunodeficiency virus (HIV), including persons diagnosed with acquired immunodeficiency syndrome (AIDS) should not receive varicella vaccine. HIV-infected children with CD4 T-lymphocyte percentage of 15% or higher, and older children and adults with a CD4 count of 200 per microliter or higher may be considered for vaccination. These persons may receive MMR and single-antigen varicella vaccines, but should not receive MMRV.

Varicella-Containing Vaccines Contraindications and Precautions

- Severe allergic reaction to vaccine component or following a prior dose
- Immunosuppression
- Pregnancy
- Moderate or severe acute illness
- Recent blood product (varicella, MMRV)
- Personal or family (i.e., sibling or parent) history of seizures of any etiology (MMRV only)

Varicella Vaccine Use in Persons with Immunosuppression

- MMRV not approved for use in persons with HIV infection
- Do not administer zoster vaccine to immunosuppressed persons

---

Women known to be pregnant or attempting to become pregnant should not receive a varicella-containing vaccine. No adverse outcomes of pregnancy or in a fetus have been reported among women who inadvertently received varicella vaccine shortly before or during pregnancy. Although the manufacturer's package insert states otherwise, ACIP recommends that pregnancy be avoided for 1 month following receipt of varicella vaccine.

The ACIP recommends prenatal assessment and postpartum vaccination for varicella. Women should be assessed during a prenatal healthcare visit for evidence of varicella immunity. Upon completion or termination of pregnancy, women who do not have evidence of varicella immunity should receive the first dose of varicella vaccine before discharge from the healthcare facility. The second dose should be administered at least 4 weeks later at the postpartum or other healthcare visit. Standing orders are recommended for healthcare settings where completion or termination of pregnancy occurs to ensure administration of varicella vaccine.

The manufacturer, in collaboration with CDC, has established a Varicella Vaccination in Pregnancy registry to monitor the maternal–fetal outcomes of pregnant women inadvertently given varicella vaccine. The telephone number for the Registry is 800-986-8999.

> **Varicella Vaccination in Pregnancy Registry**
> 800.986.8999

Vaccination of persons with moderate or severe acute illnesses should be postponed until the condition has improved. This precaution is intended to prevent complicating the management of an ill patient with a potential vaccine adverse event, such as fever. Minor illness, such as otitis media and upper respiratory infections, concurrent antibiotic therapy, and exposure or recovery from other illnesses are not contraindications to varicella vaccine. Although there is no evidence that either varicella or varicella vaccine exacerbates tuberculosis, vaccination is not recommended for persons known to have untreated active tuberculosis. Tuberculosis skin testing is not a prerequisite for varicella vaccination.

The effect of the administration of antibody-containing blood products (e.g., immune globulin, whole blood or packed red blood cells, or intravenous immune globulin) on the response to varicella vaccine virus is unknown. Because of the potential inhibition of the response to varicella vaccination by passively transferred antibodies, varicella or MMRV vaccine should not be administered for 3–11 months after receipt of antibody-containing blood products. ACIP recommends applying the same intervals used to separate antibody-containing products and MMR to varicella vaccine (see chapter 2, General Recommendations on Immunization, and Appendix A for additional details).

22

Varicella

Immune globulin should not be given for 3 weeks following vaccination unless the benefits exceed those of the vaccine. In such cases, the vaccinees should either be revaccinated or tested for immunity at least 3 months later (depending on the antibody-containing product administered) and revaccinated if seronegative.

A personal or family (i.e., sibling or parent) history of seizures of any etiology is a precaution for MMRV vaccination. Studies suggest that children who have a personal or family history of febrile seizures or family history of epilepsy are at increased risk for febrile seizures compared with children without such histories. Children with a personal or family history of seizures of any etiology generally should be vaccinated with separate MMR and varicella vaccines because the risks for using MMRV vaccine in this group of children generally outweigh the benefits.

No adverse events following varicella vaccination related to the use of salicylates (e.g., aspirin) have been reported. However, the manufacturer recommends that vaccine recipients avoid the use of salicylates for 6 weeks after receiving varicella or MMRV vaccine because of the association between aspirin use and Reye syndrome following chickenpox.

Zoster Vaccine

As with all vaccines, a severe allergic reaction to a vaccine component or following a prior dose is a contraindication to zoster vaccination. As with other live virus vaccines, pregnancy or planned pregnancy within 4 weeks and immunosuppression are contraindications to zoster vaccination.

Zoster vaccine should not be administered to persons with primary or acquired immunodeficiency. This includes persons with leukemia, lymphomas, or other malignant neoplasms affecting the bone marrow or lymphatic system. The package insert implies that zoster vaccine should not be administered to anyone who has ever had leukemia or lymphoma. However, ACIP recommends that persons whose leukemia or lymphoma is in remission and who have not received chemotherapy or radiation for at least 3 months can be vaccinated. Other immunosuppressive conditions that contraindicate zoster vaccine include AIDS or other clinical manifestation of HIV. This includes CD4 T-lymphocyte values less than 200 per mm^3 or less than 15% of total lymphocytes.

Persons receiving high-dose corticosteroid therapy should not be vaccinated. High dose is defined as 20 milligrams or more per day of prednisone or equivalent lasting two or more weeks. Zoster vaccination should be deferred for at least 1 month after discontinuation of therapy. As with other live viral vaccines, persons receiving lower doses of corticosteroids may be vaccinated. Topical, inhaled or intra-articular steroids, or long-term alternate-day treatment with low to moderate doses of short-acting systemic corticosteroids are not considered to be sufficiently immunosuppressive to contraindicate zoster vaccine.

Low doses of drugs used for the treatment of rheumatoid arthritis, inflammatory bowel disease, and other conditions, such as methotrexate, azathioprine, or 6-mercaptopurine, are also not considered sufficiently immunosuppressive to create safety concerns for zoster vaccine. Low-dose therapy with these drugs is NOT a contraindication for administration of zoster vaccine.

The experience of hematopoietic cell transplant recipients with varicella-containing vaccines, including zoster vaccine is limited. Physicians should assess the immune status of the recipient on a case-by-case basis to determine the relevant risks. If a decision is made to vaccinate with zoster vaccine, the vaccine should be administered at least 24 months after transplantation.

The safety and efficacy of zoster vaccine administered concurrently with recombinant human immune mediators and immune modulators (such as the anti–tumor necrosis factor agents adalimumab, infliximab, and etanercept) is not known. It is preferable to administer zoster vaccine before treatment with these drugs. If it is not possible to administer zoster vaccine to patients before initiation of treatment, physicians should assess the immune status of the recipient on a case-by-case basis to determine the relevant risks and benefits. Otherwise, vaccination with zoster vaccine should be deferred for at least 1 month after discontinuation of treatment.

As with all vaccines, moderate or severe acute illness is a precaution to vaccination. Current treatment with an antiviral drug active against herpesviruses, such as acyclovir, famciclovir, or valacyclovir, is a precaution to vaccination. These drugs can interfere with replication of the vaccine virus. Persons taking these drugs should discontinue them at least 24 hours before administration of zoster vaccine, and the drugs should not be taken for at least 14 days after vaccination.

Persons with a history of varicella are immune and generally maintain a high level of antibody to varicella zoster virus, a level comparable to that found in donated blood and antibody-containing blood products. Receiving an antibody-containing blood product will not change the amount of antibody in the person's blood. As a result, unlike most other live virus vaccines, recent receipt of a blood product

22

Varicella

is not a precaution for zoster vaccine. Zoster vaccine can be administered at any time before, concurrent with, or after receiving blood or other antibody-containing blood products.

Adverse Reactions Following Vaccination

Varicella Vaccine

The most common adverse reactions following varicella vaccine are local reactions, such as pain, soreness, erythema, and swelling. Based on information from the manufacturer's clinical trials of varicella vaccine, local reactions are reported by 19% of children and by 24% of adolescents and adults (33% following the second dose). These local adverse reactions are generally mild and self-limited. A varicella-like rash at injection site is reported by 3% of children and by 1% of adolescents and adults following the second dose. In both circumstances, a median of two lesions have been present. These lesions generally occur within 2 weeks, and are most commonly maculopapular rather than vesicular. A generalized varicella-like rash is reported by 4%–6% of recipients of varicella vaccine (1% after the second dose in adolescents and adults), with an average of five lesions. Most of these generalized rashes occur within 3 weeks and most are maculopapular.

Systemic reactions are not common. Fever within 42 days of vaccination is reported by 15% of children and 10% of adolescents and adults. The majority of these episodes of fever have been attributed to concurrent illness rather than to the vaccine.

Varicella vaccine is a live virus vaccine and may result in a latent infection, similar to that caused by wild varicella virus. Consequently, zoster caused by the vaccine virus has been reported, mostly among vaccinated children. Not all these cases have been confirmed as having been caused by vaccine virus. The risk of zoster following vaccination appears to be less than that following infection with wild-type virus. The majority of cases of zoster following vaccine have been mild and have not been associated with complications such as postherpetic neuralgia.

MMRV Vaccine

In MMRV vaccine prelicensure studies conducted among children 12–23 months of age, fever (reported as abnormal or elevated greater than or equal to 102°F oral equivalent) was observed 5-12 days after vaccination in 21.5% of MMRV vaccine recipients compared with 14.9% of MMR vaccine and varicella vaccine recipients. Measles-like rash was observed in 3.0% of MMRV vaccine recipients compared with 2.1% of those receiving MMR vaccine and varicella vaccine.

Varicella Vaccine Adverse Reactions

- Local reactions (pain, erythema)
  - 19% (children)
  - 24% (adolescents and adults)
- Generalized rash 3%
  - may be maculopapular rather than vesicular
  - average 5 lesions
- Systemic reactions not common
- Adverse reactions similar for MMRV

Zoster Following Vaccination

- Most cases in children
- Not all cases caused by vaccine virus
- Risk from vaccine virus less than from wild-type virus
- Usually a mild illness without complications such as postherpetic neuralgia

Two postlicensure studies indicated that among children 12 through 23 months of age, one additional febrile seizure occurred 5–12 days after vaccination per 2,300–2,600 children who had received the first dose of MMRV vaccine, compared with children who had received the first dose of MMR vaccine and varicella vaccine administered as separate injections at the same visit. Data from postlicensure studies do not suggest that children 4–6 years of age who received the second dose of MMRV vaccine had an increased risk for febrile seizures after vaccination compared with children the same age who received MMR vaccine and varicella vaccine administered as separate injections at the same visit.

Herpes Zoster Vaccine

In the largest clinical trial of zoster vaccine, local reactions (erythema, pain or tenderness, and swelling) were the most common adverse reaction reported by vaccine recipients (34%), and were reported more commonly than by placebo recipients (6%). A temperature of 101°F or higher within 42 days of vaccination occurred at a similar frequency among both vaccine (0.8%) and placebo (0.9%) recipients. No serious adverse reactions were identified during the trial.

Transmission of Varicella Vaccine Virus

Available data suggest that transmission of varicella vaccine virus is a rare event. Instances of suspected secondary transmission of vaccine virus have been reported, but in few instances has the secondary clinical illness been shown to be caused by vaccine virus. Several cases of suspected secondary transmission have been determined to have been caused by wild varicella virus. In studies of household contacts, several instances of asymptomatic seroconversion have been observed. It appears that transmission occurs mainly when the vaccinee develops a rash. If a vaccinated person develops a rash, it is recommended that close contact with persons who do not have evidence of varicella immunity and who are at high risk of complications of varicella, such as immunocompromised persons, be avoided until the rash has resolved.

Transmission of varicella due to vaccine virus from recipients of zoster vaccine has not been reported.

Vaccine Storage and Handling

Varicella-containing vaccine should be stored frozen between -58°F and +5°F (-50°C and -15°C). Manufacturer package inserts contain additional information and can be found at http://www.fda.gov/BiologicsBloodVaccines/Vaccines/ApprovedProducts/ucm093830.htm. For complete information on best practices and recommendations please

Herpes Zoster Vaccine Adverse Reactions
- Local reactions - 34% (pain, erythema)
- No increased risk of fever
- No serious adverse reactions identified

22

refer to CDC's Vaccine Storage and Handling Toolkit, http://www.cdc.gov/vaccines/recs/storage/toolkit/storage-handling-toolkit.pdf.

Varicella Zoster Immune Globulin

In March 2013, a VZIG product, VariZIG (Cangene Corporation, Winnipeg, Canada) was licensed by the FDA. It had previously been available as an investigational product. The licensed product can be requested from the sole authorized U.S. distributor, FFF Enterprises (Temecula, California), for patients who have been exposed to varicella and who are at increased risk for severe disease and complications. VariZIG can be obtained by calling FFF Enterprises at 800-843-7477 at any time or by contacting the distributor online at http://www.fffenterprises.com.

VariZIG is a purified human immune globulin preparation made from plasma containing high levels of anti-varicella antibodies (immunoglobulin class G [IgG]) that is lyophilized. When properly reconstituted, VariZIG is approximately a 5% solution of IgG that can be administered intramuscularly.

The patient groups recommended by ACIP to receive VariZIG include the following:

- Immunocompromised patients;

- Neonates whose mothers have signs and symptoms of varicella around the time of delivery (i.e., 5 days before to 2 days after);

- Preterm infants born at 28 weeks gestation or later who are exposed during the neonatal period and whose mothers do not have evidence of immunity;

- Preterm infants born earlier than 28 weeks' gestation or who weigh 1,000g or less at birth and were exposed during the neonatal period, regardless of maternal history of varicella disease or vaccination;

- and Pregnant women.

Addition information concerning the acquisition and use of this product is available in the March 30, 2012, edition of *Morbidity and Mortality Weekly Report*, available at http://www.cdc.gov/mmwr/preview/mmwrhtml/mm6112a4.htm?s_cid=mm6112a4_w.

Acknowledgement

The editors thank Dr. Cindy Weinbaum, CDC for her assistance in updating this chapter.

22

Selected References

CDC. Prevention of varicella: recommendations of the Advisory Committee on Immunization Practices (ACIP). *MMWR* 2007;56(No. RR-4):1–40.

CDC. Prevention of herpes zoster. Recommendations of the Advisory Committee on Immunization Practices. *MMWR* 2008;57(No.RR-5).

CDC. Simultaneous administration of varicella vaccine and other recommended childhood vaccines – United States, 1995-1999. *MMWR* 2001;50(No. 47):1058-61.

CDC. Use of combination measles, mumps, rubella, and varicella vaccine: recommendations of the Advisory Committee on Immunization Practices (ACIP). *MMWR* 2010;59(No. RR-3):1–12.

CDC. Immunization of health-care personnel. Recommendations of the Advisory Committee on Immunization Practices (ACIP). *MMWR* 2011;60(RR-7):1-45.

Davis MM, Patel MS, Gebremariam A. Decline in varicella-related hospitalizations and expenditures for children and adults after introduction of varicella vaccine in the United States. *Pediatrics* 2004;114:786–92.

Kuter B, Matthews H, Shinefield H, et al. Ten year follow-up of healthy children who received one or two injections of varicella vaccine. *Pediatr Infect Dis J* 2004;23:132–7.

Leung J, Harpaz R, Molinari NA, et al. Herpes zoster incidence among insured persons in the United States, 1993-2006; evaluation of impact of varicella vaccination. *Clin Infect Dis* 2011;52:332-40.

Oxman MN, Levin MJ, Johnson GR, et. al. A Vaccine to prevent herpes zoster and postherpetic neuralgia in older adults. *NEJM* 2005; 352(12): 2271-84.

Oxman MN. Zoster vaccine: current status and future prospects. *Clin Infect Dis* 2010;51:197-213.

Tseng HF, Smith N, Sy LS, Jacobsen SJ. Evaluation of the incidence of herpes zoster after concomitant administration of zoster vaccine and polysaccharide pneumococcal vaccine. *Vaccine* 2011;29:3628-32.

Seward JF, Watson BM, Peterson CL, et al. Varicella disease after introduction of varicella vaccine in the United States, 1995–2000. *JAMA* 2002;287:606–11.

22

Varicella

Seward JF, Zhang JX, Maupin TJ, Mascola L, Jumaan AO. Contagiousness of varicella in vaccinated cases: a household contact study. *JAMA* 2004;292:704–8.

Shields KE, Galil K, Seward J, et al. Varicella vaccine exposure during pregnancy: data from the first 5 years of the pregnancy registry. *Obstet Gynecol* 2001; 98:14–19.

Vazquez M, LaRuissa PS, Gershon AA, et al. Effectiveness over time of varicella vaccine. *JAMA* 2004;291:851–92.

22

APPENDIX A
Schedules and Recommendation

A

Appendix A

Immunization Schedules on the Web

www.cdc.gov/vaccines/schedules/index.htm

Childhood and Adolescent Immunization Schedule:

www.cdc.gov/vaccines/schedules/hcp/child-adolescent.html

Contains:
- Color and black & white versions
- Downloadable files for office or commercial printing
- Alternative formats (pocket size, laminated, palm, etc.)
- Simplified, parent-friendly version in English and Spanish
- Link to past years' schedules
- Interactive schedulers
- More . . .

Adult Immunization Schedule:

www.cdc.gov/vaccines/schedules/hcp/adult.html

Contains:
- Color and black & white versions
- Downloadable files
- Interactive scheduler and quiz
- Link to past years' schedules
- More . . .

Easy-to-Read Schedules for Non-Providers:

www.cdc.gov/vaccines/schedules/easy-to-read/index.html

A

Recommended Immunization Schedules for Persons Aged 0 Through 18 Years
UNITED STATES, 2015

This schedule includes recommendations in effect as of January 1, 2015. Any dose not administered at the recommended age should be administered at a subsequent visit, when indicated and feasible. The use of a combination vaccine generally is preferred over separate injections of its equivalent component vaccines. Vaccination providers should consult the relevant Advisory Committee on Immunization Practices (ACIP) statement for detailed recommendations, available online at http://www.cdc.gov/vaccines/hcp/acip-recs/index.html. Clinically significant adverse events that follow vaccination should be reported to the Vaccine Adverse Event Reporting System (VAERS) online (http://www.vaers.hhs.gov) or by telephone (800-822-7967).

The Recommended Immunization Schedules for Persons Aged 0 Through 18 Years are approved by the

Advisory Committee on Immunization Practices
(http://www.cdc.gov/vaccines/acip)

American Academy of Pediatrics
(http://www.aap.org)

American Academy of Family Physicians
(http://www.aafp.org)

American College of Obstetricians and Gynecologists
(http://www.acog.org)

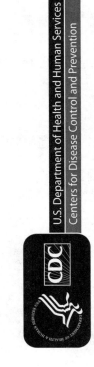

U.S. Department of Health and Human Services
Centers for Disease Control and Prevention

Figure 1. Recommended immunization schedule for persons aged 0 through 18 years – United States, 2015.

(FOR THOSE WHO FALL BEHIND OR START LATE, SEE THE CATCH-UP SCHEDULE [FIGURE 2]).

These recommendations must be read with the footnotes that follow. For those who fall behind or start late, provide catch-up vaccination at the earliest opportunity as indicated by the green bars in Figure 1. To determine minimum intervals between doses, see the catch-up schedule (Figure 2). School entry and adolescent vaccine age groups are shaded.

Vaccine	Birth	1 mo	2 mos	4 mos	6 mos	9 mos	12 mos	15 mos	18 mos	19–23 mos	2-3 yrs	4-6 yrs	7-10 yrs	11-12 yrs	13–15 yrs	16–18 yrs
Hepatitis B[1] (HepB)	1st dose	←--- 2nd dose ---→			←--- 3rd dose ---→											
Rotavirus[2] (RV) RV1 (2-dose series); RV5 (3-dose series)			1st dose	2nd dose	See footnote 2											
Diphtheria, tetanus, & acellular pertussis[3] (DTaP: <7 yrs)			1st dose	2nd dose	3rd dose			←--- 4th dose ---→				5th dose				
Tetanus, diphtheria, & acellular pertussis[4] (Tdap: ≥7 yrs)														(Tdap)		
Haemophilus influenzae type b[5] (Hib)			1st dose	2nd dose	See footnote 5		←--- 3rd or 4th dose, See footnote 5 ---→									
Pneumococcal conjugate[6] (PCV13)			1st dose	2nd dose	3rd dose		←--- 4th dose ---→									
Pneumococcal polysaccharide[6] (PPSV23)																
Inactivated poliovirus[7] (IPV: <18 yrs)			1st dose	2nd dose	←--- 3rd dose ---→							4th dose				
Influenza[8] (IIV; LAIV) 2 doses for some: See footnote 8					Annual vaccination (IIV only) 1 or 2 doses						Annual vaccination (LAIV or IIV) 1 or 2 doses		Annual vaccination (LAIV or IIV) 1 dose only			
Measles, mumps, rubella[9] (MMR)					See footnote 9		←--- 1st dose ---→					2nd dose				
Varicella[10] (VAR)							←--- 1st dose ---→					2nd dose				
Hepatitis A[11] (HepA)							←--- 2-dose series, See footnote 11 ---→									
Human papillomavirus[12] (HPV2: females only; HPV4: males and females)														(3-dose series)		
Meningococcal[13] (Hib-MenCY ≥ 6 weeks; MenACWY-D ≥9 mos; MenACWY-CRM ≥ 2 mos)			See footnote 13											1st dose		Booster

Range of recommended ages for all children

Range of recommended ages for catch-up immunization

Range of recommended ages for certain high-risk groups

Range of recommended ages during which catch-up is encouraged and for certain high-risk groups

Not routinely recommended

This schedule includes recommendations in effect as of January 1, 2015. Any dose not administered at the recommended age should be administered at a subsequent visit, when indicated and feasible. The use of a combination vaccine generally is preferred over separate injections of its equivalent component vaccines. Vaccination providers should consult the relevant Advisory Committee on Immunization Practices (ACIP) statement for detailed recommendations, available online at http://www.cdc.gov/vaccines/hcp/acip-recs/index.html. Clinically significant adverse events that follow vaccination should be reported to the Vaccine Adverse Event Reporting System (VAERS) online (http://www.vaers.hhs.gov) or by telephone (800-822-7967). Suspected cases of vaccine-preventable diseases should be reported to the state or local health department. Additional information, including precautions and contraindications for vaccination, is available from CDC online (http://www.cdc.gov/vaccines/recs/vac-admin/contraindications.htm) or by telephone (800-CDC-INFO [800-232-4636]).

This schedule is approved by the Advisory Committee on Immunization Practices (http//www.cdc.gov/vaccines/acip), the American Academy of Pediatrics (http://www.aap.org), the American Academy of Family Physicians (http://www.aafp.org), and the American College of Obstetricians and Gynecologists (http://www.acog.org).

NOTE: The above recommendations must be read along with the footnotes of this schedule.

Appendix A

FIGURE 2. Catch-up immunization schedule for persons aged 4 months through 18 years who start late or who are more than 1 month behind —United States, 2015.
The figure below provides catch-up schedules and minimum intervals between doses for children whose vaccinations have been delayed. A vaccine series does not need to be restarted, regardless of the time that has elapsed between doses. Use the section appropriate for the child's age. Always use this table in conjunction with Figure 1 and the footnotes that follow.

Vaccine	Minimum Age for Dose 1	Minimum Interval Between Doses			
		Dose 1 to Dose 2	Dose 2 to Dose 3	Dose 3 to Dose 4	Dose 4 to Dose 5
Children age 4 months through 6 years					
Hepatitis B[1]	Birth	4 weeks	8 weeks *and* at least 16 weeks after first dose. Minimum age for the final dose is 24 weeks.		
Rotavirus[2]	6 weeks	4 weeks	4 weeks[2]		
Diphtheria, tetanus, and acellular pertussis[3]	6 weeks	4 weeks	4 weeks	6 months	6 months[3]
Haemophilus influenzae type b[5]	6 weeks	4 weeks if first dose administered before the 1st birthday. 8 weeks (as final dose) if first dose was administered at age 12 through 14 months. No further doses needed if first dose was administered at age 15 months or older.	4 weeks[5] if current age is younger than 12 months **and** first dose was administered at younger than age 7 months, **and** at least 1 previous dose was PRP-T (ActHib, Pentacel) or unknown. 8 weeks (as final dose)[5] if current age is younger than 12 months **and** first dose was administered at age 7 through 11 months; OR if current age is 12 through 59 months **and** first dose was administered before the 1st birthday, **and** second dose administered at younger than 15 months; OR if both doses were PRP-OMP (PedvaxHIB; Comvax) **and** were administered before the 1st birthday. No further doses needed if previous dose was administered at age 15 months or older.	8 weeks (as final dose) This dose only necessary for children age 12 through 59 months who received 3 doses before the 1st birthday.	
Pneumococcal[6]	6 weeks	4 weeks if first dose administered before the 1st birthday. 8 weeks (as final dose for healthy children) if first dose was administered at the 1st birthday or after. No further doses needed for healthy children if first dose administered at age 24 months or older.	4 weeks if current age is younger than 12 months and previous dose given at <7 months old. 8 weeks (as final dose for healthy children) if previous dose given between 7–11 months (wait until at least 12 months old); OR if current age is 12 months or older and at least 1 dose was given before age 12 months. No further doses needed for healthy children if previous dose administered at age 24 months or older.	8 weeks (as final dose) This dose only necessary for children aged 12 through 59 months who received 3 doses before age 12 months or for children at high risk who received 3 doses at any age.	
Inactivated poliovirus[7]	6 weeks	4 weeks[7]	4 weeks[7]	6 months[7] (minimum age 4 years for final dose).	
Meningococcal[13]	6 weeks	8 weeks[13]	See footnote 13	See footnote 13	
Measles, mumps, rubella[8]	12 months	4 weeks			
Varicella[10]	12 months	3 months			
Hepatitis A[11]	12 months	6 months			
Children and adolescents age 7 through 18 years					
Tetanus, diphtheria; tetanus, diphtheria, and acellular pertussis[3]	7 years[4]	4 weeks	4 weeks if first dose of DTaP/DT was administered before the 1st birthday. 6 months (as final dose) if first dose of DTaP/DT was administered at or after the 1st birthday.	6 months if first dose of DTaP/DT was administered before the 1st birthday.	
Human papillomavirus[12]	9 years	Routine dosing intervals are recommended.[12]			
Hepatitis A[11]	Not applicable (N/A)	6 months			
Hepatitis B[1]	N/A	4 weeks	8 weeks **and** at least 16 weeks after first dose.		
Inactivated poliovirus[7]	N/A	4 weeks	4 weeks[7]	6 months[7]	
Meningococcal[13]	N/A	8 weeks[13]	See footnote 13		
Measles, mumps, rubella[8]	N/A	4 weeks			
Varicella[10]	N/A	3 months if younger than age 13 years. 4 weeks if age 13 years or older.			

NOTE: The above recommendations must be read along with the footnotes of this schedule.

Footnotes — Recommended immunization schedule for persons aged 0 through 18 years—United States, 2015

For further guidance on the use of the vaccines mentioned below, see: http://www.cdc.gov/vaccines/hcp/acip-recs/index.html.

For vaccine recommendations for persons 19 years of age and older, see the Adult Immunization Schedule.

Additional information

- For contraindications and precautions to use of a vaccine and for additional information regarding that vaccine, vaccination providers should consult the relevant ACIP statement available online at http://www.cdc.gov/vaccines/hcp/acip-recs/index.html.
- For purposes of calculating intervals between doses, 4 weeks = 28 days. Intervals of 4 months or greater are determined by calendar months.
- Vaccine doses administered 4 days or less before the minimum interval are considered valid. Doses of any vaccine administered ≥5 days earlier than the minimum interval or minimum age should not be counted as valid doses and should be repeated as age-appropriate. The repeat dose should be spaced after the invalid dose by the recommended minimum interval. For further details, see *MMWR, General Recommendations on Immunization and Reports* / Vol. 60 / No. 2; Table 1. *Recommended and minimum ages and intervals between vaccine doses* available online at http://www.cdc.gov/mmwr/pdf/rr/rr6002.pdf.
- Information on travel vaccine requirements and recommendations is available at http://wwwnc.cdc.gov/travel/destinations/list.
- For vaccination of persons with primary and secondary immunodeficiencies, see Table 13, *"Vaccination of persons with primary and secondary immunodeficiencies,"* in *General Recommendations on Immunization* (ACIP), available at http://www.cdc.gov/mmwr/pdf/rr/rr6002.pdf; and American Academy of Pediatrics. "Immunization in Special Clinical Circumstances," in Pickering LK, Baker CJ, Kimberlin DW, Long SS eds. *Red Book: 2012 report of the Committee on Infectious Diseases.* 29th ed. Elk Grove Village, IL: American Academy of Pediatrics.

1. Hepatitis B (HepB) vaccine. (Minimum age: birth)
Routine vaccination:
At birth:
- Administer monovalent HepB vaccine to all newborns before hospital discharge.
- For infants born to hepatitis B surface antigen (HBsAg)-positive mothers, administer HepB vaccine and 0.5 mL of hepatitis B immune globulin (HBIG) within 12 hours of birth. These infants should be tested for HBsAg and antibody to HBsAg (anti-HBs) 1 to 2 months after completion of the HepB series at age 9 through 18 months (preferably at the next well-child visit).
- If mother's HBsAg status is unknown, within 12 hours of birth administer HepB vaccine regardless of birth weight. For infants weighing less than 2,000 grams, administer HBIG in addition to HepB vaccine within 12 hours of birth. Determine mother's HBsAg status as soon as possible and, if mother is HBsAg-positive, also administer HBIG for infants weighing 2,000 grams or more as soon as possible, but no later than age 7 days.

Doses following the birth dose:
- The second dose should be administered at age 1 or 2 months. Monovalent HepB vaccine should be used for doses administered before age 6 weeks.
- Infants who did not receive a birth dose should receive 3 doses of a HepB-containing vaccine on a schedule of 0, 1 to 2 months, and 6 months starting as soon as feasible. See Figure 2.
- Administer the second dose 1 to 2 months after the first dose (minimum interval of 4 weeks), administer the third dose at least 8 weeks after the second dose AND at least 16 weeks after the **first** dose. The final (third or fourth) dose in the HepB vaccine series should be administered **no earlier than age 24 weeks.**
- Administration of a total of 4 doses of HepB vaccine is permitted when a combination vaccine containing HepB is administered after the birth dose.

Catch-up vaccination:
- Unvaccinated persons should complete a 3-dose series.
- A 2-dose series (doses separated by at least 4 months) of adult formulation Recombivax HB is licensed for use in children aged 11 through 15 years.
- For other catch-up guidance, see Figure 2.

2. Rotavirus (RV) vaccines. (Minimum age: 6 weeks for both RV1 [Rotarix] and RV5 [RotaTeq])
Routine vaccination:
Administer a series of RV vaccine to all infants as follows:
1. If Rotarix is used, administer a 2-dose series at 2 and 4 months of age.
2. If RotaTeq is used, administer a 3-dose series at ages 2, 4, and 6 months.
3. If any dose in the series was RotaTeq or vaccine product is unknown for any dose in the series, a total of 3 doses of RV vaccine should be administered.

Catch-up vaccination:
- The maximum age for the first dose in the series is 14 weeks, 6 days; vaccination should not be initiated for infants aged 15 weeks, 0 days or older.
- The maximum age for the final dose in the series is 8 months, 0 days.
- For other catch-up guidance, see Figure 2.

3. Diphtheria and tetanus toxoids and acellular pertussis (DTaP) vaccine. (Minimum age: 6 weeks. Exception: DTaP-IPV [Kinrix]: 4 years)
Routine vaccination:
- Administer a 5-dose series of DTaP vaccine at ages 2, 4, 6, 15 through 18 months, and 4 through 6 years. The fourth dose may be administered as early as age 12 months, provided at least 6 months have elapsed since the third dose. However, the fourth dose of DTaP need not be repeated if it was administered at least 4 months after the third dose of DTaP.

3. Diphtheria and tetanus toxoids and acellular pertussis (DTaP) vaccine (cont'd)
Catch-up vaccination:
- The fifth dose of DTaP vaccine is not necessary if the fourth dose was administered at age 4 years or older.
- For other catch-up guidance, see Figure 2.

4. Tetanus and diphtheria toxoids and acellular pertussis (Tdap) vaccine. (Minimum age: 10 years for both Boostrix and Adacel)
Routine vaccination:
- Administer 1 dose of Tdap vaccine to all adolescents aged 11 through 12 years.
- Tdap may be administered regardless of the interval since the last tetanus and diphtheria toxoid-containing vaccine.
- Administer 1 dose of Tdap vaccine to pregnant adolescents during each pregnancy (preferred during 27 through 36 weeks' gestation) regardless of time since prior Td or Tdap vaccination.

Catch-up vaccination:
- Persons aged 7 years and older who are not fully immunized with DTaP vaccine should receive Tdap vaccine as 1 dose (preferably the first) in the catch-up series; if additional doses are needed, use Td vaccine. For children 7 through 10 years who receive a dose of Tdap as part of the catch-up series, an adolescent Tdap vaccine dose at age 11 through 12 years should NOT be administered. Td should be administered instead 10 years after the Tdap dose.
- Persons aged 11 through 18 years who have not received Tdap vaccine should receive a dose followed by tetanus and diphtheria toxoid (Td) booster doses every 10 years thereafter.
- Inadvertent doses of DTaP vaccine:
  - If administered inadvertently to a child aged 7 through 10 years may count as part of the catch-up series. This dose may count as the adolescent Tdap dose, or the child can later receive a Tdap booster dose at age 11 through 12 years.
  - If administered inadvertently to an adolescent aged 11 through 18 years, the dose should be counted as the adolescent Tdap booster.
- For other catch-up guidance, see Figure 2.

5. Haemophilus influenzae type b (Hib) conjugate vaccine. (Minimum age: 6 weeks for PRP-T [ACTHIB, DTaP-IPV/Hib (Pentacel) and Hib-MenCY (MenHibrix)], PRP-OMP [PedvaxHIB or COMVAX], 12 months for PRP-T [Hiberix])
Routine vaccination:
- Administer a 2- or 3-dose Hib vaccine primary series and a booster dose (dose 3 or 4 depending on vaccine used in primary series) at age 12 through 15 months to complete a full Hib vaccine series.
- The primary series with ActHIB, MenHibrix, or Pentacel consists of 3 doses and should be administered at 2, 4, and 6 months of age. The primary series with PedvaxHib or COMVAX consists of 2 doses and should be administered at 2 and 4 months of age; a dose at age 6 months is not indicated.
- One booster dose (dose 3 or 4 depending on vaccine used in primary series) of any Hib vaccine should be administered at age 12 through 15 months. An exception is Hiberix vaccine. Hiberix should only be used for the booster (final) dose in children aged 12 months through 4 years who have received at least 1 prior dose of Hib-containing vaccine.
- For recommendations on the use of MenHibrix in patients at increased risk for meningococcal disease, please refer to the meningococcal vaccine footnotes and also to *MMWR* February 28, 2014 / 63(RR01);1-13, available at http://www.cdc.gov/mmwr/PDF/rr/rr6301.pdf.

For further guidance on the use of the vaccines mentioned below, see: http://www.cdc.gov/vaccines/hcp/acip-recs/index.html.

5. *Haemophilus influenzae* type b (Hib) conjugate vaccine (cont'd)

Catch-up vaccination:

- If dose 1 was administered at ages 12 through 14 months, administer a second (final) dose at least 8 weeks after dose 1, regardless of Hib vaccine used in the primary series.
- If both doses were PRP-OMP (PedvaxHIB or COMVAX), and were administered before the first birthday, the third (and final) dose should be administered at age 12 through 59 months and at least 8 weeks after the second dose.
- If the first dose was administered at age 7 through 11 months, administer the second dose at least 4 weeks later and a third (and final) dose at age 12 through 15 months or 8 weeks after second dose, whichever is later.
- If first dose is administered before the first birthday and second dose administered at younger than 15 months, a third (and final) dose should be given 8 weeks later.
- For unvaccinated children aged 15 months or older, administer only 1 dose.
- For other catch-up guidance, see Figure 2. For catch-up guidance related to MenHibrix, please see the meningococcal vaccine footnotes and also *MMWR* February 28, 2014 / 63(RR01);1-13, available at http://www.cdc.gov/mmwr/PDF/rr/rr6301.pdf.

Vaccination of persons with high-risk conditions:

- Children aged 12 through 59 months who are at increased risk for Hib disease, including chemotherapy recipients and those with anatomic or functional asplenia (including sickle cell disease), human immunodeficiency virus (HIV) infection, immunoglobulin deficiency, or early component complement deficiency, who have received either no doses or only 1 dose of Hib vaccine before 12 months of age, should receive 2 additional doses of Hib vaccine 8 weeks apart; children who received 2 or more doses of Hib vaccine before 12 months of age should receive 1 additional dose.
- For patients younger than 5 years of age undergoing chemotherapy or radiation treatment who received a Hib vaccine dose(s) within 14 days of starting therapy or during therapy, repeat the dose(s) at least 3 months following therapy completion.
- Recipients of hematopoietic stem cell transplant (HSCT) should be revaccinated with a 3-dose regimen of Hib vaccine starting 6 to 12 months after successful transplant, regardless of vaccination history; doses should be administered at least 4 weeks apart.
- A single dose of any Hib-containing vaccine should be administered to unimmunized* children and adolescents 15 months of age and older undergoing an elective splenectomy; if possible, vaccine should be administered at least 14 days before procedure.
- Hib vaccine is not routinely recommended for patients 5 years or older. However, 1 dose of Hib vaccine should be administered to unimmunized* persons aged 5 years or older who have anatomic or functional asplenia (including sickle cell disease) and unvaccinated persons 5 through 18 years of age with human immunodeficiency virus (HIV) infection.

Patients who have not received a primary series and booster dose or at least 1 dose of Hib vaccine after 14 months of age are considered unimmunized.

6. Pneumococcal vaccines. (Minimum age: 6 weeks for PCV13, 2 years for PPSV23)

Routine vaccination with PCV13:

- Administer a 4-dose series of PCV13 vaccine at ages 2, 4, and 6 months and at age 12 through 15 months.
- For children aged 14 through 59 months who have received an age-appropriate series of 7-valent PCV (PCV7), administer a single supplemental dose of 13-valent PCV (PCV13).

Catch-up vaccination with PCV13:

- Administer 1 dose of PCV13 to all healthy children aged 24 through 59 months who are not completely vaccinated for their age.
- For other catch-up guidance, see Figure 2.

Vaccination of persons with high-risk conditions with PCV13 and PPSV23:

- All recommended PCV13 doses should be administered prior to PPSV23 vaccination if possible.
- For children 2 through 5 years of age with any of the following conditions: chronic heart disease (particularly cyanotic congenital heart disease and cardiac failure); chronic lung disease (including asthma if treated with high-dose oral corticosteroid therapy); diabetes mellitus; cerebrospinal fluid leak; cochlear implant; sickle cell disease and other hemoglobinopathies; anatomic or functional asplenia; HIV infection; chronic renal failure; nephrotic syndrome; diseases associated with immunosuppressive drugs or radiation therapy, including malignant neoplasms, leukemias, lymphomas, and Hodgkin's disease; solid organ transplantation; or congenital immunodeficiency:
  1. Administer 1 dose of PCV13 if any incomplete schedule of 3 doses of PCV (PCV7 and/or PCV13) were received previously.
  2. Administer 2 doses of PCV13 at least 8 weeks apart if unvaccinated or any incomplete schedule of fewer than 3 doses of PCV (PCV7 and/or PCV13) were received previously.
  3. Administer 1 supplemental dose of PCV13 if 4 doses of PCV7 or other age-appropriate complete PCV7 series was received previously.
  4. The minimum interval between doses of PCV (PCV7 or PCV13) is 8 weeks.
  5. For children with no history of PPSV23 vaccination, administer PPSV23 at least 8 weeks after the most recent dose of PCV13.

6. Pneumococcal vaccines (cont'd)

- For children aged 6 through 18 years who have cerebrospinal fluid leak; cochlear implant; sickle cell disease and other hemoglobinopathies; anatomic or functional asplenia; congenital or acquired immunodeficiencies; HIV infection; chronic renal failure; nephrotic syndrome; diseases associated with treatment with immunosuppressive drugs or radiation therapy, including malignant neoplasms, leukemias, lymphomas, and Hodgkin's disease; generalized malignancy; solid organ transplantation; or multiple myeloma:
  1. If neither PCV13 nor PPSV23 has been received previously, administer 1 dose of PCV13 now and 1 dose of PPSV23 at least 8 weeks later.
  2. If PCV13 has been received previously but PPSV23 has not, administer 1 dose of PPSV23 at least 8 weeks after the most recent dose of PCV13.
  3. If PPSV23 has been received but PCV13 has not, administer 1 dose of PCV13 at least 8 weeks after the most recent dose of PPSV23.
- For children aged 6 through 18 years with chronic heart disease (particularly cyanotic congenital heart disease and cardiac failure), chronic lung disease (including asthma if treated with high-dose oral corticosteroid therapy), diabetes mellitus, alcoholism, or chronic liver disease, who have not received PPSV23, administer 1 dose of PPSV23. If PCV13 has been received previously, then PPSV23 should be administered at least 8 weeks after any prior PCV13 dose.
- A single revaccination with PPSV23 should be administered 5 years after the first dose to children with sickle cell disease or other hemoglobinopathies; anatomic or functional asplenia; congenital or acquired immunodeficiencies; HIV infection; chronic renal failure; nephrotic syndrome; diseases associated with treatment with immunosuppressive drugs or radiation therapy, including malignant neoplasms, leukemias, lymphomas, and Hodgkin's disease; generalized malignancy; solid organ transplantation; or multiple myeloma.

7. Inactivated poliovirus vaccine (IPV). (Minimum age: 6 weeks)

Routine vaccination:

- Administer a 4-dose series of IPV at ages 2, 4, 6 through 18 months, and 4 through 6 years. The final dose in the series should be administered on or after the fourth birthday and at least 6 months after the previous dose.

Catch-up vaccination:

- In the first 6 months of life, minimum age and minimum intervals are only recommended if the person is at risk of imminent exposure to circulating poliovirus (i.e., travel to a polio-endemic region or during an outbreak).
- If 4 or more doses are administered before age 4 years, an additional dose should be administered at age 4 through 6 years and at least 6 months after the previous dose.
- A fourth dose is not necessary if the third dose was administered at age 4 years or older and at least 6 months after the previous dose.
- If both OPV and IPV were administered as part of a series, a total of 4 doses should be administered, regardless of the child's current age. IPV is not routinely recommended for U.S. residents aged 18 years or older.
- For other catch-up guidance, see Figure 2.

8. Influenza vaccines. (Minimum age: 6 months for inactivated influenza vaccine [IIV], 2 years for live, attenuated influenza vaccine [LAIV])

Routine vaccination:

- Administer influenza vaccine annually to all children beginning at age 6 months. For most healthy, nonpregnant persons aged 2 through 49 years, either LAIV or IIV may be used. However, LAIV should NOT be administered to some persons, including 1) persons who have experienced severe allergic reactions to LAIV, any of its components, or to a previous dose of any other influenza vaccine; 2) children 2 through 17 years receiving aspirin or aspirin-containing products; 3) persons who are allergic to eggs; 4) pregnant women; 5) immunosuppressed persons; 6) children 2 through 4 years of age with asthma or who had wheezing in the past 12 months; or 7) persons who have taken influenza antiviral medications in the previous 48 hours. For all other contraindications and precautions to use of LAIV, see *MMWR* August 15, 2014 / 63(32);691-697 [40 pages] available at http://www.cdc.gov/mmwr/pdf/wk/mm6332.pdf.

For children aged 6 months through 8 years:

- For the 2014-15 season, administer 2 doses (separated by at least 4 weeks) to children who are receiving influenza vaccine for the first time. Some children in this age group who have been vaccinated previously will also need 2 doses. For additional guidance, follow dosing guidelines in the 2014-15 ACIP influenza vaccine recommendations, *MMWR* August 15, 2014 / 63(32);691-697 [40 pages] available at http://www.cdc.gov/mmwr/pdf/wk/mm6332.pdf.
- For the 2015-16 season, follow dosing guidelines in the 2015 ACIP influenza vaccine recommendations.

For persons aged 9 years and older:

- Administer 1 dose.

For further guidance on the use of the vaccines mentioned below, see: http://www.cdc.gov/vaccines/hcp/acip-recs/index.html.

9. **Measles, mumps, and rubella (MMR) vaccine. (Minimum age: 12 months for routine vaccination)**

Routine vaccination:
- Administer a 2-dose series of MMR vaccine at ages 12 through 15 months and 4 through 6 years. The second dose may be administered before age 4 years, provided at least 4 weeks have elapsed since the first dose.
- Administer 1 dose of MMR vaccine to infants aged 6 through 11 months before departure from the United States for international travel. These children should be revaccinated with 2 doses of MMR vaccine, the first at age 12 through 15 months (12 months if the child remains in an area where disease risk is high), and the second dose at least 4 weeks later.
- Administer 2 doses of MMR vaccine to children aged 12 months and older before departure from the United States for international travel. The first dose should be administered on or after age 12 months and the second dose at least 4 weeks later.

Catch-up vaccination:
- Ensure that all school-aged children and adolescents have had 2 doses of MMR vaccine; the minimum interval between the 2 doses is 4 weeks.

10. **Varicella (VAR) vaccine. (Minimum age: 12 months)**

Routine vaccination:
- Administer a 2-dose series of VAR vaccine at ages 12 through 15 months and 4 through 6 years. The second dose may be administered before age 4 years, provided at least 3 months have elapsed since the first dose. If the second dose was administered at least 4 weeks after the first dose, it can be accepted as valid.

Catch-up vaccination:
- Ensure that all persons aged 7 through 18 years without evidence of immunity (see MMWR 2007 / 56 [No. RR-4], available at http://www.cdc.gov/mmwr/pdf/rr/rr5604.pdf) have 2 doses of varicella vaccine. For children aged 7 through 12 years, the recommended minimum interval between doses is 3 months (if the second dose was administered at least 4 weeks after the first dose, it can be accepted as valid); for persons aged 13 years and older, the minimum interval between doses is 4 weeks.

11. **Hepatitis A (HepA) vaccine. (Minimum age: 12 months)**

Routine vaccination:
- Initiate the 2-dose HepA vaccine series at 12 through 23 months; separate the 2 doses by 6 to 18 months.
- Children who have received 1 dose of HepA vaccine before age 24 months should receive a second dose 6 to 18 months after the first dose.
- For any person aged 2 years and older who has not already received the HepA vaccine series, 2 doses of HepA vaccine separated by 6 to 18 months may be administered if immunity against hepatitis A virus infection is desired.

Catch-up vaccination:
- The minimum interval between the two doses is 6 months.

Special populations:
- Administer 2 doses of HepA vaccine at least 6 months apart to previously unvaccinated persons who live in areas where vaccination programs target older children, or who are at increased risk for infection. This includes persons travelling to or working in countries that have high or intermediate endemicity of infection; men having sex with men; users of injection and non-injection illicit drugs; persons who work with HAV-infected primates or with HAV in a research laboratory; persons with clotting-factor disorders; persons with chronic liver disease; and persons who anticipate close personal contact (e.g., household or regular babysitting) with an international adoptee during the first 60 days after arrival in the United States from a country with high or intermediate endemicity. The first dose should be administered as soon as the adoption is planned, ideally 2 or more weeks before the arrival of the adoptee.

12. **Human papillomavirus (HPV) vaccines. (Minimum age: 9 years for HPV2 [Cervarix] and HPV4 [Gardasil])**

Routine vaccination:
- Administer a 3-dose series of HPV vaccine on a schedule of 0, 1-2, and 6 months to all adolescents aged 11 through 12 years. Either HPV4 or HPV2 may be used for females, and only HPV4 may be used for males.
- The vaccine series may be started at age 9 years.
- Administer the second dose 1 to 2 months after the first dose (minimum interval of 4 weeks); administer the third dose 24 weeks after the first dose and 16 weeks after the second dose (minimum interval of 12 weeks).

Catch-up vaccination:
- Administer the vaccine series to females (either HPV2 or HPV4) and males (HPV4) at age 13 through 18 years if not previously vaccinated.
- Use recommended routine dosing intervals (see Routine vaccination above) for vaccine series catch-up.

13. **Meningococcal conjugate vaccines. (Minimum age: 6 weeks for Hib-MenCY [MenHibrix], 9 months for MenACWY-D [Menactra], 2 months for MenACWY-CRM [Menveo])**

Routine vaccination:
- Administer a single dose of Menactra or Menveo vaccine at age 11 through 12 years, with a booster dose at age 16 years.
- Adolescents aged 11 through 18 years with human immunodeficiency virus (HIV) infection should receive a 2-dose primary series of Menactra or Menveo with at least 8 weeks between doses.
- For children aged 2 months through 18 years with high-risk conditions, see below.

Catch-up vaccination:
- Administer Menactra or Menveo vaccine at age 13 through 18 years if not previously vaccinated.
- If the first dose is administered at age 13 through 15 years, a booster dose should be administered at age 16 through 18 years with a minimum interval of at least 8 weeks between doses.
- If the first dose is administered at age 16 years or older, a booster dose is not needed.
- For other catch-up guidance, see Figure 2.

Vaccination of persons with high-risk conditions and other persons at increased risk of disease:
- Children with anatomic or functional asplenia (including sickle cell disease):
  1. Menveo
     o Children who initiate vaccination at 8 weeks through 6 months: Administer doses at 2, 4, 6, and 12 months of age.
     o Unvaccinated children 7 through 23 months: Administer 2 doses, with the second dose at least 12 weeks after the first dose AND after the first birthday.
     o Children 24 months and older who have not received a complete series: Administer 2 primary doses at least 8 weeks apart.
  2. MenHibrix
     o Children 6 weeks through 18 months: Administer doses at 2, 4, 6, and 12 through 15 months of age.
     o If the first dose of MenHibrix is given at or after 12 months of age, a total of 2 doses should be given at least 8 weeks apart to ensure protection against serogroups C and Y meningococcal disease.
  3. Menactra
     o Children 24 months and older who have not received a complete series: Administer 2 primary doses at least 8 weeks apart. If Menactra is administered to a child with asplenia (including sickle cell disease), do not administer Menactra until 2 years of age and at least 4 weeks after the completion of all PCV13 doses.

- Children with persistent complement component deficiency:
  1. Menveo
     o Children who initiate vaccination at 8 weeks through 6 months: Administer doses at 2, 4, 6, and 12 months of age.
     o Unvaccinated children 7 through 23 months: Administer 2 doses, with the second dose at least 12 weeks after the first dose AND after the first birthday.
     o Children 24 months and older who have not received a complete series: Administer 2 primary doses at least 8 weeks apart.
  2. MenHibrix
     o Children 6 weeks through 18 months: Administer doses at 2, 4, 6, and 12 through 15 months of age.
     o If the first dose of MenHibrix is given at or after 12 months of age, a total of 2 doses should be given at least 8 weeks apart to ensure protection against serogroups C and Y meningococcal disease.
  3. Menactra
     o Children 9 through 23 months: Administer 2 primary doses at least 12 weeks apart.
     o Children 24 months and older who have not received a complete series: Administer 2 primary doses at least 8 weeks apart.

- For children who travel to or reside in countries in which meningococcal disease is hyperendemic or epidemic, including countries in the African meningitis belt or the Hajj, administer an age-appropriate formulation and series of Menactra or Menveo for protection against serogroups A and W meningococcal disease. Prior receipt of MenHibrix is not sufficient for children traveling to the meningitis belt or the Hajj because it does not contain serogroups A or W.
- For children at risk during a community outbreak attributable to a vaccine serogroup, administer or complete an age- and formulation-appropriate series of MenHibrix, Menactra, or Menveo.
- For booster doses among persons with high-risk conditions, refer to MMWR 2013 / 62(RR02);1-22, available at http://www.cdc.gov/mmwr/preview/mmwrhtml/rr6202a1.htm.

For other catch-up recommendations for these persons, and complete information on use of meningococcal vaccines, including guidance related to vaccination of persons at increased risk of infection, see MMWR March 22, 2013 / 62 / (RR02);1-22, available at http://www.cdc.gov/mmwr/pdf/rr/rr6202.pdf.

Appendix A

Recommended Adult Immunization Schedule
United States - 2015

The 2015 Adult Immunization Schedule was approved by the Centers for Disease Control and Prevention's (CDC) Advisory Committee on Immunization Practices (ACIP), American Academy of Family Physicians (AAFP), the American College of Physicians (ACP), the American College of Obstetricians and Gynecologists (ACOG), and the American College of Nurse-Midwives (ACNM). On February 3, 2015, the adult immunization schedule and a summary of changes from 2014 were published in the *Annals of Internal Medicine*, and a summary of changes was published in the *Morbidity and Mortality Weekly Report (MMWR)* on February 5, 2015.

All clinically significant postvaccination reactions should be reported to the Vaccine Adverse Event Reporting System (VAERS). Reporting forms and instructions on filing a VAERS report are available at www.vaers.hhs.gov or by telephone, 800-822-7967.

Additional details regarding ACIP recommendations for each of the vaccines listed in the schedule can be found at www.cdc.gov/vaccines/hcp/acip-recs/index.html.

American Academy of Family Physicians (AAFP)
www.aafp.org/

American College of Physicians (ACP)
www.acponline.org/

American College of Obstetricians and Gynecologists (ACOG)
www.acog.org/

American College of Nurse-Midwives (ACNM)
www.midwife.org/

A

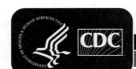

U.S. Department of Health and Human Services
Centers for Disease Control and Prevention

Recommended Adult Immunization Schedule—United States - 2015
Note: These recommendations must be read with the footnotes that follow containing number of doses, intervals between doses, and other important information.

Figure 1. Recommended adult immunization schedule, by vaccine and age group[1]

VACCINE ▼ AGE GROUP ►	19-21 years	22-26 years	27-49 years	50-59 years	60-64 years	≥ 65 years
Influenza[*,2]	1 dose annually					
Tetanus, diphtheria, pertussis (Td/Tdap)[*,3]	Substitute 1-time dose of Tdap for Td booster; then boost with Td every 10 yrs					
Varicella[*,4]	2 doses					
Human papillomavirus (HPV) Female[*,5]	3 doses					
Human papillomavirus (HPV) Male[*,5]	3 doses					
Zoster[6]					1 dose	
Measles, mumps, rubella (MMR)[*,7]	1 or 2 doses					
Pneumococcal 13-valent conjugate (PCV13)[*,8]					1-time dose	
Pneumococcal polysaccharide (PPSV23)[8]	1 or 2 doses					1 dose
Meningococcal[*,9]	1 or more doses					
Hepatitis A[*,10]	2 doses					
Hepatitis B[*,11]	3 doses					
Haemophilus influenzae type b (Hib)[*,12]	1 or 3 doses					

*Covered by the Vaccine Injury Compensation Program

For all persons in this category who meet the age requirements and who lack documentation of vaccination or have no evidence of previous infection; zoster vaccine recommended regardless of prior episode of zoster

Recommended if some other risk factor is present (e.g., on the basis of medical, occupational, lifestyle, or other indication)

No recommendation

Report all clinically significant postvaccination reactions to the Vaccine Adverse Event Reporting System (VAERS). Reporting forms and instructions on filing a VAERS report are available at www.vaers.hhs.gov or by telephone, 800-822-7967.

Information on how to file a Vaccine Injury Compensation Program claim is available at www.hrsa.gov/vaccinecompensation or by telephone, 800-338-2382. To file a claim for vaccine injury, contact the U.S. Court of Federal Claims, 717 Madison Place, N.W., Washington, D.C. 20005; telephone, 202-357-6400.

Additional information about the vaccines in this schedule, extent of available data, and contraindications for vaccination is also available at www.cdc.gov/vaccines or from the CDC-INFO Contact Center at 800-CDC-INFO (800-232-4636) in English and Spanish, 8:00 a.m. - 8:00 p.m. Eastern Time, Monday - Friday, excluding holidays.

Use of trade names and commercial sources is for identification only and does not imply endorsement by the U.S. Department of Health and Human Services.

The recommendations in this schedule were approved by the Centers for Disease Control and Prevention's (CDC) Advisory Committee on Immunization Practices (ACIP), the American Academy of Family Physicians (AAFP), the America College of Physicians (ACP), American College of Obstetricians and Gynecologists (ACOG) and American College of Nurse-Midwives (ACNM).

Figure 2. Vaccines that might be indicated for adults based on medical and other indications[1]

VACCINE ▼ INDICATION ►	Pregnancy	Immuno-compromising conditions (excluding human immunodeficiency virus [HIV]) [4,6,7,8,13]	HIV infection CD4+ T lymphocyte count [4,6,7,8,13] < 200 cells/µL	HIV infection CD4+ T lymphocyte count ≥ 200 cells/µL	Men who have sex with men (MSM)	Kidney failure, end-stage renal disease, receipt of hemodialysis	Heart disease, chronic lung disease, chronic alcoholism	Asplenia (including elective splenectomy and persistent complement component deficiencies) [8,12]	Chronic liver disease	Diabetes	Healthcare personnel
Influenza[*,2]	1 dose IIV annually	1 dose IIV annually	1 dose IIV annually	1 dose IIV or LAIV annually	1 dose IIV annually	1 dose IIV annually	1 dose IIV annually	1 dose IIV annually	1 dose IIV annually	1 dose IIV annually	1 does IIV or LAIV annually
Tetanus, diphtheria, pertussis (Td/Tdap)[*,3]	1 dose Tdap each pregnancy	Substitute 1-time dose of Tdap for Td booster; then boost with Td every 10 yrs									
Varicella[*,4]	Contraindicated		2 doses								
Human papillomavirus (HPV) Female[*,5]		3 doses through age 26 yrs	3 doses through age 26 yrs			3 doses through age 26 yrs					
Human papillomavirus (HPV) Male[*,5]		3 doses through age 26 yrs	3 doses through age 26 yrs			3 doses through age 21 yrs					
Zoster[6]	Contraindicated		1 dose								
Measles, mumps, rubella (MMR)[*,7]	Contraindicated		1 or 2 doses								
Pneumococcal 13-valent conjugate (PCV13)[*,8]		1 dose									
Pneumococcal polysaccharide (PPSV23)[8]		1 or 2 doses									
Meningococcal[*,9]		1 or more doses									
Hepatitis A[*,10]		2 doses									
Hepatitis B[*,11]		3 doses									
Haemophilus influenzae type b (Hib)[*,12]	post-HSCT recipients only	1 or 3 doses									

*Covered by the Vaccine Injury Compensation Program

For all persons in this category who meet the age requirements and who lack documentation of vaccination or have no evidence of previous infection; zoster vaccine recommended regardless of prior episode of zoster

Recommended if some other risk factor is present (e.g., on the basis of medical, occupational, lifestyle, or other indications)

No recommendation

U.S. Department of Health and Human Services
Centers for Disease Control and Prevention

These schedules indicate the recommended age groups and medical indications for which administration of currently licensed vaccines is commonly recommended for adults ages 19 years and older, as of February 1, 2015. For all vaccines being recommended on the Adult Immunization Schedule: a vaccine series does not need to be restarted, regardless of the time that has elapsed between doses. Licensed combination vaccines may be used whenever any components of the combination are indicated and when the vaccine's other components are not contraindicated. For detailed recommendations on all vaccines, including those used primarily for travelers or that are issued during the year, consult the manufacturers' package inserts and the complete statements from the Advisory Committee on Immunization Practices (www.cdc.gov/vaccines/hcp/acip-recs/index.html). Use of trade names and commercial sources is for identification only and does not imply endorsement by the U.S. Department of Health and Human Services.

Appendix A

Footnotes—Recommended Immunization Schedule for Adults Aged 19 Years or Older: United States, 2015

1. Additional information
- Additional guidance for the use of the vaccines described in this supplement is available at www.cdc.gov/vaccines/hcp/acip-recs/index.html.
- Information on vaccination recommendations when vaccination status is unknown and other general immunization information can be found in the General Recommendations on Immunization at www.cdc.gov/mmwr/preview/mmwrhtml/rr6002a1.htm.
- Information on travel vaccine requirements and recommendations (e.g., for hepatitis A and B, meningococcal, and other vaccines) is available at wwwnc.cdc.gov/travel/destinations/list.
- Additional information and resources regarding vaccination of pregnant women can be found at www.cdc.gov/vaccines/adults/rec-vac/pregnant.html.

2. Influenza vaccination
- Annual vaccination against influenza is recommended for all persons aged 6 months or older.
- Persons aged 6 months or older, including pregnant women and persons with hives-only allergy to eggs can receive the inactivated influenza vaccine (IIV). An age-appropriate IIV formulation should be used.
- Adults aged 18 years or older can receive the recombinant influenza vaccine (RIV) (FluBlok). RIV does not contain any egg protein and can be given to age-appropriate persons with egg allergy of any severity.
- Healthy, nonpregnant persons aged 2 to 49 years without high-risk medical conditions can receive either intranasally administered live, attenuated influenza vaccine (LAIV) (FluMist) or IIV.
- Health care personnel who care for severely immunocompromised persons who require care in a protected environment should receive IIV or RIV; health care personnel who receive LAIV should avoid providing care for severely immunosuppressed persons for 7 days after vaccination.
- The intramuscularly or intradermally administered IIV are options for adults aged 18 through 64 years.
- Adults aged 65 years or older can receive the standard-dose IIV or the high-dose IIV (Fluzone High-Dose).
- A list of currently available influenza vaccines can be found at www.cdc.gov/flu/protect/vaccine/vaccines.htm.

3. Tetanus, diphtheria, and acellular pertussis (Td/Tdap) vaccination
- Administer 1 dose of Tdap vaccine to pregnant women during each pregnancy (preferably during 27 to 36 weeks' gestation) regardless of interval since prior Td or Tdap vaccination.
- Persons aged 11 years or older who have not received Tdap vaccine or for whom vaccine status is unknown should receive a dose of Tdap followed by tetanus and diphtheria toxoids (Td) booster doses every 10 years thereafter. Tdap can be administered regardless of interval since the most recent tetanus or diphtheria-toxoid containing vaccine.
- Adults with an unknown or incomplete history of completing a 3-dose primary vaccination series with Td-containing vaccines should begin or complete a primary vaccination series including a Tdap dose.
- For unvaccinated adults, administer the first 2 doses at least 4 weeks apart and the third dose 6 to 12 months after the second.
- For incompletely vaccinated (i.e., less than 3 doses) adults, administer remaining doses.
- Refer to the ACIP statement for recommendations for administering Td/Tdap as prophylaxis in wound management (see footnote 1).

4. Varicella vaccination
- All adults without evidence of immunity to varicella (as defined below) should receive 2 doses of single-antigen varicella vaccine or a second dose if they have received only 1 dose.
- Vaccination should be emphasized for those who have close contact with persons at high risk for severe disease (e.g., health care personnel and family contacts of persons with immunocompromising conditions) or are at high risk for exposure or transmission (e.g., teachers; child care employees; residents and staff members of institutional settings, including correctional institutions; college students; military personnel; adolescents and adults living in households with children; nonpregnant women of childbearing age; and international travelers).
- Pregnant women should be assessed for evidence of varicella immunity. Women who do not have evidence of immunity should receive the first dose of varicella vaccine upon completion or termination of pregnancy and before discharge from the health care facility. The second dose should be administered 4 to 8 weeks after the first dose.
- Evidence of immunity to varicella in adults includes any of the following:
  — documentation of 2 doses of varicella vaccine at least 4 weeks apart;
  — U.S.-born before 1980, except health care personnel and pregnant women;
  — history of varicella based on diagnosis or verification of varicella disease by a health care provider;
  — history of herpes zoster based on diagnosis or verification of herpes zoster disease by a health care provider; or
  — laboratory evidence of immunity or laboratory confirmation of disease.

5. Human papillomavirus (HPV) vaccination
- Two vaccines are licensed for use in females, bivalent HPV vaccine (HPV2) and quadrivalent HPV vaccine (HPV4), and one HPV vaccine for use in males (HPV4).
- For females, either HPV4 or HPV2 is recommended in a 3-dose series for routine vaccination at age 11 or 12 years and for those aged 13 through 26 years, if not previously vaccinated.

- For males, HPV4 is recommended in a 3-dose series for routine vaccination at age 11 or 12 years and for those aged 13 through 21 years, if not previously vaccinated. Males aged 22 through 26 years may be vaccinated.
- HPV4 is recommended for men who have sex with men through age 26 years for those who did not get any or all doses when they were younger.
- Vaccination is recommended for immunocompromised persons (including those with HIV infection) through age 26 years for those who did not get any or all doses when they were younger.
- A complete series for either HPV4 or HPV2 consists of 3 doses. The second dose should be administered 4 to 8 weeks (minimum interval of 4 weeks) after the first dose; the third dose should be administered 24 weeks after the first dose and 16 weeks after the second dose (minimum interval of at least 12 weeks).
- HPV vaccines are not recommended for use in pregnant women. However, pregnancy testing is not needed before vaccination. If a woman is found to be pregnant after initiating the vaccination series, no intervention is needed; the remainder of the 3-dose series should be delayed until completion or termination of pregnancy.

6. Zoster vaccination
- A single dose of zoster vaccine is recommended for adults aged 60 years or older regardless of whether they report a prior episode of herpes zoster. Although the vaccine is licensed by the U.S. Food and Drug Administration for use among and can be administered to persons aged 50 years or older, ACIP recommends that vaccination begin at age 60 years.
- Persons aged 60 years or older with chronic medical conditions may be vaccinated unless their condition constitutes a contraindication, such as pregnancy or severe immunodeficiency.

7. Measles, mumps, rubella (MMR) vaccination
- Adults born before 1957 are generally considered immune to measles and mumps. All adults born in 1957 or later should have documentation of 1 or more doses of MMR vaccine unless they have a medical contraindication to the vaccine or laboratory evidence of immunity to each of the three diseases. Documentation of provider-diagnosed disease is not considered acceptable evidence of immunity for measles, mumps, or rubella.

Measles component:
- A routine second dose of MMR vaccine, administered a minimum of 28 days after the first dose, is recommended for adults who:
  — are students in postsecondary educational institutions,
  — work in a health care facility, or
  — plan to travel internationally.
- Persons who received inactivated (killed) measles vaccine or measles vaccine of unknown type during 1963–1967 should be revaccinated with 2 doses of MMR vaccine.

Mumps component:
- A routine second dose of MMR vaccine, administered a minimum of 28 days after the first dose, is recommended for adults who:
  — are students in a postsecondary educational institution,
  — work in a health care facility, or
  — plan to travel internationally.
- Persons vaccinated before 1979 with either killed mumps vaccine or mumps vaccine of unknown type who are at high risk for mumps infection (e.g., persons who are working in a health care facility) should be considered for revaccination with 2 doses of MMR vaccine.

Rubella component:
- For women of childbearing age, regardless of birth year, rubella immunity should be determined. If there is no evidence of immunity, women who are not pregnant should be vaccinated. Pregnant women who do not have evidence of immunity should receive MMR vaccine upon completion or termination of pregnancy and before discharge from the health care facility.

Health care personnel born before 1957:
- For unvaccinated health care personnel born before 1957 who lack laboratory evidence of measles, mumps, and/or rubella immunity or laboratory confirmation of disease, health care facilities should consider vaccinating personnel with 2 doses of MMR vaccine at the appropriate interval for measles and mumps or 1 dose of MMR vaccine for rubella.

8. Pneumococcal (13-valent pneumococcal conjugate vaccine [PCV13] and 23-valent pneumococcal polysaccharide vaccine [PPSV23]) vaccination
- General information
  — When indicated, only a single dose of PCV13 is recommended for adults.
  — No additional dose of PPSV23 is indicated for adults vaccinated with PPSV23 at or after age 65 years.
  — When both PCV13 and PPSV23 are indicated, PCV13 should be administered first; PCV13 and PPSV23 should not be administered during the same visit.
  — When indicated, PCV13 and PPSV23 should be administered to adults whose pneumococcal vaccination history is incomplete or unknown.
- Adults aged 65 years or older who
  — Have not received PCV13 or PPSV23: Administer PCV13 followed by PPSV23 in 6 to 12 months.
  — Have not received PCV13 but have received a dose of PPSV23 at age 65 years or older: Administer PCV13 at least 1 year after the dose of PPSV23 received at age 65 years or older.

(Continued on next page)

A

Footnotes—Recommended Immunization Schedule for Adults Aged 19 Years or Older: United States, 2015

8. Pneumococcal vaccination (continued)

— Have not received PCV13 but have received 1 or more doses of PPSV23 before age 65: Administer PCV13 at least 1 year after the most recent dose of PPSV23; administer a dose of PPSV23 6 to 12 months after PCV13, or as soon as possible if this time window has passed, and at least 5 years after the most recent dose of PPSV23.

— Have received PCV13 but not PPSV23 before age 65 years: Administer PPSV23 6 to 12 months after PCV13 or as soon as possible if this time window has passed.

— Have received PCV13 and 1 or more doses of PPSV23 before age 65 years: Administer PPSV23 6 to 12 months after PCV13, or as soon as possible if this time window has passed, and at least 5 years after the most recent dose of PPSV23.

- Adults aged 19 through 64 years with immunocompromising conditions or anatomical or functional asplenia (defined below) who

— Have not received PCV13 or PPSV23: Administer PCV13 followed by PPSV23 at least 8 weeks after PCV13; administer a second dose of PPSV23 at least 5 years after the first dose of PPSV23.

— Have not received PCV13 but have received 1 dose of PPSV23: Administer PCV13 at least 1 year after the PPSV23; administer a second dose of PPSV23 at least 8 weeks after PCV13 and at least 5 years after the first dose of PPSV23.

— Have not received PCV13 but have received 2 doses of PPSV23: Administer PCV13 at least 1 year after the most recent dose of PPSV23.

— Have received PCV13 but not PPSV23: Administer PPSV23 at least 8 weeks after PCV13; administer a second dose of PPSV23 at least 5 years after the first dose of PPSV23.

— Have received PCV13 and 1 dose of PPSV23: Administer a second dose of PPSV23 at least 5 years after the first dose of PPSV23.

- Adults aged 19 through 64 years with cerebrospinal fluid leaks or cochlear implants: Administer PCV13 followed by PPSV23 at least 8 weeks after PCV13.
- Adults aged 19 through 64 years with chronic heart disease (including congestive heart failure and cardiomyopathies, excluding hypertension), chronic lung disease (including chronic obstructive lung disease, emphysema, and asthma), chronic liver disease (including cirrhosis), alcoholism, or diabetes mellitus: Administer PPSV23.
- Adults aged 19 through 64 years who smoke cigarettes or reside in nursing home or long-term care facilities: Administer PPSV23.
- Routine pneumococcal vaccination is not recommended for American Indian/Alaska Native or other adults unless they have the indications as above; however, public health authorities may consider recommending the use of pneumococcal vaccines for American Indians/Alaska Natives or other adults who live in areas with increased risk for invasive pneumococcal disease.
- Immunocompromising conditions that are indications for pneumococcal vaccination are: Congenital or acquired immunodeficiency (including B- or T-lymphocyte deficiency, complement deficiencies, and phagocytic disorders excluding chronic granulomatous disease), HIV infection, chronic renal failure, nephrotic syndrome, leukemia, lymphoma, Hodgkin disease, generalized malignancy, multiple myeloma, solid organ transplant, and iatrogenic immunosuppression (including long-term systemic corticosteroids and radiation therapy).
- Anatomical or functional asplenia that are indications for pneumococcal vaccination are: Sickle cell disease and other hemoglobinopathies, congenital or acquired asplenia, splenic dysfunction, and splenectomy. Administer pneumococcal vaccines at least 2 weeks before immunosuppressive therapy or an elective splenectomy, and as soon as possible to adults who are newly diagnosed with asymptomatic or symptomatic HIV infection.

9. Meningococcal vaccination

- Administer 2 doses of quadrivalent meningococcal conjugate vaccine (MenACWY [Menactra, Menveo]) at least 2 months apart to adults of all ages with anatomical or functional asplenia or persistent complement component deficiencies. HIV infection is not an indication for routine vaccination with MenACWY. If an HIV-infected person of any age is vaccinated, 2 doses of MenACWY should be administered at least 2 months apart.
- Administer a single dose of meningococcal vaccine to microbiologists routinely exposed to isolates of *Neisseria meningitidis*, military recruits, persons at risk during an outbreak attributable to a vaccine serogroup, and persons who travel to or live in countries in which meningococcal disease is hyperendemic or epidemic.
- First-year college students up through age 21 years who are living in residence halls should be vaccinated if they have not received a dose on or after their 16th birthday.
- MenACWY is preferred for adults with any of the preceding indications who are aged 55 years or younger as well as for adults aged 56 years or older who a) were vaccinated previously with MenACWY and are recommended for revaccination, or b) for whom multiple doses are anticipated. Meningococcal polysaccharide vaccine (MPSV4 [Menomune]) is preferred for adults aged 56 years or older who have not received MenACWY previously and who require a single dose only (e.g., travelers).
- Revaccination with MenACWY every 5 years is recommended for adults previously vaccinated with MenACWY or MPSV4 who remain at increased risk for infection (e.g., adults with anatomical or functional asplenia, persistent complement component deficiencies, or microbiologists).

10. Hepatitis A vaccination

- Vaccinate any person seeking protection from hepatitis A virus (HAV) infection and persons with any of the following indications:

— men who have sex with men and persons who use injection or noninjection illicit drugs;

— persons working with HAV-infected primates or with HAV in a research laboratory setting;

— persons with chronic liver disease and persons who receive clotting factor concentrates;

— persons traveling to or working in countries that have high or intermediate endemicity of hepatitis A; or

— unvaccinated persons who anticipate close personal contact (e.g., household or regular babysitting) with an international adoptee during the first 60 days after arrival in the United States from a country with high or intermediate endemicity. (See footnote 1 for more information on travel recommendations.) The first dose of the 2-dose hepatitis A vaccine series should be administered as soon as adoption is planned, ideally 2 or more weeks before the arrival of the adoptee.

- Single-antigen vaccine formulations should be administered in a 2-dose schedule at either 0 and 6 to 12 months (Havrix), or 0 and 6 to 18 months (Vaqta). If the combined hepatitis A and hepatitis B vaccine (Twinrix) is used, administer 3 doses at 0, 1, and 6 months; alternatively, a 4-dose schedule may be used, administered on days 0, 7, and 21 to 30 followed by a booster dose at month 12.

11. Hepatitis B vaccination

- Vaccinate persons with any of the following indications and any person seeking protection from hepatitis B virus (HBV) infection:

— sexually active persons who are not in a long-term, mutually monogamous relationship (e.g., persons with more than 1 sex partner during the previous 6 months); persons seeking evaluation or treatment for a sexually transmitted disease (STD); current or recent injection drug users; and men who have sex with men;

— health care personnel and public safety workers who are potentially exposed to blood or other infectious body fluids;

— persons with diabetes who are younger than age 60 years as soon as feasible after diagnosis; persons with diabetes who are age 60 years or older at the discretion of the treating clinician based on the likelihood of acquiring HBV infection, including the risk posed by an increased need for assisted blood glucose monitoring in long-term care facilities, the likelihood of experiencing chronic sequelae if infected with HBV, and the likelihood of immune response to vaccination;

— persons with end-stage renal disease, including patients receiving hemodialysis, persons with HIV infection, and persons with chronic liver disease;

— household contacts and sex partners of hepatitis B surface antigen–positive persons, clients and staff members of institutions for persons with developmental disabilities, and international travelers to countries with high or intermediate prevalence of chronic HBV infection; and

— all adults in the following settings: STD treatment facilities, HIV testing and treatment facilities, facilities providing drug abuse treatment and prevention services, health care settings targeting services to injection drug users or men who have sex with men, correctional facilities, end-stage renal disease programs and facilities for chronic hemodialysis patients, and institutions and nonresidential day care facilities for persons with developmental disabilities.

- Administer missing doses to complete a 3-dose series of hepatitis B vaccine to those persons not vaccinated or not completely vaccinated. The second dose should be administered 1 month after the first dose; the third dose should be given at least 2 months after the second dose (and at least 4 months after the first dose). If the combined hepatitis A and hepatitis B vaccine (Twinrix) is used, give 3 doses at 0, 1, and 6 months; alternatively, a 4-dose Twinrix schedule, administered on days 0, 7, and 21 to 30 followed by a booster dose at month 12 may be used.
- Adult patients receiving hemodialysis or with other immunocompromising conditions should receive 1 dose of 40 mcg/mL (Recombivax HB) administered on a 3-dose schedule at 0, 1, and 6 months or 2 doses of 20 mcg/mL (Engerix-B) administered simultaneously on a 4-dose schedule at 0, 1, 2, and 6 months.

12. *Haemophilus influenzae* type b (Hib) vaccination

- One dose of Hib vaccine should be administered to persons who have anatomical or functional asplenia or sickle cell disease or are undergoing elective splenectomy if they have not previously received Hib vaccine. Hib vaccination 14 or more days before splenectomy is suggested.
- Recipients of a hematopoietic stem cell transplant (HSCT) should be vaccinated with a 3-dose regimen 6 to 12 months after a successful transplant, regardless of vaccination history; at least 4 weeks should separate doses.
- Hib vaccine is not recommended for adults with HIV infection since their risk for Hib infection is low.

13. Immunocompromising conditions

- Inactivated vaccines generally are acceptable (e.g., pneumococcal, meningococcal, and inactivated influenza vaccine) and live vaccines generally are avoided in persons with immune deficiencies or immunocompromising conditions. Information on specific conditions is available at www.cdc.gov/vaccines/hcp/acip-recs/index.html.

Appendix A

TABLE. Contraindications and precautions to commonly used vaccines in adults [1*†]

Vaccine	Contraindications	Precautions
Influenza, inactivated (IIV)[2]	• Severe allergic reaction (e.g., anaphylaxis) after previous dose of any influenza vaccine; or to a vaccine component, including egg protein	• Moderate or severe acute illness with or without fever • History of Guillain-Barré Syndrome within 6 weeks of previous influenza vaccination • Adults who experience only hives with exposure to eggs may receive RIV or, with additional safety precautions, IIV[2]
Influenza, recombinant (RIV)	• Severe allergic reaction (e.g., anaphylaxis) after previous dose of RIV or to a vaccine component. RIV does not contain any egg protein[2]	• Moderate or severe acute illness with or without fever • History of Guillain-Barré Syndrome within 6 weeks of previous influenza vaccination
Influenza, live attenuated (LAIV)[2,3]	• Severe allergic reaction (e.g., anaphylaxis) to any component of the vaccine, or to a previous dose of any influenza vaccine • In addition, ACIP recommends that LAIV not be used in the following populations: — pregnant women — immunosuppressed adults — adults with egg allergy of any severity — adults who have taken influenza antiviral medications (amantadine, rimantadine, zanamivir, or oseltamivir) within the previous 48 hours; avoid use of these antiviral drugs for 14 days after vaccination	• Moderate or severe acute illness with or without fever. • History of Guillain-Barré Syndrome within 6 weeks of previous influenza vaccination • Asthma in persons aged 5 years and older • Other chronic medical conditions, e.g., other chronic lung diseases, chronic cardiovascular disease (excluding isolated hypertension), diabetes, chronic renal or hepatic disease, hematologic disease, neurologic disease, and metabolic disorders
Tetanus, diphtheria, pertussis (Tdap); tetanus, diphtheria (Td)	• Severe allergic reaction (e.g., anaphylaxis) after a previous dose or to a vaccine component • For pertussis-containing vaccines: encephalopathy (e.g., coma, decreased level of consciousness, or prolonged seizures) not attributable to another identifiable cause within 7 days of administration of a previous dose of Tdap, diphtheria and tetanus toxoids and pertussis (DTP), or diphtheria and tetanus toxoids and acellular pertussis (DTaP) vaccine	• Moderate or severe acute illness with or without fever • Guillain-Barré Syndrome within 6 weeks after a previous dose of tetanus toxoid-containing vaccine • History of Arthus-type hypersensitivity reactions after a previous dose of tetanus or diphtheria toxoid-containing vaccine; defer vaccination until at least 10 years have elapsed since the last tetanus toxoid-containing vaccine • For pertussis-containing vaccines: progressive or unstable neurologic disorder, uncontrolled seizures, or progressive encephalopathy until a treatment regimen has been established and the condition has stabilized
Varicella[3]	• Severe allergic reaction (e.g., anaphylaxis) after a previous dose or to a vaccine component • Known severe immunodeficiency (e.g., from hematologic and solid tumors, receipt of chemotherapy, congenital immunodeficiency, or long-term immunosuppressive therapy,[4] or patients with human immunodeficiency virus [HIV] infection who are severely immunocompromised) • Pregnancy	• Recent (within 11 months) receipt of antibody-containing blood product (specific interval depends on product)[5] • Moderate or severe acute illness with or without fever • Receipt of specific antivirals (i.e., acyclovir, famciclovir, or valacyclovir) 24 hours before vaccination; avoid use of these antiviral drugs for 14 days after vaccination
Human papillomavirus (HPV)	• Severe allergic reaction (e.g., anaphylaxis) after a previous dose or to a vaccine component	• Moderate or severe acute illness with or without fever • Pregnancy
Zoster[3]	• Severe allergic reaction (e.g., anaphylaxis) to a vaccine component • Known severe immunodeficiency (e.g., from hematologic and solid tumors, receipt of chemotherapy, or long-term immunosuppressive therapy,4 or patients with HIV infection who are severely immunocompromised) • Pregnancy	• Moderate or severe acute illness with or without fever • Receipt of specific antivirals (i.e., acyclovir, famciclovir, or valacyclovir) 24 hours before vaccination; avoid use of these antiviral drugs for 14 days after vaccination
Measles, mumps, rubella (MMR)[3]	• Severe allergic reaction (e.g., anaphylaxis) after a previous dose or to a vaccine component • Known severe immunodeficiency (e.g., from hematologic and solid tumors, receipt of chemotherapy, congenital immunodeficiency, or long-term immunosuppressive therapy,[4] or patients with HIV infection who are severely immunocompromised) • Pregnancy	• Moderate or severe acute illness with or without fever • Recent (within 11 months) receipt of antibody-containing blood product (specific interval depends on product)[5] • History of thrombocytopenia or thrombocytopenic purpura • Need for tuberculin skin testing[6]
Pneumococcal conjugate (PCV13)	• Severe allergic reaction (e.g., anaphylaxis) after a previous dose or to a vaccine component, including to any vaccine containing diphtheria toxoid	• Moderate or severe acute illness with or without fever
Pneumococcal polysaccharide (PPSV23)	• Severe allergic reaction (e.g., anaphylaxis) after a previous dose or to a vaccine component	• Moderate or severe acute illness with or without fever
Meningococcal, conjugate (MenACWY); meningococcal, polysaccharide (MPSV4)	• Severe allergic reaction (e.g., anaphylaxis) after a previous dose or to a vaccine component	• Moderate or severe acute illness with or without fever
Hepatitis A	• Severe allergic reaction (e.g., anaphylaxis) after a previous dose or to a vaccine component	• Moderate or severe acute illness with or without fever
Hepatitis B	• Severe allergic reaction (e.g., anaphylaxis) after a previous dose or to a vaccine component	• Moderate or severe acute illness with or without fever
Haemophilus influenzae Type b (Hib)	• Severe allergic reaction (e.g., anaphylaxis) after a previous dose or to a vaccine component	• Moderate or severe acute illness with or without fever

1. Vaccine package inserts and the full ACIP recommendations for these vaccines should be consulted for additional information on vaccine-related contraindications and precautions and for more information on vaccine excipients. Events or conditions listed as precautions should be reviewed carefully. Benefits of and risks for administering a specific vaccine to a person under these circumstances should be considered. If the risk from the vaccine is believed to outweigh the benefit, the vaccine should not be administered. If the benefit of vaccination is believed to outweigh the risk, the vaccine should be administered. A contraindication is a condition in a recipient that increases the chance of a serious adverse reaction. Therefore, a vaccine should not be administered when a contraindication is present.

2. For more information on use of influenza vaccines among persons with egg allergies and a complete list of conditions that CDC considers to be reasons to avoid receiving LAIV, see CDC. Prevention and control of seasonal influenza with vaccines: recommendations of the Advisory Committee on Immunization Practices (ACIP) — United States, 2014–15 Influenza Season. *MMWR* 2014;63(32):691–97.

3. LAIV, MMR, varicella, or zoster vaccines can be administered on the same day. If not administered on the same day, live vaccines should be separated by at least 28 days.

4. Immunosuppressive steroid dose is considered to be ≥2 weeks of daily receipt of 20 mg of prednisone or the equivalent. Vaccination should be deferred for at least 1 month after discontinuation of such therapy. Providers should consult ACIP recommendations for complete information on the use of specific live vaccines among persons on immune-suppressing medications or with immune suppression because of other reasons.

5. Vaccine should be deferred for the appropriate interval if replacement immune globulin products are being administered. See CDC. General recommendations on immunization: recommendations of the Advisory Committee on Immunization Practices (ACIP). *MMWR* 2011;60(No. RR-2). Available at www.cdc.gov/vaccines/pubs/pinkbook/index.html.

6. Measles vaccination might suppress tuberculin reactivity temporarily. Measles-containing vaccine may be administered on the same day as tuberculin skin testing. If testing cannot be performed until after the day of MMR vaccination, the test should be postponed for at least 4 weeks after the vaccination. If an urgent need exists to skin test, do so with the understanding that reactivity might be reduced by the vaccine.

* Adapted from CDC. Table 6. Contraindications and precautions to commonly used vaccines. General recommendations on immunization: recommendations of the Advisory Committee on Immunization Practices. MMWR 2011;60(No. RR-2):40–41 and from Atkinson W, Wolfe S, Hamborsky J, eds. Appendix A. Epidemiology and prevention of vaccine preventable diseases. 12th ed. Washington, DC: Public Health Foundation, 2011. Available at www.cdc.gov/vaccines/pubs/pinkbook/index.html.

† Regarding latex allergy, consult the package insert for any vaccine administered.

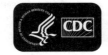

U.S. Department of Health and Human Services
Centers for Disease Control and Prevention

A

CS244083-F

Recommended and Minimum Ages and Intervals Between Doses of Routinely Recommended Vaccines[1,2,3,4]

Vaccine and dose number	Recommended age for this dose	Minimum age for this dose	Recommended interval to next dose	Minimum interval to next dose
Diphtheria-tetanus-acellular pertussis (DTaP)-1[5]	2 months	6 weeks	8 weeks	4 weeks
DTaP-2	4 months	10 weeks	8 weeks	4 weeks
DTaP-3	6 months	14 weeks	6-12 months	6 months[6]
DTaP-4	15-18 months	15 months[7]	3 years	6 months
DTaP-5	4-6 years	4 years	—	—
Haemophilus influenzae type b (Hib)-1[6,8]	2 months	6 weeks	8 weeks	4 weeks
Hib-2	4 months	10 weeks	8 weeks	4 weeks
Hib-3[9]	6 months	14 weeks	6-9 months	8 weeks
Hib-4	12-15 months	12 months	—	—
Hepatitis A (HepA)-1	12-23 months	12 months	6-18 months	6 months
HepA-2	≥18 months	18 months	—	—
Hepatitis B (HepB)-1[5]	Birth	Birth	4 weeks-4 months	4 weeks
HepB-2	1-2 months	4 weeks	8 weeks-17 months	8 weeks
HepB-3[10]	6-18 months	24 weeks	—	—
Herpes zoster (HZV)[11]	≥60 years	60 years	—	—
Human papillomavirus (HPV)-1[12]	11-12 years	9 years	8 weeks	4 weeks
HPV-2	11-12 years (+ 2 months)	9 years (+ 4 weeks)	4 months	12 weeks[13]
HPV-3[13]	11-12 years (+ 6 months)	9 years (+24 weeks)	—	—
Influenza, inactivated (IIV)[14]	≥6 months	6 months[15]	4 weeks	4 weeks
Influenza, live attenuated (LAIV)[14]	2-49 years	2 years	4 weeks	4 weeks
Measles-mumps-rubella (MMR)-1[16]	12-15 months	12 months	3-5 years	4 weeks
MMR-2[16]	4-6 years	13 months	—	—
Meningococcal conjugate (MCV)-1[17]	11-12 years	6 weeks[18]	4-5 years	8 weeks
MCV-2	16 years	11 years (+ 8 weeks)	—	—
Meningococcal polysaccharide (MPSV4)-1[17]	—	2 years	5 years	5 years
MPSV4-2	—	7 years	—	—
Pneumococcal conjugate (PCV)-1[8]	2 months	6 weeks	8 weeks	4 weeks
PCV-2	4 months	10 weeks	8 weeks	4 weeks
PCV-3	6 months	14 weeks	6 months	8 weeks
PCV-4	12-15 months	12 months	—	—
Pneumococcal polysaccharide (PPSV)-1	—	2 years	5 years	5 years
PPSV-2[19]	—	7 years	—	—
Poliovirus, Inactivated (IPV)-1[5]	2 months	6 weeks	8 weeks	4 weeks
IPV-2	4 months	10 weeks	8 weeks-14 months	4 weeks
IPV-3	6-18 months	14 weeks	3-5 years	6 months
IPV-4[20]	4-6 years	4 years	—	—
Rotavirus (RV)-1[21]	2 months	6 weeks	8 weeks	4 weeks
RV-2	4 months	10 weeks	8 weeks	4 weeks
RV-3[22]	6 months	14 weeks	—	—
Tetanus-diphtheria (Td)	11-12 years	7 years	10 years	5 years
Tetanus-diphtheria-acellular pertussis (Tdap)[23]	≥11 years	7 years	—	—
Varicella (Var)-1[16]	12-15 months	12 months	3-5 years	12 weeks[24]
Var-2[16]	4-6 years	15 months[25]	—	—

A

Appendix A

1. Combination vaccines are available. Use of licensed combination vaccines is generally preferred to separate injections of their equivalent component vaccines. When administering combination vaccines, the minimum age for administration is the oldest age for any of the individual components (*exception*: the minimum age for the first dose of MenHibrix is 6 weeks); the minimum interval between doses is equal to the greatest interval of any of the individual components.

2. Information on travel vaccines including typhoid, Japanese encephalitis, and yellow fever, is available at www.cdc.gov/travel. Information on other vaccines that are licensed in the US but not distributed, including anthrax and smallpox, is available at www.bt.cdc.gov.

3. Ages and intervals less than 4 months may be expressed in weeks. When the term "months" is used to express an age or interval, it means calendar months.

4. A hyphen used to express a range (as in "12-15 months") means "through."

5. Combination vaccines containing a hepatitis B component (Comvax, Pediarix, and Twinrix) are available. These vaccines should not be administered to infants younger than 6 weeks because of the other components (i.e., Hib, DTaP, HepA, and IPV).

6. The minimum recommended interval between DTaP-3 and DTaP-4 is 6 months. However, DTaP-4 need not be repeated if administered at least 4 months after DTaP-3. This is a special grace period (2 months long) that can be used while evaluating records retrospectively. An additional 4 days should not be added to this grace period.

7. A special grace period of 3 months, based on expert opinion, can be applied to the minimum age of 15 months when evaluating records retrospectively, which will result in an acceptable minimum age of 12 months. An additional 4 days should not be added to this grace period.

8. Children receiving the first dose of Hib or PCV vaccine at age 7 months or older require fewer doses to complete the series.

9. If PRP-OMP (Pedvax-Hib) was administered at ages 2 and 4 months, a dose at age 6 months is not required.

10. HepB-3 should be administered at least 8 weeks after HepB-2 and at least 16 weeks after HepB-1, and should not be administered before age 24 weeks.

11. Herpes zoster vaccine is recommended as a single dose for persons 60 years of age and older.

12. Bivalent HPV vaccine (Cervarix) is approved for females 9 through 25 years of age. Quadrivalent HPV vaccine (Gardasil) is approved for males and females 9 through 26 years of age.

13. The minimum age for HPV-3 is based on the baseline minimum age for the first dose (9 years) and the minimum interval of 24 weeks between the first and third doses. Dose 3 need not be repeated if it is given at least 16 weeks after the first dose (and if the intervals between doses 1 and 2 and doses 2 and 3 are maintained at 4 weeks and 12 weeks, respectively).

14. One dose of influenza vaccine per season is recommended for most people. Children younger than 9 years of age who are receiving Influenza vaccine for the first time should receive 2 doses this season. See current influenza recommendations for other factors affecting the decision to administer one vs. two doses to children younger than 9 years.

15. The minimum age for inactivated influenza vaccine varies by vaccine manufacturer and formulation. See package inserts for vaccine-specific minimum ages.

16. Combination measles-mumps-rubella-varicella (MMRV) vaccine can be used for children aged 12 months through 12 years. (See CDC. General Recommendations on Immunization: recommendations of the ACIP. *MMWR* 2011;60[No. RR-2],7.)

17. Revaccination with meningococcal vaccine is recommended for previously vaccinated persons who remain at high risk for meningococcal disease. (See CDC. Updated recommendations from the ACIP for vaccination of persons at prolonged increased risk for meningococcal disease. *MMWR* 2009;58:[1042-3])

18. Menactra can be given as young as 9 months for high-risk children. Menveo can be given as young as 2 months for high-risk children. MenHibrix can be given as young as 6 weeks for high-risk children. MenHibrix is given as a four dose series at 2 months, 4 months, 6 months and 12-18 months.

19. A second dose of PPSV 5 years after the first dose is recommended for persons ≤65 years of age at highest risk for serious pneumococcal infection, and for those who are likely to have a rapid decline in pneumococcal antibody concentration. (See CDC. Prevention of pneumococcal disease: recommendations of the ACIP. *MMWR* 1997;46[No. RR-8].)

20. A fourth dose is not needed if the third dose was administered on or after the 4th birthday and at least 6 months after the previous dose.

21. The first dose of rotavirus must be administered between 6 weeks 0 days and 14 weeks 6 days. The vaccine series should not be started after age 15 weeks 0 days. Rotavirus vaccine should not be administered to children older than 8 months 0 days, regardless of the number of doses received before that age.

22. If two doses of Rotarix are administered as age appropriate, a third dose is not necessary.

23. Only one dose of Tdap is recommended. Subsequent doses should be given as Td. For management of a tetanus-prone wound in a person who has received a primary series of a tetanus-toxoid containing vaccine, the minimum interval after a previous dose of any tetanus-containing vaccine is 5 years.

24. For persons beginning the series on or after the 13th birthday, the minimum interval from varicella-1 to varicella-2 is 4 weeks. While it is not recommended, if a child younger than 13 years receives varicella-2 at an interval of 4 weeks or longer from varicella-1, the dose does not need to be repeated.

25. A special grace period of 2 months, based on expert opinion, can be applied to the minimum age of 15 months when evaluating records retrospectively, which will result in an acceptable minimum age of 13 months. An additional 4 days should not be added to this grace period.

Adapted from Table 1, ACIP General Recommendations on Immunization.   June 2014

Summary of Recommendations for Child/Teen Immunization (Age birth through 18 years) (Page 1 of 5)

Vaccine name and route	Schedule for routine vaccination and other guidelines (any vaccine can be given with another)	Schedule for catch-up vaccination and related issues	Contraindications and precautions (mild illness is not a contraindication)
Hepatitis B (HepB) *Give IM*	• Vaccinate all children age 0 through 18yrs. • Vaccinate all newborns with monovalent vaccine prior to hospital discharge. Give dose #2 at age 1–2m and the final dose at age 6–18m (the last dose in the infant series should not be given earlier than age 24wks). After the birth dose, the series may be completed using 2 doses of single-antigen vaccine (ages 1–2m, 6–18m) or up to 3 doses of Comvax (ages 2m, 4m, 12–15m) or with 3 doses of Pediarix (ages 2m, 4m, 6m), which may result in giving a total of 4 doses of hepatitis B vaccine. • **If mother is HBsAg-positive:** Give the newborn HBIG and dose #1 within 12hrs of birth; complete series by age 6m. • **If mother's HBsAg status is unknown:** Give the newborn dose #1 within 12hrs of birth. If low birth weight (less than 2000 grams), also give HBIG within 12hrs. For infants weighing 2000 grams or more whose mother is subsequently found to be HBsAg positive, give the infant HBIG ASAP (no later than age 7d) and follow HepB immunization schedule for infants born to HBsAg-positive mothers.	• Do not restart series, no matter how long since previous dose. • 3-dose series can be started at any age. • Minimum intervals between doses: 4wks between #1 and #2, 8wks between #2 and #3, and at least 16wks between #1 and #3. **Special Notes on Hepatitis B Vaccine (HepB)** **Dosing of HepB:** Monovalent vaccine brands are interchangeable. For people age 0 through 19yrs, give 0.5 mL of either Engerix-B or Recombivax HB. **Alternative dosing schedule for unvaccinated adolescents age 11 through 15yrs:** Give 2 doses Recombivax HB 1.0 mL (adult formulation) spaced 4–6m apart. (Engerix-B is not licensed for a 2-dose schedule.) **For preterm infants:** See ACIP hepatitis B recommendations www.cdc.gov/mmwr/PDF/rr/rr5416.pdf.	**Contraindication** Previous severe allergic reaction (e.g., anaphylaxis) to this vaccine or to any of its components. **Precautions** • Moderate or severe acute illness. • For infants who weigh less than 2000 grams, see ACIP recommendations.*
DTaP, DT (Diphtheria, tetanus, acellular pertussis) *Give IM*	• Give to children at ages 2m, 4m, 6m, 15–18m, and 4–6yrs. • May give dose #1 as early as age 6wks. • May give #4 as early as age 12m if 6m have elapsed since #3. • Do not give DTaP/DT to children age 7yrs and older. • If possible, use the same DTaP product for all doses.	• #2 and #3 may be given 4wks after previous dose. • #4 may be given 6m after #3. • If #4 is given before 4th birthday, wait at least 6m for #5 (age 4–6yrs). • If #4 is given after 4th birthday, #5 is not needed.	**Contraindications** • Previous severe allergic reaction (e.g., anaphylaxis) to this vaccine or to any of its components. • For all pertussis-containing vaccines: Encephalopathy not attributable to an identifiable cause, within 7d after DTP/DTaP/Tdap. **Precautions** • Moderate or severe acute illness. • History of arthus reaction following a prior dose of tetanus or diphtheria toxoid-containing vaccine; defer vaccination until at least 10yrs have elapsed since the last tetanus toxoid-containing vaccine. • Guillain-Barré syndrome (GBS) within 6wks after previous dose of tetanus-toxoid-containing vaccine. • For DTaP only: Any of these events following a previous dose of DTP/DTaP: 1) temperature of 105°F (40.5°C) or higher within 48hrs; 2) continuous crying for 3hrs or more within 48hrs; 3) collapse or shock-like state within 48hrs; 4) seizure within 3d. • For all pertussis-containing vaccines: Progressive or unstable neurologic disorder, uncontrolled seizures, or progressive encephalopathy until a treatment regimen has been established and the condition has stabilized.
Td, Tdap (Tetanus, diphtheria, acellular pertussis) *Give IM*	• For children and teens lacking previous Tdap: Give Tdap routinely at age 11–12yrs and vaccinate older teens on a catch-up basis; then boost every 10yrs with Td. • Make special efforts to give Tdap to children and teens who are (1) in contact with infants younger than age 12m and, (2) healthcare workers with direct patient contact. • Give Tdap to pregnant adolescents during each pregnancy (preferred during 27–36 weeks' gestation), regardless of interval since prior Td or Tdap.	• Children as young as age 7yrs and teens who are unvaccinated or behind schedule should complete a primary Td series (spaced at 0, 1–2m, and 6–12m intervals); substitute Tdap for any dose in the series, preferably as dose #1. • Tdap should be given regardless of interval since previous Td.	

---

* This document was adapted from the recommendations of the Advisory Committee on Immunization Practices (ACIP). To obtain copies of these recommendations, visit CDC's website at www.cdc.gov/vaccines/hcp/ACIP-recs/index.html or visit the Immunization Action Coalition (IAC) website at www.immunize.org/acip. This table is revised periodically. Visit IAC's website at www.immunize.org/childrules to make sure you have the most current version.

Technical content reviewed by the Centers for Disease Control and Prevention www.immunize.org/catg.d/p2010.pdf • Item #P2010 (2/15)

IMMUNIZATION ACTION COALITION Saint Paul, Minnesota • 651-647-9009 • www.immunize.org • www.vaccineinformation.org

A

Summary of Recommendations for Child/Teen Immunization *(Age birth through 18 years)* (Page 2 of 5)

Vaccine name and route	Schedule for routine vaccination and other guidelines (any vaccine can be given with another)	Schedule for catch-up vaccination and related issues	Contraindications and precautions (mild illness is not a contraindication)
Rotavirus (RV) *Give orally*	• Rotarix (RV1): give at ages 2m, 4m. • RotaTeq (RV5): give at ages 2m, 4m, 6m. • May give dose #1 as early as age 6wks. • Give final dose no later than age 8m–0d.	• Do not begin series in infants older than age 14wks 6 days. • Intervals between doses may be as short as 4wks. • If prior vaccination included use of different or unknown brand(s), a total of 3 doses should be given.	**Contraindications** • Previous severe allergic reaction (e.g., anaphylaxis) to this vaccine or to any of its components. If allergy to latex, use RV5. • History of intussusception. • Diagnosis of severe combined immunodeficiency (SCID). **Precautions** • Moderate or severe acute illness. • Altered immunocompetence other than SCID. • Chronic gastrointestinal disease. • For RV1 only, spina bifida or bladder exstrophy.
Varicella (Var) (Chickenpox) *Give SC*	• Give dose #1 at age 12–15m. • Give dose #2 at age 4–6yrs. Dose #2 of Var or MMRV may be given earlier if at least 3m since dose #1. If the 2nd dose was given at least 4wks after 1st dose, it can be accepted as valid. • Give a 2nd dose to all older children/teens with history of only 1 dose. • MMRV may be used in children age 12m through 12yrs (see note below). **Note:** For the first dose of MMR and varicella given at age 12–47m, either MMR and Var or MMRV may be used. Unless the parent or caregiver expresses a preference for MMRV, CDC recommends that MMR and Var be used for the first doses in this age group.	• If younger than age 13yrs, space dose #1 and #2 at least 3m apart. If age 13yrs or older, space at least 4wks apart. • May use as postexposure prophylaxis if given within 5d. • If Var and either MMR, LAIV, and/or yellow fever vaccine are not given on the same day, space them at least 28d apart.	**Contraindications** • Previous severe allergic reaction (e.g., anaphylaxis) to this vaccine or to any of its components. • Pregnancy or possibility of pregnancy within 4wks. • Children on high-dose immunosuppressive therapy or who are immunocompromised because of malignancy and primary or acquired immunodeficiency, including HIV/AIDS (although vaccination on high-dose immunosuppressive therapy may be considered if CD4+ T-lymphocyte percentages are 15% or greater in children age 1 through 8yrs or 200 cells/μL in children age 9yrs and older) **Precautions** • Moderate or severe acute illness. • If blood, plasma, and/or immune globulin (IG or VZIG) were given in past 11m, see ACIP's *General Recommendations on Immunization* regarding time to wait before vaccinating. • Receipt of specific antivirals (i.e., acyclovir, famciclovir, or valacyclovir) 24hrs before vaccination, if possible; delay resumption of these antiviral drugs for 14d after vaccination. • For MMRV only, personal or family (i.e., sibling or parent) history of seizures. **Note:** For patients with humoral immunodeficiency or leukemia, see ACIP recommendations at www.cdc.gov/mmwr/pdf/rr/rr5604.pdf.*
MMR (Measles, mumps, rubella) *Give SC*	• Give dose #1 at age 12–15m. • Give MMR at age 6–11m if traveling internationally; revaccinate with 2 doses of MMR at age 12–15m and at least 4wks later. The dose given at younger than 12m does not count toward the 2-dose series. • Give dose #2 at age 4–6yrs. Dose #2 may be given earlier if at least 4wks since dose #1. For MMRV: dose #2 may be given earlier if at least 3m since dose #1. • Give a 2nd dose to all older children and teens with history of only 1 dose. • MMRV may be used in children age 12m through 12 years (see note above).	• If MMR and either Var, LAIV, and/or yellow fever vaccine are not given on the same day, space them at least 28d apart. • When using MMR for both doses, minimum interval is 4wks. • When using MMRV for both doses, minimum interval is 3m. • May use as postexposure prophylaxis if given within 3d.	**Contraindications** • Previous severe allergic reaction (e.g., anaphylaxis) to this vaccine or to any of its components. • Pregnancy or possibility of pregnancy within 4wks. • Severe immunodeficiency (e.g., hematologic and solid tumors; receiving chemotherapy; congenital immunodeficiency; long-term immunosuppressive therapy, or severely symptomatic HIV). Note: HIV infection is NOT a contraindication to MMR for children who are not severely immunocompromised (consult ACIP MMR recommendations [*MMWR* 2013;62 [RR–4] for details).* Vaccination is recommended if indicated for 1) children age 12m through 5yrs whose CD4+ T-lymphocyte percentage has been greater than 15% for at least 6m or 2) for children age 6yrs and older whose CD4+ T-lymphocyte counts have been 200 cells/μL or greater for at least 6m. **Precautions** • Moderate or severe acute illness. • If blood, plasma, or immune globulin given in past 11m, see ACIP's *General Recommendations on Immunization* regarding time to wait before vaccinating. • History of thrombocytopenia or thrombocytopenic purpura. • For MMRV only, personal or family (i.e., sibling or parent) history of seizures. • Need for tuberculin skin testing (TST). If TST needed, give TST before or on same day as MMR, or give TST 4wks following MMR.

Summary of Recommendations for Child/Teen Immunization *(Age birth through 18 years)* (Page 3 of 5)

February 2015

Vaccine name and route	Schedule for routine vaccination and other guidelines (any vaccine can be given with another)	Schedule for catch-up vaccination and related issues	Contraindications and precautions (mild illness is not a contraindication)
Pneumococcal conjugate (PCV13) *Give IM*	• Give at ages 2m, 4m, 6m, 12–15m (booster dose). • Dose #1 may be given as early as age 6wks. • When children are behind on PCV13 schedule, minimum interval for doses given to children younger than age 12m is 4wks; for doses given at 12m and older, it is 8wks. • For age 24 through 59m and healthy: If unvaccinated or any incomplete schedule or if 4 doses of PCV7 or any other age-appropriate complete PCV7 schedule, give 1 supplemental dose of PCV13 at least 8wks after the most recent dose. • For high-risk** children ages 2 through 5 yrs: Give 2 doses at least 8wks apart if they previously received fewer than 3 doses; give 1 dose at least 8wks after the most recent dose if they previously received 3 doses. • For high-risk** children: All recommended PCV13 doses should be given prior to PPSV vaccination. • PCV13 is not routinely given to healthy children age 5yrs and older. **** High-risk:** *For both PCV13 and PPSV,* those with sickle cell disease; anatomic or functional asplenia; chronic cardiac, pulmonary, or renal disease; diabetes; cerebrospinal fluid leaks; HIV infection; immunosuppression; diseases associated with immunosuppressive and/or radiation therapy; solid organ transplantation; or who have or will have a cochlear implant and, *for PPSV only,* alcoholism and/or chronic liver disease.	• For minimum intervals, see 3rd bullet at left. • For age 7 through 11m: If history of 0 doses, give 2 doses of PCV13, 4wks apart, with a 3rd dose at age 12–15m; if history of 1 or 2 doses, give 1 dose of PCV13 with a 2nd dose at age 12–15m at least 8wks later. • For age 12 through 23m: If unvaccinated or history of 1 dose before age 12m, give 2 doses of PCV13 8wks apart; if history of 1 dose at or after age 12m or 2 or 3 doses before age 12m, give 1 dose of PCV13 at least 8wks after most recent dose; if history of 4 doses of PCV7 or other age-appropriate complete PCV7 schedule, give 1 supplemental dose of PCV13 at least 8wks after the most recent dose. • For age 2 through 5yrs and at high risk**: If unvaccinated or any incomplete schedule of 1 or 2 doses, give 2 doses of PCV13, 1 at least 8wks after the most recent dose and another dose at least 8wks later; if any incomplete series of 3 doses, or if 4 doses of PCV7 or any other age-appropriate complete PCV7 schedule, give 1 supplemental dose of PCV13 at least 8wks after the most recent PCV7 dose. • For children ages 6 through 18yrs with functional or anatomic asplenia (including sickle cell disease), HIV infection or other immunocompromising condition, cochlear implant, or CSF leak, give 1 dose of PCV13 if no previous history of PCV13.	**Contraindication** Previous severe allergic reaction (e.g., anaphylaxis) to a PCV vaccine, to any of its components, or to any diphtheria toxoid-containing vaccine. **Precaution** Moderate or severe acute illness.
Pneumococcal polysaccharide (PPSV) *Give IM or SC*	• Give 1 dose at least 8wks after final dose of PCV13 to high-risk** children age 2yrs and older. • For children who have sickle cell disease, functional or anatomic asplenia, HIV infection, or other immunocompromising condition, give a 2nd dose of PPSV 5yrs after previous PPSV. (See ACIP pneumococcal recommendations at www.cdc.gov/mmwr/pdf/rr/rr5911.pdf.)		**Contraindication** Previous severe allergic reaction (e.g., anaphylaxis) to this vaccine or to any of its components. **Precaution** Moderate or severe acute illness.
Human papillomavirus (HPV) (HPV2, Cervarix) (HPV4, Gardasil) *Give IM*	• Give 3-dose series of either HPV2 or HPV4 to girls at age 11–12yrs on a 0, 1–2, 6m schedule. (May give as early as age 9yrs.) • Give 3-dose series of HPV4 to boys age 11–12yrs on a 0, 1–2, 6m schedule. (May give as early as age 9yrs.) • Give a 3-dose series of either HPV2 or HPV4 to all older girls/women (through age 26yrs) and 3-dose series of HPV4 to all older boys/men (through age 21yrs) who were not previously vaccinated.	Minimum intervals between doses: 4wks between #1 and #2; 12wks between #2 and #3. Overall, there must be at least 24wks between doses #1 and #3. If possible, use the same vaccine product for all doses.	**Contraindication** Previous severe allergic reaction (e.g., anaphylaxis) to this vaccine or to any of its components. **Precautions** • Moderate or severe acute illness. • Pregnancy.

Summary of Recommendations for Child/Teen Immunization *(Age birth through 18 years)*

Vaccine name and route	Schedule for routine vaccination and other guidelines (any vaccine can be given with another)	Schedule for catch-up vaccination and related issues	Contraindications and precautions (mild illness is not a contraindication)
Hepatitis A (HepA) *Give IM*	• Give 2 doses spaced 6–18m apart to all children at age 1yr (12–23m). • Vaccinate all previously unvaccinated children and adolescents age 2yrs and older who - Want to be protected from HAV infection and lack a specific risk factor. - Live in areas where vaccination programs target older children. - Travel anywhere except U.S., W. Europe, N. Zealand, Australia, Canada, or Japan. - Have chronic liver disease, clotting factor disorder, or are adolescent males who have sex with other males. - Use illicit drugs (injectable or non-injectable). - Anticipate close personal contact with an international adoptee from a country of high or intermediate endemicity during the first 60 days following the adoptee's arrival in the U.S.	• Minimum interval between doses is 6m. • Children who are not fully vaccinated by age 2yrs can be vaccinated at a subsequent visit. • Administer 2 doses at least 6 months apart to previously unvaccinated persons who live in areas where vaccination programs target older children, or who are at increased risk for infection. • Give 1 dose as postexposure prophylaxis to incompletely vaccinated children and teens age 12m and older who have recently (during the past 2wks) been exposed to hepatitis A virus.	**Contraindication** Previous severe allergic reaction (e.g., anaphylaxis) to this vaccine or to any of its components. **Precautions** • Moderate or severe acute illness.
Inactivated Polio (IPV) *Give SC or IM*	• Give to children at ages 2m, 4m, 6–18m, 4–6yrs. • May give dose #1 as early as age 6wks. • Not routinely recommended for U.S. residents age18yrs and older (except certain travelers). For information on polio vaccination for international travelers, see wwwnc.cdc.gov/travel/diseases/poliomyelitis.	• The final dose should be given on or after the 4th birthday and at least 6m from the previous dose. • If dose #3 is given after 4th birthday, dose #4 is not needed if dose #3 is given at least 6m after dose #2.	**Contraindication** Previous severe allergic reaction (e.g., anaphylaxis) to this vaccine or to any of its components. **Precautions** • Moderate or severe acute illness. • Pregnancy.
Influenza Inactivated influenza vaccine (IIV) *Give IM* ————— Live attenuated influenza vaccine (LAIV) *Give intranasally*	• Vaccinate all children and teens age 6m and older. • LAIV is preferred for healthy children ages 2 through 8yrs if immediately available; it may be given to non-pregnant people through age 49yrs who lack a contraindication or precaution. • Give 2 doses, spaced 4wks apart, to children age 6m through 8yrs who 1) are first-time vaccinees, or 2) who meet any of the additional guidance in the current year's ACIP influenza vaccine recommendations*. • For IIV, give 0.25 mL dose to children age 6–35m and 0.5 mL dose if age 3yrs and older. • If LAIV and either MMR, Var, and/or yellow fever vaccine are not given on the same day, space them at least 28d apart.		**Contraindications** • Previous severe allergic reaction (e.g., anaphylaxis) to this vaccine, to any of its components, including egg protein. Note: People age 18yrs and older with egg allergy of any severity can receive the recombinant influenza vaccine (RIV) (Flublok). RIV does not contain any egg protein. • For LAIV only: Age younger than 2yrs; pregnancy; immunosuppression (including that caused by medications or HIV); for children and teens ages 6m through 18yrs, current long-term aspirin therapy; for children age 2 through 4yrs, wheezing or asthma within the past 12m, per healthcare provider statement. Receipt of specific antivirals (i.e., amantadine, rimantadine, zanamivir, or oseltamivir) 48hrs before vaccination. Avoid use of these antiviral drugs for 14d after vaccination. For children/teens who experience only hives with exposure to eggs, give IIV with additional safety precautions (i.e., observe patients for 30 minutes after receipt of vaccine for signs of a reaction). **Precautions** • Moderate or severe acute illness. • History of Guillain-Barré syndrome (GBS) within 6wks of a previous influenza vaccination. • For LAIV only: Chronic pulmonary (including asthma in children age 5yrs and older), cardiovascular (except hypertension), renal, hepatic, neurological/neuromuscular, hematologic or metabolic (including diabetes) disorders.

Summary of Recommendations for Child/Teen Immunization *(Age birth through 18 years)*   (Page 5 of 5)

February 2015

Vaccine name and route	Schedule for routine vaccination and other guidelines (any vaccine can be given with another)	Schedule for catch-up vaccination and related issues	Contraindications and precautions (mild illness is not a contraindication)
Hib (*Haemophilus influenzae* type b) *Give IM*	• ActHib (PRP-T): give at age 2m, 4m, 6m, 12–15m (booster dose). • PedvaxHIB or Comvax (containing PRP-OMP): give at age 2m, 4m, 12–15m (booster dose). • Dose #1 of Hib vaccine should not be given earlier than age 6wks. • Give final dose (booster dose) no earlier than age 12m and a minimum of 8wks after the previous dose. • Hib vaccines are interchangeable; however, if different brands of Hib vaccines are administered for dose #1 and dose #2, a total of 3 doses is necessary to complete the primary series in infants. • For vaccination of children 12 months and older who are immunocompromised or asplenic: if previously received no doses or only 1 dose before age 12m, give 2 additional doses at least 8wks apart; if previously received 2 or more doses before age 12m, give 1 additional dose. • Hib is not routinely given to healthy children age 5yrs and older. • 1 dose of Hib vaccine should be administered to children age 5 years and older who have anatomic or functional asplenia (including sickle cell disease) and who have not received a primary series and booster dose or at least 1 dose of Hib vaccine after age 14m. • 1 dose of Hib vaccine should be administered to unvaccinated persons 5 through 18 years of age with HIV infection. • Hiberix is approved ONLY for the booster dose at age 12m through 4yrs.	**All Hib vaccines:** • If #1 was given at 12–14m, give booster in 8wks. • Give only 1 dose to unvaccinated children ages 15–59m. **ActHib:** • #2 and #3 may be given 4wks after previous dose. • If #1 was given at age 7–11m, only 3 doses are needed; #2 is given at least 4wks after #1, then final dose at age 12–15m (wait at least 8wks after dose #2). **PedvaxHIB and Comvax:** • #2 may be given 4wks after dose #1. Recipients of hematopoietic stem cell transplant should receive 3 doses of Hib vaccine at least 4wks apart, beginning 6–12m after transplant, regardless of Hib vaccination history.	**Contraindications** • Previous severe allergic reaction (e.g., anaphylaxis) to this vaccine or to any of its components. • Age younger than 6wks. **Precaution** Moderate or severe acute illness.
Meningococcal conjugate, quadrivalent (MenACWY) *Give IM* <hr> Menactra (MenACWY-D) Menveo (MenACWY-CRM) *Give IM* <hr> Hib-MenCY *Give IM* <hr> **Meningococcal polysaccharide** (MPSV4) *Give SC*	• Give a 2-dose series of quadrivalent MCV (Menactra [MenACWY-D] or Menveo [MenACWY-CRM]) with dose #1 routinely at age 11–12yrs and dose #2 at age 16yrs. • Give MenACWY to all unvaccinated teens age 13 through 18yrs. If vaccinated at age 13–15yrs, give dose #2 at age 16 through 18yrs with a minimum interval of at least 8wks between doses. • For college students, give 1 initial dose to unvaccinated first-year students age 19 through 21yrs who live in residence halls; give dose #2 if most recent dose given when younger than age 16yrs. • Give Hib-MenCY (MenHibrix) or MenACWY-CRM (Menveo) to children age 2–18m with persistent complement component deficiency or anatomic/functional asplenia; give at ages 2, 4, 6, 12–15m. • For unvaccinated or partially vaccinated children age 7–23m with persistent complement component deficiency: 1) if age 7–23m and using MenACWY-CRM (Menveo), give a 2-dose series at least 3m apart with dose #2 given after age 12m or, 2) if age 9–23m and using MenACWY-D (Menactra), give a 2-dose series at least 3m apart. • Give either brand of MenACWY to unvaccinated children age 24m and older with persistent complement component deficiency or anatomic or functional asplenia; give 2 doses, 2m apart. If MenACWY-D is given, it must be separated by 4wks from the final dose of PCV13. • Give age-appropriate series of meningococcal conjugate vaccine (brand must be licensed for age of child) to 1) children age 2m and older at risk during a community outbreak attributable to a vaccine serogroup and 2) children age 9m and older travelling to or living in countries with hyperendemic or epidemic meningococcal disease. Prior receipt of Hib-MenCY is not sufficient for children travelling to the meningitis belt or the Hajj.	• If previously vaccinated and risk of meningococcal disease persists, revaccinate with MenACWY in 3yrs (if previous dose given when younger than age 7yrs) or in 5yrs (if previous dose given at age 7yrs or older). Then, give additional booster doses every 5yrs if risk continues. • When administering MenACWY to children and teens with HIV infection, give 2 initial doses, separated by 8wks. • Minimum ages for MCV: 6wks (Hib-MenCY), 2m (MenACWY-CRM), 9m (MenACWY-D). See ACIP schedule footnotes for additional information on catch-up vaccination of high-risk persons and for Hib-MenCY.	**Contraindication** Previous severe allergic reaction (e.g., anaphylaxis) to this vaccine or to any of its components. **Precautions** Moderate or severe acute illness.

Summary of Recommendations for Adult Immunization *(Age 19 years and older)*

Vaccine name and route	People for whom vaccination is recommended	Schedule for vaccination administration (any vaccine can be given with another)	Contraindications and precautions (mild illness is not a contraindication)
Influenza Inactivated Influenza vaccine (IIV*) *Give IM or ID (intradermally)* **includes recombinant influenza vaccine (RIV)* ____ Live attenuated influenza vaccine (LAIV) *Give intranasally*	For people through age 18 years, consult "Summary of Recommendations for Child/Teen Immunization" at www.immunize.org/catg.d/ p2010.pdf. • Vaccination is recommended for all adults. • LAIV (Flumist) is approved only for healthy nonpregnant people age 2–49yrs. • Adults age 18 through 64yrs may be given any intramuscular IIV product (Fluzone, Fluvirin, Afluria, Flucelvax), or RIV (FluBlok). • Adults age 18 through 64 yrs may be given intramuscular IIV (Afluria) via jet injector (Stratis) • Adults age 65yrs and older may be given standard-dose IIV, or high-dose IIV (Fluzone High-Dose), or RIV. **Note:** Healthcare personnel who care for severely immunocompromised persons (i.e., those who require care in a protective environment) should receive IIV rather than LAIV. For information on other contraindications and precautions to LAIV, see far right column.	• Give 1 dose every year in the fall or winter. • Begin vaccination services as soon as vaccine is available and continue until the supply is depleted. • Continue to give vaccine to unvaccinated adults throughout the influenza season (including when influenza activity is present in the community) and at other times when the risk of influenza exists. • If 2 or more of the following live virus vaccines are to be given—LAIV, MMR, Var, HZV, and/or yellow fever—they should be given on the same day. If they are not, space them by at least 28d.	**Contraindications** • Previous severe allergic reaction (e.g., anaphylaxis) to this vaccine, to any of its components, including egg protein. Adults with egg allergy of any severity may receive RIV or, adults who experience only hives with exposure to eggs may receive other IIV with additional safety precautions (i.e., observe patient for 30 minutes after receipt of vaccine for signs of a reaction). • For LAIV only: pregnancy; immunosuppression; receipt of specific antivirals (i.e., amantadine, rimantadine, zanamivir, or oseltamivir) within the previous 48hrs. Avoid use of these antiviral drugs for 14d after vaccination. **Precautions** • Moderate or severe acute illness. • History of Guillain-Barré syndrome (GBS) within 6wks following previous influenza vaccination. • For LAIV only: Chronic pulmonary (including asthma), cardiovascular (except hypertension), renal, hepatic, neurologic, hematologic, or metabolic (including diabetes) disorders; immunosuppression (including that caused by medications or HIV).
Td, Tdap (Tetanus, diphtheria, pertussis) *Give IM* ____ Do not use tetanus toxoid (TT) in place of Tdap or Td.	For people through age 18 years, consult "Summary of Recommendations for Child/Teen Immunization" at www.immunize.org/catg.d/ p2010.pdf. • All people who lack written documentation of a primary series consisting of at least 3 doses of tetanus- and diphtheria-toxoid-containing vaccine. • A booster dose of Td or Tdap may be needed for wound management, so consult ACIP recommendations.* **For Tdap only:** • Adults who have not already received Tdap or whose Tdap history is not known. • Healthcare personnel of all ages. • Give Tdap to pregnant women during each pregnancy (preferred during 27—36 weeks' gestation), regardless of the interval since prior Td or Tdap.	• For people who are unvaccinated or behind, complete the primary Td series (spaced at 0, 1 to 2m, 6 to 12m intervals); substitute a one-time dose of Tdap for one of the doses in the series, preferably the first. • Give Td booster every 10yrs after the primary series has been completed. • Tdap should be given regardless of interval since previous Td.	**Contraindications** • Previous severe allergic reaction (e.g., anaphylaxis) to this vaccine or to any of its components. • For Tdap only, history of encephalopathy not attributable to an identifiable cause, within 7d following DTP/DTaP, or Tdap. **Precautions** • Moderate or severe acute illness. • Guillain-Barré syndrome within 6wks following previous dose of tetanus-toxoid-containing vaccine. • History of arthus reaction following a prior dose of tetanus- or diphtheria toxoid-containing vaccine (including MCV4); defer vaccination until at least 10yrs have elapsed since the last tetanus toxoid-containing vaccine. • For pertussis-containing vaccines only, progressive or unstable neurologic disorder, uncontrolled seizures, or progressive encephalopathy until a treatment regimen has been established and the condition has stabilized.

* This document was adapted from the recommendations of the Advisory Committee on Immunization Practices (ACIP).
To obtain copies of these recommendations, visit CDC's website at www.cdc.gov/vaccines/hcp/ACIP-recs/index.html
or visit the Immunization Action Coalition (IAC) website at www.immunize.org/acip. This table is revised periodically.
Visit IAC's website at www.immunize.org/adultrules to make sure you have the most current version.

Technical content reviewed by the Centers for Disease Control and Prevention

www.immunize.org/catg.d/p2011.pdf • Item #P2011 (2/15)

IMMUNIZATION ACTION COALITION   Saint Paul, Minnesota • 651-647-9009 • www.immunize.org • www.vaccineinformation.org

Summary of Recommendations for Adult Immunization (Age 19 years and older)

Vaccine name and route	People for whom vaccination is recommended	Schedule for vaccination administration (any vaccine can be given with another)	Contraindications and precautions (mild illness is not a contraindication)
MMR (Measles, mumps, rubella) *Give SC*	For people through age 18 years, consult "Summary of Recommendations for Child/Teen Immunization" at www.immunize.org/catg.d/p2010.pdf. • People born in 1957 or later (especially those born outside the U.S.) should receive at least 1 dose of MMR if they have no laboratory evidence of immunity to each of the 3 diseases or documentation of a dose given on or after the first birthday. • People in high-risk groups, such as healthcare personnel (paid, unpaid, or volunteer), students entering college and other post-high school educational institutions, and international travelers, should receive a total of 2 doses. • People born before 1957 are usually considered immune, but evidence of immunity (serology or documented history of 2 doses of MMR) should be considered for healthcare personnel. • Women of childbearing age who do not have acceptable evidence of rubella immunity or vaccination.	• Give 1 or 2 doses (see criteria in 1st and 2nd bullets in box to left). • If dose #2 is recommended, give it no sooner than 4wks after dose #1. • If woman of childbearing-age is found to be rubella susceptible and is not pregnant, give 1 dose of MMR; if she is pregnant, the dose should be given postpartum. This includes women who have already received 1 or 2 doses of rubella-containing vaccine. • If 2 or more of the following live virus vaccines are to be given—LAIV, MMR, Var, HZV, and/or yellow fever—they should be given on the same day. If they are not, space them by at least 28d. May use as post-exposure prophylaxis if given within 3d of exposure.	**Contraindications** • Previous severe allergic reaction (e.g., anaphylaxis) to this vaccine or to any of its components. • Pregnancy or possibility of pregnancy within 4wks. • Severe immunodeficiency (e.g., hematologic and solid tumors; receiving chemotherapy; congenital immunodeficiency; long-term immunosuppressive therapy; or severely symptomatic HIV). **Note:** HIV infection is NOT a contraindication to MMR for those who are not severely immunocompromised (i.e., CD4+ T-lymphocyte counts are greater than or equal to 200 cells/μL) for 6 months.* **Precautions** • Moderate or severe acute illness. • If blood, plasma, and/or immune globulin were given in past 11m, see ACIP's *General Recommendations on Immunization** regarding time to wait before vaccinating. • History of thrombocytopenia or thrombocytopenic purpura. **Note:** If TST (tuberculosis skin test) and MMR are both needed but not given on same day, delay TST for at least 4wks after MMR.
Varicella (chickenpox) (Var) *Give SC*	For people through age 18 years, consult "Summary of Recommendations for Child/Teen Immunization" at www.immunize.org/catg.d/p2010.pdf. • All adults without evidence of immunity. **Note:** Evidence of immunity is defined as written documentation of 2 doses of varicella vaccine; a history of varicella disease or herpes zoster (shingles) based on healthcare-provider diagnosis; laboratory evidence of immunity or confirmation of disease; and/or birth in the U.S. before 1980, with the exceptions that follow. - Healthcare personnel (HCP) born in the U.S. before 1980 who do not meet any of the criteria above should be tested or given the 2-dose vaccine series. If testing indicates they are not immune, give the 1st dose of varicella vaccine immediately. Give the 2nd dose 4–8wks later. - Pregnant women born in the U.S. before 1980 who do not meet any of the criteria above should either 1) be tested for susceptibility during pregnancy and if found susceptible, given the 1st dose of varicella vaccine postpartum before hospital discharge, or 2) not be tested for susceptibility and given the 1st dose of varicella vaccine postpartum before hospital discharge. Give the 2nd dose 4–8wks later.	• Give 2 doses. • Dose #2 is given 4—8wks after dose #1. • If dose #2 is delayed, do not repeat dose #1. Just give dose #2. • If 2 or more of the following live virus vaccines are to be given—LAIV, MMR, Var, HZV, and/or yellow fever—they should be given on the same day. If they are not, space them by at least 28d. • May use as postexposure prophylaxis if given within 5d of exposure.	**Contraindications** • Previous severe allergic reaction (e.g., anaphylaxis) anaphylactic reaction to this vaccine or to any of its components. • Pregnancy or possibility of pregnancy within 4wks. • People on long-term immunosuppressive therapy or who are immunocompromised because of malignancy and primary or acquired immunodeficiency, including HIV/AIDS (although vaccination may be considered if CD4+ T-lymphocyte counts are greater than or equal to 200 cells/μL. See *MMWR* 2007;56,RR-4). **Precautions** • Moderate or severe acute illness. • If blood, plasma, and/or immune globulin (IG or VZIG) were given in past 11m, see ACIP's *General Recommendations on Immunization** regarding time to wait before vaccinating. • Receipt of specific antivirals (i.e., acyclovir, famciclovir, or valacyclovir) 24hrs before vaccination, if possible; delay resumption of these antiviral drugs for 14d after vaccination.

Appendix A

Summary of Recommendations for Adult Immunization *(Age 19 years and older)*

Vaccine name and route	People for whom vaccination is recommended	Schedule for vaccination administration (any vaccine can be given with another)	Contraindications and precautions (mild illness is not a contraindication)
Hepatitis A (HepA) *Give IM* Brands may be used interchangeably.	For people through age 18 years, consult "Summary of Recommendations for Child/Teen Immunization" at www.immunize.org/catg.d/ p2010.pdf. • All adults who want to be protected from hepatitis A virus (HAV) infection and lack a specific risk factor. • People who travel or work anywhere EXCEPT the U.S., Western Europe, New Zealand, Australia, Canada, and Japan. • People with chronic liver disease; injecting and non-injecting drug users; men who have sex with men; people who receive clotting-factor concentrates; people who work with HAV in lab settings; food handlers when health authorities or private employers determine vaccination to be appropriate. • People who anticipate close personal contact with an international adoptee from a country of high or intermediate endemicity during the first 60 days following the adoptee's arrival in the U.S. • Postexposure: adults age 40yrs or younger with recent (within 2 wks) exposure to HAV, give HepA. For people older than age 40yrs with recent (within 2 wks) exposure to HAV, immune globulin is preferred over HepA vaccine.	• Give 2 doses, spaced 6–18m apart (depending on brand). • If dose #2 is delayed, do not repeat dose #1. Just give dose #2. For Twinrix (hepatitis A and B combination vaccine [GSK]) for patients age 18yrs and older only: give 3 doses on a 0, 1, 6m schedule. There must be at least 4wks between doses #1 and #2, and at least 5m between doses #2 and #3.	**Contraindication** Previous severe allergic reaction (e.g. anaphylaxis) to this vaccine or to any of its components. **Precautions** Moderate or severe acute illness.
Hepatitis B (HepB) *Give IM* Brands may be used interchangeably.	For people through age 18 years, consult "Summary of Recommendations for Child/Teen Immunization" at www.immunize.org/catg.d/ p2010.pdf. • All adults who want to be protected from hepatitis B virus infection and lack a specific risk factor. • Household contacts and sex partners of HBsAg-positive people; injecting drug users; sexually active people not in a long-term, mutually monogamous relationship; men who have sex with men; people with HIV; people seeking STD evaluation or treatment; hemodialysis patients and those with renal disease that may result in dialysis; diabetics younger than age 60yrs (diabetics age 60yrs and older may be vaccinated at the clinician's discretion [see ACIP recommendations*]); healthcare personnel and public safety workers who are exposed to blood; clients and staff of institutions for the developmentally disabled; inmates of long-term correctional facilities; certain international travelers; and people with chronic liver disease. **Note:** Provide serologic screening for immigrants from endemic areas. If patient is chronically infected, assure appropriate disease management. For sex partners and household contacts of HBsAg-positive people, provide serologic screening and administer initial dose of HepB vaccine at same visit.	An alternative schedule can also be used at 0, 7d, 21–30d, and a booster at 12m. Give 3 doses on a 0, 1, 6m schedule. • Alternative timing options for vaccination include 0, 2, 4m; 0, 1, 4m; and 0, 1, 2, 12m (Engerix brand only). • There must be at least 4wks between doses #1 and #2, and at least 8wks between doses #2 and #3. Overall, there must be at least 16wks between doses #1 and #3. • Give adults on hemodialysis or with other immunocompromising conditions 1 dose of 40 μg/mL (Recombivax HB) at 0, 1, 6m or 2 doses of 20 μg/mL (Engerix-B) given simultaneously at 0, 1, 2, 6m. • **Schedule for those who have fallen behind:** If the series is delayed between doses, DO NOT start the series over. Continue from where the schedule was interrupted.	**Contraindication** Previous severe allergic reaction (e.g. anaphylaxis) to this vaccine or to any of its components. **Precaution** Moderate or severe acute illness.

Summary of Recommendations for Adult Immunization (*Age 19 years and older*)

February 2015

Vaccine name and route	People for whom vaccination is recommended	Schedule for vaccination administration (any vaccine can be given with another)	Contraindications and precautions (mild illness is not a contraindication)
Zoster (shingles) (HZV) *Give SC*	• People age 60yrs and older. **Note:** Do not test people age 60yrs or older prior to zoster vaccination. Persons born in the U.S. prior to 1980 can be presumed to be immune to varicella for the purpose of zoster vaccination, regardless of their recollection of having had chickenpox.	• Give 1-time dose if unvaccinated, regardless of previous history of herpes zoster (shingles) or chickenpox. • If 2 or more of the following live virus vaccines are to be given—MMR, Var, HZV, and/or yellow fever—they should be given on the same day. If they are not, space them by at least 28d.	**Contraindications** • Previous severe allergic reaction (e.g., anaphylaxis) to any component of zoster vaccine. • Primary cellular or acquired immunodeficiency. • Pregnancy. **Precautions** • Moderate or severe acute illness. • Receipt of specific antivirals (i.e., acyclovir, famciclovir, or valacyclovir) 24hrs before vaccination, if possible; delay resumption of these antiviral drugs for 14d after vaccination.
Hib (*Haemophilus influenzae* type b) *Give IM*	For people through age 18 years, consult "Summary of Recommendations for Child/Teen Immunization" at www.immunize.org/catg.d/ p2010.pdf. • Not routinely recommended for healthy adults. • Those adults at highest risk of serious Hib disease include people who 1) have anatomic or functional asplenia, 2) are undergoing an elective splenectomy, or 3) are recipients of hematopoietic stem cell transplant (HSCT).	• Give 1 dose of any Hib conjugate vaccine to adults in categories 1 or 2 (see 2nd bullet in column to left) if no history of previous Hib vaccine. • For HSCT patients, regardless of Hib vaccination history, give 3 doses, at least 4wks apart, beginning 6–12m after transplant.	**Contraindication** Previous severe allergic reaction (e.g., anaphylaxis) to this vaccine or to any of its components. **Precautions** Moderate or severe acute illness.
Human papillomavirus (HPV) (HPV2, Cervarix) (HPV4, Gardasil) *Give IM*	For people through age 18 years, consult "Summary of Recommendations for Child/Teen Immunization" at www.immunize.org/catg.d/ p2010.pdf. • For unvaccinated females through age 26yrs: Complete a 3-dose series of HPV2 or HPV4. • For unvaccinated males through age 21yrs: Complete a 3-dose series of HPV4. • For unvaccinated males age 22 through 26yrs: Complete a 3-dose series of HPV4 for those who 1) have sex with men or 2) are immunocompromised as a result of infection (including HIV), disease, or medications, or 3) want to be protected from HPV.	• Give 3 doses on a 0, 1–2, 6m schedule. Use either HPV2 or HPV4 for women, and only HPV4 for men. • There must be at least 4wks between doses #1 and #2 and at least 12wks between doses #2 and #3. Overall, there must be at least 24wks between doses #1 and #3, and 16wks between doses #2 and #3. If possible, use the same vaccine product for all three doses.	**Contraindication** Previous severe allergic reaction (e.g., anaphylaxis) to this vaccine or to any of its components. **Precautions** • Moderate or severe acute illness. • Pregnancy.
Inactivated Polio (IPV) *Give IM or SC*	For people through age 18 years, consult "Summary of Recommendations for Child/Teen Immunization" at www.immunize.org/catg.d/ p2010.pdf. • Not routinely recommended for U.S. residents age 18yrs and older. **Note:** Adults living in the U.S. who never received or completed a primary series of polio vaccine need not be vaccinated unless they intend to travel to areas where exposure to wild-type virus is likely. Adults with documented prior vaccination can receive 1 booster dose if traveling to polio endemic areas or to areas where the risk of exposure is high.	• Refer to ACIP recommendations* regarding unique situations, schedules, and dosing information.	**Contraindication** Previous severe allergic reaction (e.g., anaphylaxis) to this vaccine or to any of its components. **Precautions** • Moderate or severe acute illness. • Pregnancy.

A

Recommended intervals between administration of immune globulin preparations and measles- or varicella-containing vaccine

Product / Indication	Dose, including mg immunoglobulin G (IgG)/kg body weight	Recommended interval before measles or varicella-containing[1] vaccine administration
Blood transfusion		
- Red blood cells (RBCs), washed	10 mL/kg (negligible IgG/kg) IV	None
- RBCs, adenine-saline added	10 mL/kg (10 mg IgG/kg) IV	3 months
- Packed RBCs (hematocrit 65%)[2]	10 mL/kg (60 mg IgG/kg) IV	6 months
- Whole blood (hematocrit 35%–50%)[2]	10 mL/kg (80-100 mg IgG/kg) IV	6 months
- Plasma/platelet products	10 mL/kg (160 mg IgG/kg) IV	7 months
Botulinum Immune Globulin Intravenous (Human)	1.5 mL/kg (75 mg IgG/kg) IV	6 months
Cytomegalovirus IGIV	150 mg/kg maximum	6 months
Hepatitis A IG		
- Contact prophylaxis	0.02 mL/kg (3.3 mg IgG/kg) IM	3 months
- International travel	0.06 mL/kg (10 mg IgG/kg) IM	3 months
Hepatitis B IG (HBIG)	0.06 mL/kg (10 mg IgG/kg) IM	3 months
IGIV		
- Replacement therapy for immune deficiencies[3]	300-400 mg/kg IV	8 months
- Immune thrombocytopenic purpura treatment	400 mg/kg IV	8 months
- Measles IG, contact prophylaxis (immunocompromised contact)	400 mg/kg IV	8 months
- Postexposure varicella prophylaxis	400 mg/kg IV	8 months
- Immune thrombocytopenic purpura treatment	1,000 mg/kg IV	10 months
Measles IG, contact prophylaxis		
- Standard (i.e., nonimmunocompromised) contact	0.5 mL/kg (80 mg IgG/kg) IM	6 months
Monoclonal antibody to respiratory syncytial virus F protein (Synagis™)[4]	15 mg/kg (IM)	None
Rabies IG (RIG)	20 IU/kg (22 mg IgG/kg) IM	4 months
Tetanus IG (TIG)	250 units (10 mg IgG/kg) IM	3 months
Varicella IG[5]	125 units/10 kg (60-200 mg IgG/kg) IM, maximum 625 units	5 months

This table is not intended for determining the correct indications and dosages for using antibody-containing products. Unvaccinated persons might not be fully protected against measles during the entire recommended interval, and additional doses of IG or measles vaccine might be indicated after measles exposure. Concentrations of measles antibody in an IG preparation can vary by manufacturer's lot. Rates of antibody clearance after receipt of an IG preparation also might vary. Recommended intervals are extrapolated from an estimated half-life of 30 days for passively acquired antibody and an observed interference with the immune response to measles vaccine for 5 months after a dose of 80 mg IgG/kg.

1 Does not include zoster vaccine. Zoster vaccine may be given with antibody-containing blood products.

2 Assumes a serum IgG concentration of 16 mg/mL.

3 Measles vaccination is recommended for children with mild or moderate immunosuppression from human immunodeficiency virus (HIV) infection, and varicella vaccination may be considered for children with mild or moderate immunosuppression from HIV, but both are contraindicated for persons with severe immunosuppression from HIV or any other immunosuppressive disorder.

4 Contains antibody only to respiratory syncytial virus.

5 Licensed VariZIG is a purified human IG preparation made from plasma containing high levels of anti-varicella antibodies (IgG).

Adapted from Table 5, ACIP General Recommendations on Immunization

June 2014

Healthcare Personnel Vaccination Recommendations

VACCINES AND RECOMMENDATIONS IN BRIEF

Hepatitis B – If previously unvaccinated, give 3-dose series (dose #1 now, #2 in 1 month, #3 approximately 5 months after #2). Give intramuscularly (IM). For HCP who perform tasks that may involve exposure to blood or body fluids, obtain anti-HBs serologic testing 1–2 months after dose #3.

Influenza – Give 1 dose of influenza vaccine annually. Inactivated injectable vaccine is given IM, except when using the intradermal influenza vaccine. Live attenuated influenza vaccine (LAIV) is given intranasally.

MMR – For healthcare personnel (HCP) born in 1957 or later without serologic evidence of immunity or prior vaccination, give 2 doses of MMR, 4 weeks apart. For HCP born prior to 1957, see below. Give subcutaneously (SC).

Varicella (chickenpox) – For HCP who have no serologic proof of immunity, prior vaccination, or diagnosis or verification of a history of varicella or herpes zoster (shingles) by a healthcare provider, give 2 doses of varicella vaccine, 4 weeks apart. Give SC.

Tetanus, diphtheria, pertussis – Give 1 dose of Tdap as soon as feasible to all HCP who have not received Tdap previously and to pregnant HCP with each pregnancy (see below). Give Td boosters every 10 years thereafter. Give IM.

Meningococcal – Give 1 dose to microbiologists who are routinely exposed to isolates of *Neisseria meningitidis* and boost every 5 years if risk continues. Give MCV4 IM; if necessary to use MPSV4, give SC.

Hepatitis A, typhoid, and polio vaccines are not routinely recommended for HCP who may have on-the-job exposure to fecal material.

Hepatitis B

Unvaccinated healthcare personnel (HCP) and/or those who cannot document previous vaccination should receive a 3-dose series of hepatitis B vaccine at 0, 1, and 6 months. HCP who perform tasks that may involve exposure to blood or body fluids should be tested for hepatitis B surface antibody (anti-HBs) 1–2 months after dose #3 to document immunity.

- If anti-HBs is at least 10 mIU/mL (positive), the vaccinee is immune. No further serologic testing or vaccination is recommended.

- If anti-HBs is less than 10 mIU/mL (negative), the vaccinee is not protected from hepatitis B virus (HBV) infection, and should receive 3 additional doses of HepB vaccine on the routine schedule, followed by anti-HBs testing 1–2 months later. A vaccinee whose anti-HBs remains less than 10 mIU/mL after 6 doses is considered a "non-responder."

For non-responders: HCP who are non-responders should be considered susceptible to HBV and should be counseled regarding precautions to prevent HBV infection and the need to obtain HBIG prophylaxis for any known or probable parenteral exposure to hepatitis B surface antigen (HBsAg)-positive blood or blood with unknown HBsAg status. It is also possible that non-responders are people who are HBsAg positive. HBsAg testing is recommended. HCP found to be HBsAg positive should be counseled and medically evaluated.

For HCP with documentation of a complete 3-dose HepB vaccine series but no documentation of anti-HBs of at least 10 mIU/mL (e.g., those vaccinated in childhood): HCP who are at risk for occupational blood or body fluid exposure might undergo anti-HBs testing upon hire or matriculation. See references 2 and 3 for details.

Influenza

All HCP, including physicians, nurses, paramedics, emergency medical technicians, employees of nursing homes and chronic care facilities, students in these professions, and volunteers, should receive annual vaccination against influenza. Live attenuated influenza vaccine (LAIV) may be given only to non-pregnant healthy HCP age 49 years and younger. Inactivated injectable influenza vaccine (IIV) is preferred over LAIV for HCP who are in close contact with severely immunosuppressed patients (e.g., stem cell transplant recipients) when they require protective isolation.

Measles, Mumps, Rubella (MMR)

HCP who work in medical facilities should be immune to measles, mumps, and rubella.

- HCP born in 1957 or later can be considered immune to measles, mumps, or rubella only if they have documentation of (a) laboratory confirmation of disease or immunity or (b) appropriate vaccination against measles, mumps, and rubella (i.e., 2 doses of live measles and mumps vaccines given on or after the first birthday and separated by 28 days or more, and at least 1 dose of live rubella vaccine). HCP with 2 documented doses of MMR are not recommended to be serologically tested for immunity; but if they are tested and results are negative or equivocal for measles, mumps, and/or rubella, these HCP should be considered to have presumptive evidence of immunity to measles, mumps, and/or rubella and are not in need of additional MMR doses.

- Although birth before 1957 generally is considered acceptable evidence of measles, mumps, and rubella immunity, 2 doses of MMR vaccine should be considered for unvaccinated HCP born before 1957 who do not have laboratory evidence of disease or immunity to measles and/or mumps. One dose of MMR vaccine should be considered for HCP with no laboratory evidence of disease or immunity to rubella. For these same HCP who do not have evidence of immunity, 2 doses of MMR vaccine are recommended during an outbreak of measles or mumps and 1 dose during an outbreak of rubella.

Varicella

It is recommended that all HCP be immune to varicella. Evidence of immunity in HCP includes documentation of 2 doses of varicella vaccine given at least 28 days apart, laboratory evidence of immunity, laboratory confirmation of disease, or diagnosis or verification of a history of varicella or herpes zoster (shingles) by a healthcare provider.

Tetanus/Diphtheria/Pertussis (Td/Tdap)

All HCPs who have not or are unsure if they have previously received a dose of Tdap should receive a dose of Tdap as soon as feasible, without regard to the interval since the previous dose of Td. Pregnant HCP should be revaccinated during each pregnancy. All HCPs should then receive Td boosters every 10 years thereafter.

Meningococcal

Vaccination with MCV4 is recommended for microbiologists who are routinely exposed to isolates of *N. meningitidis*.

REFERENCES

1 CDC. Immunization of Health-Care Personnel: Recommendations of the Advisory Committee on Immunization Practices (ACIP). *MMWR*, 2011; 60(RR-7).

2 CDC. CDC Guidance for Evaluating Health-Care Personnel for Hepatitis B Virus Protection and for Administering Postexposure Management, *MMWR*, 2013; 62(10):1–19.

3 IAC. Pre-exposure Management for Healthcare Personnel with a Documented Hepatitis B Vaccine Series Who Have Not Had Post-vaccination Serologic Testing. Accessed at www.immunize.org/catg.d/p2108.pdf.

For additional specific ACIP recommendations, visit CDC's website at www.cdc.gov/vaccines/hcp/acip-recs/index.html or visit IAC's website at www.immunize.org/acip.

Technical content reviewed by the Centers for Disease Control and Prevention

IMMUNIZATION ACTION COALITION   Saint Paul, Minnesota · 651-647-9009 · www.immunize.org · www.vaccineinformation.org

www.immunize.org/catg.d/p2017.pdf · Item #P2017 (3/15)

A

Appendix A

Vaccination of Persons with Primary and Secondary Immune Deficiencies

PRIMARY

Category	Specific Immunodeficiency	Contraindicated Vaccines[1]	Risk-Specific Recommended Vaccines[1]	Effectiveness & Comments
B-lymphocyte (humoral)	Severe antibody deficiencies (e.g., X-linked agammaglobulinemia and common variable immunodeficiency)	OPV[2] Smallpox LAIV BCG Ty21a (live oral typhoid) Yellow fever	Pneumococcal Consider measles and varicella vaccination.	The effectiveness of any vaccine is uncertain if it depends only on the humoral response (e.g., PPSV or MPSV4). IGIV interferes with the immune response to measles vaccine and possibly varicella vaccine.
	Less severe antibody deficiencies (e.g., selective IgA deficiency and IgG subclass deficiency	OPV[2] BCG Yellow fever Other live vaccines appear to be safe.	Pneumococcal	All vaccines likely effective. Immune response might be attenuated.
T-lymphocyte (cell-mediated and humoral)	Complete defects (e.g., severe combined immunodeficiency [SCID] disease, complete DiGeorge syndrome)	All live vaccines [3,4,5]	Pneumococcal	Vaccines may be ineffective.
	Partial defects (e.g., most patients with DiGeorge syndrome, Wiskott-Aldrich syndrome, ataxia-telangiectasia)	All live vaccines [3,4,5]	Pneumococcal Meningococcal Hib (if not administered in infancy)	Effectiveness of any vaccine depends on degree of immune suppression.
Complement	Persistent complement, properdin, or factor B deficiency	None	Pneumococcal Meningococcal	All routine vaccines likely effective.
Phagocytic function	Chronic granulomatous disease, leukocyte adhesion defect, and myeloperoxidase deficiency	Live bacterial vaccines[3]	Pneumococcal[6]	All inactivated vaccines safe and likely effective. Live viral vaccines likely safe and effective.

[1] Other vaccines that are universally or routinely recommended should be given if not contraindicated.
[2] OPV is no longer available in the United States.
[3] Live bacterial vaccines: BCG, and Ty21a *Salmonella typhi* vaccine.
[4] Live viral vaccines: MMR, MMRV, OPV, LAIV, yellow fever, varicella, zoster, rotavirus, and vaccinia (smallpox). Smallpox vaccine is not recommended for children or the general public.
[5] Regarding T-lymphocyte immunodeficiency as a contraindication for rotavirus vaccine, data exist only for severe combined immunodeficiency.
[6] Pneumococcal vaccine is not indicated for children with chronic granulomatous disease beyond age-based universal recommendations for PCV. Children with chronic granulomatous disease are not at increased risk for pneumococcal disease..

A

Vaccination of Persons with Primary and Secondary Immune Deficiencies

SECONDARY

Specific Immunodeficiency	Contraindicated Vaccines[1]	Risk-Specific Recommended Vaccines[1]	Effectiveness & Comments
HIV/AIDS	OPV[2] Smallpox BCG LAIV Withhold MMR and varicella in severely immunocompromised persons. Yellow fever vaccine might have a contraindication or a precaution depending on clinical parameters of immune function.[3]	Pneumococcal Consider Hib (if not administered in infancy) and Meningococcal vaccination.	MMR, varicella, rotavirus, and all inactivated vaccines, including inactivated influenza, might be effective.[4]
Malignant neoplasm, transplantation, immunosuppressive or radiation therapy	Live viral and bacterial, depending on immune status.[5,6]	Pneumococcal	Effectiveness of any vaccine depends on degree of immune suppression.
Asplenia	None	Pneumococcal Meningococcal Hib (if not administered in infancy)	All routine vaccines likely effective.
Chronic renal disease	LAIV	Pneumococcal Hepatitis B[7]	All routine vaccines likely effective.

[1] Other vaccines that are universally or routinely recommended should be given if not contraindicated.

[2] OPV is no longer available in the United States.

[3] Symptomatic HIV infection or CD4+ T-lymphocyte count of <200/mm³ or <15% of total lymphocytes for children <6 years of age is a contraindication to yellow fever vaccine administration. Asymptomatic HIV infection with CD4+ T-lymphocyte count of 200 to 499/ mm³ for persons ≥6 years of age or 15% to 24% of total lymphocytes for children <6 years of age is a precaution for yellow fever vaccine administration. Details of yellow fever vaccine recommendations are available from CDC. (CDC. Yellow Fever Vaccine: Recommendations of the ACIP. *MMWR* 2010:59 [No. RR-7].)

[4] HIV-infected children should receive IG after exposure to measles, and may receive varicella, measles, and yellow fever vaccine if CD4+ T-lymphocyte count is ≥15%.

[5] Live bacterial vaccines: BCG, and Ty21a *Salmonella typhi* vaccine.

[6] Live viral vaccines: MMR, MMRV, OPV, LAIV, yellow fever, varicella, zoster, rotavirus, and vaccinia (smallpox). Smallpox vaccine is not recommended for children or the general public.

[7] Indicated based on the risk from dialysis-based bloodborne transmission.

Adapted from Table 13, ACIP General Recommendations on Immunization.

January 2011

A

Appendix A

Guide to Contraindications and Precautions to Commonly Used Vaccines[1,*,†] (page 1 of 2)

Vaccine	Contraindications	Precautions
Hepatitis B (HepB)	• Severe allergic reaction (e.g., anaphylaxis) after a previous dose or to a vaccine component	• Moderate or severe acute illness with or without fever • Infant weighing less than 2000 grams (4 lbs, 6.4 oz)[2]
Rotavirus (RV5 [RotaTeq], RV1 [Rotarix])	• Severe allergic reaction (e.g., anaphylaxis) after a previous dose or to a vaccine component • Severe combined immunodeficiency (SCID) • History of intussusception	• Moderate or severe acute illness with or without fever • Altered immunocompetence other than SCID • Chronic gastrointestinal disease[3] • Spina bifida or bladder exstrophy[3]
Diphtheria, tetanus, pertussis (DTaP) **Tetanus, diphtheria, pertussis (Tdap)** **Tetanus, diphtheria (DT, Td)**	• Severe allergic reaction (e.g., anaphylaxis) after a previous dose or to a vaccine component • For pertussis-containing vaccines: encephalopathy (e.g., coma, decreased level of consciousness, prolonged seizures) not attributable to another identifiable cause within 7 days of administration of a previous dose of DTP or DTaP (for DTaP); or of previous dose of DTP, DTaP, or Tdap (for Tdap)	• Moderate or severe acute illness with or without fever • Guillain-Barré syndrome (GBS) within 6 weeks after a previous dose of tetanus toxoid-containing vaccine • History of Arthus-type hypersensitivity reactions after a previous dose of tetanus or diphtheria toxoid-containing vaccine; defer vaccination until at least 10 years have elapsed since the last tetanus-toxoid containing vaccine • For pertussis-containing vaccines: progressive or unstable neurologic disorder (including infantile spasms for DTaP), uncontrolled seizures, or progressive encephalopathy until a treatment regimen has been established and the condition has stabilized **For DTaP only:** • Temperature of 105° F or higher (40.5° C or higher) within 48 hours after vaccination with a previous dose of DTP/DTaP • Collapse or shock-like state (i.e., hypotonic hyporesponsive episode) within 48 hours after receiving a previous dose of DTP/DTaP • Seizure within 3 days after receiving a previous dose of DTP/DTaP • Persistent, inconsolable crying lasting 3 or more hours within 48 hours after receiving a previous dose of DTP/DTaP
Haemophilus influenzae **type b (Hib)**	• Severe allergic reaction (e.g., anaphylaxis) after a previous dose or to a vaccine component • Age younger than 6 weeks	• Moderate or severe acute illness with or without fever
Inactivated poliovirus vaccine (IPV)	• Severe allergic reaction (e.g., anaphylaxis) after a previous dose or to a vaccine component	• Moderate or severe acute illness with or without fever • Pregnancy
Pneumococcal (PCV13 or PPSV23)	• Severe allergic reaction (e.g., anaphylaxis) after a previous dose or to a vaccine component (including, for PCV13, to any diphtheria toxoid-containing vaccine)	• Moderate or severe acute illness with or without fever
Measles, mumps, rubella (MMR)[4]	• Severe allergic reaction (e.g., anaphylaxis) after a previous dose or to a vaccine component • Known severe immunodeficiency (e.g., from hematologic and solid tumors, receipt of chemotherapy, congenital immunodeficiency, or long-term immunosuppressive therapy[5] or patients with human immunodeficiency virus [HIV] infection who are severely immunocompromised)[6] • Pregnancy	• Moderate or severe acute illness with or without fever • Recent (within 11 months) receipt of antibody-containing blood product (specific interval depends on product)[7] • History of thrombocytopenia or thrombocytopenic purpura • Need for tuberculin skin testing[8]
Varicella (Var)[4]	• Severe allergic reaction (e.g., anaphylaxis) after a previous dose or to a vaccine component • Known severe immunodeficiency (e.g., from hematologic and solid tumors, receipt of chemotherapy, congenital immunodeficiency, or long-term immunosuppressive therapy[5] or patients with HIV infection who are severely immunocompromised)[6] • Pregnancy	• Moderate or severe acute illness with or without fever • Recent (within 11 months) receipt of antibody-containing blood product (specific interval depends on product)[7] • Receipt of specific antivirals (i.e., acyclovir, famciclovir, or valacyclovir) 24 hours before vaccination; avoid use of these antiviral drugs for 14 days after vaccination.
Hepatitis A (HepA)	• Severe allergic reaction (e.g., anaphylaxis) after a previous dose or to a vaccine component	• Moderate or severe acute illness with or without fever

(continued on page 2)

Technical content reviewed by the Centers for Disease Control and Prevention

IMMUNIZATION ACTION COALITION Saint Paul, Minnesota • 651-647-9009 • www.immunize.org • www.vaccineinformation.org

www.immunize.org/catg.d/p3072a.pdf • Item #P3072a (3/15)

Guide to Contraindications and Precautions to Commonly Used Vaccines[1,*,†] (page 2 of 2)

Vaccine	Contraindications	Precautions
Influenza, inactivated injectable (IIV)[9]	• Severe allergic reaction (e.g., anaphylaxis) after a previous dose of any influenza vaccine or to a vaccine component, including egg protein • In addition, ACIP recommends that LAIV not be used in the following populations: pregnant women; immunosuppressed adults; adults with egg allergy of any severity; adults who have taken influenza antiviral medications (amantadine, rimantadine, zanamivir, or oseltamivir) within the previous 48 hours; avoid use of these antiviral durgs for 14 days after vaccination	• Moderate or severe acute illness with or without fever • History of GBS within 6 weeks of previous influenza vaccination • Persons who experience only hives with exposure to eggs may receive RIV or, with additional safety precautions, IIV.[9]
Influenza, recombinant (RIV)[9]	• Severe allergic reaction (e.g., anaphylaxis) after a previous dose of RIV or to a vaccine component. RIV does not contain any egg protein.[9]	• Moderate or severe acute illness with or without fever • History of GBS within 6 weeks of previous influenza vaccination
Influenza, live attenuated (LAIV)[4,9]	• Severe allergic reaction (e.g., anaphylaxis) to any component of the vaccine, or to a previous dose of any influenza vaccine • Concomitant use of aspirin or aspirin-containing medication in children or adolescents • In addition, ACIP recommends that LAIV not be used in the following populations: pregnant women; immunosuppressed adults; adults with egg allergy of any severity; adults who have taken influenza antiviral medications (amantadine, rimantadine, zanamivir, or oseltamivir) within the previous 48 hours; avoid use of these antiviral durgs for 14 days after vaccination	• Moderate or severe acute illness with or without fever • History of GBS within 6 weeks of previous influenza vaccination • Asthma in persons age 5 years and older • Other chronic medical conditions (e.g., other chronic lung diseases, chronic cardiovascular disease [excluding isolated hypertension], diabetes, chronic renal or hepatic disease, hematologic disease, neurologic disease, and metabolic disorders)
Human papillomavirus (HPV)	• Severe allergic reaction (e.g., anaphylaxis) after a previous dose or to a vaccine component	• Moderate or severe acute illness with or without fever • Pregnancy
Meningococcal: conjugate (MenACWY), polysaccharide (MPSV4)	• Severe allergic reaction (e.g., anaphylaxis) after a previous dose or to a vaccine component	• Moderate or severe acute illness with or without fever
Zoster (HZV)[4]	• Severe allergic reaction (e.g., anaphylaxis) to a vaccine component • Known severe immunodeficiency (e.g., from hematologic and solid tumors, receipt of chemotherapy, or long-term immunosuppressive therapy[5] or patients with HIV infection who are severely immunocompromised). • Pregnancy	• Moderate or severe acute illness with or without fever • Receipt of specific antivirals (i.e., acyclovir, famciclovir, or valacyclovir) 24 hours before vaccination; avoid use of these antiviral drugs for 14 days after vaccination.

FOOTNOTES

1. Vaccine package inserts and the full ACIP recommendations for these vaccines should be consulted for additional information on vaccine-related contraindications and precautions and for more information on vaccine excipients. Events or conditions listed as precautions should be reviewed carefully. Benefits of and risks for administering a specific vaccine to a person under these circumstances should be considered. If the risk from the vaccine is believed to outweigh the benefit, the vaccine should not be administered. If the benefit of vaccination is believed to outweigh the risk, the vaccine should be administered. A contraindication increases the chance of a serious adverse reaction. Therefore, a vaccine should not be administered when a contraindication is present. Whether and when to administer DTaP to children with proven or suspected underlying neuro-logic disorders should be decided on a case-by-case basis.
2. Hepatitis B vaccination should be deferred for preterm infants and infants weighing less than 2000 g if the mother is documented to be hepatitis B surface antigen (HBsAg)-negative at the time of the infant's birth. Vaccination can commence at chronological age 1 month or at hospital discharge. For infants born to women who are HBsAg-positive, hepatitis B immunoglobulin and hepatitis B vaccine should be administered within 12 hours of birth, regardless of weight.
3. For details, see CDC. "Prevention of Rotavirus Gastroenteritis among Infants and Children: Recommendations of the Advisory Committee on Immunization Practices. (ACIP)" *MMWR* 2009;58(No. RR-2), available at www.cdc.gov/vaccines/hcp/acip-recs/index.html.
4. LAIV, MMR, varicella, or zoster vaccines can be administered on the same day. If not administered on the same day, these live vaccines should be separated by at least 28 days.
5. Immunosuppressive steroid dose is considered to be 2 or more weeks of daily receipt of 20 mg prednisone or equivalent. Vaccination should be deferred for at least 1 month after discontinuation of such therapy. Providers should consult ACIP recommendations for complete information on the use of specific live vaccines among persons on immune-suppressing medications or with immune suppression because of other reasons.

6. HIV-infected children may receive varicella and measles vaccine if CD4+ T-lymphocyte count is >15%. (Source: Adapted from American Academy of Pediatrics. Immunization in Special Clinical Circumstances. In: Pickering LK, ed. *Red Book: 2012 Report of the Committee on Infectious Diseases*. 29th ed. Elk Grove Village, IL: American Academy of Pediatrics: 2012.)
7. Vaccine should be deferred for the appropriate interval if replacement immune globulin products are being administered (see "General Recommendations on Immunization: Recommendations of the Advisory Committee on Immunization Practices (ACIP)" *MMWR* 2011;60(No. RR-2) available at www.cdc.gov/vaccines/hcp/acip-recs/index.html.)
8. Measles vaccination might suppress tuberculin reactivity temporarily. Measles-containing vaccine may be administered on the same day as tuberculin skin testing. If testing cannot be performed until after the day of MMR vaccination, the test should be postponed for at least 4 weeks after the vaccination. If an urgent need exists to skin test, do so with the understanding that reactivity might be reduced by the vaccine.
9. For more information on use of influenza vaccines among persons with egg allergies and a complete list of conditions that CDC considers to be reasons to avoid getting LAIV, see CDC. "Prevention and Control of Influenza with Vaccines: Recommendations of the Advisory Committee on Immunization Practices (ACIP) – United States, 2014–15" *MMWR* 2014;63(32):691–97.

---

* Adapted from "Table 6. Contraindications and Precautions to Commonly Used Vaccines" found in: CDC. "General Recommendations on Immunization: Recommendations of the Advisory Committee on Immunization Practices (ACIP)." *MMWR* 2011; 60(No. RR-2), p. 40–41, and from Atkinson W, Wolfe S, Hamborsky J, eds. Appendix A. *Epidemiology and Prevention of Vaccine-Preventable Diseases*.12th ed.
† Regarding latex allergy, consult the package insert for any vaccine administered.

Technical content reviewed by the Centers for Disease Control and Prevention

IMMUNIZATION ACTION COALITION   Saint Paul, Minnesota • 651-647-9009 • www.immunize.org • www.vaccineinformation.org

www.immunize.org/catg.d/p3072a.pdf • Item #P3072a (3/15)

Guide to Contraindications and Precautions to Commonly Used Vaccines in Adults[1,*,†]

Vaccine	Contraindications[1]	Precautions[1]
Influenza, inactivated (IIV) **Influenza, recombinant (RIV)**	• For IIV, severe allergic reaction (e.g., anaphylaxis) after a previous dose of any influenza vaccine; or to a vaccine component, including egg protein • For RIV, severe allergic reaction (e.g., anaphylaxis) after a previous dose of RIV or to a vaccine component. RIV does not contain egg protein[2]	• Moderate or severe acute illness with or without fever • History of Guillain-Barré Syndrome (GBS) within 6 weeks of previous influenza vaccination • Adults who experience only hives with exposure to eggs may receive RIV or, with additional safety precautions, IIV[2]
Influenza, live attenuated (LAIV)[2,3]	• Severe allergic reaction (e.g., anaphylaxis) to any component of the vaccine, or to a previous dose of any influenza vaccine • In addition, ACIP recommends that LAIV not be used in the following populations: pregnant women; immunosuppressed adults; adults with egg allergy of any severity; adults who have taken influenza antiviral medications (amantadine, rimantadine, zanamivir, or oseltamivir) within the previous 48 hours; avoid use of these antiviral durgs for 14 days after vaccination	• Moderate or severe acute illness with or without fever • History of GBS within 6 weeks of previous influenza vaccination • Asthma in persons age 5 years and older • Other chronic medical conditions (e.g., other chronic lung diseases, chronic cardiovascular disease [excluding isolated hypertension], diabetes, chronic renal or hepatic disease, hematologic disease, neurologic disease, and metabolic disorders)
Tetanus, diphtheria, pertussis (Tdap) **Tetanus, diphtheria (Td)**	• Severe allergic reaction (e.g., anaphylaxis) after a previous dose or to a vaccine component • For pertussis-containing vaccines: encephalopathy (e.g., coma, decreased level of consciousness, or prolonged seizures) not attributable to another identifiable cause within 7 days of administration of previous dose of Tdap or diphtheria and tetanus toxoids and pertussis (DTP) vaccine or diphtheria and tetanus toxoids and acellular pertussis (DTaP) vaccine	• Moderate or severe acute illness with or without fever • GBS within 6 weeks after a previous dose of tetanus toxoid-containing vaccine • History of Arthus-type hypersensitivity reactions after a previous dose of tetanus or diphtheria toxoid-containing vaccine; defer vaccination until at least 10 years have elapsed since the last tetanus toxoid-containing vaccine • For pertussis-containing vaccines: progressive or unstable neurologic disorder, uncontrolled seizures, or progressive encephalopathy until a treatment regimen has been established and the condition has stabilized
Varicella (Var)[3]	• Severe allergic reaction (e.g., anaphylaxis) after a previous dose or to a vaccine component • Known severe immunodeficiency (e.g., from hematologic and solid tumors, receipt of chemotherapy, congenital immunodeficiency, or long-term immunosuppressive therapy[4] or patients with human immunodeficiency virus [HIV] infection who are severely immunocompromised) • Pregnancy	• Moderate or severe acute illness with or without fever • Recent (within 11 months) receipt of antibody-containing blood product (specific interval depends on product)[5] • Receipt of specific antivirals (i.e., acyclovir, famciclovir, or valacyclovir) 24 hours before vaccination; avoid use of these antiviral drugs for 14 days after vaccination
Human papillomavirus (HPV)	• Severe allergic reaction (e.g., anaphylaxis) after a previous dose or to a vaccine component	• Moderate or severe acute illness with or without fever • Pregnancy
Zoster (HZV)[3]	• Severe allergic reaction (e.g., anaphylaxis) to a vaccine component • Known severe immunodeficiency (e.g., from hematologic and solid tumors, receipt of chemotherapy, or long-term immunosuppressive therapy,[4] or patients with HIV infection who are severely immunocompromised) • Pregnancy	• Moderate or severe acute illness with or without fever • Receipt of specific antivirals (i.e., acyclovir, famciclovir, or valacyclovir) 24 hours before vaccination; avoid use of these antiviral drugs for 14 days after vaccination
Measles, mumps, rubella (MMR)[3]	• Severe allergic reaction (e.g., anaphylaxis) after a previous dose or to a vaccine component • Known severe immunodeficiency (e.g., from hematologic and solid tumors, receipt of chemotherapy, congenital immunodeficiency, or long-term immunosuppressive therapy,[4] or patients with HIV infection who are severely immunocompromised) • Pregnancy	• Moderate or severe acute illness with or without fever • Recent (within 11 months) receipt of antibody-containing blood product (specific interval depends on product)[5] • History of thrombocytopenia or thrombocytopenic purpura • Need for tuberculin skin testing[6]
Pneumococcal: conjugate (PCV13), polysaccharide (PPSV23)	• Severe allergic reaction (e.g., anaphylaxis) after a previous dose or to a vaccine component (including, for PCV13, to any diphtheria toxoid-containing vaccine)	• Moderate or severe acute illness with or without fever
Meningococcal: conjugate (MenACWY), polysaccharide (MPSV4)	• Severe allergic reaction (e.g., anaphylaxis) after a previous dose or to a vaccine component	• Moderate or severe acute illness with or without fever
Hepatitis A (HepA)	• Severe allergic reaction (e.g., anaphylaxis) after a previous dose or to a vaccine component	• Moderate or severe acute illness with or without fever
Hepatitis B (HepB)	• Severe allergic reaction (e.g., anaphylaxis) after a previous dose or to a vaccine component	• Moderate or severe acute illness with or without fever
***Haemophilus influenzae* type b (Hib)**	• Severe allergic reaction (e.g., anaphylaxis) after a previous dose or to a vaccine component	• Moderate or severe acute illness with or without fever

FOOTNOTES

1. Vaccine package inserts and the full ACIP recommendations for these vaccines should be consulted for additional information on vaccine-related contraindications and precautions and for more information on vaccine excipients. Events or conditions listed as precautions should be reviewed carefully. Benefits and risks for administering a specific vaccine to a person under these circumstances should be considered. If the risk from the vaccine is believed to outweigh the benefit, the vaccine should not be administered. If the benefit of vaccination is believed to outweigh the risk, the vaccine should be administered. A contraindication increases the chance of a serious adverse reaction. Therefore, a vaccine should not be administered when a contraindication is present.
2. For more information on use of influenza vaccines among persons with egg allergies and a complete list of conditions that CDC considers to be reasons to avoid receiving LAIV, see CDC. "Prevention and Control of Seasonal Influenza with Vaccines: Recommendations of the Advisory Committee on Immunization Practices (ACIP)—United States, 2014–15 Influenza Season. *MMWR* 2014;63(32):691–97.
3. LAIV, MMR, varicella, or zoster vaccines can be administered on the same day. If not administered on the same day, these live vaccines should be separated by at least 28 days.
4. Immunosuppressive steroid dose is considered to be 2 or more weeks of daily receipt of 20 mg prednisone or the equivalent. Vaccination should be deferred for at least 1 month after discontinuation of such therapy. Providers should consult ACIP recommendations for complete information on the use of specific live vaccines among persons on immune-suppressing medications or with immune suppression because of other reasons.
5. Vaccine should be deferred for the appropriate interval if replacement immune globulin products are being administered (see Table 5 in CDC. "General Recommendations on Immunization: Recommendations of the Advisory Committee on Immunization Practices [ACIP]." *MMWR* 2011;60(No. RR-2), available at www.cdc.gov/vaccines/pubs/acip-list.htm.
6. Measles vaccination might suppress tuberculin reactivity temporarily. Measles-containing vaccine may be administered on the same day as tuberculin skin testing. If testing cannot be performed until after the day of MMR vaccination, the test should be postponed for at least 4 weeks after the vaccination. If an urgent need exists to skin test, do so with the understanding that reactivity might be reduced by the vaccine.

* Adapted from "Table 6. Contraindications and Precautions to Commonly Used Vaccines" found in: CDC. "General Recommendations on Immunization: Recommendations of the Advisory Committee on Immunization Practices (ACIP)." *MMWR* 2011;60(No. RR-2), p. 40–41, and from Atkinson W, Wolfe S, Hamborsky J, eds. Appendix A. *Epidemiology and Prevention of Vaccine-Preventable Diseases* (www.cdc.gov/vaccines/pubs/pinkbook/index.html).
† Regarding latex allergy, consult the package insert for any vaccine given.

Technical content reviewed by the Centers for Disease Control and Prevention

IMMUNIZATION ACTION COALITION Saint Paul, Minnesota • 651-647-9009 • www.immunize.org • www.vaccineinformation.org

www.immunize.org/catg.d/p3072.pdf • Item #P3072 (3/15)

A

APPENDIX B
Vaccines

Appendix B

B

U.S. Vaccines: Table 1
(For Combination Vaccines, See Table 2)

Vaccine	Trade Name	Abbreviation	Manufacturer	Type / Route	Approved	How Supplied
Adenovirus	Adenovirus Type 4 & Type 7		Barr Labs Inc.	Live Viral / Oral (tablets)	2011	two bottles: 100 tablets of each component
Anthrax	BioThrax®	AVA	Emergent BioSolutions	Inactivated Bacterial / IM	1970	multi-dose vial
DTaP	Daptacel®	DTaP	sanofi	Inactivated Bacterial / IM	2002	single-dose vial
	Infanrix®	DTaP	GlaxoSmithKline	Inactivated Bacterial / IM	1997	single-dose vial or syringe
DT	Generic	DT	sanofi	Inactivated Bacterial Toxoids / IM	1978	single-dose vial
Haemophilus influenzae type b (Hib)	ActHIB®	Hib (PRP-T)	sanofi	Inactivated Bacterial / IM	1993	single-dose vial
	Hiberix®	Hib (PRP-T)	GlaxoSmithKline	Inactivated Bacterial / IM	2009	single-dose vial
	PedvaxHIB®	Hib (PRP-OMP)	Merck	Inactivated Bacterial / IM	1989	single-dose vial
Hepatitis A	Havrix®	HepA	GlaxoSmithKline	Inactivated Viral / IM	1995	single-dose vial or syringe
	Vaqta®	HepA	Merck	Inactivated Viral / IM	1996	single-dose vial or syringe
Hepatitis B	Engerix-B®	HepB	GlaxoSmithKline	Recombinant Viral / IM	1989	single-dose vial or syringe
	Recombivax HB®	HepB	Merck	Recombinant Viral / IM	1986	single-dose vial or syringe
Herpes Zoster (Shingles)	Zostavax	HZV	Merck	Live Attenuated Viral / SC	2006	single-dose vial
Human Papillomavirus	Cervarix®	2vHPV	GlaxoSmithKline	Inactivated Viral / IM	2009	syringe
	Gardasil®	4vHPV	Merck	Inactivated Viral / IM	2006	single-dose vial or syringe
	Gardasil® 9	9vHPV	Merck	Inactivated Viral / IM	2014	single-dose vial or syringe

B

Vaccine	Trade Name	Abbreviation	Manufacturer	Type / Route	Approved	How Supplied
Influenza	Afluria®	IIV3	bioCSL	Inactivated Viral / IM	2007	multi-dose vial or syringe
	Agriflu®	IIV3	Novartis	Inactivated Viral / IM	2009	syringe
	Fluarix®	IIV3 IIV4	GlaxoSmithKline	Inactivated Viral / IM	2005 2012	syringe
	Flublok®	RIV3	Protein Sciences Corp.	Recombinant Viral / IM	2013	single-dose vial
	Flucelvax®	ccIIV3	Novartis	Inactivated Viral / IM	2012	syringe
	FluLaval®	IIV3 IIV4	GlaxoSmithKline	Inactivated Viral / IM	2006 2013	multi-dose vial or syringe
	FluMist®	LAIV4	Medimmune	Live Attenuated Viral / Intranasal (spray)	2003	single-dose intranasal sprayer
	Fluvirin®	IIV3	Novartis	Inactivated Viral / IM	1988	multi-dose vial or syringe
	Fluzone®	IIV3 IIV4	sanofi	Inactivated Viral / IM	1980	multi-dose vial or syringe
	Fluzone® High-Dose	IIV3	sanofi	Inactivated Viral / IM	2009	syringe
	Fluzone® Intradermal	IIV3	sanofi	Inactivated Viral / Intradermal	2011	single-dose microinjection system
Japanese encephalitis	Ixiaro®	JE	Valneva	Inactivated Viral / IM	2009	syringe
Measles, Mumps, Rubella	M-M-R® II	MMR	Merck	Live Attenuated Viral / SC	1978 (First MMR – 1971)	single-dose vial
Measles, Mumps, Rubella, Varicella	ProQuad®	MMRV	Merck	Live Attenuated Viral / SC	2005	single-dose vial
Meningococcal	Menomune®	MPSV4	sanofi	Inactivated Bacterial / SC	1981	single-dose vial or multi-dose vial
	Menactra®	MCV4 MenACWY	sanofi	Inactivated Bacterial / IM	2005	single-dose vial
	Menveo®	MCV4 MenACWY	GlaxoSmithKline	Inactivated Bacterial / IM	2010	single-dose vial
	Trumenba®	MenB	Pfizer	Recombinant Bacterial / IM	2014	syringe
	Bexsero®	MenB	GlaxoSmithKline	Recombinant Bacterial / IM	2015	syringe

B

Vaccine	Trade Name	Abbreviation	Manufacturer	Type / Route	Approved	How Supplied
Pneumococcal	Pneumovax® 23	PPSV23	Merck	Inactivated Bacterial / SC or IM	1983	single-dose vial, multi-dose vial, or syringe
	Prevnar 13®	PCV13	Pfizer	Inactivated Bacterial / IM	2010 (PCV7 – 2000)	syringe
Polio	Ipol®	IPV	sanofi	Inactivated Viral / SC or IM	1990 (IPV-1955)	multi-dose vial or syringe
Rabies	Imovax® Rabies		sanofi	Inactivated Viral / IM	1980	single-dose vial
	RabAvert®		GlaxoSmithKline	Inactivated Viral / IM	1997	single-dose vial
Rotavirus	RotaTeq®	RV5	Merck	Live Viral / Oral (liquid)	2006	single-dose tube
	Rotarix®	RV1	GlaxoSmithKline	Live Viral / Oral (liquid)	2008	single-dose oral applicator
Tetanus, (reduced) Diphtheria	Decavac®	Td	sanofi	Inactivated Bacterial Toxoids / IM	1955	single-dose vial or syringe
	Tenivac®	Td	sanofi	Inactivated Bacterial Toxoids / IM	2003	single-dose vial or syringe
	(Generic)	Td	Massachusetts Biological Labs	Inactivated Bacterial Toxoids / IM	1967	single-dose vial
Tetanus, (reduced) Diphtheria, (reduced) Pertussis	Boostrix®	Tdap	GlaxoSmithKline	Inactivated Bacterial / IM	2005	single-dose vial or syringe
	Adacel®	Tdap	sanofi	Inactivated Bacterial / IM	2005	single-dose vial or syringe
Typhoid	Typhim Vi®		sanofi	Inactivated Bacterial / IM	1994	multi-dose vial or syringe
	Vivotif®		PaxVax	Live Attenuated Bacterial / Oral (capsules)	1989	package of 4 capsules
Varicella	Varivax®	VAR	Merck	Live Attenuated Viral / SC	1995	single-dose vial
Vaccinia (Smallpox)	ACAM2000®		sanofi	Live Attenuated Viral / Percutaneous	2007	multi-dose vial
Yellow Fever	YF-Vax®	YF	sanofi	Live Attenuated Viral / SC	1978	multi-dose vial

B

U.S. Vaccines: Table 2
(Combination Vaccines)

Vaccine	Trade Name	Abbreviation	Manufacturer	Type / Route	Approved	How Supplied
DTaP, Polio	Kinrix®	DTaP-IPV	GlaxoSmithKline	Inactivated Bacterial & Viral / IM	2008	single-dose vial or syringe
DTaP, hepatitis B, Polio	Pediarix®	DTaP-HepB-IPV	GlaxoSmithKline	Inactivated Bacterial & Viral / IM	2002	syringe
DTaP, Polio, *Haemophilus influenzae* type b	Pentacel®	DTaP-IPV/Hib	sanofi	Inactivated Bacterial & Viral / IM	2008	single-dose vial
Haemophilus influenzae type b – hepatitis B	Comvax®	Hib-HepB	Merck	Inactivated Bacterial & Viral / IM	1996	single-dose vial
Haemophilus influenzae type b, Meningococcal	MenHibrix®	Hib-MenCY	GlaxoSmithKline	Inactivated Bacterial / IM	2012	single-dose vial
Hepatitis A, Hepatitis B	Twinrix®	HepA-HepB	GlaxoSmithKline	Inactivated/Recombinant Viral / IM	2001	single-dose vial or syringe

Abbreviations

The abbreviations on this table (Column 3) were standardized jointly by staff of the Centers for Disease Control and Prevention, ACIP Work Groups, the editor of the *Morbidity and Mortality Weekly Report* (*MMWR*), the editor of *Epidemiology and Prevention of Vaccine-Preventable Diseases* (the *Pink Book*), ACIP members, and liaison organizations to the ACIP.

These abbreviations are intended to provide a uniform approach to vaccine references used in ACIP Recommendations and Policy Notes published in the *MMWR*, the *Pink Book*, and the American Academy of Pediatrics *Red Book*, and in the U.S. immunization schedules for children, adolescents, and adults.

In descriptions of combination vaccines, dash (-) indicates: products in which the active components are supplied in their final (combined) form by the manufacturer; slash (/) indicates: products in which active components must be mixed by the user.

March 2015

Selected Discontinued U.S. Vaccines

Trade Name	Antigen(s)	Years
Acel-Imune	DTaP	1991-2001
Attenuvax	Measles (live)	
Attenuvax-Smallpox	Measles-Smallpox	1967
b-CAPSA-1	Hib (polysaccharide)	1985-89
Biavax	Rubella-Mumps (live)	
BioRab	Rabies	1988-2007
Cendevax	Rubella (live)	1969-79
Certiva	DTaP	1998-2000
Decavac	Td	1953-2012
Dip-Pert-Tet	DTP	
Diptussis	Diphtheria-Pertussis	1949-55
Dryvax	Vaccinia	1944-2008
Ecolarix	Measles-Rubella (live)	
Flu Shield	Influenza	
Fluogen	Influenza	
generic	Tetanus-Toxoid (adsorbed)	1937-2014
Heptavax-B	Hepatitis B (plasma derived)	1981-90
HIB-Immune	Hib (polysaccharide)	1985-89
HibTITER	Hib (conjugate)	1990-2007
HIB-Vax	Hib (polysaccharide)	1985-89
JE-VAX	Japanese Encephalitis	1992-2011
Liovax	Smallpox	
Lirubel	Measles-Rubella (live)	1974-78
Lirugen	Measles (live)	1965-76
Lymerix	Lyme Disease	1998-2002
M-Vac	Measles	1963-79
M-M-Vax	Measles-Mumps (live)	1973
Meningovax	Meningococcal	
Meruvax II	Rubella (live)	1969-79
Mevilin-L	Measles (live)	

Appendix B

Trade Name	Antigen(s)	Years
MOPV	Polio (live, oral, monovalent, types I, II, & III)	
Mumpsvax	Mumps (live)	
OmniHIB	Hib (conjugate)	
Orimune	Polio (live, oral)	1961-2000
Perdipigen	Diphtheria/Pertussis	1949-55
Pfizer-Vax Measles-K	Measles (inactivated)	1963-68
Pfizer-Vax Measles-L	Measles (live)	1965-70
Pnu-Imune	Pneumococcal (polysaccharide 14- or 23-valent)	1977-83
Poliovax	Polio (inactivated)	1988-91
Prevnar	Pneumococcal (conjugate 7-valent)	2000-2011
ProHIBIT	Hib (conjugate)	1987-2000
Purivax	Polio (inactivated)	1956-65
Quadrigen	DTP-Polio	1959-68
Rabies Iradogen	Rabies	1908-57
RotaShield	Rotavirus (live oral)	1998-99
Rubelogen	Rubella (live)	1969-72
Rubeovax	Measles (live)	1963-71
Serobacterin	Pertussis	1945-54
Solgen	DTP	1962-77
Tetra-Solgen	DTP-Polio	1959-68
Tetramune	DTP-Hib	
Tetravax	DTP-Polio	1959-65
Topagen	Pertussis (intranasal)	
Tri-Immunol	DTP	
Tridipigen	DTP	
TriHIBit	DTaP/Hib	1996-2011
Trinfagen No. 1	DT-Polio	Early 1960s
Trinivac	DTP	1952-64
Tripedia	DTaP	1992-2011
Wyvac	Rabies	1982-85

March 2013

Vaccine Excipient & Media Summary
Excipients Included in U.S. Vaccines, by Vaccine

This table includes not only vaccine ingredients (e.g., adjuvants and preservatives), but also substances used during the manufacturing process, including vaccine-production media, that are removed from the final product and present only in trace quantities. In addition to the substances listed, most vaccines contain Sodium Chloride (table salt).

Last Updated February 2015

All reasonable efforts have been made to ensure the accuracy of this information, but manufacturers may change product contents before that information is reflected here. If in doubt, check the manufacturer's package insert.

Vaccine	Contains	Source: Manufacturer's P.I. Dated
Adenovirus	sucrose, D-mannose, D-fructose, dextrose, potassium phosphate, plasdone C, anhydrous lactose, micro crystalline cellulose, polacrilin potassium, magnesium stearate, cellulose acetate phthalate, alcohol, acetone, castor oil, FD&C Yellow #6 aluminum lake dye, human serum albumin, fetal bovine serum, sodium bicarbonate, human-diploid fibroblast cell cultures (WI-38), Dulbecco's Modified Eagle's Medium, monosodium glutamate	March 2011
Anthrax (Biothrax)	aluminum hydroxide, benzethonium chloride, formaldehyde, amino acids, vitamins, inorganic salts and sugars	May 2012
BCG (Tice)	glycerin, asparagine, citric acid, potassium phosphate, magnesium sulfate, Iron ammonium citrate, lactose	February 2009
DT (Sanofi)	aluminum potassium sulfate, peptone, bovine extract, formaldehyde, thimerosal (trace), modified Mueller and Miller medium, ammonium sulfate	December 2005
DTaP (Daptacel)	aluminum phosphate, formaldehyde, glutaraldehyde, 2-Phenoxyethanol, Stainer-Scholte medium, modified Mueller's growth medium, modified Mueller-Miller casamino acid medium (without beef heart infusion), dimethyl 1-beta-cyclodextrin, ammonium sulfate	October 2013
DTaP (Infanrix)	formaldehyde, glutaraldehyde, aluminum hydroxide, polysorbate 80, Fenton medium (containing bovine extract), modified Latham medium (derived from bovine casein), modified Stainer-Scholte liquid medium	November 2013
DTaP-IPV (Kinrix)	formaldehyde, glutaraldehyde, aluminum hydroxide, Vero (monkey kidney) cells, calf serum, lactalbumin hydrolysate, polysorbate 80, neomycin sulfate, polymyxin B, Fenton medium (containing bovine extract), modified Latham medium (derived from bovine casein), modified Stainer-Scholte liquid medium	November 2013
DTaP-HepB-IPV (Pediarix)	formaldehyde, gluteraldehyde, aluminum hydroxide, aluminum phosphate, lactalbumin hydrolysate, polysorbate 80, neomycin sulfate, polymyxin B, yeast protein, calf serum, Fenton medium (containing bovine extract), modified Latham medium (derived from bovine casein), modified Stainer-Scholte liquid medium, Vero (monkey kidney) cells	November 2013
DTaP-IPV/Hib (Pentacel)	aluminum phosphate, polysorbate 80, formaldehyde, sucrose, gutaraldehyde, bovine serum albumin, 2-phenoxethanol, neomycin, polymyxin B sulfate, Mueller's Growth Medium, Mueller-Miller casamino acid medium (without beef heart infusion), Stainer-Scholte medium (modified by the addition of casamino acids and dimethyl-beta-cyclodextrin), MRC-5 (human diploid) cells, CMRL 1969 medium (supplemented with calf serum), ammonium sulfate, and medium 199	October 2013
Hib (ActHIB)	ammonium sulfate, formalin, sucrose, Modified Mueller and Miller medium	January 2014
Hib (Hiberix)	formaldehyde, lactose, semi-synthetic medium	March 2012
Hib (PedvaxHIB)	aluminum hydroxphosphate sulfate, ethanol, enzymes, phenol, detergent, complex fermentation medium	December 2010

B

Vaccine	Contains	Source: Manufacturer's P.I. Dated
Hib/Hep B (Comvax)	yeast (vaccine contains no detectable yeast DNA), nicotinamide adenine dinucleotide, hemin chloride, soy peptone, dextrose, mineral salts, amino acids, formaldehyde, potassium aluminum sulfate, amorphous aluminum hydroxyphosphate sulfate, sodium borate, phenol, ethanol, enzymes, detergent	December 2010
Hib/Mening. CY (MenHibrix)	tris (trometamol)-HCl, sucrose, formaldehyde, synthetic medium, semi-synthetic medium	2012
Hep A (Havrix)	aluminum hydroxide, amino acid supplement, polysorbate 20, formalin, neomycin sulfate, MRC-5 cellular proteins	December 2013
Hep A (Vaqta)	amorphous aluminum hydroxyphosphate sulfate, bovine albumin, formaldehyde, neomycin, sodium borate, MRC-5 (human diploid) cells	February 2014
Hep B (Engerix-B)	aluminum hydroxide, yeast protein, phosphate buffers, sodium dihydrogen phosphate dihydrate	December 2013
Hep B (Recombivax)	yeast protein, soy peptone, dextrose, amino acids, mineral salts, potassium aluminum sulfate, amorphous aluminum hydroxyphosphate sulfate, formaldehyde, phosphate buffer	May 2014
Hep A/Hep B (Twinrix)	formalin, yeast protein, aluminum phosphate, aluminum hydroxide, amino acids, phosphate buffer, polysorbate 20, neomycin sulfate, MRC-5 human diploid cells	August 2012
Human Papillomavirus (HPV) (Cerverix)	vitamins, amino acids, lipids, mineral salts, aluminum hydroxide, sodium dihydrogen phosphate dehydrate, 3-O-desacyl-4' Monophosphoryl lipid A, insect cell, bacterial, and viral protein	November 2013
Human Papillomavirus (HPV) (Gardasil)	yeast protein, vitamins, amino acids, mineral salts, carbohydrates, amorphous aluminum hydroxyphosphate sulfate, L-histidine, polysorbate 80, sodium borate	June 2014
Human Papillomavirus (HPV) (Gardasil 9)	yeast protein, vitamins, amino acids, mineral salts, carbohydrates, amorphous aluminum hydroxyphosphate sulfate, L-histidine, polysorbate 80, sodium borate	December 2014
Influenza (Afluria)	beta-propiolactone, thimerosol (multi-dose vials only), monobasic sodium phosphate, dibasic sodium phosphate, monobasic potassium phosphate, potassium chloride, calcium chloride, sodium taurodeoxycholate, neomycin sulfate, polymyxin B, egg protein, sucrose	December 2013
Influenza (Agriflu)	egg proteins, formaldehyde, polysorbate 80, cetyltrimethylammonium bromide, neomycin sulfate, kanamycin, barium	2013
Influenza (Fluarix) Trivalent and Quadrivalent	octoxynol-10 (Triton X-100), α-tocopheryl hydrogen succinate, polysorbate 80 (Tween 80), hydrocortisone, gentamicin sulfate, ovalbumin, formaldehyde, sodium deoxycholate, sucrose, phosphate buffer	June 2014
Influenza (Flublok)	monobasic sodium phosphate, dibasic sodium phosphate, polysorbate 20, baculovirus and host cell proteins, baculovirus and cellular DNA, Triton X-100, lipids, vitamins, amino acids, mineral salts	March 2014
Influenza (Flucelvax)	Madin Darby Canine Kidney (MDCK) cell protein, MDCK cell DNA, polysorbate 80, cetyltrimethlyammonium bromide, β-propiolactone, phosphate buffer	March 2014
Influenza (Fluvirin)	nonylphenol ethoxylate, thimerosal (multidose vial–trace only in prefilled syringe), polymyxin, neomycin, beta-propiolactone, egg proteins, phosphate buffer	February 2014
Influenza (Flulaval) Trivalent and Quadrivalent	thimerosal, formaldehyde, sodium deoxycholate, egg proteins, phosphate buffer	February 2013
Influenza (Fluzone: Standard (Trivalent and Quadrivalent), High-Dose, & Intradermal)	formaldehyde, octylphenol ethoxylate (Triton X-100), gelatin (standard trivalent formulation only), thimerosal (multi-dose vial only) , egg protein, phosphate buffers, sucrose	2014

B

Vaccine	Contains	Source: Manufacturer's P.I. Dated
Influenza (FluMist) Quadrivalent	ethylene diamine tetraacetic acid (EDTA), monosodium glutamate, hydrolyzed porcine gelatin, arginine, sucrose, dibasic potassium phosphate, monobasic potassium phosphate, gentamicin sulfate, egg protein	July 2013
Japanese Encephalitis (Ixiaro)	aluminum hydroxide, Vero cells, protamine sulfate, formaldehyde, bovine serum albumin, sodium metabisulphite, sucrose	May 2013
Meningococcal (MCV4-Menactra)	formaldehyde, phosphate buffers, Mueller Hinton agar, Watson Scherp media, Modified Mueller and Miller medium, detergent, alcohol, ammonium sulfate	April 2013
Meningococcal (MCV4-Menveo)	formaldehyde, amino acids, yeast extract, Franz complete medium, CY medium	August 2013
Meningococcal (MPSV4-Menomune)	thimerosal (multi-dose vial only), lactose, Mueller Hinton casein agar, Watson Scherp media, detergent, alcohol	April 2013
Meningococcal (MenB – Bexsero)	aluminum hydroxide, *E. coli*, histidine, sucrose, deoxycholate, kanomycin	2015
Meningococcal (MenB – Trumenba)	polysorbate 80, histodine, *E. coli*, fermentation growth media	October 2015
MMR (MMR-II)	Medium 199 (vitamins, amino acids, fetal bovine serum, sucrose, glutamate) , Minimum Essential Medium, phosphate, recombinant human albumin, neomycin, sorbitol, hydrolyzed gelatin, chick embryo cell culture, WI-38 human diploid lung fibroblasts	June 2014
MMRV (ProQuad)	sucrose, hydrolyzed gelatin, sorbitol, monosodium L-glutamate, sodium phosphate dibasic, human albumin, sodium bicarbonate, potassium phosphate monobasic, potassium chloride, potassium phosphate dibasic, neomycin, bovine calf serum, chick embryo cell culture, WI-38 human diploid lung fibroblasts, MRC-5 cells	March 2014
Pneumococcal (PCV13 – Prevnar 13)	casamino acids, yeast, ammonium sulfate, Polysorbate 80, succinate buffer, aluminum phosphate, soy peptone broth	January 2014
Pneumococcal (PPSV-23 – Pneumovax)	phenol	May 2014
Polio (IPV – Ipol)	2-phenoxyethanol, formaldehyde, neomycin, streptomycin, polymyxin B, monkey kidney cells, Eagle MEM modified medium, calf serum protein, Medium 199	May 2013
Rabies (Imovax)	Human albumin, neomycin sulfate, phenol red indicator, MRC-5 human diploid cells, beta-propriolactone	April 2013
Rabies (RabAvert)	β-propiolactone, potassium glutamate, chicken protein, egg protein, neomycin, chlortetracycline, amphotericin B, human serum albumin, polygeline (processed bovine gelatin), sodium EDTA, bovine serum	March 2012
Rotavirus (RotaTeq)	sucrose, sodium citrate, sodium phosphate monobasic monohydrate, sodium hydroxide, polysorbate 80, cell culture media, fetal bovine serum, vero cells *[DNA from porcine circoviruses (PCV) 1 and 2 has been detected in RotaTeq. PCV-1 and PCV-2 are not known to cause disease in humans.]*	June 2013
Rotavirus (Rotarix)	amino acids, dextran, sorbitol, sucrose, calcium carbonate, xanthan, Dulbecco's Modified Eagle Medium (potassium chloride, magnesium sulfate, ferric (III) nitrate, sodium phosphate, sodium pyruvate, D-glucose, concentrated vitamin solution, L-cystine, L-tyrosine, amino acids solution, L-glutamine, calcium chloride, sodium hydrogenocarbonate, and phenol red) *[Porcine circovirus type 1 (PCV-1) is present in Rotarix. PCV-1 is not known to cause disease in humans.]*	May 2014
Smallpox (Vaccinia – ACAM2000)	human serum albumin, mannitol, neomycin, glycerin, polymyxin B, phenol, Vero cells, HEPES	September 2009

B

e	Contains	Source: Manufacturer's P.I. Dated
...ecavac)	aluminum potassium sulfate, peptone, formaldehyde, thimerosal, bovine muscle tissue (US sourced), Mueller and Miller medium, ammonium sulfate	March 2011
Td (Tenivac)	aluminum phosphate, formaldehyde, modified Mueller-Miller casamino acid medium without beef heart infusion, ammonium sulfate	April 2013
Td (Mass Biologics)	aluminum phosphate, formaldehyde, thimerosal (trace), ammonium phosphate, modified Mueller's media (containing bovine extracts)	February 2011
Tdap (Adacel)	aluminum phosphate, formaldehyde, glutaraldehyde, 2-phenoxyethanol, ammonium sulfate, Stainer-Scholte medium, dimethyl-beta-cyclodextrin, modified Mueller's growth medium, Mueller-Miller casamino acid medium (without beef heart infusion)	March 2014
Tdap (Boostrix)	formaldehyde, glutaraldehyde, aluminum hydroxide, polysorbate 80 (Tween 80), Latham medium derived from bovine casein, Fenton medium containing a bovine extract, Stainer-Scholte liquid medium	February 2013
Typhoid (inactivated – Typhim Vi)	hexadecyltrimethylammonium bromide, formaldehyde, phenol, polydimethylsiloxane, disodium phosphate, monosodium phosphate, semi-synthetic medium	March 2014
Typhoid (oral – Ty21a)	yeast extract, casein, dextrose, galactose, sucrose, ascorbic acid, amino acids, lactose, magnesium stearate. gelatin	September 2013
Varicella (Varivax)	sucrose, phosphate, glutamate, gelatin, monosodium L-glutamate, sodium phosphate dibasic, potassium phosphate monobasic, potassium chloride, sodium phosphate monobasic, potassium chloride, EDTA, residual components of MRC-5 cells including DNA and protein, neomycin, fetal bovine serum, human diploid cell cultures (WI-38), embryonic guinea pig cell cultures, human embryonic lung cultures	March 2014
Yellow Fever (YF-Vax)	sorbitol, gelatin, egg protein	May 2013
Zoster (Shingles – Zostavax)	sucrose, hydrolyzed porcine gelatin, monosodium L-glutamate, sodium phosphate dibasic, potassium phosphate monobasic, neomycin, potassium chloride, residual components of MRC-5 cells including DNA and protein, bovine calf serum	February 2014

A table listing vaccine excipients and media *by excipient* can be found in:

Grabenstein JD. *ImmunoFacts: Vaccines and Immunologic Drugs* – 2013 (38th revision). St Louis, MO: Wolters Kluwer Health, 2012.

Latex in Vaccine Packaging

"If a person reports a severe (anaphylactic) allergy to latex, vaccines supplied in vials or syringes that contain natural rubber, or whose product information does not say "not made with natural rubber latex" should not be administered unless the benefit of vaccination outweighs the risk for a potential allergic reaction. In these cases, providers should be prepared to treat patients who are having an allergic reaction. For latex allergies other than anaphylactic allergies (e.g., a history of contact allergy to latex gloves), vaccines supplied in vials or syringes that contain dry natural rubber or rubber latex may be administered." (ACIP *General Recommendations on Immunization*. 2011)

The following table is accurate, to the best of our knowledge, as of February 2015. **If in doubt, check the package insert for the vaccine in question.**

Vaccine		Latex?	Source: Manufacturer's PI Dated:
Adenovirus (Adenovirus Type 4 and Type 7)		NO	March 2011
Anthrax (Biothrax)		YES – Vial	May 2012
Comvax		YES – Vial	December 2010
DTaP	Daptacel	NO	October 2013
	Infanrix	YES – Syringe NO – Vial	November 2013
DT (Sanofi)		YES	December 2005
Hib	Hiberix	YES – Syringe Tip Cap	March 2012
	PedvaxHIB	YES – Vial	December 2010
	ActHIB	YES – Diluent vial NO – Lyophilized vaccine vial	January 2014
Hepatitis A	Havrix	YES – Syringe NO – Vial	December 2013
	Vaqta	YES – Vial YES – Syringe	February 2014
Hepatitis B	Engerix-B	YES – Syringe NO – Vial	December 2013
	Recombivax HB	YES – Vial YES – Syringe	May 2014
HPV	Gardasil	NO	June 2014
	Gardasil 9	NO	December 2014
	Cervarix	YES	November 2013
Influenza	Afluria	NO	December 2013
	Agriflu	YES – Syringe Tip Cap	2013
	Fluarix	NO	June 2014
	Fluarix Quadrivalent	NO	June 2014
	Flublok	NO	March 2014
	Flucelvax	YES – Syringe Tip Cap	March 2014
	FluLaval	NO	February 2013
	FluMist Quadrivalent	NO	July 2013
	Fluvirin	YES – Syringe Tip Cap NO– Vial	February 2014

B

Vaccine		Latex?	Source: Manufacturer's PI Dated:
Influenza (cont'd)	Fluzone	NO	2014
	Fluzone High-Dose	NO	2014
	Fluzone Intradermal	NO	2014
	Fluzone Quadrivalent	NO	2014
Japanese Encephalitis (Ixiaro)		NO	May 2013
Kinrix		YES – Syringe NO – Vial	November 2013
MMR (M-M-R II)		NO	June 2014
MMRV (ProQuad)		NO	March 2014
Meningococcal	Menomune	YES	April 2013
	Menactra	NO	April 2013
	Menveo	NO	August 2013
	Bexsero	YES – Syringe Tip Cap	2015
	Trumenba	NO	October 2014
MenHibrix		NO	2012
Pediarix		YES – Syringe NO – Vial	November 2013
Pentacel		NO	October 2013
Pneumococcal	Pneumovax 23	NO	May 2014
	Prevnar 13	NO	January 2014
Polio (IPOL)		NO	May 2013
Rabies	Imovax Rabies	NO	April 2013
	RabAvert	NO	March 2012
Rotavirus	RotaTeq	NO	June 2013
	Rotarix	YES – Oral Applicator of Diluent	May 2014
Td	Decavac	YES – Syringe NO – Vial	March 2011
	Tenivac	NO	April 2013
	Mass Biologics	NO	February 2011
Tdap	Adacel	YES – Syringe Tip Cap NO – Vial	March 2014
	Boostrix	YES – Syringe NO – Vial	February 2014
Twinrix		YES – Syringe NO – Vial	August 2012
Typhoid	Typhim Vi	NO	March 2014
	Vivotif Berna	NO	September 2013
Varicella (Varivax)		NO	March 2014
Vaccinia (Smallpox) (ACAM2000)		NO	September 2009
Yellow Fever (YF-Vax)		YES – Vial	May 2013
Zoster (Shingles) (Zostavax)		NO	February 2014

February 2015

THIMEROSAL TABLE
(updated 12/11/13)

Institute for Vaccine Safety

www.vaccinesafety.edu

Vaccine	Brand Name		Manufacturer	Thimerosal Concentration	Mercury Mcg/0.5 mL
Anthrax	BioThrax		BioPort Corp	0	0
DTaP	Daptacel		sanofi pasteur	0	0
	Infanrix		GlaxoSmithKline	0	0
	Tripedia		sanofi pasteur	*̲	*̲
DTaP+HepB+IPV	Pediarix		GlaxoSmithKline	0	0
DTaP+IPV	Kinrix		GlaxoSmithKline	0	0
DTaP+IPV+Hib	Pentacel		sanofi pasteur	0	0
DT	Diphtheria & Tetanus Toxoids Adsorbed USP		sanofi pasteur	*̲	*̲
Td	Decavac		sanofi pasteur	*̲	*̲
	Tetanus and Diphtheria Toxoids Adsorbed		Mass Biolocial Labs	*̲	*̲
Tdap	Adacel		sanofi pasteur	0	0
	Boostrix		GlaxoSmithKline	0	0
Tetanus Toxoid	Generic		sanofi pasteur	.01%	25
Hib	ActHib		sanofi pasteur	0	0
	Hiberix		GlaxoSmithKline	0	0
	PedvaxHIB		Merck	0	0
Hib+HepB	Comvax		Merck	0	0
Hepatitis A	Havrix		GlaxoSmithKline	0	0
	Vaqta		Merck	0	0
Hepatitis B	Engerix-B		GlaxoSmithKline	0	0
	Recombivax HB		Merck	0	0
Hep A+B	Twinrix		GlaxoSmithKline	0	0
HPV	Cervarix		GlaxoSmithKline	0	0
	Gardasil		Merck	0	0
Influenza 2013/14 Formula	Afluria	single dose	CSL Limited for Merck	0	0
		multi-dose		0.01%	24.5
	Agriflu		Novartis	0	0
	Fluarix	Trivalent & Quadrivelent	GlaxoSmithKline	0	0
	Flublok		Protein Sciences Corp	0	0
	Flucelvax		Novartix	0	0
	FluLaval		GlaxoSmithKline	.01%	25
	FluMist Quadravelent		MedImmune	0	0
	Fluvirin	prefilled syringe	Novartis	*̲	*̲ 25
		multi-dose		0.01%	
	Fluzone	single dose	sanofi pasteur	0	0
		multi-dose		0.01%	25
		High Dose		0	0
		Intradermal		0	0
		Quadrivalent		0	0
Japanese Encephalitis	Ixiaro	commercial | military	Intercell Bio	0	0
	JE-Vax		sanofi pasteur	0.007%	
Meningococcal	Menactra		sanofi pasteur	0	0
	Menomune-A/C/Y/W-135	single dose	sanofi pasteur	0	0
		multi-dose		0.01%	24.5
	Menveo		Novartis	0	0

B

MMR	M-M-R II	Merck	0	0
MMR+Varicella	ProQuad	Merck	0	0
Pneumococcal	Pneumovax 23	Merck	0	0
	Prevnar	Wyeth-Ayerst	0	0
	Prevnar 13	Wyeth-Ayers	0	0
Polio	IPOL	sanofi pasteur	0	0
Rabies	Imovax	sanofi pasteur	0	0
	RabAvert	Chiron	0	0
Rotavirus	Rotarix	GlaxoSmithKline	0	0
	RotaTeq	Merck	0	0
Typhoid Fever	Typhim Vi	sanofi pasteur	0	0
	Vivotif	Berna Biotch	0	0
Varicella Zoster	Varivax	Merck	0	0
	Zostavax	Merck	0	0
Yellow Fever	YF-VAX	sanofi pasteur	0	0

* This product should be considered equivalent to thimerosal-free products. This vaccine may contain trace amounts (<0.3 mcg) of mercury left after postproduction thimerosal removal; these amounts have no biological effect. JAMA 1999;282(18) and JAMA 2000;283(16).

Institute for Vaccine Safety

Johns Hopkins Bloomberg
School of Public Health
www.vaccinesafety.edu

B

Foreign Language Terms
Aids to translating foreign immunization records.

Table 1:   **Disease, Vaccine, and Related Terms.** This table lists terms for vaccine-preventable diseases and vaccines, and other terms that might be found on an immunization record, by language.

Table 2:   **Trade Names.** This table lists the names of specific vaccines that are used, or have been used, internationally, along with the manufacturer and country or region where the vaccine is produced or used, when known.

These tables have been adapted from (among other sources)
lists developed by
the Minnesota Department of Health Immunization Program
(now maintained by the Immunization Action Coalition)
and
Washington State Department of Health.

See also:
http://www.immunize.org/izpractices/p5121.pdf

These lists are not comprehensive. We have checked sources,
but we cannot claim complete accuracy.

B

Foreign Vaccines
Table 1: Disease, Vaccine, and Related Terms

Albanian	
Difteria	Diphtheria
Fruthi	Measles
Pertusisi	Pertussis
Tetanozi	Tetanus

Arabic	
Alhasiba	Rubella
As'al	Pertussis
Athab	Mumps
Difteria	Diphtheria
El Safra	Hepatitis
Has 'ba	Measles
Shel'el	Polio

Bosnian	
Beseže	BCG
Detepe	DPT
Difterija	Diphtheria
Dječja paraliza	Polio
Gripa	Influenza
Ljudski papilloma virus	Human Papillomavirus
Male boginje	Rubella
Ospice	Chickenpox
Rubeola	Measles
Tuberkuloza	Tuberculosis
Upala pluća	Pneumonia
Veliki boginje	Smallpox
Veliki kašalj	Pertussis
Zauške	Mumps
Žutica	Hepatitis

Chinese	
疫苗	Vaccine
麻疹	Measles
腮腺炎	Mumps
白	Diphtheria
流感 or 流行性感冒	Influenza
乙	B

Croatian	
Beseže	BCG
Detepe	DTP
Difterija	Diphtheria
Dječje paralize	Polio
Gripe	Influenza
Haemophilus influenzae tipa b	*Haemophilus influenzae* type b
Hri pavac	Pertussis

Kašalj hripavac	Pertussis
Meningokoknog konjugirati	Meningococcal Conjugate
Ospice	Measles
Pneumokoka konjugirano	Pneumococcal Conjugate
Rotavirusa	Rotavirus
Rubeola	Rubella
Šindra	Shingles (Herpes Zoster)
Tetanusa	Tetnaus
Tuberculosa	Tuberculosis
Upala pluća	Pneumonia
Veliki boginje	Smallpox
Vodene kozice	Varicella
Zapaljenje	Hepatitis
Zaušnjaci	Mumps
Žutica	Hepatitis

Czech	
Davivy Kasel	Pertussis
Difterie	Diphtheria
Hepatitida	Hepatitis
Parotitida	Mumps
Pertuse	Pertussis
Poliomyelitis	Polio
Plané Nestovice	Chickenpox
Spalnicky	Measles
Subinuira	Influenza
Zardenky	Rubella
Zaškrt	Diphtheria
Zlutá Zimnice	Yellow Fever

Danish	
Bornelammelse	Polio
Difteritis	Diphtheria
Faaresyge (Fåresyge)	Mumps
Kighoste	Pertussis
Leverbetaendelse	Hepatitis
Meslinger	Measles
MFR	MMR
Rode Hunde	Rubella
Stivkrampe	Tetanus

Dutch	
BMR	MMR
Bof	Mumps
Difterie	Diphtheria
DKTP	DTP
Gelekoorts	Yellow Fever
Gordelroos	Varicella

Griep	Influenza
Humaan papillovirus	Human papillomavirus
Kinderverlamming	Polio
Kinkhoest	Pertussis
Longontsteking	Pneumonia
Mazelen	Measles
Meningokokken conjugaat	Meningococcal Conjugate
Pneumokokken conjugaat	Pneumococcal conjugaat
Pokken	Smallpox
Rode hond	Rubella
Stijfkramp	Tetanus
Tering	Tuberculosis
Waterpekkea	Chickenpox

Ethiopian (Oromiffaa)

Cufaa	Tetanus
Difteeriyaa	Diphtheria
Gifira	Measles
Gifira farangli	Rubella
Laamsheesaa	Polio
Qakkee	Pertussis
Shimbiraa	Hepatitis

Finnish

Hinkuyska	Pertussis
Jaykkakouristus	Tetanus
Kurkkumata	Diphtheria
Lapsihalvaus	Polio
Sikotauti	Mumps
Tuhkarokko	Measles
Vihurirokko	Rubella

French

Coqueluche	Pertussis
Diphtérie	Diphtheria
DTC, DT Coq	DTP
DTCP	DTP +Polio
Fievre jaune	Yellow Fever
Grippe	Influenza
l'Haemophilus b	Hib
Oreillons	Mumps
Poliomyélite	Polio
ROR	MMR
Rougeole	Measles
Rubéole	Rubella
Tétanos	Tetanus
Tuberculose	Tuberculosis
Variole	Smallpox

German

Diphtherie	Diphtheria
FSME	Tick-borne encephalitis
Gelbfieber	Yellow Fever

Grippe	Influenza
Keuchhusten	Pertussis
Kinderlähmung	Polio
Masern	Measles
Pocken	Smallpox
Röteln	Rubella
Starrkramph	Tetanus
Tuberkulose	Tuberculosis
Wundstarrkrampf	Tetanus
Zei Genpeter	Mumps

Greek

Δινθγρίτιδα, Τέτανος και Κοκκύτης	DTP
Ο Αιμόνιλος της γρίππης τύπου B	Hib
Μηνιγγοκοκκική Ασθένγα ομάδας C	Meningococcal C
Ιλαρά - Μαγουλάδγς – Ερυθρά	MMR
Πολιομυγλίτιδα	Polio
Τέτανος και Δινθγρίτιδα	Td

Haitian Creole

Difteri	Diphtheria
Epatit	Hepatitis
Flou	Influenza
Koklich	Pertussis
Lawoujβl, Laroujβl	Measles
Malmouton	Mumps
Polyo	Polio
Ribeyβl	Rubella
Saranpyon	Varicella
Tetanβs	Tetanus

Hmong

Hawb pob	Pertussis
Kabmob siab hom B	Hepatitis B
Kub cer	Diphtheria
Qhua Maj	Rubella
Qhua Pias	Measles
Qog	Mumps
Tuag tes tuag taw	Polio
Ua npuag	Tetanus

Indonesian

Batuk rejan	Pertussis
Beguk	Mumps
Biring Peluh	Rubella
Campak	Measles
Difteri	Diphtheria
Penyakit lumpuh	Polio
Radang hati	Hepatitis

Italian

Antipolio inattivato	IPV
Difterite	Diphtheria
Emofilo b	Hib
Epatite	Hepatitis
Febbre Giallo	Yellow Fever

Morbillo	Measles
MPR (morbillo, parotite, rosolia)	MMR
Parotite	Mumps
Pertosse	Pertussis
Poliomielite	Polio
Polmonite	Pneumonia
Rosolia	Rubella
Tetano	Tetanus
Tosse Asinina	Pertussis
Tubercolosi	Tuberculosis
Vaioloso	Smallpox

Japanese	
A 型肝炎	Hepatitis A
B 型肝炎	Hepatitis B
Fushin (風疹)	Rubella
Hashika (麻疹 or はしか)	Measles
Hashofu (破傷風)	Tetanus
Hyakaseki (百日咳)	Pertussis
Jifuteria (ジフテリア)	Diphtheria
Otafukukuaze (流行性耳下腺炎 or おたふくかぜ)	Mumps
Sh naimahi (ポリオ)	Polio
三種混合	DTaP
水痘 or みずぼうそう	Varicella
肺炎球菌	Pneumococcal
インフルエンザ菌	Hib
日本脳炎	Japanese Encephalitis
インフルエンザ	Influenza
ツベルクリン	PPD
追加接種	Booster

Malay	
Batok rejan	Pertussis
Penyaakit bengok	Mumps
Sakit champak	Measles
Sakit rengkong	Diphtheria

Norwegian	
Difteri	Diphtheria
Kikhoste	Pertussis
Kopper	Smallpox
Kusma	Mumps
Leverbetennelse	Hepatitis
Meslinger	Measles
Poliomyelitt	Polio
Rρde hunder	Rubella
Stivkrampe	Tetanus
Vannkopper	Varicella

Polish	
Błonicy, Błonica, Błonnica	Diphtheria
Dyfteria	Diphtheria
Gruzlica	Tuberculosis
Grypa	Influenza
Haemophilus influenza typu b	*Haemophilus influenzae* Type b
Koklusz	Pertussis
Krztuscowi, Krztuścowi, Krztusiec	Pertussis
Meningokokom sprzężenia	Meningococcal Conjugate
Odra	Measles
Ospa	Smallpox
Ospa Wietrzna	Chickenpox
Paraliz dzieciecy	Polio
Pojar German	Rubella
Pojarul, Pojarului	Measles
Półpasiec	Shingles (Herpes Zoster)
Przeciwko błonicy	Diphtheria
Przypominajace	Booster
Rotavirusy	Rotavirus
Rozyczka	Rubella
Skoniugowanej szczepionki pnuemokokowej	Pneumococcal Conjugate
Swinka	Mumps
Tezec, Tężcowi	Tetanus
Wirus brodawczaka ludzkiego	Human Papillomavirus
Wirusowemu zapaleniu wątroby typu A	Hepatitis A
Wirusowemu zapaleniu wątroby typu B	Hepatitis B
Zapalenie pluc	Pneumonia
Zapalenie watroby	Hepatitis
Zólta Goraczka	Yellow Fever

Portuguese	
Cachumba (papeira)	Mumps
Coqueluche	Pertussis
Difteria	Diphtheria
Febre Amarela	Yellow Fever
Gripe	Influenza
Hepatite	Hepatitis
Paralisia infantil	Polio
Parotidite epidémica	Mumps
Poliomielite	Polio
Rúbéola	Rubella
Sarampo	Measles
Tetânica, Tétano	Tetanus
Triplice	DTP
VAHB	Hepatitis B Vaccine
VAP	Polio Vaccine
Varicela	Chickenpox
VAS	Measles Vaccine
VASPR	MMR
VAT	Tetanus Vaccine

B

Romanian	
AR	Measles
Conjugate meningococice	Meningococcal Conjugate
Difteria (Difteriei)	Diphtheria
Di Te	DT
Di-Te-Per	DTP
Febra Galbena	Yellow Fever
Gripa	Influenza
Haemophilus influenza tip b boala	*Haemophilus influenzae* type b
Hepatita	Hepatitis
Holera	Cholera
Oreion, Oreionul, Oreionului	Mumps
Papilomavirus uman	Human papillomavirus
Pneumococic conjugat	Pneumococcal Conjugate
Pneumoniei	Pneumonia
Pojar German	Rubella
Pojarul	Measles
Poliomielita, Poliomielitic	Polio
Rubeolei, Rubeola	Rubella
Rujeola, Rujeolei	Measles
Și varicelă	Varicella
Tetanos,Tetanosul, Tetanosului	Tetanus
Tuberculozei	Tuberculosis
Tuse convulsiva, Tusei convulsive	Pertussis
Varicelă, Varicelei	Varicella
Variola, Variolei	Smallpox

Russian	
Бцр	BCG
АКДС	DTP
Дифтерит, Дифтерия	Diphtheria
Гемоифлюс инфлюзнцы типа Б, Гемофільной инфекции типа Б	Hib
Гепатит	Hepatitis
Вирус папилломы человека	Human Papillomavirus
Грипп	Influenza
Корь	Measles
Свинка, Паротит	Mumps
Коклюша	Pertussis
Лневмокковоя конъюгированной	Pneumococcal conjugate
Воспале лёгких Пневмония	Pneumonia
Полиомиелит	Polio
Ротавірусной	Rotavirus
Краснуха	Rubella
Опоясьвывающий лишай	Shingles (Herpes Zoster)

Оспа	Smallpox
Столбняк, Столбняка	Tetanus
Туберкулез, Туберкулес	Tuberculosis
Ветрянка, Ветрянкая Оспа (Вітрянка)	Varicella
Манту	Mantoux (TB Test)
Вакцина	Vaccine
Вакцинация	Series
Ревакцинация	Booster
Подпись	Signature
Серия, доза	Series, Dose

Samoan	
Mami	Mumps
Misela	Measles
Rupela	Rubella

Serbian	
Beseže	BCG
Detepe	DTP
Difterija, ДиФтрије	Diphtheria
Хаемопхилус ИнФлуензае Тип Б болести	Haemophilus influenza type b
Хепатитиса А	Hepatitis A
Хепатитиса В	Hepatitis B
Људски Папилома Вирус	Human Papillomavirus
Мале богиње	Measles
Менингококне Коњуговано	Meningococcal Conjugate
Dječja paraliza	Polio
Gripa, Грип	Influenza
Hri pavac	Pertussis
Male boginje	Rubella
Pljuskavice, Kozice	Varicella
Upala pluća	Pneumonia
Veliki boginje	Smallpox
Veliki kašalj, Великог	Pertussis
Zapaljenje	Hepatitis
Zaušnjaci, Заушке	Mumps
Žutica	Hepatitis

Slovak	
Chrípka	Influenza
Čierny kašeľ	Pertussis
Detská obrna	Poliomyelitis
Diftéria	Diphtheria
DiTePe	DTP
Haemophilus influenza typ b ochorenia	*Haemophilus Influenzae* type b
Hepatitida	Hepatitis
Kiahne	Smallpox
Konjugovaná pneumokoková	Pneumococcal Conjugate
Krzamak	Measles

B

Appendix B

L'udský papillomavirus	Human papillomavirus
Meningokokove j konjugovanou	Meningococcal Conjugate
Morbilli, Osýpky	Measles
Ovčim kiahňam, Ovčie kiahne	Varicella
Parotitis	Mumps
Pásového oparu, Pásový opar	Shingles
Polyomyelitida	Polio
Priusnica	Mumps
Rubeola, Ruzienka	Rubella
Tuberkulóza	Tuberculosis
Zápal□plüc	Pneumonia
Záškrt	Diphtheria
Spanish	
Antineumocócica conjugada	Pneumococcal conjugate
Cólera	Cholera
Coqueluche	Pertussis
Difteria	Diphtheria
Doble Antigen	Td (Mexico)
Doble Viral	Measles-Rubella (Mexico)
Duple	DT (Cuba)
Gripe	Influenza
Hemófilo tipo b, Haemophilus influenzae tipo b	Haemophilus influenza type b
Hemófilo tipo b	Hib
Herpes	Shingles (Herpes Zoster)
Meningococo Conjugada	Meningococcal conjugate
Numonía	Pneumonia
Paperas, Parotiditis	Mumps
Poliomielitis	Polio
Pulmonía	Pneumonia
Rubéola	Rubella
Sarampión, Sarampión Comun	Measles
Sarampión Aleman	Rubella
SRP	MMR
Tetánica, Tétano, Tétanos	Tetanus
Tos Ferina	Pertussis
Tuberculínica	Tuberculosis
Varicela	Varicella
Viruela	Smallpox
Virus del Papilloma Humano	Human Papillomavirus
Zona de Matojos	Shingles (Herpes Zoster)
Somali	
Bus-buska	Varicella
Cagaarshowga	Hepatitis
Cuno xanuun	Diphtheria

Dabayl	Polio
Duf	Polio
Furuq	Smallpox
Gowracato	Diphtheria
Gurra dhaabsis	Mumps
Hablobaas	Varicella
Haemophilus nooca b	Hib
Infilowense	Influenza
Jadeeco	Measles
Jadeeco been, Jadeeco jarmalka	Rubella
Joonis	Hepatitis
Kix	Pertussis
Qaamow-Qashiir	Mumps
Qaaxo-Tiibi	Tuberculosis
Qanja Barar	Mumps
Sambabaha	Pneumonia
Tallaakla Qaaxada	BCG
Taytano	Tetanus
Wareento	Pneumonia
Xiiqdheer	Pertussis
Swedish	
Bältros, Herpes Zoste	Shingles (Herpes Zoster)
Difteri	Diphtheria
Duplex	DT
Gula Febern	Yellow Fever
Haemophilus influenzae typ b	Haemophilus influenza type b
Hepatit A	Hepatitis A
Hepatit B	Hepatitis B
Influensa	Influenza
Kikhosta	Pertussis
Kolera	Cholera
Konjugerat Pneumokock	Pneumococcal conjugate
Mänskliga papillovirus	Human papillomavirus
Mässling, Masslingormerly	Measles
Meningokockinfektion Konjugatet	Meningococcal conjugate
MPR	MMR
Påssjuka, Pässjura	Mumps
Polio	Polio
Röda Hund, Röda Hund	Rubella
Smittkopper, Smittkoppor	Smallpox
Stelkramp	Tetanus
Trippel	DTP
Tuberkulos	Tuberculosis
Vattkopper	Varicella
Tagalog	
Beke	Mumps
Dipterya	Diphtheria

Pertusis	Pertussis
Polyo	Polio
Tetano	Tetanus
Tigdas	Measles
Turkish	
Boğmaca	Pertussis
Çocuk Felci	Polio
DBT	DPT
Difteri	Diphtheria
Erken Yaz-Beyin Iltihabı'na	Tick-borne encephalitis
Grip	Influenza
KKK	MMR
Kabakulak	Mumps
Kızamık	Measles
Kımamıkçık	Rubella
Meningekoklar	Meningococcal
Kuduz	Rabies
Pnömokoklar	Pneumococcal
Su Çiçeği	Varicella
Tetanos	Tetanus
Ukranian	
Дифтерії	Diphtheria
Гемофілъної інфекції Типу В Захворювань	Haemophilus influenzae type b
Гепатиту S	Hepatitis A
Гепатиту В	Hepatitis B
Вірус Паппіломи Людини	Human Papillomavirus
Грипу	Influenza
Менінгококова Сполучених	Meningococcal Conjugate
Кір	Mumps
Кашлюку	Pertussis
Пневмококковой Конъюгированной	Pneumococcal Conjugate
Поліо, Поліомієліту	Polio
Ротавірусної	Rotavirus
Оперізуючий Герпес (Оиерізуючий лЛишай)	Shingles (Herpes Zoster)
Стовбняк, Правця	Tetanus
Вітряної Віспи (Вітрянка)	Varicella
Vietnamese	
Bach Hâu	Diphtheria
Bai liet	Polio
Ban Đo	Rubella
Dai	Rabies
Ho GB	Pertussis
Quai Bi	Mumps
SBi Uon Ván	Tetanus
So'i	Measles
Sot TΛ LiΛt	Polio
Thuong hBn	Typhoid

Uon ván	Tetanus
ViΛm gan siΛu vi B (VGSV B)	Hepatitis B
VNNB	Japanese encephalitis

May 2012

Foreign Language Terms
Table 2: Product Names

Trade Name/ Abbreviation	Component(s)	Manufacturer, Country
6 in 1	Diphtheria, tetanus, pertussis, polio, Hib, hepatitis B	GSK, Ireland
ADC-M (АДС-М)	Td	Russia
A.D.T.	Diphtheria, tetanus (adsorbed)	Commonwealth, Australia
A.K.D.S.	Diphtheria, tetanus, pertussis	UK
ACVax	Meningococcal (polysaccharide A & C)	GSK, UK
ACWYVax	Meningococcal (polysaccharide A, C, Y, W135)	GSK, UK
Acelluvax	Pertussis (acellular)	Chiron, Italy
ACTAcel	Diphtheria, tetanus, pertussis, Hib	Sanofi Pasteur, Argentina
Adifteper	Diphtheria, tetanus, pertussis	Ism, Italy
Adinvira A+B	Influenza (whole virus)	Imuna
Adiugrip	Influenza	Sanofi Pasteur
Admun	Influenza (whole virus)	Duncan
Admune GP	Influenza (whole virus)	Duncan
Agrippal	Influenza	Novartis
AH	Hepatitis B	(Romania)
Aimmugen	Hepatitis A (inactivated)	Chemo-Sero-Therapeutic Resh Inst. Japan
Aldiana	Diphtheria (adsorbed)	Sevac, Czech Republic
Alditeana	Diphtheria, tetanus (adsorbed)	Sevac, Czech Republic
Alditerpera	Diphtheria, tetanus (adsorbed), pertussis	Sevac, Czech Republic
Almevax	Rubella	Evans
Alorbat	Influenza (whole virus)	Asta Pharma
Alteana Sevac	Tetanus	Institute of Sera and Vaccines
AM-BC	Meningococcal B & C	Cuba
Amaril	Yellow Fever	Sanofi Pasteur, France
AmBirix	Hepatitis A, Hepatitis B	GSK, Europe
AMC	Hib (polysaccharide)	Cuba
Anadifterall	Diphtheria (adsorbed)	Chiron, Italy
Anatetall	Tetanus (adsorbed)	Chiron, Italy
Anatoxal Di Te	Diphtheria, tetanus	Berna Biotech, Europe
Anatoxal Di Te per	Diphtheria, tetanus, pertussis	Berna Biotech, Europe
AP	Polio	(Romania)
AS	Measles	Cuba
Arilvax	Yellow fever	MEDI, UK
ATPA	Tetanus toxoid	(Romania)
AVAC-1, AVA	Anthrax	(for U.S. military use)
AVAXIM	Hepatitis A	Aventis Pasteur, France

B

Trade Name/ Abbreviation	Component(s)	Manufacturer, Country
B-Hepavac II	Hepatitis B	Merck, Singapore
Begrivac	Influenza (split virus)	Novartis
Betagen	Hepatitis B	Sanofi Pasteur
Biaflu Zonale	Influenza (whole virus)	Farmabiagini, Italy
Biken-HB	Hepatitis B	Biken, Japan
Bilive	Hepatitis A/Hepatitis B (recombinant)	Sinovac, China
Bimmugen	Hepatitis B (recombinant, adsorbed, yeast derived)	Chemo-Sero-Therapeutic Resh Inst., Japan
Biviraten Berna	Measles, mumps (live)	Berna Biotech, Switzerland
Buccopol Berna	Polio (oral)	Berna Biotech, Europe
BVAC	Botulinum antitoxin	(for U.S. military use)
B-Vaxin	Hepatitis B	Laboratorios Pablo Cassara, Argentina
C.D.T.	Diphtheria, tetanus (pediatric, adsorbed)	Commonwealth, Australia
CEF	Measles (Schwarz strain)	Chiron, Italy
Cacar	Smallpox	Indonesia
Campak Kerig	Measles	Pasteur Institute, Indonesia
Celluvax	Pertussis (acellular)	Chiron, Italy
Chiromas	Influenza (same as Fluad)	Novartis, Spain
Cinquerix	Diphtheria, tetanus, pertussis, Hib, polio	GSK, Europe
Cocquelucheau	Pertussis (adsorbed)	Sanoti Pasteur, France
Cuadruple	Diphtheria, tetanus, pertussis, Hib	Mexico
D-Immun	Diphtheria	Osterreichisches Institut, Austria
D.S.D.P.T.	Diphtheria, tetanus, pertussis (adsorbed)	Dong Shin Pharm, Korea
D.T. Bis Rudivax	Diphtheria, tetanus, rubella	Sanofi Pasteur, France
Di Anatoxal	Diphtheria	Berna Biotech, Europe
Di Te Per Pol Impfstoff	Diphtheria, tetanus, pertussis, polio	Berna Biotech, Switzerland
Di-Te-Pol SSI	Diphtheria, tetanus, polio	Statens Seruminstitut, Denmark
Dif-Tet-All	Diphtheria, tetanus	Chiron, Italy
Diftavax	Diphtheria, tetanus	Sanofi Pasteur
Ditanrix	Diphtheria, tetanus	GSK, Europe
DiTe Anatoxal	Diphtheria, tetanus (adsorbed)	Berna Biotech, Switzerland
Ditoxim	Diphtheria, tetanus (adsorbed)	Dong Shin Pharm, Korea
Double Anigen B.I.	Diphtheria, tetanus	Bengal Immunity Co., India
DT Adulte	Diphtheria, tetanus (adult)	Sanofi Pasteur, France
DT Bis	Diphtheria, tetanus (booster)	Sanofi Pasteur, France
DT Coq	Diphtheria, tetanus, pertussis	Sanofi Pasteur, France
DT Polio	Diphtheria, tetanus, polio	Sanofi Pasteur, France
DT TAB	Diphtheria, tetanus *Salmonella typhi, Paratyphi* A & B	Sanofi Pasteur, France
DT Vax	Diphtheria, tetanus (pediatric)	Sanofi Pasteur, France
DT Wellcovax	Diphtheria, tetanus (pediatric)	Chiron, UK
Dual Antigen Sii	Diphtheria, tetanus (adsorbed)	Serum Institute of India (Sii)
Dultavax	Diphtheria, tetanus, polio (booster)	Aventis Pasteur, France
Dupla	Diphtheria, tetanus	Instituto Butantan, Brazil
Duplex	Diphtheria, tetanus	Sweden

B

Trade Name/ Abbreviation	Component(s)	Manufacturer, Country
Easyfive	DTwP-Hib-HepB	India
Ecolarix	Measles, rubella (Schwarz & RA 27/3)	GSK, Europe
Elvarix	Influenza (split virus)	VEB, Sachsesches Serumwerk Dresden
EMAV	Meningococcal serogroup A	China
Encepur	Tick-borne encephalitis	Chiron, Europe
Enivac-HB	Hepatitis B (recombinant DNA)	Centro de Ingenieria Genetica Y Biotecnologia, Cuba
Enterovaccino	Typhoid (IM)	Isi
Enzira	Influenza	CSL
Eolarix	Measles, rubella (Schwartz & RA 27/3)	GSK, Europe
Epaxal Berna	Hepatitis A – virosomal vaccine	Berna Biotech, Switzerland
Ervax	Rubella (live)	GSK, Mexico
Ervevax RA 27/3	Rubella (live)	GSK, Belgium
Esavalenti	(Hexavalent) Diphtheria, tetanus, pertussis, polio, Hib, hepatitis B	Italy
Euvax-B	Hepatitis B (recombinant DNA)	LG Chemical, South Korea
Fendrix	Hepatitis B (dialysis formulation)	GSK, Europe
Fluad	Influenza (adults $\geq$65)	Novartis, Europe, Asia, NZ
Flubron	Influenza (whole virus)	Pfizer
Flugen	Influenza	UK
Fluvax	Influenza	CSL, Australia
Fluvirine	Influenza	CellTech Pharma SA
FOH-M	Polio (inactivated)	Russia
FrocuoOke	Polio (inactivated)	Russia
FSME-IMMUNE	Tick-borne encephalitis	Baxter, Austria
FSPD	Measles	Russia
Funed-CEME	Diphtheria, tetanus, pertussis	Belo Horizonte, Brazil
Gen H-B-Vax	Hepatitis B	Merck-Behringwerke
GenHevac B Pasteur	Hepatitis B	Sanofi Pasteur
Gene Vac-B	Hepatitis B	Serum Institute of India (Sii)
Gripax	Influenza (whole virus)	Hebrew University
Gripe	Influenza (whole virus)	Spain
Gripguard	Influenza (same as Fluad)	Novartis, France
Gripovax	Influenza (whole virus)	GSK
Gunevax	Rubella	Chiron, Italy
H-Adiftal	Diphtheria	Ism, Italy
H-Adiftetal	Diphtheria, tetanus	Ism, Italy
H-Atetal	Tetanus	Ism, Italy
HarPaBreHnr B CtauOHAP	Rubella	Russia
HAVPur	Hepatitis A	Chiron, Germany
HB Vax Pro	Hepatitis B	SP
HBY	Hepatitis B (recombinant)	KGC, Japan

B

Trade Name/ Abbreviation	Component(s)	Manufacturer, Country
HDCV	Human Diploid Cell Rabies Vaccine	
Heberbiovac HB	Hepatitis B	Heberbiotec, Cuba
Hepabest	Hepatitis A	Sanofi Pasteur, Mexico
Hepacare	Hepatitis B (recombinant)	Chiron, Europe
Hepaccine-B	Hepatitis B (plasma derived)	Chiel Jedang, South Korea
Hepagene	Hepatitis B	Chiron, Europe
Hepativax	Hepatitis B	Sanofi Pasteur, Mexico
Hepatyrix	Hepatitis A, typhoid	GSK
Hepavax-B	Hepatitis B (plasma derived)	Korea Green Cross, South Korea
Hepavax-Gene	Hepatitis B (recombinant DNA)	Korea Green Cross, South Korea
Hepcare	Hepatitis B	Chiron, Europe
Heprecomb	Hepatitis B (yeast derived)	Berna Biotech, Switzerland
Hevac B	Hepatitis B (plasma derived)	Sanofi Pasteur, France
Hexamune	Diphtheria, Tetanus, (acellular) Pertussis, Hib, hepatitis B, polio	Aventis, Latin America
Hexavac (Hexavax)	Diphtheria, tetanus, pertussis, polio, hepatitis B, Hib	Sanofi Pasteur, Europe or Mexico
Hiberix	Hib conjugate	GSK
HIBest	Hib	Sanofi Pasteur
Hinkuys karokoe	Pertussis (adsorbed)	Natl. Public Health Institute, Finland
HIS	Influenza	Serbian Institute, Yugoslavia
IBV	Polio (inactivated)	Statens Seruminstitut, Denmark
Immravax	Measles, mumps, rubella	Sanofi Pasteur, Europe
Immugrip	Influenza	Pierre Fabre Médicament
Immunil	Pneumococcal (polysaccharide)	Sidus
Imovax Parotiditis	Mumps	Sanofi Pasteur, Europe
Imovax Polio	Polio	Sanofi Pasteur, Europe
Imovax Sarampion	Measles	Sanofi Pasteur, Europe
Imovas D.T.	Diphtheria, tetanus (adult)	Sanofi Pasteur, Europe
Imovas Gripe	Influenza	Sanofi Pasteur, Europe
Imovax D.P.T.	Diphtheria, tetanus, pertussis	Sanofi Pasteur Mexico
Imovax R.O.R.	Measles, rubella, mumps (live)	Sanofi Pasteur, Europe
Imovax Rubeola	Measles	Sanofi Pasteur, Europe
Imovax Mumps	Mumps	Sanofi Pasteur, Europe
Imovax Oreillons	Mumps	Sanofi Pasteur, Europe
Imovax Rage	Rabies	Sanofi Pasteur, Europe
Imovax Tetano	Tetanus	Sanofi Pasteur, Europe
Infanrix Hexa	Diphtheria, tetanus, pertussis, polio, Hib, hepatitis B	GSK, France
Infanrix Penta	Diphtheria, tetanus, pertussis, hepatitis B, polio	GSK, Europe
Infanrix Quinta	Diphtheria, tetanus, pertussis, polio, Hib	GSK, Europe
Infanrix Tetra	Diphtheria, tetanus, pertussis, polio	GSK, Europe
Inflexal	Influenza	Swiss Serum and Vaccine Institute

B

Appendix B

Trade Name/ Abbreviation	Component(s)	Manufacturer, Country
Influmix	Influenza (whole virus)	Schiapparelli
Influpozzi Zonale	Influenza (whole virus)	Ivp
Influsplit SSW	Influenza (split virus)	VEB Sachsecsches Serumwerk Dresden
Influvac	Influenza	Solvay-Pharma
Influvirus	Influenza	Ism, Italy
Invirin	Influenza (whole virus)	GSK
Ipad TP	Tetanus, polio	Sanofi Pasteur, France
IPV-Virelon	Polio (inactivated)	Chiron, Europe
Isiflu Zonale	Influenza (whole virus)	Isi, Italy
Istivac	Influenza	Sanofi Pasteur, Europe
Kaksoisrokote Dubbelvaccin	Diphtheria, tetanus (pediatric)	Natl. Public Health Institute, Finland
Kikhoste-Vaksine	Pertussis	Statens Institutt for Folkehelse, Norway
Koplivac	Measles (Edmonston strain)	Philips-Duphar, Australia
Kotipa	Cholera, typhoid, paratyphoid	Perum Bio Farma, Indonesia
Krztuscowi	Pertussis	Poland
Ksztu	Pertussis	Poland
Lancy Vaxina	Smallpox	Swiss Serum and Vaccine Institute, Switzerland
Lavantuu Tirokote	Typhoid	Central Pub Health La, Finland
Liomorbillo	Measles	
Liovaxs	Smallpox	Chiron, Italy
Lirugen	Measles	Sanofi Pasteur
LM – 3 RIT	Measles, mumps, rubella (live)	Dong Shin Pharm, Korea
LM – 2 RIT	Measles, mumps (live)	Dong Shin Pharm, Korea
Lteanas Imuna	Tetanus (adsorbed)	Imuna sp., Slovakia
Lyssavac N	Rabies	Berna Biotech, Europe
M-M-Rvax	Measles, mumps, rubella	Chiron, Europe
M-M-Vax	Measles, mumps	Merck, Europe
M-Vac	Measles (live)	Serum Institute of India (Sii)
Massern-Impfstoff SSW	Measles (live)	Chiron, Germany
Massling	Measles	Sweden
MDPH-PA	Anthrax	
Measavac	Measles (Edmonston strain)	Pfizer, UK
MenAfriVac	Meningococcal A Conjugate	Africa
Mencevax A	Meningococcal Group A (polysaccharide)	SmithKline/RIT, Belgium
Mencevax ACWY	Meningococcal quadravalent	GSK
Mengivax A/C	Meningococcal Groups A & C (conjugate)	Sanofi Pasteur, Europe
Meningitec	Meningococcal Group C (conjugate)	Wyeth, UK, Australia
Meningtec	Meningococcal Group C (conjugate)	Wyeth, Canada
Meninvact	Meningococcal Group C (conjugate)	Sanofi Pasteur
Menjugate	Meningococcal Group C (conjugate)	Novartis
Menpovax 4	Meningococcal Groups A, C, Y & W135 (polysaccharide)	Chiron, Europe
Menpovax A+C	Meningococcal Groups A & C	Chiron, Italy

Trade Name/ Abbreviation	Component(s)	Manufacturer, Country
MeNZB	Meningococcal Group B	Novartus, New Zealand
Mesavac	Measles (Edmonston strain)	Pfizer, UK
Mevilin-L	Measles (Schwarz strain)	Chiron, UK
MFV	Influenza (whole virus)	Servier, UK
MFV-Ject	Influenza (whole virus)	Sanofi Pasteur, Europe
Miniflu	Influenza	Schiapparelli, Italy
Mo-Ru Viraten	Measles, rubella	Berna Biotech, Canada
Moniarix	Pneumococcal 17-valent (polysaccharide)	GSK, Europe
Monovax / Monovac	BCG	Sanofi Pasteur, France
Mopavac	Measles, mumps (live)	Sevac, Czech Republic
Morbilvax	Measles (live)	Chiron, Italy
Morubel	Measles, rubella (live)	Chiron, Italy
Moruman Berna	Measles immunoglobulin	Berna, Switzerland
Morupar	Measles, mumps, rubella (live)	Chiron, Italy
Movivac	Measles (live)	Sevac, Czech Republic
Mumaten	Mumps (live)	Berna Biotech, Switzerland
Munevan	Influenza (whole virus)	Medeva
Mutagrip	Influenza	Sanofi Pasteur, Germany
Nasoflu	Influenza	GSK, Europe
Neis Vac-C	Meningococcal Group C (conjugate)	Baxter, Europe & Canada
Neumo Imovax	Pneumococcal 23-valent (polysaccharide)	Sanofi Pasteur, Mexico
Neotyf	Typhoid (live, oral)	Chiron, Italy
Nilgrip	Influenza	CSL
Nivgrip	Influenza (whole virus)	Nicolau Institute of Virology, Romania
NorHOMHerHTA	Polio (inactivated)	Russia
Nothav	Hepatitis A	Chiron, Italy
Okavax	Varicella (live)	Biken / Sanofi Pasteur, Japan & Europe
Optaflu	Influenza (cell culture-based)	Novartis, Europe, Iceland, Norway
Oral Virelon	Polio (oral)	Chiron, Germany
Pariorix	Mumps (live)	GSK, Mexico & Europe
Pavivac	Mumps (live)	Sevac, Czech Republic
Pediacel	Diphtheria, tetanus, acellular pertussis, Hib, polio	Europe
Penta	Diphtheria, tetanus, acellular pertussis, Hib, polio	Sanofi Pasteur, Europe
PENT-HIBest	Diphtheria, tetanus, pertussis, polio, Hib	Sanofi Pasteur
Pentacel	Diphtheria, tetanus, pertussis, polio, Hib	Sanofi Pasteur, Canada
Pentacoq	Diphtheria, tetanus, pertussis, polio, Hib	Sanofi Pasteur
PentAct-HIB	Diphtheria, tetanus, pertussis, polio, Hib	Sanofi Pasteur, Europe
Pentavac	Diphtheria, tetanus, pertussis, polio, Hib	Sanofi Pasteur
Pentavalente	Diphtheria, tetanus, pertussis, hepatitis B, Hib	Mexico (Prior to July 2007)
Pentavalente Acelular	Diphtheria, tetanus, pertussis, polio, Hib	Mexico (August 2007 to present)

B

Appendix B

Trade Name/ Abbreviation	Component(s)	Manufacturer, Country
Pentavalenti	Diphtheria, tetanus, pertussis, polio, Hib **OR** Diphtheria, tetanus, pertussis, polio, hepatitis B	Italy
Pentaxim	Diphtheria, tetanus, pertussis, polio, Hib	Aventis Pasteur, France
Pluserix	Measles, rubella	GSK, Mexico & Europe
Pneumopur	Pneumococcal 23-valent (polysaccharide)	Chiron, Europe
POLIAcel	Diphtheria, tetanus, pertussis, polio, Hib	Sanofi Pasteur, Argentina
Poliomyelite	Polio (inactivated)	France
Polioral	Polio (live, oral, trivalent)	Novartis
Polio Sabin	Polio (oral)	GSK, Europe
Poloral	Polio (oral)	Swiss Serum and Vaccine Institute
Prevenar	Pneumococcal 7-valent (conjugate)	Wyeth, France
Previgrip	Influenza	Chiron, France
Primavax	Diphtheria, tetanus, hepatitis B	Sanofi Pasteur, Europe
Priorix	Measles, mumps, rubella (live)	GSK, Europe & Australia
Priorix-Tetra	Measles, mumps, rubella, varicella (live)	GSK, Europe
Probivac-B	Hepatitis B	Probiomed, Mexico
Procomvax	Hib, hepatitis B	Sanofi Pasteur, Europe
PRS	MMR	Cuba
PRV	Pentavalent Rotavirus Vaccine	Palau
Pulmovax	Pneumococcal 23-valent (polysaccharide)	Merck
Q-Vac	Diphtheria, tetanus, pertussis, hepatitis B	Serum Institute of India (Sii)
Quadracel	Diphtheria, tetanus, acellular pertussis, polio	Sanofi Pasteur, Mexico
QUADRAcel/Hibest	Diphtheria, tetanus, acellular pertussis, polio, Hib	Sanofi Pasteur, Argentina
Quadravax	Diphtheria, tetanus, pertussis, polio	GSK
Quadruple	Diphtheria, tetanus, pertussis, Hib	Mexico
Quatro-Virelon	Diphtheria, tetanus, pertussis, polio	Chiron, Europe
Quinivax-IN	Diphtheria, tetanus, pertussis, polio, Hib	Valda Laboratori, Europe
Quintuple	Diphtheria, tetanus, pertussis, polio, Hib	GSK, Mexico
Quinvaxem	Diphtheria, tetanus, pertussis, Hib, Hepatitis B	Novartis/Crucell
R-HB Vaccine	Hepatitis B (recombinant)	Mitsubishi Chem Corp, Japan
R-Vac	Rubella (live)	Serum Institute of India (Sii)
Rabdomune	Rabies	Impdfstofwerke, Germany
Rabipur	Rabies	Chiron, Germany
Rabivac	Rabies	Chiron, Germany
Rasilvax	Rabies	Chiron, Italy
RDCV	"Rabies Diploid Cell Vaccine"	
Refortrix	Diphtheria, tetanus (adult)	GSK
Repevax	Diphtheria, tetanus, pertussis, polio	Sanofi Pasteur
Revaxis	Tetanus, diphtheria, polio (adult)	Sanofi Pasteur (Europe)
Rimevax	Measles (live, Schwarz strain)	GSK, Mexico & Europe
Rimparix	Measles, mumps (live)	GSK, Europe
RIT-LM-2	Measles, mumps (live)	Dong Shin Pharm, Korea
RIT-LM-3	Measles, mumps, rubella (live)	Dong Shin Pharm, Korea

B

Trade Name/ Abbreviation	Component(s)	Manufacturer, Country
Rorvax	Measles, mumps, rubella (live)	Sanofi Pasteur, Europe & Brazil
Rosovax	Rubella	Ism, Italy
Rouvax	Measles (live)	Sanofi Pasteur, Europe
Rubavax	Rubella (live)	Sanofi Pasteur, UK
Rubeaten	Rubella (live)	Berna Biotech, Europe
Rubellovac	Rubella (live)	Chiron, Germany
Rubilin	Rubella (live)	Chiron, UK
Rudi-Rouvax	Measles, rubella (live)	Sanofi Pasteur, France
Rudivax	Rubella (live)	Sanofi Pasteur, France
Sahia	Polio (live oral)	Multiple manufacturers
Sampar	Plague	Sanofi Pasteur, Indonesia
Sandovac	Influenza	Sandoz, Austria
Serap	Diphtheria, tetanus, pertussis	Perum Bio Farma, Indonesia
Shanvac-B	Hepatitis B	Shantha, India
SMBV	Rabies	Sanofi Pasteur, Europe
Sii Rabivax	Rabies	Serum Institute of India (Sii)
Sii Triple Antigen	Diphtheria, tetanus, pertussis	Serum Institute of India (Sii)
Stamaril	Yellow fever (live)	Sanofi Pasteur, Europe
Streptopur	Pneumococcal 23-valent (polysaccharide)	Chiron, Europe
Subinvira	Influenza (split virus)	Imuna, Czech Republic
Synflorix	Pneumococcal (10-valent, conjugate)	GSK, Europe, Australia
T. Polio	Tetanus, polio	SP (Canada)
T.A.B.	Typhoid, paratyphoid (A & B)	- Institute Pasteur, Tunisia - Egypt - Pharmaceutical Industries Corp., Burma
T-Immun	Tetanus (adsorbed)	Baxter, Germany
T-Vaccinol	Tetanus	Roehm Pharma, Germany
T-Wellcovax	Tetanus	Wellcopharm, Germany
Tanrix	Tetanus	GSK, Europe
Td-Pur	Tetanus, diphtheria (adult)	Chiron, Europe
Td-Virelon	Tetanus, diphtheria, polio	Chiron, Europe
Te Anatoxal	Tetanus	Berna Biotech, Switzerland
Telvaclptap	Tetanus	Yugoslavia
Tet-Aktiv	Tetanus	Tropon-Cutter, Germany
Tet-Tox	Tetanus	CSL Limited, Australia
Tetagrip	Tetanus, influenza	SP, France
Tetamun SSW	Tetanus (fluid, nonadsorbed)	Veb Sachsisches Serumwerk, Germany
Tetamyn	Tetanus	Bioclon, Mexico
Tetano-difter	Tetanus, diphtheria	Celltech Pharma
Tetanol	Tetanus (adsorbed)	Chiron, Sanofi Pasteur, Europe & Mexico
Tetanovac	Tetanus	Sanofi Pasteur, Mexico
Tetasorbat SSW	Tetanus (adsorbed)	Veb Sachsisches Serumwerk, Germany
Tetatox	Tetanus (adsorbed)	Berna Biotech, Italy
Tetavax	Tetanus (adsorbed)	Sanofi Pasteur, Europe
Tetracoq 05	Diphtheria, tetanus, pertussis, polio	Sanofi Pasteur, France

B

Appendix B

Trade Name/ Abbreviation	Component(s)	Manufacturer, Country
TetrAct-HIB	Diphtheria, tetanus, pertussis, Hib	Sanofi Pasteur, Europe
Tetravac Acellulaire	Diphtheria, tetanus, acellular pertussis, polio	Sanofi Pasteur, Europe
Tetravalenti	Diphtheria, tetanus, pertussis, hepatitis B	Italy
Tetraxim	Tetanus, diphtheria, pertussis, polio	Sanofi Pasteur, Europe
Theracys	BCG	Aventis Pasteur, Canada
Ticovac	Tick-borne encephalitis	Baxter SA
Tifovax	Typhoid (Vi polysaccharide)	Sanofi Pasteur, Mexico
Titifica	Typhoid and paratyphoid	Italy
TOPV	Polio (oral, trivalent)	Multiple manufacturers
Trenin DPT Behring	Diphtheria, tetanus, pertussis	Chiron Behring GmbH, Germany
Tresivac	Measles, mumps, rubella (live)	Serum Institute of India (Sii)
Triacel	Diphtheria, tetanus, acellular pertussis	Sanofi Pasteur, Europe & Mexico
Triacelluvax	Diphtheria, tetanus, acellular pertussis	Chiron, Europe
Trimovax	Measles, mumps, rubella (live)	Sanofi Pasteur,
Tripacel	Diphtheria, tetanus, acellular pertussis	Sanofi Pasteur, Europe
Triple antigen	Diphtheria, tetanus, pertussis	- Chowgule & Co., India - CSL Limited, Australia
Triple Sabin	Polio (live, oral)	Mexico
Triple	Diphtheria, tetanus, pertussis	Cuba, Mexico
Triple viral	Measles, mumps, rubella	- Mexico - Immunology Institute, Croatia
Triple Virica	Measles, mumps, rubella	Dominican Republic
Triplice (VT)	Diphtheria, tetanus, pertussis	Instituto Butantan, Brazil
Triplice Viral (VTV)	Measles, mumps, rubella	Instituto Butantan, Brazil
Triplovax	Measles, mumps, rubella	Sanofi Pasteur, Europe & Brazil
Tritanrix	Diphtheria, tetanus, whole-cell pertussis	GSK
Tritanrix-HB	Diphtheria, tetanus, whole-cell pertussis, hepatitis B	GSK, Mexico
Tritanrix-HB-Hib	Diphtheria, tetanus, whole-cell pertussis, hepatitis B, Hib	GSK
Trivacuna Leti	Diphtheria, tetanus (adsorbed), pertussis	Laboratory Leti, Spain
Trivax	Diphtheria, tetanus (plain), pertussis	Chiron, UK
Trivax-AD	Diphtheria, tetanus (adsorbed), pertussis	Chiron, UK
Trivax-Hib	Diphtheria, tetanus, pertussis, Hib	GSK, Europe
Trivb	Diphtheria, tetanus, pertussis	Brazil
Triviraten	Measles, mumps, rubella (live)	Berna Biotech, Switzerland
Trivivac	Measles, mumps, rubella (live)	Sevac, Czech Republic
Trivivax	Measles, mumps, rubella	Sanofi Pasteur, Mexico
Tussitrupin Forte	Pertussis	Staatliches Institut, Germany
Tuvax	BCG	Japan BCG Laboratory, Japan
Tyne	BCG	Sweden
Typherix	Typhoid (Vi polysaccharide)	GSK, Europe & Australia
Typhopara-typhoidique	Typhoid and paratyphoid	France

B

Trade Name/ Abbreviation	Component(s)	Manufacturer, Country
Typhoral-L	Typhoid (Ty21a oral)	Berna Biotech, Germany
Typh-Vax	Typhoid	CSL Limited, Australia
VAA	Yellow fever (vaccine anti-amaril)	Democratic Republic of Congo
Va-Diftet	Diphtheria, tetanus	Finlay Vacunas y Sueros, Cuba
Va-Mengoc-BC	Meningococcal Groups B & C	Finlay Vacunas y Sueros, Cuba
Vac-DPT	Diphtheria, tetanus, pertussis	Bioclon, Mexico
Vaccin Difteric Adsorbit	Diphtheria (adsorbed)	Cantacuzino Institute, Romania
Vaccin Rabique Pasteur	Rabies	Pasteur Vaccins
Vaccin Combinat Diftero-Tetanic	Diphtheria, tetanus (adsorbed)	Cantacuzino Institute, Romania
Vaccin tuberculeux attenue lyophilize	BCG	Sanofi Pasteur, France
Vaccinum Morbillorum Vivum	Measles (live)	Moscow Research Institute, Russia
Vacina Dupla	Diphtheria, tetanus	Instituto Butantan, Brazil
Vacina Triplice	Diphtheria, tetanus, pertussis	Instituto Butantan, Brazil
Vacina Triplice Viral	Measles, mumps, rubella	Brazil
Vacuna Doble	Tetanus, diphtheria	Instituto Biologico Argentino
Vacunol	Tetanus	Temis-Lostato, Brazil
Vaksin Sampar	Plague	Perum Bio Farma, Indonesia
Vaksin Cacar	Smallpox	Indonesia
Vaksin Serap	Diphtheria, tetanus, pertussis	Perum Bio Farma, Indonesia
Vaksin Campak Kerig	Measles (live)	Perum Bio Farma, Indonesia
Vaksin Kotipa	Cholera, typhoid, paratyphoid A, B & C	Perum Bio Farma, Indonesia
Vamoavax	Measles, mumps (live)	Institute of Immunology, Croatia
Varicella-RIT	Varicella	GSK, Europe
Varicellon	Zaricella zoster immunoglobulin	Behringwerke Aktiengesellischaft, Germany
Varie	Smallpox (lyophilized)	Institute of sera and Vaccine, Czech Republic
Varilrix	Varicella (live, Oka strain)	GSK, Australia, New Zealand
Varirix	Varicella (live, Oka strain)	GSK, Europe & Mexico
VAT	Tetanus (vaccin anatoxine tetanique)	Francophone Africa
Vax-Tet	Tetanus	Finlay Vacunas & Sueros, Cuba
Vaxem-Hib	Hib (polysaccharide)	Chiron, Europe
Vaxicoq	Pertussis (adsorbed)	Sanofi Pasteur, France
Vaxigrip	Influenza	Sanofi Pasteur, Europe & Australia
Vaxihaler-Flu	Influenza (inhaler)	Riker, UK
Vaxipar	Mumps (live)	Chiron, Italy
VCDT	Diphtheria, tetanus (pediatric)	Cantacuzino Institute, Romania
VDA Vaccin Difteric Adsorbit	Diphtheria	Cantacuzino Institute, Romania
Verorab	Rabies (purified vero cell)	Sanofi Pasteur, France

B

Appendix B

Trade Name/ Abbreviation	Component(s)	Manufacturer, Country
ViATIM	Hepatitis A, typhoid	Sanofi Pasteur, UK
Vibriomune	Cholera	Duncan Flockhart, UK
Viralinte	Hepatitis B	Ivax Pharmaceuticals, Mexico
Virelon C	Polio (inactivated)	Chiron, Germany
Virelon T 20	Polio (live, oral trivalent)	Chiron, Germany
Virivac	Measles, mumps, rubella (live)	Merck, Finland
Virovac Massling, Perotid, Rubella	Measles, mumps, rubella	Sweden
Vopix	Polio (oral)	PT Biofarma, Indonesia
VPH	Human Papillomavirus	Spanish
V T (Vacine Triplice)	Diphtheria, tetanus, pertussis	Instituto Butantan, Brazil
V T V (Vacina Triplice Viral)	Measles, mumps, rubella	Brazil
V V R	Measles (live)	Cantucuzino Institute, Romania
Welltrivax Trivalente	Diphtheria, tetanus, pertussis	Spain
X-Flu	Influenza	CSL
Zaantide	Diphtheria antitoxin	Imunoloski Zavod, Croatia
Zaantite	Tetanus antitoxin	Imunoloski Zavod, Croatia
Zaditeadvax	Diphtheria, tetanus	Imunoloski Zavod, Croatia
Zaditevax	Diphtheria, tetanus	Imunoloski Zavod, Croatia
Zamevax A+C	Meningococcal Groups A & C (polysaccharide)	Imunoloski Zavod, Croatia
Zamovax	Measles (live)	Imunoloski Zavod, Croatia
Zamruvax	Measles, rubella (live)	Imunoloski Zavod, Croatia
Zapavax	Mumps	Imunoloski Zavod, Croatia
Zaruvax	Rubella (live)	Imunoloski Zavod, Croatia
Zatetravax	Diphtheria, tetanus, pertussis, parapertussis	Imunoloski Zavod, Croatia
Zatevax	Tetanus	Imunoloski Zavod, Croatia
Zatribavax	Diphtheria, tetanus, pertussis	Imunoloski Zavod, Croatia
Zatrivax	Measles, mumps, rubella (live)	Imunoloski Zavod, Croatia

March 2015

B

APPENDIX C
Vaccine Information Statements

C

Appendix C

It's Federal Law!

You must give your patients current Vaccine Information Statements (VISs)

> **To obtain current VISs in more than 30 languages, visit the Immunization Action Coalition's website at www.immunize.org/vis**

As healthcare professionals understand, the risks of serious consequences following vaccination are many hundreds or thousands of times less likely than the risks associated with the diseases that the vaccines protect against. Most adverse reactions from vaccines are mild and self-limited. Serious complications are rare, but they can have a devastating effect on the recipient, family members, and the providers involved with the care of the patient. We must continue the efforts to make vaccines as safe as possible.

Equally important is the need to furnish vaccine recipients (or the parents/legal representatives of minors) with objective information on vaccine safety and the diseases that the vaccines protect against, so that they are actively involved in making decisions affecting their health or the health of their children. When people are not informed about vaccine adverse events, even common, mild events, they can lose their trust in healthcare providers and vaccines. Vaccine Information Statements (VISs) provide a standardized way to present objective information about vaccine benefits and adverse events.

What are VISs?

VISs are developed by the staff of the Centers for Disease Control and Prevention (CDC) and undergo intense scrutiny by panels of experts for accuracy. Each VIS provides information to properly inform the adult vaccine recipient or the minor child's parent or legal representative about the risks and benefits of each vaccine. VISs are not meant to replace interactions with healthcare providers, who should answer questions and address concerns that the recipient or the parent/legal representative may have.

Use of the VIS is mandatory!

Before a healthcare provider vaccinates a child or an adult with a dose of any vaccine containing diphtheria, tetanus, pertussis, measles, mumps, rubella, polio, hepatitis A, hepatitis B, *Haemophilus influenzae* type b (Hib), influenza, pneumococcal conjugate, meningococcal, rotavirus, human papillomavirus (HPV), or varicella (chickenpox) vaccine, the provider is required by the National Childhood Vaccine Injury Act (NCVIA) to provide a copy of the VIS to either the adult recipient or to the child's parent/legal representative.

How to get VISs

All available VISs can be downloaded from the website of the Immunization Action Coalition at www.immunize.org/vis or from CDC's website at www.cdc.gov/vaccines/hcp/vis/index.html. Ready-to-copy versions may also be available from your state or local health department.

You can find VISs in more than 30 languages on the Immunization Action Coalition website at www.immunize.org/vis. To find VISs in alternative formats (e.g., audio, web-video), go to: www.immunize.org/vis/vis_sources.asp

Most current versions of VISs

As of June 11, 2014, the most recent versions of the VISs are as follows:

Adenovirus	6/11/14	Meningococcal	10/14/11
Anthrax	3/10/10	Multi-vaccine	unavailable
Chickenpox	3/13/08		Expected mid-2014
DTaP	5/17/07	PCV13	2/27/13
Hib	2/4/14	PPSV	10/6/09
Hepatitis A	10/25/11	Polio	11/8/11
Hepatitis B	2/2/12	Rabies	10/6/09
HPV-Cervarix	5/3/11	Rotavirus	8/26/13
HPV-Gardasil	5/17/13	Shingles	10/6/09
Influenza	7/26/13	Td	2/4/14
Japanese enceph.	1/24/14	Tdap	5/9/13
MMR	4/20/12	Typhoid	5/29/12
MMRV	5/21/10	Yellow fever	3/30/11

> **According to CDC, every time one of these vaccines is given — regardless of what combination vaccine it is given in — regardless of whether it is given by a public health clinic or a private provider — regardless of how the vaccine was purchased — and regardless of the age of the recipient — the appropriate VIS must be given out prior to the vaccination.**
>
> Source: www.cdc.gov/vaccines/hcp/vis/about/facts-vis.html

(Page 1 of 2)

C

Appendix C

Top 10 Facts about VISs

Fact 1 **It's federal law!**
Federal law requires that VISs must be used for the following vaccines when vaccinating patients of ALL ages:

- DTaP (includes DT)
- Td and Tdap
- Hib
- hepatitis A
- hepatitis B
- HPV
- influenza (inactivated and live vaccines)
- MMR and MMRV
- meningococcal
- pneumococcal conjugate
- polio
- rotavirus
- varicella

According to CDC, every time one of these vaccines is given — regardless of what combination vaccine it is given in — regardless of whether it is given by a public health clinic or a private provider — regardless of how the vaccine was purchased — and regardless of the age of the recipient — the appropriate VIS must be given out prior to the vaccination. There are also VISs for vaccines not covered by NCVIA: anthrax, Japanese encephalitis, pneumococcal polysaccharide, rabies, shingles, smallpox, typhoid, and yellow fever. CDC recommends the use of VISs whenever these vaccines are given. The VIS must always be used if vaccine was purchased under CDC contract.

> By using the VISs with your patients, you are helping to develop a better educated patient population and you are doing the right thing.

Fact 2 **VISs are required for both public and private sectors**
Federal law requires use of VISs in both the public and private sector settings and regardless of the source of payment for the vaccine.

Fact 3 **VIS must be provided *before* vaccine is administered to the patient**
The VIS provides information about the disease and the vaccine and should be given to the patient before vaccine is administered. It is also acceptable to hand out the VIS well before administering vaccines (e.g., at a prenatal visit or at birth for vaccines an infant will receive during infancy), as long as you still provide the VIS right before administering vaccines.

Fact 4 **You must provide a current VIS for each dose of vaccine**
The most current VIS must be provided before each dose of vaccine is given, including vaccines given as a series of doses. If five doses of a single vaccine are required, the patient (parent/legal representative) must have the opportunity to read the information on the VIS before each dose is given.

Fact 5 **You must provide VISs for combination vaccines too**
There is a VIS available for MMRV (ProQuad). An alternative VIS — the multi-vaccine VIS — is an option to providing single-vaccine VISs when administering one or more of these routine birth-through-6-month vaccines: DTaP, hepatitis B, Hib, pneumo-

coccal (PCV), polio (IPV), or rotavirus (RV). The multi-vaccine VIS can also be used when giving combination vaccines (e.g., Pediarix, Pentacel, Comvax) or when giving two or more routine vaccines at other pediatric visits (e.g., 12–15 months, 4–6 years). However, when giving combination vaccines for which no VIS exist (e.g., Twinrix), give out all relevant single VISs. For example, before administering Twinrix give your patient the VISs for both hepatitis A and hepatitis B vaccines.

Fact 6 **VISs are available in other formats, including more than 30 languages**
You may use laminated copies of VISs for patients and parents to read and return before leaving the clinic, but you must **also** offer the patient (parent/legal representative) a printed copy of the VIS to take home.

If they prefer to download the VIS onto a mobile device, direct them to CDC's VIS Mobile Downloads web page: http://m.cdc.gov/VIS

To download VISs in other languages, visit www.immunize.org/vis

Fact 7 **Federal law does not require signed consent in order for a person to be vaccinated**
Signed consent is not required by federal law (although some states may require them).

Fact 8 **To verify that a VIS was given, providers must record in the patient's chart (or permanent office log or file) the following information:**
- The published date of the VIS
- The date the VIS is given to the patient
- Name, address (office address), and title of the person who administers the vaccine
- The date the vaccine is administered
- The vaccine manufacturer and lot number of each dose administered

Fact 9 **VISs should not be altered before giving them to patients**
Providers should not change a VIS or write their own VISs. It is permissible to add a practice's name, address, or phone number to an existing VIS. Providers are encouraged to supplement the VIS with additional patient-education materials.

Fact 10 **Provide VISs to all patients**
For patients who don't read or speak English, the law requires that providers ensure all patients (parent/legal representatives) receive a VIS, regardless of their ability to read English. If available, provide a translation of the VIS in the patient's language.

Translations of VISs in more than 30 languages are available from IAC. Go to www.immunize.org/vis for VISs in multiple languages as well as in other formats.

Immunization Action Coalition • Saint Paul, Minnesota • (651) 647-9009 • www.immunize.org • www.vaccineinformation.org

Instructions for the Use of
Vaccine Information Statements

Required Use

1. Provide a Vaccine Information Statement (VIS) when a vaccination is given.

As required under the National Childhood Vaccine Injury Act (42 U.S.C. §300aa-26), all health care providers in the United States who administer, to any child or adult, any of the following vaccines — diphtheria, tetanus, pertussis, measles, mumps, rubella, polio, hepatitis A, hepatitis B, *Haemophilus influenzae* type b (Hib), trivalent influenza, pneumococcal conjugate, meningococcal, rotavirus, human papillomavirus (HPV), or varicella (chickenpox) — shall, prior to administration of each dose of the vaccine, provide a copy to keep of the relevant current edition vaccine information materials that have been produced by the Centers for Disease Control and Prevention (CDC):

- to the parent or legal representative[1] of any child to whom the provider intends to administer such vaccine, or

- to any adult[2] to whom the provider intends to administer such vaccine.

If there is not a single VIS for a combination vaccine, use the VISs for all component vaccines.

VISs should be supplemented with visual presentations or oral explanations as appropriate.

> [1] "Legal representative" is defined as a parent or other individual who is qualified under State law to consent to the immunization of a minor child or incompetent adult.
>
> [2] In the case of an incompetent adult, relevant VISs shall be provided to the individual's legal representative. If the incompetent adult is living in a long-term care facility, all relevant VISs may be provided at the time of admission, or at the time of consent if later than admission, rather than prior to each vaccination.

2. Record information for each VIS provided.

Health care providers shall make a notation in each patient's permanent medical record at the time vaccine information materials are provided, indicating:

(1) the edition date of the Vaccine Information Statement distributed, and
(2) the date the VIS was provided.

This recordkeeping requirement supplements the requirement of 42 U.S.C. §300aa-25 that all health care providers administering these vaccines must record in the patient's permanent medical record (or in a permanent office log):

(3) the name, address and title of the individual who administers the vaccine,
(4) the date of administration, and
(5) the vaccine manufacturer and lot number of the vaccine used.

Applicability of State Law

Health care providers should consult their legal counsel to determine additional State requirements pertaining to immunization. The Federal requirement to provide the vaccine information materials supplements any applicable State laws.

Availability of Copies

Copies are available in English and many other languages from CDC's website at **www.cdc.gov/vaccines/pubs/vis**. Single camera-ready copies may also be available from State health departments.

Current VIS Editions

DTaP/DT: 5/17/07	Meningococcal: 10/14/11[†]
Hib: 2/4/14[†]	Pneumococcal (PCV13): 2/27/13[†]
Hepatitis A: 10/25/11[†]	Polio: 11/8/11[†]
Hepatitis B: 2/2/12[†]	Rotavirus: 8/26/13[†]
HPV (Cervarix): 5/3/11[†]	Td: 2/4/14[†]
HPV (Gardasil): 5/17/13[†]	Tdap: 5/9/13[†]
Influenza (inactivated): 8/19/14[†]	Varicella: 3/13/08[†]
Influenza (live): 8/19/14[†]	Multi-Vaccine*: 10/22/14[†]
MMR: 4/20/12[†]	
MMRV: 5/21/10[†]	

*An optional alternative when two or more routine childhood vaccines (i.e., DTaP, hepatitis B, Hib, pneumococcal, or polio) are administered at the same visit.

†Interim

Reference 42 U.S.C. §300aa-26
October 22, 2014

C

Appendix C

Vaccine Information Statements: Frequently Asked Questions

Are VISs "informed consent" forms?

No. People sometimes use the term "informed consent" loosely when referring to VISs.

There is no Federal requirement for informed consent. VISs are written to fulfill the information requirements of the National Childhood Vaccine Injury Act (NCVIA). But because they cover both benefits and risks associated with vaccinations, they provide enough information that anyone reading them should be adequately informed. Some states have informed consent laws. Check your state medical consent law to determine if there are any specific informed consent requirements relating to immunization. VISs may be used for informed consent as long as they conform to the appropriate state laws.

Should the VISs be used for adults getting vaccines as well as for children?

Yes. Anyone receiving a covered vaccine should be given the appropriate VIS. VISs for vaccines that may be administered to both children and adults are worded so they may be used by both. Apart from legal requirements, it is good practice to give the appropriate VIS every time a vaccine is administered, to anyone of any age.

The law states that vaccine information materials be given to a child's legal representatives. How is "legal representative" defined?

A "legal representative" is a parent or other individual who is qualified under state law to consent to the immunization of a minor. There is not an overriding Federal definition.

Must the patient, parent, or legal representative physically take away a copy of each VIS, or can we simply let them read a copy and make sure they understand it?

Ideally each VIS should be taken home. They contain information that may be needed later (e.g., information about what to do in the case of an adverse reaction). Patients may choose not to take the VIS, but the provider should offer them the opportunity to do so. VISs are available electronically, and may be taken away in electronic form.

When do providers have to start using a new VIS?

The date for a new VISs required use is announced when the final draft is published in the Federal Register. Ideally, providers will begin using a new VIS immediately, particularly if the vaccine's contraindications or adverse event profile have changed since the previous version.

How should we comply with the law for patients who cannot read the VISs (e.g., those who are illiterate or blind)?

The NCVIA allows providers to supplement the VISs with "visual presentations" or "oral explanations" as needed. VISs can be read to illiterate or blind patients, or videotapes can be used as supplements. At least one CD-ROM is being produced on which users can hear the VIS's read. The VISs available on CDC's website are compatible with screen reader devices.

Why are the dates on some of the VISs several years old? Are they obsolete? Why can't they be updated every year?

VISs are updated only when they need to be. For instance, a VIS would be updated if there were a change in ACIP recommendations that affects the vaccine's adverse event profile, indications, or contraindications. **VISs posted on the CDC website are always the current versions.** Annually changing the dates on VISs that haven't changed otherwise could be confusing, because there would be multiple VISs in circulation that were identical but would have different dates.

Sometimes a VIS will contain a recommendation that is at odds with the manufacturer's package insert. Why?

VISs are based on recommendations of the Advisory Committee on Immunization Practices (ACIP), the committee that advises CDC on immunization policy. The ACIP's recommendations occasionally differ from those made by the manufacturer. These differences may involve adverse events. Package inserts generally tend to include all adverse events that were temporally associated with a vaccine during clinical trials, whereas ACIP tends to recognize only those shown to be causally linked to the vaccine. ACIP may also harmonize recommendations for similar vaccines produced by different manufacturers, for which approved indications differ slightly.

What is the reading level of VISs?

VIS's generally test at about a 10th grade reading level, according to Fletch-Kincaid. However, traditional "grade level" measures may be misleading for VISs. VISs are carefully written to be accessible to a diverse audience while remaining technically accurate. Several representative VISs have been subjected to focus group testing among low-literacy parents in a variety of racial and ethnic groups (some not native English speakers), and were generally judged to be easy to read and understand. VISs are always reviewed for readability, within the constraints imposed by the need for technical accuracy.

Questions concerning the Pediatric Multi-Vaccine VIS:

May the existing, single-vaccine VISs still be used?

Yes. The Multi-Vaccine VIS is an optional alternative to existing VISs. Providers wishing to continue using the individual VISs may do so. These will continue to be updated when recommendations change.

C

May the Multi-Vaccine VIS be used with combination vaccines, such as Pediarix or Comvax?

Yes. Just check the appropriate boxes on the first page as you would if you were administering the individual vaccines.

When we record the edition date of the VISs on the patient's medical record, do we record the date on the Multi-Vaccine VIS or the dates on the individual VISs?

Record the date of the Multi-Vaccine VIS for each vaccine given. If there is ever a question, this will make it clear that this VIS was used, and not the individual VISs.

Can the Multi-Vaccine VIS be used for children older than 6 months, or for adolescents or adults getting any of these vaccines?

It may be used for older children getting two or more of these vaccines during the same visit (e.g., a 12-month old getting Hib and PCV or a 4-year old getting DTaP and IPV). It should not be used for adolescents or adults.

Can the Multi-Vaccine VIS be used for catch-up doses?

Yes, as long as the doses are given to children as part of the primary series or routine pediatric boosters.

If a single-vaccine VIS is updated before the Multi-Vaccine VIS, may the multi continue to be used for that vaccine?

Sometimes there can be delays in updating a VIS. If an individual VIS for a vaccine covered on the multi gets updated before the multi does, the multi may still be used. You may give the patient the new single VIS at the same time, or explain verbally or with other written materials any changes. This is most important if the changes involve contraindications or adverse events; *in these cases be certain the patient gets up-to-date information*. It is less important if the update reflects other changes, such as changes in the routine schedule.

Questions concerning use of VISs for minors when the legal representative is not present at the time of vaccination:

C

When parents/legal representatives are not present at the time of vaccination of a minor (e.g., school-located vaccination clinics held during school hours, school-based health centers), several challenges arise related to provision of Vaccine Information Statements (VISs). Please see the questions and answers below for guidance on how to address these challenges:

How early can VISs be provided to parents/legal representatives prior to vaccination?

The National Childhood Vaccine Injury Act requires that a current VIS be provided to parents/legal representatives *prior to vaccination*. Although the Act does not specify the amount of time allowed between VIS provision and vaccination, they must be provided as close to the time of vaccination as is programmatically feasible and reasonable, keeping in mind that VISs are designed to inform vaccine recipients (or their parents/legal representatives) about the risks and benefits of specific vaccines, as well as medical eligibility, prior to vaccine receipt. For example, providing VISs several weeks prior to a scheduled school-located vaccination clinic may be reasonable. However, providing VISs several months prior to vaccination (e.g., providing them in July for a January vaccination clinic or at the end of one school year for a vaccination clinic the next school year) is not acceptable as parents/legal representatives may not have retained the VISs to review just prior to vaccination, the VIS may have since been revised, and a student's medical eligibility may have changed during that time.

Is there a requirement to verify that parents/legal representatives have actually received and reviewed the VIS?

Yes. The mandatory instructions for use of the VIS require providers to make a notation in the patient's medical record or permanent office log regarding provision of the VIS. If VISs (paper or electronic) are not provided to parents/legal representatives at the time of vaccination, parents/legal representatives must acknowledge in writing (or electronically) receipt and review of the current VIS. This can be accomplished by including a written statement that the parent/legal representative received and reviewed the current edition of the VIS, with the edition date specified, on the medical consent form authorizing vaccination. The parent's/legal representative's signature (or electronic signature if allowed under state law) then verifies receipt/review. Where allowed under the applicable state medical consent law, such verification/consent can be accomplished through electronic means. The signed verification of receipt/review of the VIS must be retained by the clinic/health care provider in the same manner and for the same timeframe as other medical consents are required to be retained by health care providers under the state's medical consent law.

What if the VIS is updated after it has been provided to parents/legal representatives but before vaccination occurs?

The VIS provided to parents/legal representatives must be current at the time of vaccination. If a VIS is updated and becomes effective after a previous version has been provided to parents/legal representatives, the parents/legal representatives must be notified of the updated VIS, a current VIS must be redistributed prior to vaccination, and verification of receipt/review of the current VIS must be obtained. Programs may wish to consider requiring parents/legal representatives to re-consent to vaccination in such a situation.

Appendix C

What are the acceptable methods of VIS provision to parents/legal representatives?

If the parent/legal representative is present at the time of vaccination, the VIS (paper or electronic) must be provided to the parent/legal representative before the child is vaccinated. If the parent/legal representative is not present, provision of the VIS prior to vaccination must be coupled with a method to verify parent/legal representative receipt of the VIS, in addition to parent/legal representative consent to vaccination in compliance with the applicable state medical consent law. Some examples of methods of VIS provision are as follows*:

- Providing a physical copy of the VIS to the parent/legal representative;
- Providing a link to the VIS in a physical letter sent to the parent/legal representative;
- Providing the VIS as an attachment or weblink contained within an email sent to the parent/legal representative.

*As noted above, if not provided directly to the parent/legal representative at the time of vaccination, the VIS must be provided prior to vaccination along with a requirement to acknowledge receipt/review of the VIS. This requirement can be accomplished by adding a written statement that the parent/legal representative received and reviewed the current edition of the VIS, with the edition date specified, on the medical consent form authorizing vaccination. Where allowed under the applicable state medical consent law, such verification/consent can be accomplished through electronic means.

Our state allows parents/legal representatives to provide a single, one-time consent for vaccines that require multiple doses given over weeks or months. In this case, do we have to provide a VIS prior to every dose administered?

Yes. Since a child's medical condition might change between doses, a VIS must be provided prior to administration of each dose to allow the parent to review the child's situation and determine whether or not to withdraw consent for additional doses. However, an additional acknowledged verification of receipt/review of the VIS and consent to vaccination for the following doses is not required if a single consent for a vaccine series is authorized under the applicable state medical consent law. In that instance, the original verification of receipt/review of the VIS and consent to the vaccination series sent prior to administration of the first dose must comply with any state medical consent requirement related to providing a process through which the parent/legal representative may later withdraw consent for additional doses, if such a requirement exists.

C

CDC's Vaccine Information Statement Webpage

http://www.cdc.gov/vaccines/hcp/vis/index.html

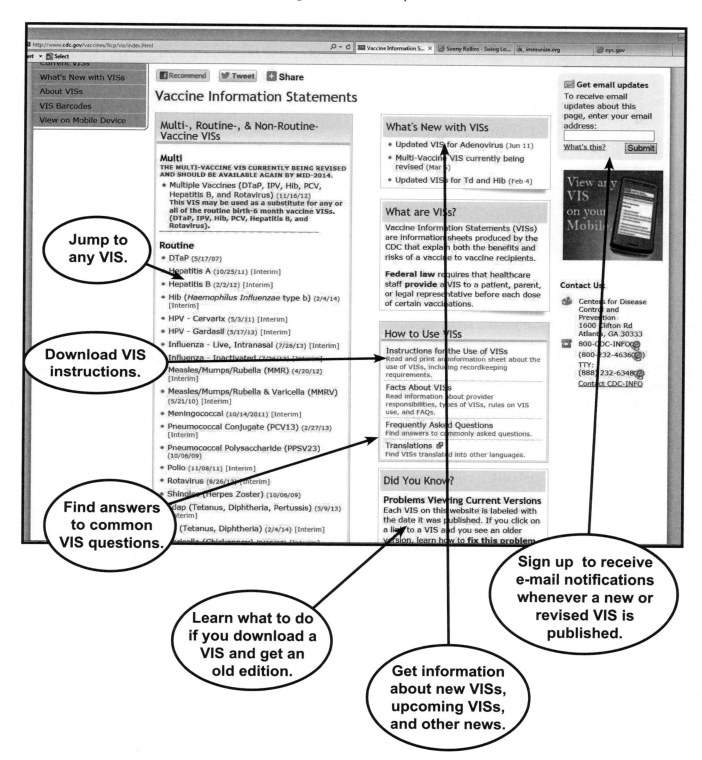

Appendix C

APPENDIX D
Vaccine Safety

D

Appendix D

D

The Vaccine Adverse Event Reporting System (VAERS)

VAERS is a national vaccine safety surveillance program co-sponsored by the Centers for Disease Control and Prevention (CDC) and the Food and Drug Administration (FDA). VAERS collects and analyzes information from reports of adverse events following receipt of US-licensed vaccines. In recent years, VAERS has received approximately 30,000 US reports annually, most of which describe mild adverse events like fever and injection site reactions. Very rarely, people experience serious adverse events following immunization. By monitoring such events, VAERS can help to identify important new safety concerns.

VAERS is a spontaneous reporting system, meaning that reports about adverse events can be submitted voluntarily by anyone. VAERS has limitations as a surveillance system: data may, and often do, include incorrect and incomplete information. Underreporting, or failure to report events, is another limitation. Serious medical events are more likely to be reported than minor ones. Importantly, VAERS cannot determine cause and effect. The report of an adverse event to VAERS does not indicate that a vaccine caused the event. It only indicates that the event occurred sometime after vaccine receipt. VAERS accepts all reports without judging whether or not the event was caused by the vaccine. More information on the limitations of VAERS data can be found at: http://vaers.hhs.gov/data/index

WHO CAN REPORT? Anyone can submit a VAERS report. Most reports are sent in by vaccine manufacturers and health care providers, but vaccine recipients, parents/guardians, and others may also submit reports.

WHAT SHOULD BE REPORTED? VAERS encourages reporting of any clinically significant adverse event that occurs after the administration of any vaccine licensed in the United States.

The National Childhood Vaccine Injury Act of 1986 requires health care providers to report:
- Any health event listed by the vaccine manufacturer as a contraindication to subsequent doses of the vaccine,
- Any event listed in the Reportable Events Table that occurs within the specified time period after the vaccination.

A copy of the Reportable Events Table can be found on the following page, or at http://vaers.hhs.gov/resources/VAERS_Table_of_Reportable_Events_Following_Vaccination.pdf.

HOW TO REPORT There are three ways to report to VAERS:

- **Online.** Complete a VAERS online form at https://vaers.hhs.gov/esub/step1.
  Before you begin, review the Instructions for Completing the VAERS On-Line Form at http://vaers.hhs.gov/esub/help. The VAERS On-Line form must be completed in a single sitting (i.e., you cannot save your work and return later to finish). Information supplied on this form is transmitted securely to VAERS.

- **Fax.** Download a VAERS form at http://vaers.hhs.gov/resources/vaers_form.pdf, or request a form by sending an e-mail to info@vaers.org, by calling 800-822-7967, or by faxing a request to 877-721-0366. Review the Instructions for Completing the VAERS Paper Form at http://vaers.hhs.gov/helpinstructions. Fax the completed form to 877-721-0366.

- **Mail.** Download a VAERS form at http://vaers.hhs.gov/resources/vaers_form.pdf, or request a form by sending an e-mail to info@vaers.org, by calling 800-822-7967, or by faxing a request to 877-721-0366. Review the Instructions for Completing the VAERS Paper Form at http://vaers.hhs.gov/helpinstructions. Mail the completed form to VAERS, P.O. Box 1100, Rockville, MD 20849-1100. A pre-paid postage stamp is included on the back of the form.

For more information, visit the VAERS website at http://vaers.hhs.gov .

Updated March 18, 2013

D

Appendix D

VAERS Table of Reportable Events Following Vaccination*

Vaccine/Toxoid	Event and Interval from Vaccination
Tetanus in any combination: DTaP, DTP, DTP-Hib, DT, Td, TT, Tdap, DTaP-IPV, DTaP-IPV/Hib, DTaPHepB-IPV	A. Anaphylaxis or anaphylactic shock (7 days) B. Brachial neuritis (28 days) C. Any acute complications or sequelae (including death) of above events (interval - not applicable) D. Events described in manufacturer's package insert as contraindications to additional doses of vaccine (interval - see package insert)
Pertussis in any combination: DTaP, DTP, DTP-Hib, Tdap, P, DTaP-IPV, DTaP-IPV/Hib, DTaP-HepB-IPV	A. Anaphylaxis or anaphylactic shock (7 days) B. Encephalopathy or encephalitis (7 days) C. Any acute complications or sequelae (including death) of above events (interval - not applicable) D. Events described in manufacturer's package insert as contraindications to additional doses of vaccine (interval - see package insert)
Measles, mumps and rubella in any combination: MMR, MR, M, MMRV, R	A. Anaphylaxis or anaphylactic shock (7 days) B. Encephalopathy or encephalitis (15 days) C. Any acute complications or sequelae (including death) of above events (interval - not applicable) D. Events described in manufacturer's package insert as contraindications to additional doses of vaccine (interval - see package insert)
Rubella in any combination: MMR, MMRV, MR, R	A. Chronic arthritis (42 days) B. Any acute complications or sequelae (including death) of above event (interval - not applicable) C. Events described in manufacturer's package insert as contraindications to additional doses of vaccine (interval - see package insert)
Measles in any combination: MMR, MMRV, MR, M	A. Thrombocytopenic purpura (7-30 days) B. Vaccine-strain measles viral infection in an immunodeficient recipient (6 months) C. Any acute complications or sequelae (including death) of above events (interval - not applicable) D. Events described in manufacturer's package insert as contraindications to additional doses of vaccine (interval - see package insert)

Oral Polio (OPV)	A. Paralytic polio
	  o in a non-immunodeficient recipient (30 days)
	  o in an immunodeficient recipient (6 months)
	  o in a vaccine-associated community case (interval - not applicable)
	B. Vaccine-strain polio viral infection
	  o in a non-immunodeficient recipient (30 days)
	  o in an immunodeficient recipient (6 months)
	  o in a vaccine-associated community case (interval - not applicable)
	C. Any acute complication or sequelae (including death) of above events (interval - not applicable)
	D. Events described in manufacturer's package insert as contraindications to additional doses of vaccine (interval - see package insert)

Inactivated Polio: IPV, DTaP-IPV, DTaP-IPV/HIB, DTaP-HepB-IPV	A. Anaphylaxis or anaphylactic shock (7 days) B. Any acute complication or sequelae (including death) of the above event (interval - not applicable) C. Events described in manufacturer's package insert as contraindications to additional doses of vaccine (interval - see package insert)
Hepatitis B in any combination: HepB, HepA-HepB, DTaP-HepB-IPV, Hib-HepB	A. Anaphylaxis or anaphylactic shock (7 days) B. Any acute complications or sequelae (including death) of the above event (interval - not applicable) C. Events described in manufacturer's package insert as contraindications to additional doses of vaccine (interval - see package insert)
Hemophilus influenzae type b in any combination (conjugate): Hib, Hib-HepB, DTP-Hib, DTaP-IPV/Hib	Events described in manufacturer's package insert as contraindications to additional doses of vaccine (interval – see package insert)
Varicella in any combination: VAR, MMRV	Events described in manufacturer's package insert as contraindications to additional doses of vaccine (interval – see package insert)
Rotavirus (monovalent or pentavalent) RV1, RV5	Events described in manufacturer's package insert as contraindications to additional doses of vaccine (interval – see package insert)
Pneumococcal conjugate (7-valent or 13-valent) PCV7, PCV13	Events described in manufacturer's package insert as contraindications to additional doses of vaccine (interval – see package insert)

D

The Vaccine Injury Compensation Program (VICP)

The VICP is a no-fault alternative to the traditional tort system for resolving vaccine injury claims. It was established as part of the National Childhood Vaccine Injury Act of 1986, after a rash of lawsuits against vaccine manufacturers and healthcare providers threatened to cause vaccine shortages and reduce vaccination rates.

The VICP is administered jointly by the U.S. Department of Health and Human Services (HHS), the U.S. Court of Federal Claims (the Court), and the U.S. Department of Justice (DOJ). The VICP is located in the HHS, Health Resources and Services Administration (HRSA), Healthcare Systems Bureau, Division of Vaccine Injury Compensation.

Briefly, an individual claiming a vaccine-related injury or death files a petition for compensation with the Court, and may be represented by an attorney. A HHS physician reviews the petition to determine whether it meets the medical criteria for compensation. A recommendation is provided to the Court. The HHS position is presented before a "special master," who makes the decision for compensation under the VICP. A decision may be appealed to a judge of the Court, then to the Federal Circuit Court of Appeals, and eventually to the U.S. Supreme Court.

A petitioner may file a claim in civil court against the vaccine company and/or the vaccine administrator only after first filing a claim under the VICP and then rejecting the decision of the Court.

Who Can File a Claim?

- You may file a claim if you received a vaccine covered by the VICP and believe that you have been injured by this vaccine.
- You may also file a claim if you are a parent or legal guardian of a child or disabled adult who received a vaccine covered by the VICP and believe that the person was injured by this vaccine.
- You may file a claim if you are the legal representative of the estate of a deceased person who received a vaccine covered by the VICP and believe that the person's death resulted from the vaccine injury.
- You may file a claim if you are *not* a United States citizen.
- Some people who receive vaccines outside of the U.S. may be eligible for compensation. See the VICP website for more details.
- **In addition**, to be eligible to file a claim, the effects of the person's injury must have:
  1. lasted for more than 6 months after the vaccine was given; or
  2. resulted in a hospital stay **and** surgery; or
  3. resulted in death.

There is no age restriction on who may file a claim. Anyone receiving a vaccine covered by the VICP, no matter their age, can file a claim or have one filed on their behalf.

To learn how to file a claim, see the VICP website at http://www.hrsa.gov/vaccinecompensation/fileclaim.html.

Vaccines covered by VICP are diphtheria, tetanus, pertussis, Hib, hepatitis A, hepatitis B, human papillomavirus, trivalent influenza, measles, mumps, rubella, meningococcal, polio, pneumococcal conjugate, rotavirus, and varicella, in any combination. (Additional vaccines may be added in the future.)

D

Appendix D

The **Vaccine Injury Table** makes it easier for some people to get compensation. The Table lists and explains injuries and conditions that are presumed to be caused by vaccines. It also lists time periods in which the first symptom of these injuries and conditions must occur after receiving the vaccine. If the first symptom of these injuries/conditions occurs within the listed time periods, it is presumed that the vaccine was the cause of the injury or condition unless another cause is found. For example, if a patient received the tetanus vaccine and had a severe allergic reaction (anaphylaxis) within 4 hours after receiving the vaccine, then it is presumed that the tetanus vaccine caused the injury, if no other cause is found.

If an injury or condition is not on the Table or if it did not occur within the time period on the Table, the petitioner must prove that the vaccine caused the injury or condition. Such proof must be based on medical records or opinion, which may include expert witness testimony.

A copy of the Vaccine Injury Table is on the following page, or can be found online at http://www.hrsa.gov/vaccinecompensation/vaccinetable.html. A comprehensive explanation of terms used in the table accompanies the online version.

March 2013

For more information, visit the VICP website at http://www.hrsa.gov/vaccinecompensation.

D

National Childhood Vaccine Injury Act: Vaccine Injury Table

Vaccine	Illness, disability, injury or condition covered	Time period for first symptom or manifestation of onset or of significant aggravation after vaccine administration
I. Vaccines containing tetanus toxoid (e.g., DTaP, DTP, DT, Td, or TT)	A. Anaphylaxis or anaphylactic shock	4 hours
	B. Brachial Neuritis	2-28 days
	C. Any acute complication or sequela (including death) of an illness, disability, injury, or condition referred to above which illness, disability, injury, or condition arose within the time period prescribed	Not applicable
II. Vaccines containing whole cell pertussis bacteria, extracted or partial cell pertussis bacteria, or specific pertussis antigen(s) (e.g., DTP, DTaP, P, DTP-Hib)	A. Anaphylaxis or anaphylactic shock	4 hours
	B. Encephalopathy (or encephalitis)	72 hours
	C. Any acute complication or sequela (including death) of an illness, disability, injury, or condition referred to above which illness, disability, injury, or condition arose within the time period prescribed	Not applicable
III. Measles, mumps, and rubella vaccine or any of its components (e.g., MMR, MR, M, R)	A. Anaphylaxis or anaphylactic shock	4 hours
	B. Encephalopathy (or encephalitis)	5-15 days (not less than 5 days and not more than 15 days
	C. Any acute complication or sequela (including death) of an illness, disability, injury, or condition referred to above which illness, disability, injury, or condition arose within the time period prescribed	Not applicable
IV. Vaccines containing rubella virus (e.g., MMR, MR, R)	A. Chronic arthritis	7-42 days
	B. Any acute complication or sequela (including death) of an illness, disability, injury, or condition referred to above which illness, disability, injury, or condition arose within the time period prescribed	Not applicable
V. Vaccines containing measles virus (e.g., MMR, MR, M)	A. Thrombocytopenic purpura	7-30 days
	B. Vaccine-Strain Measles Viral Infection in an immunodeficient recipient	6 months
	C. Any acute complication or sequela (including death) of an illness, disability, injury, or condition referred to above which illness, disability, injury, or condition arose within the time period prescribed	Not applicable
VI. Vaccines containing polio live virus (OPV)	A. Paralytic Polio - in a non-immunodeficient recipient - in an immunodeficient recipient - in a vaccine associated community case	30 days 6 months Not applicable
	B. Vaccine-Strain Polio Viral Infection - in a non-immunodeficient recipient - in an immunodeficient recipient - in a vaccine associated community case	30 days 6 months Not applicable
	C. Any acute complication or sequela (including death) of an illness, disability, injury, or condition referred to above which illness, disability, injury, or condition arose within the time period prescribed	Not applicable

D

Vaccine	Illness, disability, injury or condition covered	Time period for first symptom or manifestation of onset or of significant aggravation after vaccine administration
VII. Vaccines containing polio inactivated virus (e.g., IPV)	A. Anaphylaxis or anaphylactic shock	4 hours
	B. Any acute complication or sequela (including death) of an illness, disability, injury, or condition referred to above which illness, disability, injury, or condition arose within the time period prescribed	Not applicable
VIII. Hepatitis B vaccines	A. Anaphylaxis or anaphylactic shock	4 hours
	B. Any acute complication or sequela (including death) of an illness, disability, injury, or condition referred to above which illness, disability, injury, or condition arose within the time period prescribed	Not applicable
IX. Haemophilus influenzae type B polysaccharide conjugate vaccines	No condition specified	Not applicable
X. Varicella vaccine	No condition specified	Not applicable
XI. Rotavirus vaccine	No condition specified	Not applicable
XII. Pneumococcal conjugate vaccines	No condition specified	Not applicable
XIII. Hepatitis A vaccines	No condition specified	Not applicable
XIV. Trivalent influenza vaccines	No condition specified	Not applicable
XV. Meningococcal vaccines	No condition specified	Not applicable
XVI. Human papillomavirus (HPV) vaccines	No condition specified	Not applicable
XVII. Any new vaccine recommended by the Centers for Disease Control and Prevention for routine administration to children, after publication by the Secretary of a notice of coverage*	No condition specified	Not applicable

*Now includes all vaccines against seasonal influenza (except trivalent influenza vaccines, which are already covered), effective November 12, 2013.

D

Countermeasures Injury Compensation Program (CICP)

Overview

The Countermeasures Injury Compensation Program (CICP) is a Federal program that provides benefits to individuals who are seriously injured as a result of the administration or use of a covered countermeasure. CICP also provides death benefits to certain survivors if death directly resulted from receipt of a covered countermeasure. Covered countermeasures may include vaccines, antivirals, drugs, biologics, or medical devices used to prevent, treat, or diagnose an illness that the Secretary of the United States Department of Health and Human Services (the Secretary) declares to be an actual or potential public health emergency. Examples of currently covered countermeasures are pandemic influenza vaccines including the 2009 pandemic H1N1 influenza vaccine, antivirals (e.g., Tamiflu®, Relenza®, peramivir), ventilation assistance devices (e.g., mechanical ventilators), and respiratory protection devices (e.g., N-95 masks) used to treat, diagnose or prevent pandemic influenza. In addition, countermeasures, including vaccines, used to diagnose, treat or prevent smallpox, anthrax, botulism, and acute radiation syndrome are currently covered. Adverse events during pre-licensure testing may be covered as well.

This Program was established by the Public Readiness and Emergency Preparedness Act of 2005 (PREP Act), 42 U.S.C. § 247d-6e. The PREP Act also confers broad liability protections covering the manufacture, testing, development, distribution, or use of the designated covered countermeasure.

Filing Deadline and Application and Review Process

Individuals have one (1) year from the date the vaccine or other covered countermeasure was administered or used to request compensation benefits. If their injury is added to a Countermeasures Injury Table, then they may also have one year from the effective date of the Table addition to file. To file a claim, individuals must submit a Request for Benefits Form and the Authorization for Use or Disclosure of Health Information Form to request medical records from each health care provider who treated the injured person. In addition, medical records from one year before the injury to the present time must be submitted. Health care providers should send medical records directly to the Program. All documents should be sent to:

Health Resources and Services Administration
Countermeasures Injury Compensation Program
5600 Fishers Lane, Room 11C-26
Rockville, MD 20857

After an individual has submitted a complete Request for Benefits package, CICP medical staff reviews it to determine if the individual is eligible for compensation. An individual may be eligible for compensation if compelling, reliable, valid, medical and scientific evidence exists demonstrating that the injury for which compensation is sought was caused by the administration or use of a covered countermeasure and no other more likely cause of the injury is found. If an individual is found eligible for compensation, the type and amount of benefits are determined by the Program. If an individual is not eligible for compensation, he/she may request the Associate Administrator of the Healthcare Systems Bureau, HRSA, to reconsider the Program's decision. The Associate Administrator will convene an independent panel to review the Program's decision, make its own findings, and make a recommendation. The Associate Administrator will review this recommendation and make a final decision.

D

Appendix D

Benefits Available

Eligible individuals may be compensated for reasonable and necessary unreimbursable medical expenses and for lost employment income at the time of the injury. Death benefits may be paid to certain survivors of covered countermeasures recipients who have died as a direct result of the covered countermeasure injury. The U.S. Department of Health and Human Services is the payer of last resort. Therefore, payments are reduced by those of other third party payers.

Contact Information
Website: http://www.hrsa.gov/cicp/
E-mail: CICP@hrsa.gov
Phone: 1-855-266-CICP (2427)

Updated March 18, 2013

D

APPENDIX E

Data and Statistics

E

Appendix E

Reported Cases and Deaths from Vaccine Preventable Diseases, United States, 1950-2013

Year	Diphtheria Cases	Diphtheria Deaths	Tetanus Cases	Tetanus Deaths	Pertussis Cases	Pertussis Deaths	Polio (paralytic) Cases	Polio (paralytic) Deaths
1950	5,796	410	486	336	120,718	1,118	33,300[†]	1,904
1951	3,983	302	506	394	68,687	951	28,386[†]	1,551
1952	2,960	217	484	360	45,030	402	57,879[†]	3,145
1953	2,355	156	506	337	37,129	270	35,592[†]	1,450
1954	2,041	145	524	332	60,886	373	18,308	1,368
1955	1,984	150	462	265	62,786	467	13,850	1043
1956	1,568	103	468	246	31,732	266	7,911	566
1957	1,211	81	447	279	28,295	183	2,499	221
1958	918	74	445	303	32,148	177	3,697	255
1959	934	72	445	283	40,005	269	6,289	454
1960	918	69	368	231	14,809	118	2,525	230
1960	617	68	379	242	11,468	76	988	90
1962	444	41	322	215	17,749	83	762	60
1963	314	45	325	210	17,135	115	396	41
1964	293	42	289	179	13,005	93	106	17
1965	164	18	300	181	6,799	55	61	16
1966	209	20	235	158	7,717	49	106	9
1967	219	32	263	144	9,718	37	40	16
1968	260	30	178	66	4,810	36	53	24
1969	241	25	192	89	3,285	13	18	13
1970	435	30	148	79	4,249	12	31	7
1971	215	13	116	64	3036	18	17	18
1972	152	10	128	58	3,287	6	29	2
1973	228	10	101	40	1,759	5	7	10
1974	272	5	101	44	2,402	14	7	3
1975	307	5	102	45	1,738	8	13	9
1976	128	7	75	32	1,010	7	10	16
1977	84	5	87	24	2,177	10	19	16
1978	76	4	86	32	2,063	6	8	13

†Total reported cases (i.e., including non-paralytic)

E

Appendix E

Year	Diphtheria		Tetanus		Pertussis		Polio (paralytic)	
	Cases	Deaths	Cases	Deaths	Cases	Deaths	Cases	Deaths
1979	59	1	81	30	1,623	6	22	1
1980	3	1	95	28	1,730	11	9	2
1981	5	0	72	31	1,248	6	10	0
1982	2	1	88	22	1,895	4	12	0
1983	5	0	91	22	2,463	5	13	0
1984	1	0	74	20	2,276	7	9	0
1985	3	0	83	23	3,589	4	8	0
1986	0	0	64	22	4,195	6	10	0
1987	3	1	48	16	2,823	1	9	0
1988	2	0	53	17	3,450	4	9	0
1989	3	0	53	9	4,157	12	11	0
1990	4	1	64	11	4,570	12	6	0
1991	5	0	57	11	2,719	0	10	1
1992	4	1	45	9	4,083	5	6	0
1993	0	0	48	11	6,586	1	4	0
1994	2	0	51	9	4,617	8	8	0
1995	0	1	41	5	5,137	6	7	1
1996	2	0	36	1	7,796	4	7	0
1997	4	0	50	4	6,564	6	6	0
1998	1	1	34	7	6,279	5	3	0
1999	1	1	40	7	7,288	7	2	0
2000	1	0	35	5	7,867	12	0	0
2001	2	0	37	5	7,580	17	0	0
2002	1	0	25	5	9,771	18	0	0
2003	1	1	20	4	11,647	11	0	0
2004	0	0	34	4	25,827	16	0	0
2005	0	0	27	1	25,616	31	1[§]	0
2006	0	0	41	4	15,632	9	0	0
2007	0	0	28	5	10,454	9	0	0
2008	0	0	19	3	13,278	20	0	0
2009	0	0	18	6	16,858	15	1[§]	0
2010	0	0	26	3	27,550	26	0	0
2011	0	NA	36	NA	18,719	NA	0	NA
2012	1	NA	37	NA	48,277	NA	0	NA
2013	0	NA	26	NA	28,639	NA	1[§]	NA

§ Vaccine-associated/derived paralytic polio.

Year	Measles Cases	Measles Deaths	Mumps Cases	Mumps Deaths	Rubella Cases	Rubella Deaths	CRS Cases
1950	319,124	468	NR		NR		NR
1951	530,118	683	NR		NR		NR
1952	683,077	618	NR		NR		NR
1953	449,146	462	NR		NR		NR
1954	682,720	518	NR		NR		NR
1955	555,156	345	NR		NR		NR
1956	611,936	530	NR		NR		NR
1957	486,799	389	NR		NR		NR
1958	763,094	552	NR		NR		NR
1959	406,162	385	NR		NR		NR
1960	441,703	380	NR	42	NR	12	NR
1961	423,919	434	NR	53	NR	14	NR
1962	481,530	408	NR	43	NR	8	NR
1963	385,156	364	NR	48	NR	16	NR
1964	458,083	421	NR	50	NR	53	NR
1965	261,904	276	NR	31	NR	16	NR
1966	204,136	261	NR	43	46,975	12	NR
1967	62,705	81	NR	37	46,888	16	NR
1968	22,231	24	152,209	25	49,371	24	NR
1969	25,826	41	90,918	22	57,686	29	62
1970	47,351	89	104,953	16	56,552	31	67
1971	75,290	90	124,939	22	45,086	20	44
1972	32,275	24	74,215	16	25,507	14	32
1973	26,690	23	69,612	12	27,804	16	30
1974	22,094	20	59,128	6	11,917	15	22
1975	24,374	20	59,647	8	16,652	21	32
1976	41,126	12	38,492	8	12,491	12	22
1977	57,345	15	21,436	5	20,395	17	29
1978	26,871	11	16,817	3	18,269	10	30
1979	13,597	6	14,255	2	11,795	1	57
1980	13,506	11	8,576	2	3,904	1	14
1981	3,124	2	4,941	1	2,077	5	10

Appendix E

Year	Measles		Mumps		Rubella		CRS
	Cases	Deaths	Cases	Deaths	Cases	Deaths	Cases
1982	1,714	2	5,270	2	2,325	4	13
1983	1,497	4	3,355	2	970	3	7
1984	2,587	1	3,021	1	752	1	2
1985	2,822	4	2,982	0	630	1	2
1986	6,282	2	7,790	0	55	1	13
1987	3,655	2	12,848	2	306	0	3
1988	3,396	3	4,866	2	225	1	2
1989	18,193	32	5,712	3	396	4	2
1990	27,786	64	5,292	1	1,125	8	32
1991	9,643	27	4,264	1	1,401	1	34
1992	2,237	4	2,572	0	160	1	11
1993	312	0	1,692	0	192	0	4
1994	963	0	1,537	0	227	0	7
1995	309	2	906	0	128	1	3
1996	508	1	751	1	238	0	2
1997	138	2	683	0	181	0	9
1998	100	0	666	1	364	0	9
1999	100	2	387	1	267	0	6
2000	86	1	338	2	176	0	8
2001	116	1	266	0	23	2	3
2002	44	0	270	1	18	0	1
2003	56	1	231	0	7	0	4
2004	37	0	258	0	10	1	0
2005	66	NA	314	0	11	0	1
2006	55	0	6,584	1	11	0	1
2007	43	0	800	0	11	1	0
2008	140	0	454	2	16	0	0
2009	71	NA	1991	2	3	2	2
2010	63	NA	2,612	2	5	2	0
2011	220	NA	404	NA	4	NA	0
2012	55	NA	229	NA	9	NA	3
2013	187	NA	584	NA	9	NA	1

E

Year	Hepatitis A Cases	Hepatitis A Deaths	Hepatitis B Cases	Hepatitis B Deaths	Haemophilus Cases	Haemophilus Deaths	Varicella Cases	Varicella Deaths
1966	32,859	NA	1,497	NA	NR	NR	NR	NA
1967	38,909	NA	2,458	NA	NR	NR	NR	NA
1968	45,893	NA	4,829	NA	NR	NR	NR	NA
1969	48,416	NA	5,909	NA	NR	NR	NR	NA
1970	56,797	NA	8,310	NA	NR	NR	NR	NA
1971	59,606	NA	9,556	NA	NR	NR	NR	NA
1972	54,074	NA	9,402	NA	NR	NR	164,114	122
1973	50,749	NA	8,451	NA	NR	NR	182,927	138
1974	40,358	NA	10,631	NA	NR	NR	141,495	106
1975	35,855	NA	13,121	NA	NR	NR	154,248	83
1976	33,288	NA	14,973	NA	NR	NR	183,990	106
1977	31,153	NA	16,831	NA	NR	NR	188,396	89
1978	29,500	NA	15,016	NA	NR	NR	154,089	91
1979	30,407	129	15,452	260	NR	NR	199,081	103
1980	29,087	112	19,015	294	NR	NR	190,894	78
1981	25,802	93	21,152	394	NR	NR	200,766	84
1982	23,403	83	22,177	375	NR	NR	167,423	61
1983	21,532	82	24,318	438	NR	NR	177,462	57
1984	22,040	77	26,115	465	NR	NR	221,983	53
1985	23,210	80	26,611	490	NR	NR	178,162	68
1986	23,430	65	26,107	557	NR	NR	183,243	47
1987	25,280	77	25,916	595	NR	NR	213,196	89
1988	28,507	70	23,177	621	NR	NR	192,857	83
1989	35,821	88	23,419	711	NR	NR	185,441	89
1990	31,441	76	21,102	816	NR	NR	173,099	120
1991	24,378	71	18,003	912	2,764	17	147,076	81
1992	23,112	82	16,126	903	1,412	16	158,364	100
1993	24,238	95	13,361	1041	1,419	7	134,722	100
1994	26,796	97	12,517	1120	1,174	5	151,219	124
1995	31,582	142	10,805	1027	1,180	12	120,624	115
1996	31,032	121	10,637	1082	1,170	7	83,511	81

Appendix E

Year	Hepatitis A		Hepatitis B		Haemophilus		Varicella	
	Cases	Deaths	Cases	Deaths	Cases	Deaths	Cases	Deaths
1997	30,021	127	10,416	1,030	1,162	7	98,727	99
1998	23,229	114	10,258	1,052	1,194	11	82,455	81
1999	17,047	134	7,694	832	1,309	6	46,016	48
2000	13,397	106	8,036	886	1,398	6	27,382	44
2001	10,609	83	7,843	769	1,597	11	22,536	26
2002	8,795	76	7,996	762	1,743	7	22,841	32
2003	7,653	54	7,526	685	2,013	5	20,948	16
2004	5,970	58	6,741	643	2,085	11	26,659	19
2005	4,488	43	5,119	642	2,304	4	32,242	13
2006	3,579	34	4,713	700	2,436	4	48,445	18
2007	2,979	34	4,519	719	2,541	10	40,146	6
2008	2,585	37	4,033	671	2,886	3	30,386	18
2009	1,987	26	3,405	597	3,022	7	20,480	22
2010	1,670	29	3,374	588	3,151	4	15,427	15
2011	1,398	NA	2,903	NA	3,539	NA	14,513	5
2012	1,562	NA	2,895	NA	3,418	NA	13,447	3
2013	1,781	NA	3.050	NA	3,792	NA	11,359	NA

Notes
NA - Not Available
NR - Not nationally reportable
CRS: Congenital Rubella Syndrome

Prior to 1966, hepatitis A and B were not separated from other types of hepatitis. Prior to 1978, deaths from hepatitis A and B were not separated from deaths from other types of hepatitis.

Haemophilus (Hi) reporting includes all serotypes and all ages. In 2013, 31 cases of invasive Hi type b disease were reported among children younger than 5 years of age.

Varicella was removed from the nationally notifiable disease list in 1991. In 2012, varicella cases were reported from 39 states, the District of Columbia, New York City, Guam, Puerto Rico, the Northern Mariana Islands and the U.S. Virgin Islands.

Sources:
Cases: Final totals of nationally reportable infectious diseases are reported in *Morbidity and Mortality Weekly Report* (*MMWR*). Tables are published for the previous year in August or September of the following year. Final totals for 2013 were published in *MMWR* 2014;63(32):702-715. CDC also publishes a more comprehensive surveillance document, the annual *Summary of Notifiable Diseases*. The most current annual summary was published on July 5, 2013 for calendar year 2011. This document and annual summaries for previous years are available on the MMWR website at http://www.cdc.gov/mmwr/.

Deaths: National Center for Health Statistics Mortality Report for respective years.

September 2014

Impact of Vaccines in the 20th & 21st Centuries

Comparison of 20th Century Annual Morbidity & Current Morbidity

Disease	20th Century Annual Morbidity*	2013 Reported Cases†	% Decrease
Smallpox	29,005	0	100%
Diphtheria	21,053	0	100%
Pertussis	200,752	28,639	86%
Tetanus	580	26	96%
Polio (paralytic)	16,316	1	>99%
Measles	530,217	187	>99%
Mumps	162,344	584	>99%
Rubella	47,745	9	>99%
CRS	152	1	99%
Haemophilus influenzae	20,000 (est.)	31§	>99%

Sources:

* *JAMA.* 2007;298(18):2155-2163
† CDC. *MMWR* August 15, 2014;63(32);702-715. (MMWR 3013 final data)
§ *Haemophilus influenzae* type b (Hib) <5 years of age. An additional 10 cases of Hib are estimated to have occurred among the 185 reports of Hi (<5 years of age) with unknown serotype.

Comparison of Pre-Vaccine Era Estimated Annual Morbidity with Current Estimate

Disease	Pre-Vaccine Era Annual Estimate	2013 Estimate (unless otherwise specified)	% Decrease
Hepatitis A	117,333*	2,890†	98%
Hepatitis B (acute)	66,232*	18,800†	72%
Pneumococcus (invasive) All ages <5 years of age	63,067* 16,069*	33,500ⁿ 1,900§	47% 88%
Rotavirus (hospitalizations <3 years of age)	62,500‡	12,500**	80%
Varicella	4,085,120*	167,490††	96%

Sources:

* *JAMA.* 2007;298(18):2155-2163
† CDC. Viral Hepatitis Surveillance – United States, 2011
ⁿ CDC. Active Bacterial Core surveillance Provisional Report; *S. pneumonia* 2013.
§ CDC. Unpublished, Active Bacterial Core surveillance
‡ CDC. *MMWR.* February 6, 2009 / 58(RR02); 1-25
** New Vaccine Surveillance Network 2013 data (unpublished); U.S. rotavirus disease now has biennial pattern
†† CDC. Varicella Program 2013 data (unpublished)

September 2014

E

Vaccine Coverage Levels – United States, 1962-2012

Year	DTP 3+	DTP4+	Polio 3+	MMR*	Hib3+	Var	PCV3+	HepB3+	Rota	Combined 4-3-1	Combined 4-3-1-3
1962	67.3										
1963	71.4										
1964	74.6										
1965	72.7										
1966	74.0										
1967	77.9			60.0							
1968	76.8			61.5							
1969	77.4			61.4							
1970	76.4			58.4							
1971	77.8			62.2							
1972	74.1			62.8							
1973	71.7		59.5	61.0							
1974	72.4		60.0	63.4							
1975	73.2		63.6	65.5							
1976	72.7		61.3	66.3							
1977	69.6		62.6	65.0							
1978	66.6		59.5	63.6							
1979	64.4		59.7	66.5							
1080	66.0		58.9	66.6							
1981	68.1		59.2	66.8							
1982	67.1		57.0	67.6							
1983	65.4		56.9	66.3							
1984	65.0		53.2	65.8							
1985	63.6		53.6	61.2							
1986†											
1987†											
1988†											
1989†											
1990†											
1991	68.8		53.2	82.0							
1992	83.0	59.0	72.4	82.5	28.2			8.0		68.7	55.3
1993	88.2	72.1	78.9	84.1	55.0			16.3		67.1	
1994	93.0	77.7	83.0	89.0	86.0			37.0		75.0	
1995	94.7	78.5	87.9	87.6	91.7			68.0		76.2	74.2
1996	95.0	81.1	91.1	90.7	91.7	16.0		81.8		78.4	76.5
1997	95.5	81.5	90.8	90.5	92.7	25.9		83.7		77.9	76.2
1998	95.6	83.9	90.8	92.0	93.4	43.2		87.0		80.6	79.2
1999	95.9	83.3	89.6	91.5	93.5	57.5		88.1		79.9	78.4
2000	94.1	81.7	89.5	90.5	93.4	67.8		90.3		77.6	76.2
2001	94.3	82.1	89.4	91.4	93.0	76.3		88.9		78.6	77.2
2002	94.9	81.6	90.2	91.6	93.1	80.6	40.8	88.9		78.5	77.5
2003	96.0	84.8	91.6	93.0	93.9	84.8	68.1	92.4		82.2	81.3
2004	95.9	85.5	91.6	93.0	93.5	87.5	73.2	92.4		83.5	82.5
2005	96.1	85.7	91.7	91.5	93.9	87.9	82.8	92.9		83.1	82.4
2006	95.8	85.2	92.9	92.4	93.4	89.3	87.0	93.4		83.2	82.3
2007	95.5	84.5	92.6	92.3	92.6	90.0	90.0	92.7		82.8	81.1
2008		84.6	93.6	92.1	90.9	90.7	80.1§	93.5			
2009	94.0	83.9	92.8	90.0	92.1	89.6	92.6	92.4	43.9	81.5	
2010	95.0	84.4	93.3	91.5	90.4	90.4	92.6	91.8	59.2	82.0	78.8
2011	95.5	84.6	93.9	91.6	94.0	90.8	93.6	91.1	67.3	82.6	81.9
2012	94.3	82.5	92.8	90.8	80.9‡	90.2	92.3	89.7	68.6	80.5	76.0

*Previously reported as measles-containing vaccine (MCV)
†No national coverage data were collected from 1986 through 1990.
§In 2008, data are for PCV4+.
‡Full series of Hib: ≥3 or ≥4 doses depending on product received (includes primary series plus booster dose)

Combined 4-3-1: Four or more doses of DTP/DTaP/DT, three or more doses of poliovirus vaccine, and one or more doses of any measles-containing vaccine.

Combined 4-3-1-3: Four or more doses of DTP/DTaP/DT, three or more doses of poliovirus vaccine, one or more doses of any measles-containing vaccine, and three or more doses of *Haemophilus influenzae* type b vaccine.

Data prior to 1993 were collected by the National Health Interview Survey and represent 2-year-old children. Data from 1993 forward are from the National Immunization Survey and represent 19-35 month-old children. Different methods were used for the two surveys.

Data are available for vaccines and combinations of vaccines not reflected on this table. For more information about annual coverage figures from 1994 to the present, see http://www.cdc.gov/vaccines/stats-surv/nis/default.htm.

July 2014

APPENDIX F

Immunization Resources

F

Appendix F

CDC Contact Information & Resources

Telephone
Immunization Call Center
800-232-4636 (800-CDC-INFO)
Contact CDC-INFO between 8:00am and 8:00pm (ET) Monday through Friday, in English or Spanish, with questions concerning immunizations or vaccine-preventable diseases, to find the location of immunization clinics near you, or to order single copies of immunization materials from the National Center for Immunization and Respiratory Diseases (NCIRD).

E-Mail
nipinfo@cdc.gov
Healthcare providers can submit immunization or vaccine-preventable disease related questions to this e-mail address. You will get an answer from a CDC immunization expert, usually within 24 hours.

Internet
CDC Vaccines: http://www.cdc.gov/vaccines*
Vaccine Safety: http://www.cdc.gov/od/science/iso or
http://www.cdc.gov/vaccines/vac-gen/safety/default.htm
Hepatitis: http://www.cdc.gov/hepatitis
Influenza: http://www.cdc.gov/flu
Human Papillomavirus: http://www.cdc.gov/std/hpv
Smallpox: http://emergency.cdc.gov/agent/smallpox/index.asp
Travelers' Health: http://wwwn.cdc.gov/travel
Vaccine Storage & Handling Toolkit: http://www.cdc.gov/vaccines/recs/storage/toolkit/
ACIP Recommendations: http://www.cdc.gov/vaccines/pubs/ACIP-list.htm
Vaccines for Children (VFC) Program: http://www.cdc.gov/vaccines/programs/vfc/index.html

(For specific information on other vaccine-preventable diseases,
visit the main CDC website at http://www.cdc.gov and use the "A-Z Index.")

*Calendar of upcoming events, online access to CDC publications, online publications ordering, vaccine safety information, current pediatric and adult immunization schedules, downloadable Comprehensive Clinic Assessment Software Application (CoCASA), Frequently Asked Questions, PowerPoint slide presentations, links to other immunization sites, and much more.

NCIRD Training & Education Resources. Download NCIRD's curriculum brochure:
http://www.cdc.gov/vaccines/ed/downloads/curric-brochure.pdf

F

Publications may be ordered through NCIRD's Online Publications Order Form:
http://wwwn.cdc.gov/pubs/CDCInfoOnDemand.aspx

Selected Online Resources

There are many useful online resources dealing with various aspects of vaccination. Here are a few of them:

The Military Vaccine Agency (MILVAX)
http://www.vaccines.mil/
Information about vaccination in the military.

The National Vaccine Injury Compensation Program
http://www.hrsa.gov/vaccinecompensation/index.html
All about the program, and instructions for filing a claim for compensating injuries believed to have been caused by a vaccine.

The Vaccine Adverse Event Reporting System (VAERS)
http://vaers.hhs.gov/index
Information about reporting an adverse event following vaccination.

U.S. Food & Drug Administration (FDA) "Vaccines, Blood & Biologics"
http://www.fda.gov/BiologicsBloodVaccines/Vaccines/default.htm
Information about recent and pending vaccine approvals, links to manufacturers' package inserts, and much more.

Immunization Action Coalition (IAC)
http://www.immunize.org
Find hundreds of free downloadable materials for both providers and patients and other useful information. You can subscribe to their three publications (*Needle Tips*, *Vaccinate Adults*, and *Vaccinate Women*) at www.immunize.org/subscribe, or find manufacturers' vaccine package inserts at http://www.immunize.org/packageinserts/.

California Department of Public Health EZIZ Materials
http://www.eziz.org/resources/materials_home.html
Their specialty is Administration and Storage & Handling materials.

Children's Hospital of Philadelphia Vaccine Education Center
http://www.chop.edu/service/vaccine-education-center/home.html
Download print materials for parents, including information on current safety topics. Also find a separate information page describing each vaccine.

Alliance for Immunization in Michigan (AIM) Toolkit
http://www.aimtoolkit.org
Among other features, their "Quick Look Handouts" are useful job aids for immunization providers.

Vaccinate Your Baby
http://www.vaccinateyourbaby.org/
Includes videos, news, links to other credible sites, even a smartphone app for reminding parents to schedule vaccine visits.

Institute for Vaccine Safety
http://www.vaccinesafety.edu
Provides information about vaccine safety concerns and objective and timely information to physicians and health-care providers and to parents.

Healthmap Vaccine Finder
http://flushot.healthmap.org/
HealthMap Vaccine Finder is a free, online service where users can search for locations that offer immunizations.

Contact Information:
Selected Vaccine Manufacturers & Distributors

Manufacturer/Website	Phone Number	Products
bioCSL http://www.biocsl-us.com/	844-275-2461	Afluria
Biotest Pharmaceuticals www.biotestpharma.com/products/	800-458-4244	Bivigam (IGIV), Nabi-HB (HBIG)
Emergent Biosolutions www.emergentbiosolutions.com	866-300-7602	BioThrax, HepaGam B (HBIG), VARIZIG (VZIG)
GlaxoSmithKline www.gskvaccines.com	866-475-8222	Bexsero, Boostrix, Cervarix, Engerix-B, Fluarix, Flulaval, Havrix, Hiberix, Infanrix, Kinrix, Menveo, MenHibrix, RabAvert, Rotarix, Pediarix, Twinrix
Massachusetts Biological Labs www.umassmed.edu/massbiolabs/index.aspx	617-474-3000	IGIM, Td
MedImmune, Inc. www.medimmune.com	877-633-4411	FluMist
Merck & Co., Inc. http://www.merck.com/product/vaccines/home.html	800-444-2080	BCG, Comvax, Gardasil, Gardasil 9, M-M-R II, PedvaxHIB, Pneumovax 23, ProQuad, Recombivax HB, RotaTeq, Vaqta, Varivax, Zostavax
Novartis Vaccines www.novartisvaccines.com/us/index.shtml	877-683-4732	Agriflu, Flucelvax, Fluvirin, (distributer for Ixiaro)
PaxVax http://www.paxvax.com/	858-450-9595	Vivotif
Pfizer www.pfizerpro.com/	800-438-1985	Prevnar 13, Trumenba
Protein Sciences Corp. http://www.proteinsciences.com/	800-488-7099	FluBlok
sanofi Pasteur www.vaccineshoppe.com	800-822-2463	ACAM2000, ActHIB, Adacel, Daptacel, Decavac, DT, Fluzone, Imovax Rabies, Ipol, Menactra, Menomune, Pentacel, Tenivac, Typhim Vi, YF Vax
Talecris Biotherapeutics www.talecris.com/talecris-biotherapeutics-us-home.htm	800-520-2807	HBIG, IGIM, RIG, TIG

March 2015

F

National Center for Immunization and Respiratory Diseases

Immunization Grantees

States, D.C. & IHS

Alabama

Alabama Dept. of Public Health
State Immunization Program
The RSA Tower,
201 Monroe St., Suite 1460
P.O. Box 303017
Montgomery, Alabama 36104

Phone 334-206-5023 / Fax 334-206-2044

Program Manager: Cindy Lesinger
cindy.lesinger@adph.state.al.us

Alaska

Alaska Dept. of Health and Social Services
Immunization Program
3601 C Street, Suite 540
Anchorage, Alaska 99503

Phone 907-269-8006 / Fax 907-562-7802

Program Manager: Gerri Yett
gerri.yett@alaska.gov

Arizona

Arizona Dept of Health Services
Immunization Program Office
150 N. 18th Ave, Suite 120
Phoenix, Arizona 85007-3233

Phone 602-364-3639 / Fax 602-364-3285

Program Manager: Dana Goodloe
Dana.Goodloe@azdhs.gov

Arkansas

Arkansas Department of Health
Immunization Section
4815 West Markham, Mail Slot 48
Little Rock, AR 72205-3867

Phone 501-661-2169 / Fax 501-661-2300

Program Manager: Hilda Douglas
Hilda.douglas@arkansas.gov

California

California Dept. of Public Health
Division of Communicable Disease Control
Center for Infectious Diseases
850 Marina Bay Parkway, Building P
Richmond, California 94804-6403

Phone 510-620-3748/ Fax 510-620-3774

Program Manager: Maria Volk (acting)
maria.volk@cdph.ca.gov

Colorado

Colorado Dept. of Pub. Hlth & Environment
DCEED-IMM-A3
4300 Cherry Creek Drive South
Denver, Colorado 80246-1530

Phone 303-692-6242 / Fax 303-691-6118

Program Manager: Lynn Trefren
lynn.trefren@ state.co.us

Connecticut

Connecticut State Dept. of Public Health
Immunization Program
P.O. Box 340308
410 Capitol Ave. MS #11 MUN
Hartford, CT 06134-0308

Phone 860-509-7929 / Fax 860-509-7945

Program Manager: Michael Bolduc (interim)
michael.bolduc@ct.gov

Delaware

Division of Public Health
Thomas Collins Building, Suite 4
540 South DuPont Highway
Dover, Delaware 19901

Phone 302-744-1181 / Fax 302-739-2555

Program Manager: James Talbott
James.Talbott@state.de.us

District of Columbia

DC Department of Health
Child, Adolescent and School Health Bureau
6323 Georgia Avenue, Suite 305
Washington, DC 20011

Phone 202-576-9336 / Fax 202-576-9322

Program Manager: Nancy Ejuma
Nancy.ejuma@dc.gov

Florida

Florida Dept. of Health
Bureau of Immunization
4052 Bald Cypress Way Bin A-11
Tallahassee, Florida 32399-1719

Phone 850-245-4331 / Fax 850-922-4195

Program Manager: Robert Griffin (interim)
Robert.Griffin@FLHealth.gov

Georgia

Georgia Department of Community Health
Division of Public Health
2 Peachtree Street, NW, Ste. 13-276
Atlanta, GA 30303

Phone 404-657-3157 / Fax 404-344-1463

Program Manager: Sheila Lovett (interim)
Sheila.lovett@dhr.state.ga.us

Hawaii

Hawaii Dept. of Health
Immunization Branch
1250 Punchbowl Street,
Kinau Hale, 4th Floor
Honolulu, HI 96813

Phone 808-586-8328 / Fax 808-586-8347

Program Manager: Ronald Balajadia
Ronald.balajadia@doh.hawaii.gov

Idaho

Idaho Dept. of Health/Welfare
Immunization Program
4th Floor, 450 West State Street
Boise, Idaho 83720

Phone 208-334-5942 / Fax 208-334-4914

Program Manager: Mitch Scoggins
scogginm@dhw.idaho.gov

Illinois

Illinois Dept. of Public Health
Immunization Program
525 West Jefferson St.
Springfield, Illinois 62761

Phone 217-785-1455 / Fax 217-524-0967

Program Manager: William Moran
William.moran@illinois.gov

Indiana

Indiana State Dept. of Health
Immunization Program
2 North Meridian Street, 6-A
Indianapolis, Indiana 46204-3003

Phone 317-233-7010 / Fax 317-233-3719

Program Manager: David McCormick
DMcCormick@isdh.IN.gov

Iowa

Iowa Dept. of Public Health
Bureau of Immunization and TB
321 E. 12th Street
Des Moines, IA 50319-0075

Phone: 515-281-7228 / Fax 800-831-6292

Program Manager: Bethany Kintigh
Bethany.Kintigh@idph.iowa.gov

Kansas

Kansas Dept. of Health & Envir.
1000 SW Jackson, Suite 210
Topeka, Kansas 66612-1274

Phone 785-296-0687 / Fax 785-296-6510

Program Manager: Tim Budge
TBudge@kdheks.gov

Kentucky

Kentucky Cabinet for Health and Family Services
Dept. for Public Health
Division of Epidemiology and Health Planning
Immunization Program
275 East Main Street, HS2E-B
Frankfort, KY 40621-0001

Phone 502-564-4478 x 4257 / Fax 502-564-4760

Program Manager: Margaret C. Jones
MargaretC.Jones@ky.gov

Louisiana

Louisiana Department of Health and Hospitals
Immunization Program
1450 L and A Road, Suite 107
Metairie, Louisiana 70001

Phone 504-838-5300 / Fax 504-838-5206

Program Manager: Ruben Tapia
Ruben.Tapia@la.gov

Maine

Maine Center for Disease Control and Prevention,
Immunization Program
Key Plaza, 9th Floor
286 Water Street
Augusta, Maine 04330

Phone 207-287-2541 / Fax 207-287-8127

Program Manager: Tonya Philbrick
Tonya.Philbrick@maine.gov

Maryland

Maryland Dept. of Health and Mental Hygiene
Center for Immunization
201 W. Preston Street, Suite 318
Baltimore, Maryland 21201

Phone 410-767-6672 / Fax 410-333-5893

Program Manager: Gregory Reed
Greg.Reed@maryland.gov

Massachusetts

Division of Epidemiology and Immunization
Massachusetts Department of Public Health
305 South Street - Room 559
Jamaica Plain, MA 02130-3597

Phone 617-983-6880 / Fax 617-983-6840

Program Manager: Pejman Talebian
Pejman.Talebian@state.ma.us

F

Michigan

Michigan Dept. of Community Health
Division of Immunization
210 Townsend Street
P.O. Box 30195
Lansing, MI 48913

Phone 517-335-8159 / Fax 517-335-9855

Program Manager: Bob Swanson
SwansonR@Michigan.gov

Nevada

Nevada Dept of Health and Human Services
Immunization Program
4150 Technology Way, Suite 210
Carson City, NV 89706

Phone 775-684-3209 / Fax 775-684-8338

Program Manager: Karissa L. Loper
kloper@health.nv.gov

Minnesota

Minnesota Dept. of Health
Immunization, TB and International Health
625 N. Robert Street, P.O. Box 64975
St. Paul, Minnesota 55164-0975

Phone 651-201-5545 / Fax 651-201-5501

Program Manager: Margaret Roddy
Margaret.Roddy@state.mn.us

New Hampshire

New Hampshire Dept of Health/Human Svc
Immunization Program
29 Hazen Drive
Concord, New Hampshire 03301

Phone 603-271-4482 / Fax 603-271-3850

Program Manager: Colleen Haggerty (interim)
Colleen.M.Haggerty@dhhs.state.nh.us

Mississippi

Mississippi State Dept. of Health
Bureau of Immunization
570 Woodrow Wilson Blvd.
PO Box 1700
Jackson, Mississippi 39215-1700

Phone 601-576-7734 / Fax 601-576-7686

Program Manager: Latrina McLenton
Latrina.mcclenton@msdh. ms.gov

New Jersey

New Jersey Dept of Health and Senior Svc
Vaccine Preventable Disease Program
P.O. Box 369
135 E. State Street
Trenton, New Jersey 08625-0369

Phone 609-826-4861 / Fax 609-826-4866

Program Manager: Steven Bors
steven.bors @doh.state.nj.us

Missouri

Bureau of Immunization Assessment & Assurance
Missouri Dept of Health and Senior Services
930 Wildwood Drive, PO Box 570
Jefferson City, MO 65102

Phone 573- 751-6124 / Fax 573-526-0238

Program Manager: Cathy Sullivan
cathy.sullivan@health.mo.gov

New Mexico

New Mexico Dept of Health, Immunization Program
Runnels Building – Suite S1200
1190 St. Francis Drive
Santa Fe, New Mexico 87502-6110

Phone 505-476-1778 / Fax 505-476-3638

Program Manager: Daniel Burke (interim)
Daniel.burke@state.nm.us

Montana

DPHHS Immunization Program
Health Policy and Services Division
P.O. Box 202951
1400 Broadway Room C-211
Helena, Montana 59601-2951

Phone 406-444-0065 / Fax 406-444-2920

Program Manager: Bekki Wehner
bwehner@mt.gov

New York

New York State Dept of Health
Division of Epidemiology, Bureau of Immunization
Corning Tower, Rm 503, ESP
Albany, New York 12237

Phone 518-473-4437 / Fax 518-474-1495

Program Manager: Elizabeth Rausch-Phung, MD
Elizabeth.rausch-phung@health.ny.gov

Nebraska

Nebraska Dept. of Health and Human Svc.
Immunization Services
P.O. Box 95026
Lincoln, Nebraska 68509-5026

Phone 402-471-2139 / Fax 402-471-6426

Program Manager: Sara Morgan
sara.morgan@nebraska.gov

North Carolina

North Carolina Dept. of Health/Hum Svcs
Immunization Branch
1917 Mail Service Center
5601 Six Forks Road
Raleigh, North Carolina 27699-1917

Phone 919-707-5551 / Fax 919-870-4824

Program Manager: Wendy Holmes
wendy.holmes@dhhs.nc.gov

F

North Dakota

North Dakota Department of Health
Division of Disease Control
2635 East Main Avenue
P.O. Box 5520
Bismarck, North Dakota 58501-5044

Phone 701-328-4556 / Fax 701-328-2499

Program Manager: Molly Howell
mahowell@nd.gov

Ohio

Ohio Department of Health
Immunization Program
35 East Chestnut Street
Columbus, Ohio 43215

Phone 614-466-0239 / Fax 614-728-4279

Program Manager: John Joseph
John.joseph@odh.ohio.gov

Oklahoma

Oklahoma State Dept of Health
Immunization Service
1000 N.E. 10th Street
Oklahoma City, Oklahoma 73117-1299

Phone 405-271-4073 / Fax 405-271-6133

Program Manager: Lori Linstead
loril@health.ok.gov

Oregon

Oregon State Health Division
Immunization Program Suite 370
800 NE Oregon Street
Portland, Oregon 97232

Phone 971-673-0318 / Fax 971-673-0278

Program Manager: Aaron Dunn
aaron.dunn@dhsoha.state.or.us

Pennsylvania

Pennsylvania Dept of Health
Division of Immunizations
625 Forster Street
Harrisburg, Pennsylvania 17120

Phone 717-787-56813 / Fax 717-705-5513

Program Manager: Cindy Findley
cfindley@state.pa.us

Rhode Island

Rhode Island Department of Health
Immunization Program
3 Capitol Hill, Room 309
Providence, Rhode Island 02908-5097

Phone 401-222-5922 / Fax 401-222-1442

Program Manager: Tricia Washburn
Tricia.Washburn@health.ri.gov

South Carolina

SC Department of Health and Environmental Control
Immunization Division
1751 Calhoun Street
Columbia, SC 29201-2606

Phone 803- 898-0435/ Fax 803-898-0326

Program Manager: Leanne S. Bailey
baileyls@dhec.sc.gov

South Dakota

South Dakota Dept. of Health
Immunization Program
615 East 4th Street
Pierre, South Dakota 57501

Phone 605-773-5323 / Fax 605-773-5509

Program Manager: Tim Heath
Tim.Heath@state.sd.us

Tennessee

State Immunization Program
Tennessee Department of Health
3rd Floor, Andrew Johnson Tower
710 James Robertson Parkway
Nashville, TN 37243

Phone: 615-741-7247 / Fax: 615-532-8526

Program Manager: Catherine Haralson
catherine.d.haralson@tn.gov

Texas

Texas Department of State Health Services
Immunization Branch
P.O. Box 149347, MC 1946
Austin, Texas 78714-9347

Phone 512-776-6215 / Fax 512-776-7176

Program Manager: Kelly Patson
kelly.patson@dshs.texas.gov

Utah

Utah Dept of Health
CFHS/Immunization
288 North 1460 West St.
P.O. Box 142001
Salt Lake City, Utah 84114-2001

Phone 801-538-6905 / Fax 801-538-9440

Program Manager: Linda Abel
label@utah.gov

Vermont

Vermont Department of Health
Immunization Program
P.O. Box 70
108 Cherry Street
Burlington, Vermont 05402-0070

Phone 802-652-4185 / Fax 802-863-7395

Program Manager: Christine Finley
Christine.Finley@state.vt.us

F

Appendix F

Virginia

Virginia State Dept of Health
Division of Immunization
109 Governor Street, Room 314 West
Richmond, Virginia 23219

Phone 804-864-8087/ Fax 804-864-8089

Program Manager: James Farrell
James.Farrell@vdh.virginia.gov

Washington

Washington State Dept of Health
Immunization and CHILD Profile Section
P.O. Box 47843
310 Israel Road SE
Turnwater, Washington 98501

Phone 360-236-3568 / Fax 360-236-3590

Program Manager: Michele Roberts
Michele.roberts@doh.wa.gov

West Virginia

West Virginia Dept of Health/Human Svc
Bureau for Public Health
Division of Immunization Services
350 Capitol Street, Room 125
Charleston, West Virginia 25301-3715

Phone 304-356-4035/ Fax 304-558-6335

Program Manager: Jeff Neccuzi
jeffrey.j.neccuzi@wv.gov

Wisconsin

Wisconsin Division of Public Health
Immunization Program
1 West Wilson Street
P.O. Box 2659
Madison, Wisconsin 53701-2659

Phone 608-266-1339 / Fax 608-267-9493

Program Manager: Dan Hopfensperger
Dan.Hopfensperger@dhs.wisconsin.gov

Wyoming

Immunization Section
Community and Public Health Division
Wyoming Department of Health
6101 Yellowstone Rd. Suite 420
Cheyenne, WY 82002

Phone 307-777-2413/ Fax 307-777-3615

Program Manager: Lisa Wordeman
lisa.wordeman@ wyo.gov

Indian Health Service

IHS Division of Epidemiology
5300 Homestead Road, NE
Albuquerque, NM 87110

Phone 505-248-4374 / Fax 505-248-4393

Program Manager: Amy Groom
Amy.Groom@ihs.gov

F

Territories

American Samoa

ASG Department of Health
American Samoa Immunization Program
LBJ Tropical Medical Center
Pago Pago, American Samoa 96799

Phone 011-684-699-8464 / Fax 011 684-699-8467

Program Manager: Yolanda Masuno Faleafaga
y3masunu@gmail.com

Commonwealth of the Northern Mariana Islands

Division of Public Health
CHC Building
Lower Navy Hill
P.O. Box 500409
Saipan, MP 96950

Phone 670-236-8733 / Fax 670-236-8700

Program Manager: Jeremy Sasamoto
jsasamoto@gmail.com

Guam

Immunization Program
Dept. of Public Health and Social Services
123 Chalan Kareta
Mangilao, Guam 96913-6304

Phone 671-735-7143 / Fax 671-734-1475

Program Manager: Annette L. Aguon
annette.aguon@dphss.guam.gov

Palau

Bureau of Public Health, Ministry of Health
Palau Immunization Program
Republic of Palau
P.O. Box 6027
Koror, Palau 96960

Phone 680-488-2212, ext 300 / Fax 680-488-4800

Program Manager: Merlyn Basilius
mbasilius@gmail.com

Marshall Islands

Ministry of Health
Immunization Program
Amata Kabua Blvd.
PO Box 16
Majuro, Marshall Islands 96960

Phone 692-625-8457 / Fax 692-625-4543

Program Manager: Daisy Pedro
dnk_pedro@yahoo.com

Puerto Rico

Puerto Rico Health Department
Immunization Program/PASET
P.O. Box 70184
San Juan, Puerto Rico 00936

Phone 787-265-2929 ext 3327 / Fax 787-274-6807

Program Manager: Angel M. Rivera, MD
anrivera@salud.gov.pr

Federated States of Micronesia

FSM Division of Health and Social Affairs
Immunization Program
P.O. Box PS-70
Palikir, Pohnpei, Micronesia 96941

Phone 691-320-2619 / Fax 011 691-320-5263

Program Manager: Louisa Helgenberger
lahelgenberger@fsmhealth.fm

Virgin Islands

VI Department of Health
1303 Hospital Ground, Suite 10
St. Thomas, VI 00802-6722

Phone 340-776-1155 / Fax 340-774-5813

Program Manager: Gail A. Jackson
Gail.Jackson@usvi-doh.org

Appendix F

Cities

Chicago

Chicago Dept of Public Health
Immunization Program
Westside Center for Disease Control
2160 West Ogden Avenue
Chicago, Illinois 60612

Phone 312-746-6120 / Fax 312-746-6388

Program Manager: Maribel Chavez-Torres
Maribel.chavez-torres@cityofchicago.org

Houston

Houston Dept. of Health and Human Svc.
8000 N. Stadium Drive, 5th Floor
Houston, TX 77054

Phone 832-393-4640 / Fax 832-393-5241

Program Manager: Omar Salgado
omar.salgado@houstontx.gov

New York City

New York City Dept of Health and Mental Hygiene
Bureau of Immunization
42-09 28th Street, Room 5-97, CN-21
Long Island City, New York 11101-4132

Phone 347-396-2471 / Fax 347-396-2558

Program Manager: Jane R. Zucker, MD
jzucker@health.nyc.gov

San Antonio

San Antonio Metropolitan Health District
332 W. Commerce, Suite 108
San Antonio, TX 78205

Phone 210- 207-8794 / Fax 210-207-8882

Program Manager: Kenya Wilson (interim)
Kenya.wilson@sanantoni Add o.gov

Philadelphia

Philadelphia Dept. of Health
Division of Disease Control
500 South Broad Street
Philadelphia, Pennsylvania 19146-1613

Phone 215-685-6603 / Fax 215-685-6806

Program Manager: James Lutz
James.Lutz@phila.gov

March, 2015

F